Contents

THIRD EDITION

Conversational Spanish for Health Professionals

Essential Expressions, Questions, and Directions for Medical Personnel to Facilitate Conversation with Spanish-Speaking Patients and Coworkers

ROCHELLE K. KELZ, Ph.D.

Dean of Arts & Sciences
Associate Professor of Romance Languages
Indiana University Kokomo
Kokomo, Indiana

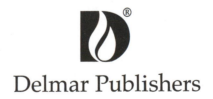

Delmar Publishers

I(T)P® International Thomson Publishing

Albany • Bonn • Boston • Cincinnati • Detroit • London • Madrid
Melbourne • Mexico City • New York • Pacific Grove • Paris • San Francisco
Singapore • Tokyo • Toronto • Washington

Notice to the Reader

Cover Design: Charles Cummings Advertising/Art Inc.

Delmar Staff:
Publisher: Susan Simpfenderfer
Acquisitions Editor: Marlene McHugh Pratt
Production Manager: Linda Helfrich
Project Editor: William Trudell
Developmental Editor: Jill Rembetski
Art & Design Coordinator: Rich Killar
Editorial Assistant: Maria Perretta

COPYRIGHT © 1999 By Rochelle Kelz, Ph.D.

The ITP logo is a trademark under license

Delmar Publishers
3 Columbia Circle, Box 15015
Albany, New York 12212-5015

International Thomson Publishing Europe
Berkshire House
168-173 High Holborn
London, WC1V7AA
United Kingdom

Nelson ITP, Australia
102 Dodds Street
South Melbourne,
Victoria, 3205 Australia

Nelson Canada
1120 Birchmont Road
Scarborough, Ontario
M1K 5G4, Canada

International Thomson Publishing France
Tour Maine-Montparnasse
33 Avenue du Maine
75755 Paris Cedex 15, France

International Thomson Editores
Seneca 53
Colonia Polanco
11560 Mexico D.F. Mexico

International Thomson Publishing GmbH
Königswinterer Strasβe 418
53227 Bonn
Germany

International Thomson Publishing Asia
60 Albert Street
#15-01 Albert Complex
Singapore 189969

International Thomson Publishing Japan
Hirakawa-cho Kyowa Building, 3F
2-2-1 Hirakawa-cho, Chiyoda-ku,
Tokyo 102, Japan

ITE Spain/Paraninfo
Calle Magallanes, 25
28015-Madrid, Espana

Printed in Canada

Library of Congress Cataloging-in-Publication Data

Kelz, Rochelle K.
    Conversational Spanish for health professionals: essential expressions, questions, and directions for medical personnel to facilitate conversation with Spanish-speaking patients and coworkers / Rochelle K. Kelz. — 3rd ed.
        p.   cm.
    Includes bibliographical references and index.
    1. Spanish language—Conversation and phrase books (for medical personnel) 2. Medicine—Terminology. I. Title.
PC4120.M3K4   1998
468.3'421'02461—dc21

98-32215
CIP

Preface

The Hispanic or *Latino* population in the United States continues to grow at an astounding rate. As a consequence of this population boom, most health care providers come into regular, daily contact with Hispanics who are overrepresented in a variety of health concerns. These health concerns derive from language barriers, inadequate insurance coverage, socioeconomic factors, cultural patterns of behavior, and too few Hispanic health care providers.

In order to effectively serve this population, health care providers must be able to communicate with those individuals seeking assistance. Communication of simple facts can be difficult for non-Spanish-speaking health professionals, and miscommunication can have deadly consequences. Being bilingual can prove a vital link in a hospital setting. In my own experience, I was able to clear the channels of communication for a frightened, non-English-speaking mother whose ill newborn had been separated from her. This mother believed that the staff had killed her child. By explaining to her what had happened, I was able to alleviate the woman's distress.

It is important to bridge the language barrier that can hamper the health care offered to Hispanics/ *Latinos* and to learn how to conduct patient histories and physical exams in Spanish. Role-playing and vignettes are part of the process used to help students learn to interact with patients and eradicate feelings of seclusion. This text is designed to meet the needs of those professionals working in hospitals, clinics, dental offices, physicians' offices, pharmacies, outpatient facilities, etc. as well as the needs of students in medical, nursing, pharmacy, dental, and other allied health schools. The Spanish expressions used in this text are, for the most part, those used in United States communities with significant Spanish-speaking populations and in Spanish-speaking countries close to the United States.

Conversational Spanish for Health Professionales responds to requests for a more compact work with updated materials, exercises, activities, and opportunities for partner and group work. The title has been changed to more accurately reflect its usefulness to all types of health providers, not just those in medicine. It is an adaptation of **Conversational Spanish for Medical Personnel**, the result of discussion, planning, and ongoing collaboration between students, instructors, and the author. Supported by carefully integrated supplementary materials, the book is the result of years of research, development, class testing, and revision. Its new format makes locating material easier than ever. Now health professionals can easily find areas of conversation that are specifically related to their daily needs.

I appreciate your support and ongoing communication, and look forward to your reactions to this adapted text, which many of you may find better suits the goals of your program.

Highlights of Conversational Spanish for Health Professionals

- For the convenience of the health provider, every chapter is given in a bilingual format, thus eliminating the time-consuming need to consult a dictionary for unknown words or phrases.
- Whenever possible, questions have been selected which will elicit a "yes" or "no" response from the patient.
- Conversation is presented which deals with topics familiar to those in the medical, dental, or health care settings. Repetition enables the provider to enhance his or her retention.
- The organization of Chapters 5-10 follows the actual physical workup and examination.
- Cultural notes are presented throughout the text, thus, enabling the provider to better serve the patient.
- Class-room tested information gap activities in which students simulate realistic situations appear in this edition. Students work in pairs and supply one another with needed information.

GRAMMAR PRESENTATION

Earlier editions of *Conversational Spanish for Medical Personnel* contained an extensive chapter devoted to comprehensive grammar explanations. This has been eliminated from this new text in order to make space for an abundance of new material. Instructors and students should consult any first year grammar text of their choice. I recognize that this may not perfectly fit every individual's (teaching or learning) needs, but I hope that the additional chapters containing new and improved ideas and materials allow everyone to find something of need and value.

CHAPTER ORGANIZATION

Conversational Spanish for Health Professionals contains sixteen chapters, topically organized and designed to encourage communication and insight into the language and culture of over 300 million people.

Chapter 1, **Hispanics and Their Health,** presents a brief overview of the demographics and cultural differences in the health perceptions of many Spanish-speaking patients. This chapter will assist the provider in becoming more culturally aware and sensitive to Spanish-speaking patients.

Chapter 2 provides detailed information about the **Pronunciation of Spanish** along with many exercises for practice.

Chapter 3 presents **Anatomic and Physiological Vocabulary** and illustrations as well as numerous exercises that will enable retention of this information.

Chapter 4, **Numerical Expressions,** presents the terminology of numbers, time, and other matters that are essential for mastery by providers as they work with the Spanish-speaking.

Chapter 5 contains **Conversations for Administrative Personnel.** Included are general questions pertaining to overall health, payment and insurance, information for admission, emergency room reports, and other useful conversations.

Chapter 6, **Basic Preliminary Conversations,** contains extensive new material along with expanded and improved original dialogues. Conversations designed for the ambulance, others to greet and welcome patients, and still others useful for admitting the patient to the room are some of the topics.

Chapter 7 begins the format of the **Medical History: Present Illness and Past History.**

Chapter 8 continues with **Review of Systems,** a format familiar to providers.

Chapter 9 provides conversation to elicit **Personal, Social, and Family History.**

Chapter 10 contains extensive new material as it prepares the provider to do the actual **Physical Examination.**

Chapter 11 prepares the provider with the words and structures for **Labor & Delivery, Surgery, Medication, Diet, Treatments, Drug Overdose, and Accidental Poisonings.**

Chapter 12 provides specific instructions for breast self-examination, testicular self-examination, the use of condoms, and tests such as IVPs in this section about **Medical Therapy, Laboratory Tests, and Patient Instructions.**

Chapter 13 is a completely new chapter containing **Dental Conversations.** It covers dental subjects such as the initial visit, dental X-rays, caries, prophies, brushing and flossing, endodontia, periodontia, oral surgery, reconstructive dentistry, pediatric dentistry, and orthodontia.

Chapter 14 contains sample hospital **Authorizations and Signature** forms along with key vocabulary and idioms for that purpose. Included are authorizations for surgery, blood transfusions, abortions, sterilization, and others, as well as consents for anesthesia, liability releases for emergency, inpatient or outpatient treatment, living will, durable power of attorney for health care, and a patient authorization to the hospital for other releases of information.

Chapter 15 contains **Readings for Health Professionals.** This includes a variety of pertinent bilingual readings on taking a temperature, diabetes, gallstones, kidney stones, instructions for an MRI, post-op oral surgery instructions, and instructions for oral care after a pulpotomy.

Chapter 16 provides **Crucial Vocabulary for Health Professionals** by category. This section is designed to serve as a quick and handy reference.

The book concludes with an English-Spanish Vocabulary Appendix, a Spanish-English Vocabulary Appendix, an Answer Key, and finally, an appendix of Selected Bibliography.

ACKNOWLEDGEMENTS

Book writing often feels like a lonely process. Nonetheless, the process seems less lonely because of my contact with many Spanish-speaking colleagues and friends. I wish that I could thank personally all of the individuals—colleagues and students of mine, healthcare professionals and patients from almost all parts of the Spanish-speaking world—from whom I have learned so much. Their experience, advice, and wisdom are an important foundation for this work.

As with the two earlier editions, I owe much to many. Thank you again to all who helped me in the two prior editions—your contribution still lingers in this work. However, I want to particularly mention those who have made more recent contributions. They are Dottie Winterton, Gail Shay and Larry Thacker. Also, I owe a debt of thanks to Jill Rembetski, my developmental editor, who waded through my manuscript, improving it greatly with her editorial suggestions. Thanks also to Chad Thomas, Aleida Ruelas-Hertel, Jodi Gaherty, and the rest of the staff at Carlisle Publishers Services for their work on the production of this book.

I would also like to thank all the colleagues and readers in the United States and around the Spanish-speaking world who have provided valuable comments and suggestions and noted earlier errors which have now been corrected.

Finally, on a more personal note, I want to thank the members of my family for their support and their patience with my long absences: Dr. Sam and Florence, Melissa and Dr. Max, and the newest member, Dr. Rachel. I owe more than I can say to my spouse and closest colleague, Arnold Abrams, without whom my sanity and health would be significantly diminished. I dedicate this edition to you. Thank you for your critiques, your support, and your love.

RECONOCIMIENTOS

Muchas veces parece un proceso solitario el escribir un libro. Sin embargo, el proceso me parece menos solitario a causa de mi contacto con muchos colegas y amigos de habla español. Ojalá que pudiese darles las gracias personalmente a todos los individuos—colegas, y estudiantes míos, profesionales en el cuidado de la salud y pacientes de casi todos los países de habla español—de quienes he aprendido tanto. Su experiencia, consejo, y sabiduría forman la base para esta obra.

Como en el caso de las dos ediciones anteriores, debo mucho a muchos. A las personas que me han ayudado con las dos ediciones anteriores—su contribución todavía persiste en esta obra. No obstante, quiero mencionar especialmente a los que han contribuido más recientemente. Son Dottie Winterton, Gail Shay and Larry Thacker. A Jill Rembetski mi redactor, quien leyó mi manuscrito, le tengo que estar agradecida por mejorarlo mucho con sus sugerencias editoriales. Gracias también a Chad Thomas, Aleida Ruelas-Hertel, Jodi Gaherty y el resto del equipo de trabajo de Carlisle Publishers Services por su colaboración en la producción de este libro.

También quisiera dar las gracias a todos los colegas y lectores de los Estados Unidos y del mundo de habla español quienes me han enviado sus comentarios, observaciones, y sugerencias así como mención de unos errores anteriores, los que ya corregí.

Finalmente, hablando personalmente, quiero ofrecer mis más profundas gracias a los miembros de mi familia por su apoyo y su paciencia durante mis ausencias extendidas: El Dr. Sam y Florence, Melissa y el Dr. Max, y la más reciente adición, la Dra. Rachel. No hay palabras que puedan expresar mi apreciación a mi esposo y colega más intimo, Arnold Abrams, sin quien sufrirían tanto mi sanidad como mi salud. Te dedico esta edición a ti. Gracias por tu crítica, tu apoyo, y tu amor.

"Errors, like straws, upon the surface flow; He who would search for pearls must dive below."

John Dryden

Hispanics and Their Health
Hispanos y su salud

The United States has long been considered a melting pot, a nation of nations. As the second largest minority in the United States, the Hispanic population (on the U.S. mainland) was estimated to number 29.7 million in 1997 and is projected to reach 36.1 million by the turn of the century.[1] As a consequence of this population boom, most health care providers now come into regular, daily contact with Hispanics who are overrepresented in a variety of health concerns. These health concerns derive from language barriers, inadequate insurance coverage, socioeconomic factors, cultural patterns of behavior, and too few Hispanic health care providers.

To effectively serve this population, health care providers must first understand certain facts about the Hispanics in addition to their language: who they are; what language barriers exist; and what their ethnic backgrounds, beliefs, basic values, attitudes, expectancies, social behaviors, and approaches to health are. They must also seek to understand the cultural differences many Hispanics encounter when seeking health care services in the United States. Health care providers need to exercise cultural sensitivity in their delivery of such services.

LA RAZA, LATINO, OR HISPANIC?

¿LA RAZA, LATINO, O HISPANO?

More than semantics are involved in the issue of classification and subclassification of Hispanic populations. Poorly defined groupings can produce programs that do not respond to actual needs and cultural sensitivities. Incorrect ethnic labeling can and may obscure the diversity of social histories and cultural identities that characterize these populations and, in turn, can influence health behaviors, the way care is accessed, and ultimately, health outcomes.[2] Probably the most far-reaching implications of how to refer to this large group have to do with the sense of shared identity among Hispanic communities and the public perception of what such an identity means in the broad context of social affiliation in American society.[3]

This population continues to search for a single term that is acceptable to all. Prior to 1978, Hispanics were generally described as "Spanish-speaking" people. This label was/is not completely accurate because many Hispanics do not speak Spanish, or at least cannot use it fluently. It also does not take into consideration the large number of non-Hispanics who do speak Spanish.

To describe Hispanics as having "Spanish surnames" does not take into account the number of Hispanic people who do not have such names. For example, large numbers of immigrants left Europe and settled throughout Central and South America during the middle of the twentieth century. They, their children, and their grandchildren have become "Hispanicized" and are today considered Hispanic despite their surnames. Additionally, because of intermarriage in the United States, many individuals who have been raised as Hispanic do not have surnames that reflect this characteristic.

The terms *la Raza*, *Latino*, and *Hispano* have been suggested by different Hispanic groups in various parts of the country. Generally speaking, these terms describe persons who can trace their ancestry to Spain or to the Spanish-speaking regions of the Caribbean or Latin America. The fact that there is no term that has everyone's acceptance further emphasizes their diversity. These terms are usually considered to be synonymous, however, and this author will use them interchangeably.

La Raza is a term that Mexican scholar José Vasconcelos coined early in the twentieth century to reflect the diversity of the people of Latin America. It reflects the mixture inherent in the Hispanic people who are a blend of many of the world's races, cultures, and religions. It is meant as an inclusive concept, meaning that Hispanics share a common heritage and destiny with all other peoples of the world. Some have translated this term into English as "the people," or "the Hispanic people of the New World"; it should not be used, however, as a term meant to exclude others as what might happen when it is mistranslated as "The Race." Nonetheless, for some people this term has a negative connotation, a reference to the colonial experience and Spain's conquest of Latin America.

The term *Latino* has been suggested as a "better" label (Hayes-Bautista & Chapa, 1987; Pérez-Stable, 1987) because the ethnic components of the Hispanic-American population are mostly Mexican, Puerto Rican, Cuban, and Central and South American. The term is gaining acceptance in the Northeast and on the West Coast. Hispanics are *Latinos*, but *Latinos* are not necessarily Hispanics. (*Latinos* have their origin in countries where the languages derive from Latin.[4]) Some individuals resent being classified in this manner, primarily because they perceive the term to be imposed on them whereas others have assimilated and acculturated to such an extent that despite their Spanish surnames, they do not consider themselves Hispanics.[5]

Those who do accept the term *Latino* usually consider it an umbrella term and after admitting that they are Latinos, will provide a more specific ethnic identification by giving their national origin. For example, many Puerto Ricans frequently refer to themselves as *"Boricuas"* or *"Boriqueños,"* derivatives of *Boriquén*, the name used by the Taínos, the first natives of that island, for Puerto Rico. (After the Spanish-American War of 1898, Spain gave Puerto Rico to the United States. In 1953 Puerto Rico became a free state associated with the United States although its inhabitants have been U.S. citizens since 1917.[6]) Puerto Ricans, especially those born on the mainland, frequently call themselves *"Nuyoricans"* or *"New York Ricans"* since New York City has the largest Puerto Rican population (1,086,601 in 1990 and approximately 1,850,000 in 1996) outside of Puerto Rico.[7] Persons of Mexican origin may prefer the terms **"Mexican American"** or **"Chicano."** The latter term has a political empowerment connotation.[8] For Cubans living in the United States, who number 2 million, more than 600,000 of whom live in the city of Miami, the term **"Cuban Americans"** is often used when referring to those of second generation and beyond. The more recently arrived Cubans who left Cuba from Mariel Bay in 1980 are customarily called *"Marielitos."* This classification of Hispanics into subcategories based primarily on national origin is useful to health care practitioners who can distinguish between access to care issues likely to be experienced by Puerto Rican communities covered by U.S. entitlement programs and those faced by Central and South Americans, some of whom may be fleeing a war-torn countryside, and who, because of these circumstances, might be undocumented.

Currently, Hispanic or *Hispano* is the most widely used term. It derives from the Latin word for Spain (*Hispania*) which also describes the entire Iberian Peninsula and refers to the Spanish-speaking people of different races and eighteen separate nationalities in the Americas, and Puerto Rico. The appropriateness of the term is validated by the Royal Academy of Spanish Language which uses the word *"Hispanoamericanos"* to refer to those individuals born in Spanish-speaking countries south of the Río Grande. The federal government coined the term *"Hispanic,"* which the U.S. Office of Management and Budget (OMB) then adopted as the phrase *"Hispanic Origin"* in 1978. Origin can be viewed as the ancestry, nationality group, lineage, or country of birth of the person, the person's parents, or ancestors before their arrival in the United States.[9] The U.S. government made the assumption that the only commonality among these differing countries was the tenuous connection to the Spanish language and/or culture. The term is most widespread among the more acculturated, economically successful *Latinos* in the United States and is often used by *Latino* political or professional organizations. Finally, it is the term which the U.S. federal government, its agencies, and many state and local organizations use when capturing data about populations.

Nevertheless, it must be emphasized that Hispanics are not all alike. Actually, most Hispanics are racially mixed, a combination of European White, African Black, and American Indian/Native American.[10] They come from a diversity of backgrounds and have very different sets of behaviors and values. Most Hispanics are also Roman Catholics, but not all. Some Hispanics are U.S. citizens; others are not. Some are recent arrivals to the United States while others have been in this country for many generations. Many Hispanics are monolingual in English, others speak only Spanish, and still others are bilingual in English and Spanish. There are diverse levels of assimilation, acculturation, and socioeconomic status, and diversity in the way in which they deal with their illnesses and their use of health services.

HISPANIC POPULATION

POBLACION HISPANA

Since the mid-1970s large numbers of immigrants have come to the United States in search of refuge and opportunities (see Figures 1–1 and 1–2). Because of political unrest abroad and changes in U.S. immigration policies, more than 7 million immigrants arrived here during the 1980s, surpassing any decade since 1900 to 1910. In 1992, more than 1 million legal immigrants and refugees entered the United States. Most were Spanish speaking from El Salvador, Mexico, Cuba, Puerto Rico, and other Latin American countries, although large groups also came from the Philippines, Cambodia, Laos, Taiwan, South Korea, Vietnam, Eastern Europe, and the former Soviet republics. In 1997, the biggest influx of foreign born was from Central and South America and the Caribbean.[11] These immigrants have generally headed for America's large urban centers.

Immigration, as experienced by the Hispanic population, is different in many respects from the immigration experienced by European descended population groups on the Atlantic coast during the nineteenth and early twentieth centuries.[12] There are also different immigration rates within the Hispanic

1993 Composition of Legally Admitted Immigrant Flows within the United States to Seven Major Metropolitan Areas   FIGURE **1.1**

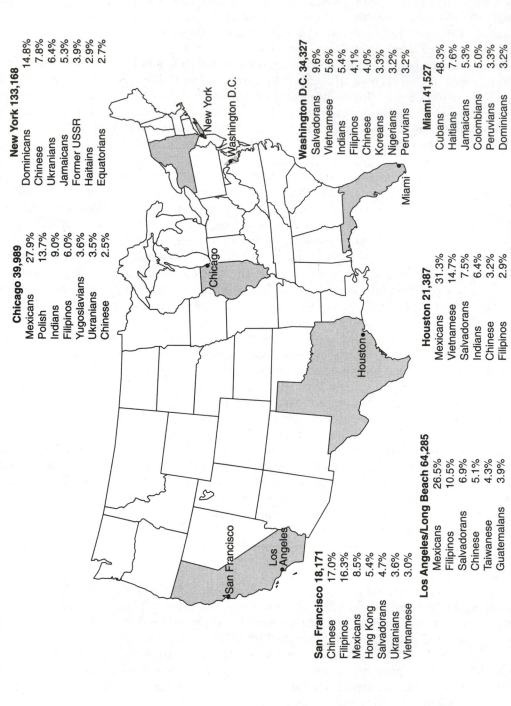

New York 133,168

Dominicans	14.8%
Chinese	7.8%
Ukranians	6.4%
Jamaicans	5.3%
Former USSR	3.9%
Haitains	2.9%
Equatorians	2.7%

Chicago 39,989

Mexicans	27.9%
Polish	13.7%
Indians	9.0%
Filipinos	6.0%
Yugoslavians	3.6%
Ukranians	3.5%
Chinese	2.5%

Washington D.C. 34,327

Salvadorans	9.6%
Vietnamese	5.6%
Indians	5.4%
Filipinos	4.1%
Chinese	4.0%
Koreans	3.3%
Nigerians	3.2%
Peruvians	3.2%

Miami 41,527

Cubans	48.3%
Haitians	7.6%
Jamaicans	5.3%
Colombians	5.0%
Peruvians	3.3%
Dominicans	3.2%

Houston 21,387

Mexicans	31.3%
Vietnamese	14.7%
Salvadorans	7.5%
Indians	6.4%
Chinese	3.2%
Filipinos	2.9%

San Francisco 18,171

Chinese	17.0%
Filipinos	16.3%
Mexicans	8.5%
Hong Kong	5.4%
Salvadorans	4.7%
Ukranians	3.6%
Vietnamese	3.0%

Los Angeles/Long Beach 64,285

Mexicans	26.5%
Filipinos	10.5%
Salvadorans	6.9%
Chinese	5.1%
Taiwanese	4.3%
Guatemalans	3.9%

Source: U.S. Immigration and Naturalization Service. *1993 Statistical Yearbook* (Washington, D.C.: U.S. Government Printing Office, 1994).

1996 Composition of Legally Admitted Immigrant Flows within the United States to Seven Major Metropolitan Areas   FIGURE **1.2**

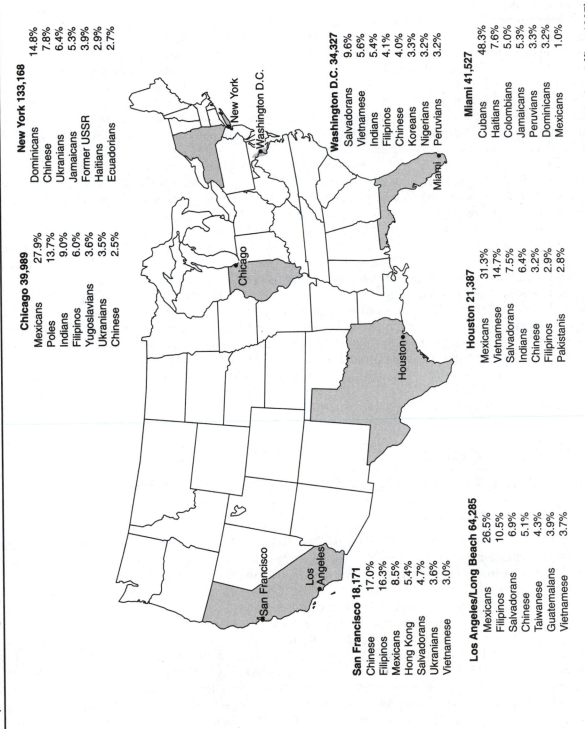

New York 133,168

Dominicans	14.8%
Chinese	7.8%
Ukranians	6.4%
Jamaicans	5.3%
Former USSR	3.9%
Haitians	2.9%
Ecuadorians	2.7%

Chicago 39,989

Mexicans	27.9%
Poles	13.7%
Indians	9.0%
Filipinos	6.0%
Yugoslavians	3.6%
Ukranians	3.5%
Chinese	2.5%

Washington D.C. 34,327

Salvadorans	9.6%
Vietnamese	5.6%
Indians	5.4%
Filipinos	4.1%
Chinese	4.0%
Koreans	3.3%
Nigerians	3.2%
Peruvians	3.2%

Miami 41,527

Cubans	48.3%
Haitians	7.6%
Colombians	5.0%
Jamaicans	5.3%
Peruvians	3.3%
Dominicans	3.2%
Mexicans	1.0%

Houston 21,387

Mexicans	31.3%
Vietnamese	14.7%
Salvadorans	7.5%
Indians	6.4%
Chinese	3.2%
Filipinos	2.9%
Pakistanis	2.8%

San Francisco 18,171

Chinese	17.0%
Filipinos	16.3%
Mexicans	8.5%
Hong Kong	5.4%
Salvadorans	4.7%
Ukranians	3.6%
Vietnamese	3.0%

Los Angeles/Long Beach 64,285

Mexicans	26.5%
Filipinos	10.5%
Salvadorans	6.9%
Chinese	5.1%
Taiwanese	4.3%
Guatemalans	3.9%
Vietnamese	3.7%

Source: U.S. Immigration and Naturalization Service. *1996 Statistical Yearbook* (Washington, D.C.: U.S. Government Printing Office, 1997).

population which divide and define this population into subgroups. The immigration variable for Hispanics is more complex than just the status of being foreign born; it also includes the dimensions of permanence and documentation.

The Hispanic population in the United States has witnessed tremendous growth since 1960 when it accounted for almost 6% of the population. By 1980 Hispanics were the second largest ethnic minority in the United States accounting for over 6% of the total U.S. population (14.6 million). Following the 1990 census, a post-enumeration survey conducted by the Census Bureau indicated that from 4.2% to 7.3% of the U.S. Hispanic population may not have been counted by the 1990 census. That percentage increased to 9% by 1993 and has climbed steadily to 11.1% of the total population of the United States, representing more than 29.7 million people of Hispanic origin in 1997. This figure does not include the 3.6 million who reside in the Commonwealth of Puerto Rico. In comparison, Whites and Blacks constituted 71.9% and 12.8%, respectively, of the total population.[13] Hispanics have become the dominant minority, outnumbering Blacks in New York, Los Angeles, San Diego, Phoenix, San Francisco, and Denver; they are the majority in San Antonio, Texas. All areas of the United States, however, have experienced significant Hispanic growth in the last several years.[14] According to government projections, Hispanics will eclipse Blacks as the nation's largest minority group in the year 2010.[15, 16] Furthermore, the Census Bureau predicts that by 2050, the U.S. population will be almost evenly divided between minorities and non-Hispanic Whites. Hispanics are projected to have 24.5% of the total U.S. population in 2050.

A recent study demonstrated that "fully 50% of America's Hispanics considered themselves Hispanic first and American second."[17] These foreign-born Hispanics are more dependent on Spanish than ever; the proximity of their homelands is causing a growing number of Hispanics to consider themselves temporary expatriates in the United States, not permanent Americans; fewer Hispanics than ever before equate making it in America with becoming part of America's cultural mainstream. Additionally, both the proximity and number of Spanish countries near the United States create a constant awareness of the heritage.[18] Hispanic immigrants are a major cultural and linguistic group that, unlike earlier groups, are not assimilating but are acculturating. As the twenty-first century approaches, America is considered a place where ethnic culture and linguist groups maintain their level of identity.

Nonetheless, the majority of the Hispanic population was born in the United States and retains U.S. citizenship. According to 1996 data, over three-fifths (62.1%) of U.S. Hispanics were native born and less than two-fifths (38.0%) were foreign born. In that same year, however, 69.0% of the Hispanic population were U.S. citizens.[19]

DEMOGRAPHIC PROFILE OF THE U.S. HISPANIC POPULATION

EL PERFIL DEMOGRAFICO DE LOS HISPANOS EN LOS EEUU

DIVERSITY *DIVERSIDAD*

Hispanics are an ethnically and racially diverse population. Although the entire population is classified as "Hispanic," ethnomedical researchers have identified five distinct categories of Hispanics: Mexican Americans, Puerto Ricans, Cuban Americans, Central or South Americans, and "Other."[20] Mexican Americans—the largest subgroup—initially came from northern Mexico, hence the reference in Spanish to *un norteño* when referring to a Mexican living in the United States.[21] Recent immigration patterns indicate that people are coming from deep in the interior of Mexico.

The region which is now Florida, a word which means "flowery" in Spanish, was settled in the 16th century by the Spaniards, who founded the city of St. Augustine, the oldest permanent settlement in the United States, in 1565. Many Mexican-American families have lived in the southwestern United States long before the English-speaking population arrived. Names of states (Montana [mountain], Colorado [red], Nevada [snowy]), cities (Los Angeles [the angels], Los Alamos [the poplars], Las Vegas [the fertile plains], Santa Fe [holy faith]), and names of landmarks (the Alamo, the misssion at San Juan Capistrano, the *Camino Real* highway, the "mission style" of architecture, Mendocino National Forest), mountains (Tula Rosa, Escudilla, and Mangas Mountains and the San Andreas Fault), and rivers (the Brazos, Misisipi, Nueces, and Río Grande Rivers) speak to their historical presence. Additional immigration occurred following the 1910 Mexican Revolution. In fact, the majority of the Hispanic population in the Southwest probably can be traced to these settlers. The establishment of Chicago as a railroad hub for the nation and the need for migrant workers resulted in the diffusion of this population of Mexican ancestry into the Midwest in general and Chicago in particular. Immigration from Mexico has continued in ever growing numbers since the 1960s. Mexican Americans, who constitute approximately 64% of the U.S. Hispanic population,[22] are found in large numbers in California and Texas although they are also found in northern cities such as Chicago, Detroit, and Toledo.[23]

Soon after Spain ceded Puerto Rico to the United States in 1898, Puerto Ricans began settling on the mainland. They initially came to New York City in the 1920s in small numbers, but after World War II, New York witnessed a large migration of Puerto Ricans. By the 1950s, they began moving in significant numbers to adjacent states. By the 1960s, Puerto Ricans began moving westward in significant numbers. Puerto Ricans, who form 10.4% of the Hispanic population, are concentrated primarily in New York, but are found in many cities in Connecticut, Massachusetts, New Jersey, and Pennsylvania as well as in Illinois, Ohio, southern Florida, and on the West Coast.[23, 24]

During the nineteenth century, Cuban settlements occurred in the Tampa (Florida) and New York areas. Nonetheless, it was not until Fidel Castro came into power that the "great Cuban immigration" occurred. Subsequent smaller waves of immigration have been ongoing. Cubans, comprising 4.2% of the Hispanic population, are found primarily in Florida.[23, 25] However, there are also major Cuban communities in New York, northern New Jersey, Chicago, New Orleans, Atlanta, and Los Angeles.[23]

Since the 1960s, there has been large-scale immigration to the United States from many different areas of Latin America. Central and South America are the fastest growing sources of Hispanics in the United States. Almost one-tenth of El Salvador's population has immigrated to the United States since the 1970s and currently reside in Los Angeles, New York City, Washington, D.C., and the San Francisco Bay Area. Significant numbers of immigrants from Guatemala and Nicaragua have also followed the patterns set by those from El Salvador, although their numbers have not been as great. The *Nicaragüenses* form a sizeable community in Miami. At present the largest single Hispanic source of immigrants to New York City are *Dominicanos*, and there are still large numbers of *Colombianos* living both in Miami and New York City.[23, 26] Immigrants from other countries in Latin America are found in all U.S. (Hispanic) communities.

GEOGRAPHIC DISTRIBUTION   *DISTRIBUCION GEOGRAFICA*

Geographically, Hispanics are found all over the United States—in all fifty states, the U.S. territories, and the Commonwealth of Puerto Rico—but, as noted, the geographic distribution of the Hispanic subgroups varies greatly. Nonetheless, they are clustered tightly in a few regions, rather than being found evenly distributed throughout the country. About 60% of all Hispanics, the largest concentrations of Hispanics in percentage terms, live in five southwestern states (Arizona, California, Colorado, New Mexico, and Texas), and 86% of these persons are of Mexican origin. About 30% of all Hispanics reside in California, 22% in Texas, 8% in Arizona, Colorado, and New Mexico, 12% in New York, and 27% throughout the rest of the United States. In 1995, the five states with the largest absolute numbers of Hispanics—74% of the nation's Hispanic population—were California, whose Hispanic population was estimated to be 8.9 million (34.3% of the total U.S. Hispanic population); Texas, with 5.0 million (19.3%); New York, 2.5 million (9.6%); Florida, 1.9 million (7.2%); and Illinois, 1.1 million (4.0%).[27] These figures reflect migration patterns to border states and to areas where air travel was easy and economical. Even the most populous region in the United States, the central region, has one of the smallest populations of Hispanics in absolute numbers as well as the smallest percentage of Hispanics.[28] Of all U.S. Hispanics, 90% are urbanites,[29] even though the majority of the Hispanic population live in select states. Chicago has proportions of Hispanic populations in its metropolitan area that seem reflective of the national trend: Mexicans, 65%; Puerto Ricans, 22.6%; Central Americans, 3.6%; and Cubans, 2.0%.[30]

CHARACTERISTICS OF THE U.S. HISPANIC POPULATION

CARACTERISTICAS DE LA POBLACION HISPANA VIVIENDO EN LOS EEUU

AGE   *EDAD*

The U.S. Hispanic population has grown faster than the overall U.S. population since 1990. The number of Hispanics increased 25.3% from 1990 to 1996, compared with 6.4% for the overall U.S. population. The Census Bureau estimates that the Hispanic population will increase 27.5% between 1996 and 2005, to 36.1 million, while during that same period the non-Hispanic Black population will increase 11.2%, to 35.5 million.[31] The rapid growth in the Hispanic component of the population nationwide has been fueled by significant immigration, high fertility rates, and their youth. Immigration accounts for one-third of this population explosion.[32] On average, Hispanics reflect larger families than either non-Hispanic Whites or African Americans, and they are relatively young. Overall, Hispanics are much younger than non-Hispanics, and a large proportion are children. Almost 30% (29.8%) of the Hispanic population is under age 15, compared with 21.5% of the non-Hispanic population. In 1996, for example, more than one-third (35.2%) of Hispanics were under age 18, compared with one-quarter (24.9%) of Whites and nearly one-third (32.0%) of Blacks. In 1996 the median age for Hispanics was estimated at 26.4 years, while the median age estimates for Whites and Blacks were 35.7 years and 29.5 years, respectively.[33]

BIRTH RATE   *EL INDICE DE NATALIDAD*

Another consequence of the youth of Hispanics is their growing birth rate. The fertility rate of Hispanic women is 46% higher than the rate for non-Hispanic women.[34] From 1990 to 1996, Hispanic women between the ages of 15 and 44 were estimated to average 106.3 births per 1,000 women annually, compared with 67.7 births for the total population, up from the 1985 statistics which showed 97 births per 1,000 Hispanic women compared with 65 births per 1,000 for the total population.[35] Furthermore, 17.4% of all Hispanic births were to teenage mothers in 1995, compared with 12.8% of all births.[36] Mexican-American and "other Hispanic" women are largely responsible for this high birth rate (111 per 1,000 and 109 per 1,000 respectively).[37] The Puerto Rican birth rate is comparable to the average of non-Hispanics (68 births per 1,000), while that of Cuban Americans is lower (54 births per 1,000). Also, the average size of the Hispanic family is 4.4 people compared with the average size of the non-Hispanic family, which is 3.5 people. As this young, "fertile" group moves into the reproductive years, the Hispanic population is expected to sustain growth in the near future. Births will account for about two-thirds of the projected Hispanic increase. In general, Hispanics experience fewer premature births and low perinatal mortality than the rest of the population. The Census Bureau says that the number of Hispanic births will double by mid-century. Hispanic women age 14 to 49 currently bear an average of 2.9 children apiece over a lifetime, the highest rate of any major ethnic or racial group. This is in sharp contrast to the birth rate for non-Hispanic women, which is 1.9 children.[38]

SENIORS   *ANCIANOS*

Since 1970 there has been a significant growth (61%) in the number of Hispanics age 65 and older. While there are still about twice as many non-Hispanics (12.8%) who are 65 years of age or older compared with Hispanics (5.7%), the Bureau of the Census projects that over the next 20 years the increase in the total number of Hispanics in this category will account for 25% of the total Hispanic population growth.[39]

LANGUAGE   *IDIOMA*

Spanish is used by every one of the twenty Spanish-speaking nationalities comprising the U.S. Hispanic population. As a living language, it is constantly changing. Approximately 60% of contemporary Spanish vocabulary is derived from Latin. The other 40% comes from a variety of other languages including Arabic, Basque, Greek, and the languages of Native Americans (Nahuatl from Mexico, Mayan from Mexico and Guatemala, Quechua from Ecuador, the Southern Andes, Argentina, and other areas). Each country where Spanish is spoken has nationality colorations related to pronunciation, cadence, and the meaning of individual words, just as there are colorations among English speakers. An example can be found in the different ways of saying "bus." In most of the Spanish-speaking world people say *el autobús, el ómnibus,* or just *el bus.* Nonetheless, in Guatemala and El Salvador the word is *camioneta;* in Chile it is *micro,* in Panama, *chiva* and in Argentina *colectivo;* in Puerto Rico, Cuba, and the Canary Islands of Spain, the word is *la guagua;* and in Mexico people say *el camión.* Uncertainty results when people from the rest of Latin America or Spain hear the Mexicans speak of being hit by *el camión.* Listeners from Venezuela may think that the person was struck by a truck (the meaning in most places) when in reality the speaker meant a bus. Likewise, when someone says, *"Me robaron la guagua,"* it is not clear if the bus was stolen or if a small baby (the translation of *guagua* in Chile) was kidnapped!

PRIDE *ORGULLO*

The Anglo world tends to view all speakers of Spanish as the same; nevertheless, individual Spanish speakers tend to maintain a fierce sense of national and/or regional pride and identity, which is passed down from one generation to the next. When asked about their origin, someone whose ancestors came from Spain may respond, "*Soy madrileño/madrileña* (I am from Madrid)," someone else might say, "*Soy de Jalisco* (I am from Jalisco)," and still another, "*Soy habanero/habanera* (I am from Havana)" rather than saying, "*Soy español/española* (I am a Spaniard)," "*Soy mexicano/mexicana* (I am Mexican)," or "*Soy cubano/cubana/Soy de Cuba* (I am Cuban/I am from Cuba)."

NAMES *NOMBRES*

Hispanics also maintain certain traditions inherited from Spain concerning their names. Persons of Spanish or Hispanic descent often have several given or first names or **nombres de pila (nombres de bautismo)**. There are many compound first names such as Juan Carlos, María Rosa, José Antonio. It is common for Hispanics to be named after saints in the Catholic Church, after Jesus Christ, after Joseph and Mary, or after the places where, or the people to whom, the Virgin Mary appeared. Boys might be named *Jesús, José Asunción,* or *José María. María* is frequently used as the second part in compound male names (as are *Jesús* and *Jesús María*): *José María, Ramón María, Tomás María.* Girls are commonly named *María de Jesús* or *María Josefina.* In fact, the name *María* is especially frequent in compound names honoring special venerations to the Virgin Mary. Girls bearing one of these compound names are usually known by the latter part of the compound: *María de la Concepción* (Mary of the Immaculate Conception) is known as *Concepción, María de la Luz* (Mary of the Light) as *Luz, María del Pilar* (Mary of the Pillar) as *Pilar.* Girls are often given names of virtues, such as *Consuelo* (Consolation), *Esperanza* (Hope), and *Mercedes* (Mercy).

Nicknames are used in Spanish as in English and may be quite different from the original name: Dolores is known as Lola, Francisco as Paco, José as Pepe. It is quite common to use nicknames that refer to physical characteristics which may or may not be accurate, but which are used among close relatives and friends to express affection. *Gordo* or *Gordito* ("Fatty") might be used for a skinny male; *Negrita* ("Blacky") might be the nickname of a blond girl.

Hispanics retain both paternal and maternal surnames (*el apellido*). The paternal surname precedes the maternal one. Neither is ever considered to be a middle name. Only in the case of an illegitimate child is the maternal surname alone used. Sometimes these family names are connected by the conjunction *y* (and), or by a hyphen; generally they are not. Occasionally, the maternal family name is abbreviated, in which case the first initial of the mother's last name follows the father's last name. In cases when the paternal family name is extremely common (the Spanish equivalent of Smith or Jones), it is either abbreviated or omitted.[40] Thus, in the case of *Jaime José Alfredo Fernández y García,* the first three names are given names, *Fernández* is the surname of the father and *García* is the surname of the mother. In addition, the following variations may be found: *Jaime José Alfredo Fernández García; Jaime José Alfredo Fernández G.; Jaime José Alfredo Fernández; Jaime José Alfredo F. García; Jaime José Alfredo García; Jaime José Alfredo Fernández-García.*

An Hispanic woman upon her marriage drops her mother's maiden name and replaces it with that of her husband, prefixed by *de.* Thus, *María Fernández y Montero* becomes *María Fernández de González* upon her marriage to *Juan Carlos González y Ortiz.* Should her husband die, she is known as *María Fernández Vda. de González* (*Vda.* is *viuda,* which means widow).

A number of Spanish surnames include the preposition *de,* with or without the definite article *el/la/los/las.* At one time the preposition *de* indicated nobility, but no such distinction is made now and the use of *de* is optional. However, some families still retain it as part of the surname: *del Campo, de la Torre, de la Rosa.* Likewise, many Spanish surnames end in *-ez,* a suffix originally added to the father's first name to denote "son of," much the same way that the suffix was used in English. Compare Ericson, the son of Eric with Fernández, *el hijo de Fernando* (son of Fernando).

Proper alphabetizing of Spanish surnames requires knowledge of the differences between the English and Spanish alphabets, the former having twenty-six letters, the latter, prior to 1994, having thirty, but currently having twenty-eight as the result of an effort to join the technology age. For alphabetizing purposes, surnames precede proper names. Compound surnames are arranged according to the first surname. For those names with a lower case *de, del, de la,* or *de los,* these are placed after the name: *Ríos,*

Fernando de los. Uppercase prepositions, which generally indicate surnames of French, Italian, or Portuguese origin, precede the surname: *Da Rosa, Carlos.* Names of married women are arranged according to the maiden name.

FAMILY   *LA FAMILIA*

The concept of family and kinship relations is determined culturally. The Hispanic family is significantly larger than the U.S. "nuclear family" and has traditionally been viewed as one of the greatest strengths of the Hispanic community. Hispanics tend to live in family households rather than alone or with nonrelatives. Within this unit, Hispanic families exhibit interdependence, affiliation, and cooperation. It is not at all unusual to find grandmothers involved in the daily care and raising of their grandchildren. It is an expectation, not an intrusion, that several generations live together under one roof. Although customs are changing, it is also still an expectation that single, adult children live at home while they attend college, or until they take a job away from home, or until they marry. Even after children leave home, family ties remain strong. When family members travel, they are expected to stay with relatives rather than in hotels. Close friends are often made "family" members and welcomed by other extended family members. Consider the greetings, *"Mi casa es su casa"* and *"Está en su casa."*

Practices involving how children are raised differ greatly. A large circle of family members is always present to assist with the children. Some live in the home, others (aunts, uncles, and cousins) live in close proximity. Babysitters are quite uncommon for the most part. Children, including babies and toddlers, commonly accompany their families to restaurants, church, movies, or anywhere else the adults go without regard to the hour. The younger generation quickly learns to behave appropriately, especially when constantly reminded to *Pórtate bien* and Hispanic adults tend to be rather tolerant of occasional commotion and slight noise.

Hispanic families are somewhat larger than other U.S. families. Every major Hispanic-origin group shows a substantially larger household size than the total U.S. mean of 2.8 persons per household. The average household size for the U.S. Hispanic population is 3.7 persons. The larger Hispanic household size is culturally related to the extended-family tradition and the prevalence of the Catholic religion, which prohibits most forms of birth control. Although the majority of Hispanics are Christian, not all are Catholic. Fundamentalist denominations, such as Protestants and Pentecostals, have been particularly successful in attracting U.S. Hispanics who find Catholicism somewhat outmoded in its doctrines. Churches serving U.S. Hispanics, however, provide an atmosphere of community participation. It is an accepted fact of Hispanic life in the United States that priests and ministers offer advice and counsel about educational, political, and social issues concerning human rights.

On average, there are differences in family size among the major Hispanic subgroups. Mexican Americans have the largest household size (3.9 persons), particularly in small towns or rural areas, followed in order by Puerto Ricans, Central Americans, and Cubans, who show the smallest number of persons in the household (3.3 persons). In addition to having the smallest family size of any of the Hispanic groups, Cubans have the highest median age, the highest educational and income level, followed in order by Latin-American immigrants, Mexicans, and Puerto Ricans. Nonetheless, families are changing. Although Hispanics remain less likely to be divorced than the general population,[41] the number of Hispanic single-parent households is increasing, as is the percentage of Hispanic children under 18 living with one rather than both parents.[42]

ECONOMIC STATUS   *POSICION ECONOMICA*

Nearly two-thirds (62.6%) of the total Hispanic population 16 years and over, or 12.7 million, were employed in 1997. In other words, the majority of those eligible for employment, 90.8%, were in the labor force and working in 1997. Nevertheless, unemployment rates for Hispanics age 16 and over were considerably higher in March 1997 (9.2%) than for non-Hispanic Whites (4.8%), but lower than for Blacks (11.2%).[43] Most Hispanics work in white-collar jobs including managerial, administrative support, and professional specialties. In 1996, about 28% of Hispanic males were employed in blue-collar, agricultural, and service industries. There are no accurate data on Hispanic migrant and/or seasonal farm workers. Workers in such occupations have less flexibility to schedule medical appointments and take medications during the time they are on the job. Employed Hispanics are more likely to work in labor-intensive, and less lucrative, occupations than non-Hispanics. They also are more likely to earn less than non-Hispanic Whites, even among year-round, full-time workers. Hispanics have been called "working poor." In 1997, the median weekly earnings for Hispanic full-time workers was $351, compared with $519 for Whites and $400 for Blacks. In 1996, the real per capita income for Hispanics was $10,048, compared with $19,181 for Whites and $11,899 for Blacks. Real median household income for households maintained by a person(s) of Hispanic origin was $24,906 in 1996, compared with $37,161 for comparable households of Whites and $23,482 of Blacks.[44]

The Commerce Department's Census Bureau, using many different measures of poverty, concluded that "being poor in America is a transitory condition for many and a chronic condition for a small percentage of the population. Most people who experience poverty generally escape it within a few months."[45] This is not the case for Hispanics who are more likely to live below the poverty level than non-Hispanics. In 1996, approximately 36.5 million people, representing 13.7% of the nation's population, lived below the official average poverty threshold, which, for a family of four, was $16,036. Poverty rates for Hispanic families and their children remain disproportionately high. As a result of their low income, about one-fourth of all Hispanic families in the United States were living below the poverty level in 1996.[46] Although the Hispanic population was only 11.1% of the total population in 1997, about three of ten individuals (29.9%) living in poverty in the United States were of Hispanic origin. Despite this fact, Hispanic Americans even with this low median income are the richest Hispanics in the world.

Income affects health insurance coverage. Health insurance is tied to economic status and to health care coverage in the workplace. Among the various race and ethnic groups, persons of Hispanic origin were the most likely not to be covered by health insurance benefits in the workplace throughout 1996. They were less likely to have private or government health insurance than Whites or Blacks, but more likely to be covered by Medicaid than Whites. Some Hispanics who have access to group health insurance cannot afford the premiums to cover themselves and their families. In 1995, 33.3% of all Hispanics were not covered by health insurance. This can be sharply contrasted to the smaller percentages of Whites (14.2%) and Blacks (21.0%) who did not have health insurance coverage. Among the Hispanic subgroups, Puerto Ricans and Cuban Americans are twice as likely to be uninsured as the non-Hispanic Whites, and Mexican Americans under 65 years of age are more than three times as likely to be uninsured. Higher percentages of Hispanic children (28.9%) were found lacking any form of health insurance than White (13.9%) and Black (18.8%) children.[47]

EDUCATIONAL STATUS *ESTADO EDUCACIONAL*

The inadequate educational attainment of Hispanics remains a serious concern. Hispanics have a much smaller percentage of high school and college graduates than Whites or Blacks.[48] Many Hispanics live at or below the poverty level[49] and are not academically prepared to meet the challenges of today, much less those of tomorrow. Almost from the beginning, Hispanic youngsters are less likely than their peers to take advantage of educational opportunities. For instance, of children enrolled in Head Start in 1991, 14.2% were Hispanic and 38.0% were Black, despite the fact that Hispanic and Black children are similarly represented among preschool children living in poverty. By 1997 that percentage had improved to 26.1% for Hispanics and slightly declined for Blacks (36.1%).[50] Half of Hispanic youth leave school without obtaining a diploma. Nearly half a million Hispanic youngsters dropped out of high school in 1995 alone.[51] In 1996 over one-half (53.1%) of Hispanics 25 years old and over had graduated from high school in sharp contrast to over four-fifths (82.8%) of Whites and almost three-fourths (74.3%) of Blacks in that same age category. Although approximately one of ten Hispanics (10%) earned a bachelor's degree or better in 1997, one of four (24.3%) Whites and one of seven (13.6%) Blacks had completed college.[52] There are not enough Hispanic students preparing themselves for professions. The American Council for Education's study, *Minorities in Higher Education*, clearly indicates that they "are grossly under-represented at every rung of the educational ladder." According to the National Science Foundation, Blacks and Hispanics comprise less than 8% of college graduates with science or engineering degrees. Almost worse is the fact that there are not enough Hispanics among those responsible for health care. Too few Hispanics are studying medicine in the United States. In recent years the Association of American Medical Schools has reported an enrollment of only about half the proportion of Hispanics in the national population.

SIMILARITIES   *SEMEJANZAS*

Although each of the Hispanic subgroups in the United States has its own distinctiveness, certain generalizations can be made about cultural and sociodemographic similarities that are shared by all Hispanic groups living in the United States which distinguish them from the general population. All groups share the common colonial experience with Spain as well as the virtual elimination of the native population.[53] Another commonality has to do with an uneasiness toward the "Yankees" (*los yanquis*), Imperialism, and the Yankees' attitudes toward Latin America that have prevailed for almost 200 years in Latin America. All groups have a connection to the Spanish language, which permits them to easily communicate with each other providing a sense of unity. Finally, they share common values which originated in Spain: the large, extended family, the definitions of respect and honor, the social stratifications based on class and profession, and the distrust of government in general.

RECAP   *RECAPITULACION*

The sociodemographic commonalities, listed in table format, pertain to age, socioeconomic welfare, educational attainment, and language background.

1. *Age:* They are very young. The median age in 1996 for all U.S. Hispanics was 26.4 years compared with 35.7 years for Whites and 29.5 for Blacks. The median age for Mexican Americans was 23.9 years, for Puerto Ricans it was 26.7 years, for Central and South Americans it was 27.4 years, but for Cuban Americans it was 42.9 years.[22] The youthfulness of this population will help shape the U.S. demographics in the future.

2. *Housing:* They reside primarily in urban areas. According to the Bureau of the Census about half of all Hispanics live in the central areas of large cities and 87% are urban residents. Nonetheless, Hispanics are less likely to own their residence than other ethnic or racial groups.[54]

3. *Family Composition:* Over half of Hispanic households are married-couple family households (54.8%), thus continuing the two-parent family as the most common family structure. Nonetheless, single Hispanic females head nearly one-fifth (19.2%) of Hispanic households compared with 9.6% of White households and 31.9% of Black households. The average number of persons per Hispanic household is 3.5 compared with 2.6 persons per non-Hispanic household.[55]

4. *Economic Status:* (a) The median family Hispanic income continues to be significantly below that of White families and has been declining since 1990. In 1995, it was $24,570 ($42,646 for Whites and $25,970 for Blacks). More than one of four (26.5%) Hispanic families live in poverty compared with 10.2% of non-Hispanic families.[56] (b) This level of poverty cannot be attributed, however, to low participation in the labor force. A significant segment of Hispanics are participating in the labor force. In 1996, 60.6% of the Hispanic population 16 years old and over were employed compared with 64.1% of Whites and 57.4% of Blacks. Hispanics are generally employed in manual labor and service occupations as well as in managerial, administrative support, and professional specialties. In 1996, the Hispanic unemployment rate was 8.9% compared with 4.7% for White workers and 10.5% for Black workers. In 1997, those figures increased to 9.2% for Hispanic workers, 4.8% for White workers, and 11.2% for Black workers. The earnings level of Hispanics makes them considered the "working poor" as evidenced from a comparison of only households with a working individual. Hispanics were more likely to live in poverty (22.0%) than were Black (21.1%) or White (7.3%) households.[57]

5. *Educational Status:* The average educational level of Hispanics continues to be less than that of the United States as a whole, although it has been steadily improving. In 1997, over one-half (55%) of Hispanics 25 years old and older had graduated from high school compared with 1980 figures when only 44% of the Hispanic population had completed twelfth grade.[58]

6. *Language Preference:* The vast majority of Hispanics who speak Spanish are also proficient in English. In 1990, 91.5% of the 17.3 million persons 5 years old and over who spoke Spanish at home also spoke English.[59]

There are certain attitudinal and cultural similarities shared by all U.S. Hispanic groups:[60]

1. They maintain close family ties and paternal leadership characteristics, valuing the tradition of extended family.
2. They take tremendous pride in themselves and in their heritage and culture.
3. Hispanics have a high regard for the work ethic and for advancement through individual initiative and achievement.
4. Hispanics tend to be fiscally conservative in nature, but will spend money on family-oriented outlays.
5. About 85% of all Hispanics are Roman Catholics, although this figure is declining.
6. Hispanics respond best to audio and visual images rather than to lengthy details.
7. Home and neighborhood are very important.

8. The vast majority of Hispanics are tied culturally to the language, even if they are not fluent in Spanish. Hispanics consider their language the most important part of their tradition to preserve.

9. Hispanics have a strong need to be "recognized," while simultaneously evidencing pride and self-esteem in being American.

LANGUAGE BARRIERS

BARRERAS DEL IDIOMA

As the population of the United States becomes ever more diverse and the number of languages spoken increases, there are ever increasing numbers of patients who speak no English. This communication gap can form an impenetrable wall between practitioner and patient and undermine both quality and dignity of treatment. It is almost impossible to effectively treat and diagnose people when one is unable to communicate with them.

Hispanics living in the United States are heterogeneous linguistically: there are Hispanics who speak only Spanish, mostly Spanish, fluent Spanish and English, mostly English, and only English. Because a large portion of Hispanics living in the United States is immigrant, language becomes an important factor for those immigrants seeking health services due to their inability to speak, read, or write in the English language.[61] The number of people in the country with limited or no proficiency in English is growing. According to the U.S. Census Bureau, more than 31 million people in the United States speak a language other than English at home. This equates to 14% of people in the United States over age 5 who speak a language other than English at home, up from 11% in 1980.[62] The Association of State and Territorial Health Officials estimates that approximately 6% of the U.S. population age 5 and over have limited English proficiency skills.[63] In the 1990 census, about 15 million Americans, or 6% of the population, said that they had significant problems communicating in English, up from the 4.9% in 1980. Demographers say that the percentage of limited English proficient individuals is increasing and with this increase, the challenge to provide services, including education, law enforcement, and medical care.

Immigrants must learn a difficult language—English—and new customs while meeting the everyday needs of food, shelter, and income. Economic insecurity and physical and emotional stress have long been characteristic of immigrant life. Nonetheless, becoming ill can turn the existing stress into health and economic catastrophe, especially when English language skills are limited. These individuals must then deal with the increased stress of an illness while attempting to deal with the complexities of the U.S. health care system. Because of the vast array of public and private health care providers and the costly fee-for-service method of payment in the United States, most immigrants find private care unaffordable and public care often limited and unaccessible.[64] Non-English-speaking patients generally avoid the offices of physicians who do not understand their language or customs, but they do visit hospitals and large clinics. Nowhere is the need for translation greater than in health care, where a miscommunication could make the difference between good care and bad, or possibly even between life and death!

Health care providers tend to be Caucasian and English speaking, whereas patients increasingly come from varied ethnic and racial groups.[65] Health care programs developed for one group (e.g., Puerto Ricans) cannot be transferred to another ethnic group (e.g., Mexicans) without modifications for cultural differences. Health care providers, patient education classes, and health literature and information must be bilingual. Language barriers and inadequate medical interpreting not only increase uncertainty for immigrants seeking care for an illness, but they discourage people with limited or no English from seeking preventive care. In fact, many Hispanics use home remedies or *curanderos* (faith healers) until the medical problem reaches a serious stage. It is well documented that when these individuals with limited or no English skills cannot communicate with health care providers, they frequently stop seeking care; however, neither they nor their children stop getting sick.[66]

Unfortunately, there are all too many anecdotes which detail the health care problems that arise between patient and practitioner when the patient has limited English proficiency skills. It is not unusual to hear of erroneous or delayed diagnosis and treatment because an interpreter cannot be found to speak with the patient. Serious problems and misunderstandings also arise when practitioners enlist relatives or untrained hospital janitors or clerks to translate complex medical information for a non-English-speaking patient. Furthermore, this practice infringes on their right to be adequately informed of their conditions and treatment plans. Relatives and friends acting as interpreters may withhold information, either to keep doctors from learning embarrassing or damaging facts, or to protect patients from bad news. Practitioners must be attuned to the need for culturally appropriate communication when the only bilingual translator available is a child related to the patient. Too often, patients, wishing to save their children from trauma, or too embarrassed to discuss private concerns in front of them, may withhold critical information, thus compromising their care. A husband who abused his wife would not be likely to explain her injuries accurately. When nonmedical hospital personnel are pressed into being interpreters, they have, in all likelihood, a limited familiarity with medical terms and usually bring to the task their own judgments.[67] One Spanish-speaking woman recently miscarried at the county hospital in Chicago. Because there were no available translators, she mistakenly believed that she was intentionally given medication that caused her to abort.[68] In Houston another patient, a Mexican peasant, invented vague symptoms because she was too embarrassed to describe her real problem—a rectal fistula—while her son was translating. Consequently, she was misdiagnosed.[69] Still another expectant Hispanic mother, who spoke no English, learned in her ninth month of pregnancy when she went to a new facility for a checkup that she was carrying an anencephalic baby, a child with a fatal birth defect—a fact that medical personnel elsewhere thought they had conveyed months earlier.[70] Elsewhere, parents of a Guatemalan child with ear infections administered the oral medication in their child's ears because they misunderstood the hospital staff's instructions.[71] Other non-health-related issues must also be considered.

HEALTH PROBLEMS AND RISKS

PROBLEMAS Y RIESGOS DE SALUD

Most ethnomedical research on the Hispanic population in the United States has focused on Mexican Americans, individuals born and raised in Mexico prior to relocating to the U.S., and Chicanos, individuals of Mexican descent, born and raised in the U.S., with more limited attention directed toward Puerto Ricans and Cubans. Those Hispanics who trace their origin to Central and South America, and who now constitute about 20% of the persons of Hispanic heritage in the United States, have been studied to an even lesser extent.

Until very recently, public interest in and research on Hispanics and their health risks have been limited. Therefore, the limited data available make it very difficult to properly address the health problems of the Hispanic population in the United States. We now know that there are positive and disturbing factors to consider with regard to Hispanic health. Data show that Hispanic adults are less likely to see a physician than any other racial or ethnic group.[72] This lack of access complicates chronic illnesses such as diabetes, AIDS, cancer, heart disease, and cirrhosis.

Available data establish that diabetes mellitus is one of the most serious and significant health threats to this population. Studies indicate that Mexican Americans are known to have a prevalence of type II diabetes three times that of the general population.[73] Another study suggests that one of four Mexican Americans (23.9%) and Puerto Ricans (26.1%) 45 years old and over suffer from diabetes. It also reveals that one-third (33.3%) of Hispanics 65 years old and over are diabetic compared with 17.0% of non-Hispanic Whites.[74] Despite all known facts, there is a lack of screening for early detection of diabetes in the Hispanic population.

Other factors of chronic illness present among Hispanic adults are diet and exercise. Low levels of physical activity and high fat consumption are associated with diabetes and cardiovascular disease. Mexican-American men are more likely than non-Hispanic Black and non-Hispanic White men to have high serum cholesterol levels (20.3% compared with 16.6% and 19.1%).[75] However, Mexican-American women are not as likely as non-Hispanic Black and non-Hispanic White women to have high serum cholesterol levels (19.4%, 20.7%, and 20.0%, respectively).[73] Despite this fact, more Hispanics are overweight than non-Hispanic Whites, especially women.

HIV/AIDS is a continually emerging threat to Hispanics. Along with diabetes, HIV/AIDS has been one of two exceptionally serious health crises for the Hispanic community. There is also a disproportionate number of Hispanics who have reported cases of AIDS. Although only 11% of the total U.S. population,[76] Hispanics accounted for 18% of the 641,086 cumulative reported AIDS cases and 21% of the 60,634 new AIDS cases through December 1997.[77] This cumulative incidence for Hispanic adults is three times that of non-Hispanic Whites. These rates are likely underestimates because many Hispanic men who have sex with men do not self-identify as gay/bisexual.[78] This percentage does not include Hispanics who are HIV positive, nor does it include those Hispanics who have been diagnosed with AIDS, but whose cases have not yet been reported to public health officials.[79] In the same way, although Hispanic children comprise only 14.5% of the total childhood-age population, they accounted for 23.2% of all pediatric AIDS cases through December 1997.[80] The incidence of AIDS among Hispanic children is more than five times the incidence among non-Hispanic White children. The majority of Hispanic children with AIDS contracted it perinatally when born to a mother who was an IV drug user or having sex with an IV drug user.[81]

The HIV/AIDS risk among Hispanics varies depending on the level of acculturation,[82] lifestyle, where they were born, and where they live in the United States. The prevalence of this disease among Hispanics varies by region. Puerto Rican–born Hispanics living in the Northeast and Hispanics born in the Dominican Republic have the highest rates.[83] They reflect the geography of injection drug use in the United States.[84] In the West and Southwest, where many Hispanics of Mexican and Central or South American origin live, much lower rates of HIV are reported.[85]

Most HIV and AIDS cases among Hispanics have been among men. The majority of them have been gay, bisexual, and injection drug users. In 1997, 34% of all AIDS cases among Hispanic men occurred in men who have sex with men, 30% occurred among injection drug users, 4% occurred among men who have sex with men and inject drugs, and 8% were due to heterosexual contact. Among Hispanic women, most cases have been the result of heterosexual exposures, although drug use also plays a major role in the spread of infection to women.[86]

Cultural influences such as *machismo, familismo,* and homophobia may be internalized by Hispanic gay men and make safer sex practices difficult. *Machismo* dictates that intercourse is a way to prove masculinity.[87] For gay Hispanics, *familismo,* the importance of the family as a social unit and source of support, can create conflict because families perceive homosexuality as sinful. Familial support is often achieved through silence about sexual preference, which instills low self-esteem and personal shame among Hispanic gay men.[88] Hispanics have been slowly overcoming a well-known resistance to acknowledging homosexuality in their communities, the use of intravenous drugs, shared needles, and unprotected sex and are attempting to educate themselves on the issue of AIDS transmission and prevention. Nonetheless, although there is now material available in Spanish, AIDS facts targeting middle-class Cuban males produce little effect on Puerto Rican teenagers using intravenous drugs. Each subgroup must be specifically targeted and addressed in a culturally effective way.

As a rule, Hispanics have a lower incidence of certain chronic diseases such as heart disease and cancer.[89] Although national mortality data for coronary heart disease (CHD) are unavailable, certain data are based on regional studies of Puerto Ricans in New York, and Mexican Americans in Texas and Los Angeles County. The findings indicate that Mexican Americans appear to have lower mortality rates from CHD than Whites in those regions.[90] Because of the higher prevalence of so many CHD risk factors such as diabetes, obesity, and lower socioeconomic levels, this lower rate was unexpected.[91] National mortality data for cancer are also unavailable. Studies by the Surveillance, Epidemiology, and End Results (SEER) Program of the National Cancer Institute have been limited to Hispanics living in the Commonwealth of Puerto Rico and in New Mexico. Findings indicate a lower overall incidence of cancer for Hispanics in the two areas studied than for Whites (246 cases compared with 335/100,000). These findings also indicate that Hispanics have a high incidence of cancer of the cervix, pancreas, prostate, and stomach. Hispanics have twice the rate of cervical and stomach cancers as found among Whites.[92] The most common cancer among Hispanic men is cancer of the prostate, which occurs in nearly 59 of 100,000 cases.[93] Breast and colorectal cancers, the most common cancers among women, are considerably less prevalent among Hispanics than among Whites and Blacks.[94] However, Puerto Rican women are at a disproportionately high risk for breast and cervical cancer. The fact that the vast majority have little or no access to preventive health care means that they are not seen until they seek care through emergency rooms when their condition has reached advanced stages. This fact suggests that their care will be more costly than if they had been seen routinely and that their prognosis is less favorable than that of other female groups.[95]

Alcohol use among Hispanics is estimated between two and three times the national average, which accounts for high morbidity and mortality due to a heightened incidence of cirrhosis of the liver and chronic liver disease.[96] Arterial hypertension is another serious health problem of Hispanics. According to Dr. Antonia Novello, a former surgeon general of the United States, hypertension appears to be more prevalent among Hispanics than non-Hispanic Whites.[2, 97] In general, the lower the socioeconomic status, the more likely hypertension exists among Hispanics—even when controlling for female obesity.[98] Even more distressing are the high levels of unrecognized and untreated hypertension in Hispanic populations. Hispanics who are economically disadvantaged exhibit a higher risk for unrecognized and untreated hypertension.

Hispanic men are more likely to have undiagnosed, untreated, or uncontrolled hypertension than the national average. Hispanic females are more likely than Hispanic men to be aware of their condition, although fewer receive treatment for it, and very few have it controlled.[99]

Hispanics are less likely to smoke or use illicit drugs than non-Hispanics.[100] In 1996, 24.7% of Hispanics 12 years old and over smoked, compared with 29.8% of Whites and 30.4% of Blacks.[73] Increases in cigarette smoking have resulted in a doubling of the rate of lung cancer among Hispanic women. Pregnant Hispanic women are less likely to smoke, making their youngsters far less likely to have been exposed to secondhand smoke prenatally. By the time that those same children were of preschool age, however, they were more likely to be exposed to smoke postnatally.[101] The 1996 statistics bear out that Hispanics are less likely to use illicit drugs than non-Hispanics: 5.2% of Hispanics used illicit drugs, compared with 6.1% of Whites and 7.5% of Blacks.[102] Hispanic adolescents, however, are more likely than their peers to abuse illicit drugs.[103]

Infant mortality is a commonly used indicator of a population's health status, and refers to deaths occurring in children during the first year of life. The rate is defined as the number of deaths per 1,000 live births. There is a relatively low infant mortality rate, even though Hispanic mothers are more than three times as likely as non-Hispanic White mothers (11.0% and 3.2%, respectively) and as likely as non-Hispanic Black mothers (10.7%) to have late or no prenatal care.[104] These percentages vary, however, within the Hispanic subgroups. Mexican-American mothers are the least likely to seek prenatal care (12.2%) and Cuban-American mothers are the most likely. In fact, the percentage of Cuban-American mothers receiving late or no prenatal care resembles that for non-Hispanic White mothers (2.4% and 3.2%, respectively).[104] In 1995, the infant mortality rate was 6.1 of 1,000 live births for Hispanics, 6.3 of 1,000 for White infants, and 15.1 of 1,000 for Black infants. Within the Hispanic subgroups, Cuban-American mothers had the lowest such rate (5.9 of 1,000 live births) whereas Puerto Ricans had the highest infant mortality rate (9.0 of 1,000 live births), although Puerto Ricans are the most likely to have access to prenatal care services.[104, 105]

Data about the age of the mother and the infant's birthweight are derived from birth certificates and surveys, which have the same limitations as data on death certificates.[106] Puerto Rican mothers have the highest rate of low-birth-weight births at 9.4%, close to the 13.6% rate of non-Hispanic Black mothers. Cuban-American, Mexican-American, and Central- and South-American mothers also have levels of low-birth-weight births (5.6%, 5.6%, and 5.9%, respectively) similar to those of non-Hispanic White mothers (5.7%).[104]

That these numbers clearly reflect the low perinatal mortality and fewer premature births is obvious, but they leave some questions about why this is possible, considering that 39% of Hispanics are uninsured and, therefore, less likely to seek medical attention, compared with 14% of non-Hispanic Whites.[107] A recent study found that 44% of Hispanic mothers who had inadequate prenatal care reported that the reason they did not see a doctor on a monthly basis during their last pregnancy was because there was "no need; I was healthy."[108] It is necessary to remember that many Hispanics define illness as having actual symptoms and not feeling well.[109] With that in mind, it is explainable, if not understandable, why the prenatal visits were so late or even nonexistent. Culturally, if these women felt healthy, they saw no reason to seek medical attention. One can also speculate that Hispanic women of childbearing age are less likely to use alcohol or abuse illicit drugs than their non-Hispanic counterparts.[110] Additionally, it is evident that Hispanic mothers tend to eat healthier than non-Hispanic women.[111] One study underscores the fact that immigrant Hispanic mothers had healthier live babies, smaller percentages of low-birth-weight births, and less infant mortality than did Hispanic mothers who had been born somewhere in the United States.[112]

The lack of access to preventive care services begun during the prenatal period continues to characterize Hispanic childhood. The health and well-being of Hispanic children are at greatest risk during both the preschool- and adolescent-age periods. Hispanic youngsters are also less likely than other groups of children to see a physician when ill. Figures indicate that among Hispanic children, there is a higher incidence of childhood diseases which are preventable by immunization such as measles,[113] lead poisoning,[114] and infectious diseases. Also, the severity of illness appears to be greater among Hispanic children than among their White peers for diseases such as pneumonia[115] and chronic illnesses including asthma[116] and bronchitis. Childhood injuries and violent deaths are much higher than in other racial or ethnic groups.[117] Hispanic adolescents are at risk of alcoholism and other substances,[118] unprotected sex,[119] and suicide.[120] The incidence of these risks is tied to a lack of access to early prevention services.

It is important to study health issues by Hispanic subgroups. Health differences exist between U.S.-born and foreign-born Hispanics from the same subgroup. For instance, health problems experienced by Chicanos and Mexican Americans are very different than those experienced in Mexico. The California Hispanic population serves as an epidemiological linkage between Mexico and the United States. Income and education are two important causes for these epidemiological differences. With assimilation, the U.S.-born Hispanics will resemble the U.S. population more and more with regard to education, employment, family relations, diet, child rearing practices, and so forth. It is well documented that the health of an infant reflects the general physical environment associated with the parents' income, education, breastfeeding practices, and preventive health measures. Diarrhea and pneumonia are almost nonexistent as a cause of death in California, for instance, but are major causes of early childhood death in Jalisco, Mexico. Because a child is not yet capable of taking care of him or herself, the parents' involvement in the child's health is vital. Research makes it clear that many early childhood health conditions are influenced by the parents' lack of education and/or income.

Proper diet and proper health care seem to be largely unavailable to the nation's 6 million plus seasonal and migrant farmworkers—many of whom are illegal aliens and two-thirds of whom are of Mexican origin. Illegals have been frightened of seeking fundamental health services such as immunizations, dental care, and prenatal care for expectant mothers. In the latter instance, without such attention, pregnant women run a higher-than-average risk of delivering a child who is mentally or physically impaired.

More research needs to be collected about other health concerns of the Hispanic community. As a result of their diet and lifestyle, gastrointestinal problems are common among Hispanics. The high incidence rate of gallstones is a health issue of major concern for the Hispanic population. Other problems include dental caries; periodontitis,[121] which is frequently associated with diabetes; illness from chronic and acute pesticide exposure;[122] depression; tuberculosis; and proper nutrition, especially during childhood.[123]

HISPANIC FOLK MEDICINE

REMEDIOS CASEROS HISPANOS

Random House Webster's College Dictionary (2nd ed., New York: Random House, 1997) defines folk medicine as "the ordinary person's concept of health, illness, and healing; it is the treatment of disease practiced traditionally among the common people stressing the use of herbs and other natural substances; the health practices arising from cultural traditions, from the empirical use of native remedies, especially food substances, or from superstition." Folk medicine can refer to any disease-and-cure concept from a honey-lemon-tequila mixture to cure a cough, to the causes, cures, and classifications of major disease symptoms and magic. Another definition is "a syndrome in which members of a particular group claim to suffer and for which their culture provides an etiology, diagnosis, preventive measure and regimen of healing."[124] These illnesses have a high degree of psychological and/or religious overtones. Inherent in the healing is the involvement of the family. For Hispanics, the extended family not only passes cultural beliefs and practices from generation to generation, but also provides an important source of support. In fact, researchers believe that the close family ties are an important factor in the lower utilization of mental health services by Hispanics as compared with other groups.[125] Generally people improve because of their personal faith in their remedies, their religion, and familial commitment. Such practices, though often considered as limited in value and frequently scoffed at by the medical profession, are readily accessible, practical, and tend to validate one's belief system. Many people have used some form of *remedios caseros*, or folk medicine, when they resort to home remedies. (The term *folk medicine* is an expression that can be used with an entire range of illnesses and diseases, from the non-life-threatening disease-and-cure concepts, such as combining equal parts of honey, lemon, and tequila together to cure a cough to the causes, cures, and classifications of major disease symptoms and magic.) Such remedies frequently help people treat minor illnesses which do not require a doctor's care, and they are especially useful when access to medical care is limited.

Without adequate access to health care, some Hispanics seek the services of folk healers either instead of, or in addition to, mainstream health care. Although Hispanics' reliance on folk medicine is limited, health providers must be aware of the possibility of its use.[126] To understand why people turn to folk medicine, it is helpful to know how they define *disease*. Most researchers note that there is no single theory of disease common to all Hispanics, yet certain cultural attitudes about health and illness are particular to many of them. Education and acculturation have produced some change in the medical beliefs held by many Spanish-speaking and Hispanic-American individuals. Nonetheless, while it is common to think that only the poor or unacculturated people will practice folk medicine, it should be noted that even the most sophisticated, educated Hispanic sometimes relies on *curanderismo*, or folk medicine, although the individual may not admit it to others.

A recent study entitled, "Utilization of *Curanderos* by Mexican Americans," suggests that folk systems of care are not necessarily the primary choice of Hispanics seeking health services.[127] Nonetheless, many Hispanics clearly utilize home remedies as evidenced by the sizeable number of small stores selling such items wherever large Hispanic communities exist. One must review this finding in the context of family and community—two values that are extremely important to all Hispanic subgroups. The family[128] and community[129] provide an element of *personalismo*, which is important to Hispanic patients, whereas the Anglo emphasis on the individual does not consider the patient in the larger context of family and community.

In terms of their views about medicine, Hispanics fall into three categories. At one extreme are the conservatives, who retain strong social and cultural ties to their country of origin. They have strong faith in the traditional folk medical beliefs and practices, and magic and religion assume great importance in their world. At the other extreme are the highly assimilated, whose faith in traditional cures is replaced by reliance on modern medicine. Magic and religion have little importance in their world. Most Hispanics, however, belong to the transitional group and their cultural beliefs reflect a very heterogeneous mixture of traditional folk beliefs and Anglo-American traits.

For many, folk beliefs and practices provide a culturally acceptable explanation for the unusual happenings within and around the patient.[130] Most Spanish-speaking people do not recognize illness in the absence of symptoms. When they feel well and are pain free, they believe they are well and will usually deny or delay acceptance of diagnosis and treatment of the early stages of diseases such as diabetes mellitus, hypertension, and tuberculosis. There is thus some problem accepting the Anglo germ theory of disease. If these germs or *animalitos* cannot be seen, they cannot exist.[131] Many believe that health is a gift from God and that there is very little that can be done to avoid illness.[132] For some Hispanics, being sick is considered a punishment. To help the illness disappear, these people will do penance. This may vary from keeping a *promesa* (promise) made to a patron saint, to making a long pilgrimage to a church, or even to "walking" on their knees several blocks to church.

All cultures have systems for classifying diseases on the basis of etiology, symptoms, and treatments. Among the people of Latin-American heritage, beliefs about health and illness have important sociocultural significance. Hispanics view the problems of health and illness as manifestations of closely linked physiologic and behavioral disturbance. Many folk beliefs are prompted by a physical image, such as when pregnant women carry keys to ensure that their baby will remain firmly "locked" in the womb. Many beliefs have an association with the etymology of the Spanish word for the particular affliction, which also often serves to reinforce that same belief. An example of the relationship of language origin to disease would be the use of the word *eclipsado*. The word, which literally means "eclipsed," refers to a child born with a harelip. This word acknowledges that the condition is (thought to be) caused when a pregnant woman views a lunar eclipse during her pregnancy. A synonym is *comido de la luna*, "eaten by the moon," which compares the disfigurement with the devouring of the sun by the moon during an eclipse. Other examples are plentiful.

Knowledge of the patient's existing beliefs and practices in medicine is extremely important; nonetheless, "an unsystematic collection of scraps of information may lead to an exaggerated respect for taboos and an underestimation of the importance of features of the society which may throw a medical program out of gear."[133] Most Hispanics share their Anglo neighbors' views on health and illness; occasionally, however, some will expand on these concepts by including some or all of the following perspectives: (1) a *religious* perspective in which God sends man illness and suffering because of failure to live a good, spiritual life; (2) a *sociological* perspective, which attributes illness to an excessive adherence to the overly materialistic Anglo lifestyle; (3) a *supernaturalistic* perspective, which is based on the power of mind over matter and the acceptance of good and evil spiritual influences; and (4) a *naturalistic* perspective, which acknowledges the importance of maintaining the body in a state of harmony and balance and holds that nature provides cures in the form of foods, herbs, and so forth.[134]

Researchers who have studied the principal features of folk medicine in Latin American countries and among Hispanics in the United States point to the eclectic nature of Latin American folk medicine. Folk concepts of disease are strongly rooted in Hispanic society, dating back hundreds of years to widely separated sources: medieval Spain; some (Meso-) American Indian tribes whose highly sophisticated native system of medicine linked health to religion; homeopathic therapy, which involves taking small amounts of herbs and/or drugs that, in larger, more concentrated doses, would cause symptoms similar to those of a specific disease; a potpourri of spiritual beliefs ranging from Christianity to spiritism which attribute the causes and cures of specific diseases to supernatural intervention; Anglo folk medicine and patent medicines; "scientific" medical sources; and the same holistic health care practices gaining popularity in the United States.[135] An important characteristic of this belief system is its capacity to assimilate practices from various folk and "scientific" medical traditions. This eclectic belief system in the causes of illness permits them to make judgments about a disease and to make choices in selecting a practitioner to cure them. Though not limited to folk diseases, the popular belief that certain diseases are thought to be caused by outside forces best cured by folk healers leads many Hispanics to seek nonscientific help. Each of the three major Hispanic groups in the United States—Mexican, Puerto Rican, and Cuban—has a preference for a specific type of folk healing.

In Mexican, Mexican-American, and Chicano communities, *curanderismo* (lay/folk healing) is prevalent. Studies have shown that 90% of folk medicine adherents do not use the services of a *curandero*,[136] or lay healer, but obtain their remedies from a hierarchy of lay healers. Hispanics look to kin, friends, and employers for consultative and prescriptive advice. Women treat most minor ailments for their family and are frequently consulted by neighbors as "home medical specialists" and are referred to respectfully as *señora* (ma'am) or *abuela* (grandmother). If the patient's condition requires more knowledge, other "home medical specialists" are sought such as the *yerbero/yerbera* (herbalist), the *partera* (midwife, who also treats problems with young children), or the *sobador/sobadora* (the folk practitioner who is adept at massage). If none of the lay healers can solve the problem, the patient is referred to the *curandero/curandera*.

Curanderos are highly respected, trusted members of the community. They do not accept direct remuneration for their services, but most accept gifts. Their healing consists primarily of prayers, usually before an altar in their home; they also prescribe remedies which assist in the recuperation to full health. Although *curanderos* are acknowledged experts in folk illnesses, they prescribe remedies for medical problems, too. Curing often draws on a wide range of treatment sources, including patent remedies, herbs, over-the-counter medicines, and prescription medicines. Herbalists or *curanderos* regularly prescribe treatments for people suffering from upper respiratory infections or rheumatism, for example. Sample "drugs" prescribed by an herbalist for a URI may include restricting dairy products and refined carbohydrates, quantities of vitamins C, B, and zinc; chamomile to calm restlessness, catmint to reduce nasal congestion, elderflower to reduce catarrhal symptoms, and echinacea to increase immunity. A *curandero* may suggest *salvia* (sage) tea as a tonic; *gordolobo* (mullein) tea as an antispasmodic; *orégano de la sierra* (oregano) tea for relief of a sore throat; and *eucalipto* (eucalyptus) tea as a mild bronchodilator. For patients seeking relief from rheumatism, a *curandero* may suggest using different poultices including *arnica* (arnica), *gobernadora* (chaparral), and *romero* (rosemary). An herbalist may prescribe using celery seed (a uricosuric agent); willow bark (an antiinflammatory); ginger (a circulatory "stimulant"), and devil's claw (to reduce inflammation and discomfort). Most *curanderos* recognize their limitations and will refer all serious illnesses—gynecologic and genitourinary problems, persistent digestive disorders, problems thought to be of the heart and blood—to a medical specialist or the hospital.[137]

In Puerto Rican communities, *espiritismo* (spiritism/spiritualism) is the folk healing practice of choice, and relies on the belief that evil spirits cause illness and emotional and social problems.[138] *Espiritismo* maintains that an invisible, spirit-filled world surrounds the visible world. Spirits can penetrate the visible world and attach themselves to human beings, sometimes causing illness. The practitioner is called an *espiritista*, a "spiritualist." The *espiritista* is considered to be a psychic, a person who is able to identify illnesses and their sources, communicate with these spirits, and treat the ailments. Many feel that the *espiritista* experiences the patient's pain in exactly the same location in his or her own body. Relief is found through a ritualistic cleansing process known as a *barrida* (sweeping), which rids the body of the evil spirit. Music, herbs and potions, movements, and other paraphernalia are used. This belief is also prevalent in the Caribbean. *Espiritistas* play an important role in rural areas where they are sought after to cure *un mal puesto*, a term which covers a wide gamut of symptoms and diseases, including tuberculosis, insanity, and other chronic illnesses attributed to witchcraft. Another common folk illness for some Puerto Ricans is *ataque* (attack). The syndrome is characterized by mutism, hyperventilation, violence, bizarre behavior, hyperkinesis, and uncommunicativeness. The symptoms occur as a response to shocking or unexpected news. It is viewed as a severe expression of shock, anxiety, or sadness. *Causa* (cause) is an ailment whose origin the *espiritista* must determine. If it is deemed to the result of a material *causa*, a physician will be contacted.

If the problem is determined to have a spiritual *causa,* a spiritualist is consulted. Also popular in Puerto Rico are *sobadoras* (female healers) who are similar to *curanderos.* They use oils (*aceite de culebra* [snake oil] and *aceite de olivo* [olive oil]) in their treatments of patients. They combine massage with listening skills.

Santería, the belief in the power of the saints to speak and cure through living persons, is practiced in Cuban and Cuban-American communities although the belief is also found elsewhere in the Caribbean. This Afro-Cuban belief combines Catholic saints and African Yoruban *Orichas* (spirits/deities). Although related to *espiritismo,* the *santeros/santeras* are the medium through whom a saint speaks or cures. Cuban home altars often contain *jimaguas,* African spirit dolls. *Santería* also uses herbs and potions. People consult a *santero/santera* to diagnose and treat a *bilongo* (hex). A *bilongo* can cause any illness, but only *santeros* can eliminate it.

Any of these traditional folk healers—*curanderos, espiritistas,* or *santeros*—may also serve as an acceptable alternative source for dealing with psychological and physical problems. These folk healers often provide marital, familial, or other personal counseling. Ethnomedical investigations about Hispanic illness referral systems have shown that folk curers are consulted only after the curing resources of the family have been exhausted.[139] If folk curers are consulted, it is always before official scientific doctors. The physician is consulted only after the folk curer fails. This combined use of household curing and physicians may be partly related to financial circumstances. When it becomes economically possible for Hispanics living in the United States to get care from health facilities and medical institutions, they quickly avail themselves of this care.[140]

A widespread Hispanic custom exists of borrowing prescriptions that are proven effective for relatives and friends and using leftover medicines for symptoms that seem similar.[141] Friends and relatives returning from "back home" replenish supplies of antibiotics and other drugs administered only by physician's prescription in the United States, but sold readily over-the-counter elsewhere.[142] Often Hispanics medicate themselves without any understanding of the limitations or risks involved. Home remedies such as tea or oil with honey are often taken as complements to drugstore medicines. Like other groups, Hispanic continuance or stoppage of medication may be based on the expectation of observable results. Many will discontinue medication if they do not see an immediate improvement of their symptoms. Others will take their medicine only until they get well, rather than for long-term therapeutic purposes, which reflects the belief that taking too much medication could be harmful.[143]

Many choices of remedies are offered by folk healers. Although they may use the same herbs, *curanderos* and *yerberos* (herbalists)[144] may use them differently. The following is a listing of folk remedies that are in common use throughout the United States and Hispanic America today.

TABLE 1.1: COMMON HISPANIC FOLK REMEDIES   *REMEDIOS CASEROS COMUNES*

English Name	Spanish Name	Use
Aloe Vera	*Zabila*	External—cuts, burns Internal—purgative, immune stimulant
Arnica Flower Tea	*Té de arnica*	To treat internal blows, bronchitis, pneumonia, and as a muscular tonic
Black Sage Tea/Wormwood	*Estafiate/Té de estafiate*	Parasites, colic, indigestion, diarrhea, and cramps, *bilis,* and *empacho*
Borage Tea	*Té de borraja*	Problems with coughs, urination, and perspiration, prevention of infection from chickenpox and measles.
Bricklebush	*Rodigiosa*	Adult onset diabetes, gallbladder disease
Chamomile	*Agua de manzanilla/Manzanilla*	Menstruation, diarrhea, nausea, flatus, colic, anxiety, and as an eyewash
Chaparral	*Gobernadora*	Arthritis (poultice); tea for cancer, venereal disease, tuberculosis, cramps, *pasmo,* analgesic
Cinnamon Tea	*Té de canela*	Coughs, tonic for anemia, aids digestion and prevents gas
Corn Tassel Tea	*Té de barba de elote*	Kidney problems, gallstones, and swollen legs from pregnancy or gout

(continued on the next page)

English Name	Spanish Name	Use
Croton Tea	*Té de pionillo*	Tea or a vaginal douche to treat *frío en la matriz*, "cold womb," and to help with diabetes, inflammation of the kidneys, and bladder problems
Damiana Tea	*Damiana/Té de damiana*	Tea or a vaginal douche to treat *frío en la matriz*, "cold womb," & to help with chickenpox, diabetes, inflammation of the kidneys, & bladder problems, or as an aphrodisiac
Desert Milkweed Tea	*Té de hierba del indio*	Kidney disorders
Elderberry Tea	*Té de negrita*	Colic
Eucalyptus (Vicks VapoRub)	*Eucalipto*	Coryza, asthma, bronchitis, tuberculosis
Fennel Tea	*Té de hinojo*	Gas, infants' colic, and vomiting
Garlic	*Ajo*	Hypertension, antibiotic, cough syrup, *tripa ida*
Herb Rose Tea	*Té de rosa de castilia*	Colic, *empacho*, an eyewash for conjunctivitis
Lavender Tea	*Té de flor de sauz y hojas de alhucema*	For measles and fever
Lead/Mercury Oxides	*Azarcón/Greta*	For *empacho*, teething
Limberbush Tea	*Té de sangre de drago*	Anemia
Linden Flowers	*Tilia/ Té de flores de tilo*	Calm nerves, fitful coughs & fevers caused by infections, as a sedative & diaphoretic, & for hypertension
Mallow Tea	*Té de malva*	Dysentery and children's stomachaches
Mormon Tea	*Té de canutillo*	Anemia
Mullein	*Gordolobo*	Cough suppressant, asthma, coryza, tuberculosis
Orange Blossom Tea	*Té de azahar*	Heart and nerve conditions
Orange Leaves Tea	*Té de naranja*	Colic
Oregano	*Orégano*	Coryza, expectorant, menstrual difficulties, worms
Parsley Tea	*Té de osha*	Helps cure kidney infections
Passion Flower	*Pasionara*	Anxiety and hypertension
Peppermint	*Yerba buena or Hierbabuena*	Dyspepsia, flatus, colic, *susto*
Rosemary Tea	*Té de romero*	Regulates menstruation and stimulates digestion
Rue Tea	*Ruda/Té de ruda*	Alleviates high blood pressure, headaches, antispasmodic, as an insect repellent *empacho*, and for menstrual problems, difficult deliveries, abortions, & abortifacient.
Sage	*Saliva*	Prevent hair loss, coryza, diabetes
Sapodilla	*Zapote blanco*	Insomnia, hypertension, malaria
Sarsaparilla Tea	*Té de cocolmeca or Té de zarzaparrilla*	Kidney problems, gout, psoriasis, syphilis, rheumatism
Spasm Herb Tea	*Té de hierba del pasmo*	*Pasmo*
Spearmint Tea	*Té de yerbabuena or Té de menta verde*	Colic
Spider Milkweed Tea	*Té de inmortal*	Stomachaches
Strong Tea	*Té cargado or Té fuerte*	Stomachaches
Swamp Root Tea	*Té de hierba del manzo*	Stomachaches
Tansy Mustard Herb Tea	*Té de pamita*	Fights intestinal infections, dysentery, & regulates menstruation
Trumpet Flowers	*Tronadora*	Adult onset diabetes, gastric symptoms, chickenpox
Wild Marjoram Tea	*Té de orégano*	Fights intestinal infections, dysentery, and regulates menstruation
Wormseed Tea	*Té de epazote/Té de México*	Parasites and helps menstruation
Other herbs used medicinally as a tea	*Té de baquena*	Help people with kidney stones
	Té de careaquillo	Colds
	Té de mavi	Colds
	Té de quinino de pobre	Diabetes
	Té de sacabuche	Indigestion/stomach disorders
	Tisana	Anemia

With regard to etiologic factors, many ethnomedical researchers follow Lyle Saunders, who classifies diseases by origin: empirical, magical, and psychological.[145] Empirical or "natural" diseases are those in which a known external factor operates directly on the organism to produce the illness. Magical diseases are those in which the cause lies beyond empirical knowledge and cannot be verified easily. Psychological diseases are those in which a strong emotional experience causes the appearance of the disease symptoms. In addition, Margaret Clark has grouped folk illnesses according to their origins: diseases of hot and cold imbalance, diseases of dislocation of internal organs (i.e., *caída de la mollera*), diseases of emotional origin (i.e., *susto*), diseases of magical origin (i.e., *mal ojo*), and a residual category containing "standard scientific" diseases such as *empacho*.[146] Many of these theories overlap; additionally, individuals often attempt to use *remedios caseros* for various scientific diseases.

One syndrome that has continued to exist in Hispanic folk medicine today is related to the hot and cold theory of disease.[147] Many illnesses are directly attributed to imbalances of "hot" and "cold" principles. The theory of hot and cold is one of the most prevalent medical beliefs in Latin America, dating back to medieval Spain. The Spaniards subscribed to the Hippocratic theory of a healthy balance between hot and cold body essences (humors); health maintenance required the proper mixture of hot and cold foods, just as good health required the avoidance of exposure to extreme temperatures with the proper mixture of hot and cold body humors.[148] This theory arbitrarily assigns "hot" and "cold" qualities to foods. Temperature or vasodilation and a high metabolic rate are considerations in labeling an illness or body condition "hot." Select examples of hot diseases or states include acid indigestion, diabetes, diarrhea, hypertension, pregnancy, rashes, ulcers, and the folk diseases *bilis*, *ojo*, and *susto*.[149] Vasoconstriction and a low metabolic rate are characteristic of cold diseases or states. Some examples are arthritis, colic, common colds, coryza, hay fever, menstrual periods and especially menstrual cramps, pneumonia, and the folk diseases *empacho* and *frío de la matriz*.

New foods and drugs are incorporated into the system according to the effect they have on the body. Penicillin often seems to cause a rash and is thus considered "hot." Calcium, which might cause muscular spasms, would be considered "cold."[150] This belief in hot and cold theory is gradually becoming modified so that it is less at odds with "modern" scientific ideas—alcohol rubs ("cold") or cool baths to reduce high fevers. Generally Hispanics do not think about the principles of hot and cold unless they are ill or are in some other type of vulnerable state. During this state, thoughts may turn to treatment designed to restore harmony and balance. Thus, "hot" diseases are treated with "cold" remedies, and "cold" diseases are treated with "hot" remedies. For example, many modern-day Hispanics suffer from hypertension, a "hot" illness. When questioned about the cause, the majority of Hispanics seem to believe that their hypertension is due to *corajes* (anger) or *susto* (fear); others ascribe its etiology to "thick blood." Consequently, they turn to cool remedies such as bananas and lemon juice for treatment as well as teas of passion flowers (*pasionara*), linden (*tilia*), or *zapote blanco*. Another example of a "hot" illness is diabetes mellitus. Although individuals with classic symptoms of diabetes would be wise to see a physician, all too often they doctor with the natural herbal medicines prescribed by *curanderos*. Although most *curanderos* encourage consultation with a physician for these symptoms, they also frequently prescribe various remedies. For instance, treatment may be started with *maturique* root infusion for about one week for people who are extremely hyperglycemic. For maintenance therapy, trumpet flower-herb or root infusion (*tronadora*), brickle bush (*prodigiosa*) tea, or sage (*salvia*) tea are used. Other options include cactus (*nopal*), aloe vera juice, or bitter gourd. None of these treatments has proven totally safe or effective. Today most people know nothing about hot/cold diseases and hot/cold herbs, and although they often talk about the heat and coldness of foods, medicines, or body states, people now generally think in terms of the actual temperature of foods rather than in terms of the qualities of hot and cold. For that reason, there is a slight decrease in the therapeutic use of foods to treat hot and cold disorders than a decade ago. Now such disorders are often treated with herbal remedies or with topical applications.[151]

Another syndrome involves diseases of dislocation of internal organs. *Caída de la mollera* or *mollera caída*, "fallen fontanelle," occurs in infants. The symptoms are insomnia, loss of appetite, excessive crying, severe diarrhea, vomiting, and fever. A diagnosis is made by feeling the top of the baby's head to detect a depression of the anterior fontanelle. The child is treated by having the adult insert both thumbs into the infant's mouth and gently push upward on the palate. The baby may be held upside down by the ankles, allowing gravity to help push the fontanelle back into place. An alternative treatment utilizes suction. Yet another treatment places a poultice of herbs and raw eggs, or fresh soap shavings, over the fontanelle in an attempt to "pull" the fontanelle up into place. Prayers, usually in sets of three, accompany these remedies. Should none of these cures prove to be effective, *curanderos* will refer the mother to a physician or clinic for treatment. Clinically, this illness resembles dehydration.[152]

Health care practitioners seeing infants suffering from this disease would be wise to suggest that the mother give herbal teas as a remedy, a medicine that she would find culturally acceptable, rather than boiled water. This would provide a compromise to the two modes of treatment; it would also substitute the more scientific solution to the problem without demeaning the other method.

Diseases of emotional origin include a number of illnesses not commonly recognized by health care practitioners. Common emotional illnesses of natural origin are *bilis* (anger, literally "bile") and *susto* or *espanto* (fright). *Bilis* has nothing to do with the bile produced by the gallbladder; rather it is an illness to which adults are susceptible. It is caused by strong anger or *coraje,* which then produces an excess of yellow stomach bile. The symptoms are diarrhea, vomiting, sometimes a yellowish complexion, chronic fatigue, and acute nervous tension. Herbal teas made of rosemary, chamomile, and camphor leaf or a combination of cassia bark, lemon shoots, cinnamon bark, toasted walnut, and whiskey are among some of the recognized treatments.[153]

Susto, or spirit loss due to fright, is one of the most common forms of folk illness in all of Latin America. It is caused by any natural fright, such as almost being hit by a truck or being badly frightened by a snake. *Susto* occurs when an individual is unable to cope with personal experiences. *Espanto* is a more severe form of fright, generally attributed to an encounter with the supernatural, such as seeing a ghost. It should be noted that if a pregnant woman is *asustada* or *espantada* (frightened), her baby will be born with *susto* or *espanto.*[154]

The child who suffers from *auto* often has horrible nightmares about the fright that caused the illness and often cries, whines, has insomnia, loss of appetite, and is irritable. The adult suffering from this disease also shows similar symptoms: nightmares, general malaise, loss of interest in things, dyspnea, indigestion, palpitations, depression, and anorexia. The patient may develop sores on the body and experience great pain. Some patients have an irregular pulse. Some *curanderos* believe that fright can lead to heart trouble (a heart attack), peptic ulcers, and even mental retardation.[155]

Advanced fright sickness is known as *susto pasado.* Its symptoms are prolonged exhaustion and coughing, in addition to the abovementioned symptoms. Margaret Clark describes a popular cure that uses two branches of sweet pepper trees and incantations by a *curandero.*[156] The *curandero* spends much time with the patient, familiarizing himself with the social and familial problems that the patient is experiencing. Then the *curandero* is able to provide not only a ritual cure, but also an emotional support system to help overcome the patient's fear. William Holland describes a different cure, which consists of inserting a piece of garlic into the anus on nine consecutive nights, accompanied by prayers.[157]

Diseases of magical origin include many supernatural folk diseases. *Mal (de) ojo,* or evil eye, is the most supernatural ailment that afflicts children primarily, but adults may be susceptible to it as well. The symptoms of *mal ojo* include vomiting, listlessness, excessive crying, trembling, aches and pains, and even rashes. It occurs in children to whom affectionate overtures have been made, without physical contact. The possessor of the evil eye projects evil into whomever or whatever he or she admires. Touching the person or thing removes the harmful force of the *mal ojo* if the individual with the evil eye is known.[158] Most Hispanics touch a child's head after admiring the child's beauty. Wearing a red ribbon or red clothes usually protects susceptible individuals from the damaging forces of the evil eye.[159] If that person is a stranger or is unavailable, *mal ojo* is treated by a spiritualistic "sweeping" of the afflicted person's body with an egg, accompanied by prayer.[160]

Hechicería, or bewitchment, describes any chronic or unexplained illness. Symptoms include strange, erratic behavior, hallucinations, constant fear, nervousness, and insomnia.[161]

Demencia, or "insanity," is considered an illness brought about by witchcraft. A witch casts an evil element into the *aire* (air), directed at a susceptible individual. Persons suffering from *demencia* exhibit amnesia, guilt or persecution complexes, and hallucinations.[162]

Visiones, or visions, is a milder mental disturbance caused by witches. The patient sees visions of the witch and his or her client, who often leave teeth marks or scratches on the patient's body.[163]

Miedo, or fear, is a still milder mental disturbance caused by witches. The patient imagines that he sees frightful things that "normal" people cannot see.[164]

There are also many "standard scientific diseases." Health practitioners should be aware of disorders of the blood, disorders classified as obstructions of the genitourinary and gastrointestinal tracts, and strong emotional experiences linked with cardiac functioning. Disorders of the blood are often associated with behavioral concerns in Hispanic folk medicine. A major diagnostic tool of emergent illness is *la debilidad de la sangre* (weakness of the blood). The Hispanic recognizes pale color, sallow skin, or weight loss as symptoms of weak blood. *Decaimiento* (feelings of malaise and low spirits) among adults is attributed to weak blood. Among children, correct conduct and academic progress are considered to depend on qualities of the blood.[165] Hispanics take vitamins, tonics, iron, and laxatives—all of which they purchase as over-the-counter medicine—for weaknesses of the blood.

Many of the illnesses associated with obstructions of the gastrointestinal and genitourinary tracts are folk diseases and are usually treated within the household or by a folk practitioner.[166] Many are concerned about cleansing the stomach and purifying the digestive and biliary juices. They believe that it is necessary to periodically purge the stomach and intestinal tract. *Empacho*, correctly termed *impacción*, is the recognized folk disease that results when the stomach is not "clean." *Empacho* is said to be a form of bowel obstruction; however, it applies to any stomach disorder, especially if gas is present. A large ball or knot in the stomach, which produces swelling or lumps in the legs, are symptoms of *empacho*. The disease is most common among children, but attacks adults as well. An herb tea made of mint, chamomile, and *epazote*, followed by a strong physic, cures the disease. *Empacho* may be caused by a poor diet or by eating foods that are not easily tolerated.[167]

Diseases of the heart that are associated with a strong emotional experience reflect a mixture of both folk and scientific medicine. Many Hispanics use the terminology of professional health care workers, such as *palpitaciones* (palpitations) and *presión alta* (high blood pressure), while retaining folk concepts of etiology and prevention. (These symptoms are typically associated with nerves or anxiety, not the heart.) These disorders are treated by physicians.

Melarchic(h)o, which corresponds to a reactive depression, is an illness that occurs following the death of a loved one. Symptoms include tearfulness, anorexia, insomnia, and listlessness.[168]

Mal aire, or bad air, is thought to be the result of evil spirits that dwell in the air, particularly the night air, and have the power to cause the victim to fall ill. Night air (*sereno*) is especially dangerous to children. It frequently causes pus to form in a baby's eyes or make them run. Symptoms of *mal aire* include back pain, muscle contractions, and muscle paralysis. Pneumonia may ensue, as may tuberculosis. The treatment involves eliminating the bad air by massage or by cupping.[169]

Aire, or air, applies to earaches, colds, stiff necks, headaches, and even dizziness. *Aire* occurs when air enters the body through one of its openings. Severe cases of *aire* often produce paralysis, twisted mouth, or some form of mental incapacity.[170]

Congestión is another folk-defined disease. It is a vulgar term that applies equally to a headache, a pain in the chest, a stomachache, or general body aches. It also applies to food poisoning, allergic reactions, and breathing problems—asthma, pneumonia, and obstructions of the throat. It has even been used to refer to heart attacks, convulsions, seizures, tetanus, meningitis, polio, and emboli. *Congestión* is caused by eating the "wrong" food, by a cold, or by not following the prescribed postpartum *dieta*.[171]

Latido, pulsing, or palpitations of the heart, is an abdominal disease. It is caused by abstaining from food for a long time. In its advanced stages, this serious, often fatal disease is accompanied by high fever, cough, and even blood-tinged sputum. It is characterized by severe emaciation, which makes it possible to feel the normal pulsation of the abdominal aorta upon deep palpitation.[172] Ralph Beals reported that "the disease may be caused if the person arrives somewhere very agitated and drinks cold water or something cold, like *fresca*."[173]

Fiebre, or fever, technically refers to an elevation of body temperature to a point higher than normal. In rural areas *fiebre* refers to a number of illnesses that cause a rise in body temperature: malaria, typhoid fever, typhus, hepatitis, pneumonia, rheumatic fever, postpartum fever, and brucellosis.[174]

Bolitas, or "little balls" (lumps) that occur in the extremities, are considered to be dislocated nerves. They are treated with massage or physical manipulation.

Chipil (literally "cry-baby") occurs when a nursing mother becomes pregnant before weaning her infant. The contaminated milk causes digestive disturbances and anger in the child, who often shows an inability to suck and cries excessively. Herbal teas and affection are the best cure.[175]

Nervios, or nerves, is an ailment believed to be caused by sexual perversions such as fellatio and cunnilingus, as well as by premature ejaculation.[176]

Dolor de ijar, or loin pain, occurs in women in the stomach, abdomen, or waist. Among the causes of this disease are urinary tract infections, ovarian or cervical cysts, appendicitis, and severe bowel cramps.[177]

Dolor de costado, or side pain, refers to any passing pain that begins suddenly. In rural areas this may refer to appendicitis, gallbladder problems, tuberculosis, or a liver involvement due to amoebic dysentery.[178]

The most common techniques of curing consist of "cupping" (*ventosas*); massage (*sobadas*); oral administration of herbal teas; topical application of herbs, oils, liniments; the use of purges; recitation of prayer; and floral offerings either to God or to the saints. Any or all of these techniques can be used to treat a particular disease. As mentioned, Hispanics are influenced by a combination of Spanish medicine based on ancient and medieval concepts, spiritualism, indigenous beliefs, patent remedies, homeopathic therapy, and the professional biomedical traditions.

HISPANIC UTILIZATION OF ANGLO HEALTH CARE FACILITIES

UTILIZACION HISPANA DE PLANTELES DE SALUD ANGLOSAJONES

Many commonplace problems plague Hispanics living in the United States: cultural insensitivity, poverty, a general lack of health insurance coverage, language barriers, long waits, and rising medical and dental costs. Hispanics seeking medical attention suffer from the pain and drain of illness as well as from perceived unfeeling bureaucratic abuses.

Very few hospitals or clinics in the United States have well-established professionally staffed interpreting services, although efforts are slowly being made by the federal government to change this problem. Most facilities frequently use nonprofessionals as interpreters, a practice that can create problems as previously enumerated. Hispanics in the United States speak many different dialects of Spanish. Consequently, symptoms of illness, parts of the body, and physiological functions are only a few areas in which dialects differ in vocabulary. *Constipación* could mean a "cold," "nasal congestion," or "intestinal congestion." A problem with the *empeine* could refer to the "instep," "ringworm," or the "groin."

Most Hispanic immigrants are from Mexico, and most are young adults in their early 20s to late 30s. The very young and the very old rarely immigrate. A significant but unknown number of the Hispanic population are undocumented, which poses obstacles to health care services and programs and also affects the type of health care services used by Hispanics. In one of the most extensive studies done on the differences between documented and undocumented Hispanics, Leo R. Chavez et al. found that the utilization pattern for documented Hispanics showed U.S. doctors were used by 32.9%, U.S. clinics by 28.0%, U.S. hospitals by 23.2%, and Mexican health care by 16.0%. For undocumented Hispanics, the utilization pattern differed: U.S. clinics were used by 38.1%, U.S. doctors by 28.2%, U.S. hospitals by 20.5%, and Mexican health care by only 13.1%. Also found were statistically significant sex differences in utilization patterns, with women more likely to use clinics and private practitioners than men, whereas men were twice as likely as women to use Mexican-style health services.[179] Chavez explains women's use pattern as reflective of their health care needs of obstetrical, gynecological, and child health services. In addition, Chavez et al. report that for their sample of San Diego documented and undocumented Hispanics who delivered in the United States within the last 5 years the percentage of undocumented mothers with "inadequate" prenatal care, defined by the Center for Health Statistics of the California Department of Health Services as no care or care which began in the third trimester is 3.6% of the legally immigrated mothers and 11.5% of the undocumented mothers. Only 3.8% of the women in the general maternal population in San Diego County received inadequate care well below the rate exhibited in the study. However, the study showed hospitals provided most of the prenatal care that these women received. Hospitals provided 29.3% of the care, U.S. private physicians provided 16.2%, and community clinics, 12.5%. One quarter (25.6%) of the women elected prenatal care in Mexico rather than use a U.S.-based provider.[180] Permanence and documentation status may affect a woman's ability to obtain prenatal care, for example. Immigration factors may also affect the medical and personal behavior factors (such as diet), which also may influence the birth outcomes.

Furthermore, Hispanics who receive most of their medical or health care services from large public hospitals in large urban areas in the United States rarely have continuity of health care because these facilities have rotating staffs.

CULTURAL DIFFERENCES

DIFERENCIAS CULTURALES

Language difficulties frequently mask other communications problems that health care professionals do not recognize, resulting in many misconceptions about the U.S. Hispanic population as a whole. American cultural expectations are often different from those of Spanish speakers who sometimes believe questions and a display of fear show a lack of respect and trust for the physicians and nurses. Also, many Spanish speakers will refuse to accept help from outsiders, including welfare, baby-sitters, even extra attention from the nursing staff. This attitude reflects the cultural belief that assistance from family and neighbors is acceptable because it can be repaid, unlike assistance from these "outsiders" whom the recipients have no way of paying back in kind. Pride is a very important consideration.

People from different cultures perceive the world differently and express those perceptions using language, thus the strong bond between culture and language. Meaning comes from people's perceptions rather than the literal words. One salient difference can be seen in the English word *family* which is expressed in Spanish by *familia*. These cognates are influenced by cultural factors. For Anglos, the word usually refers to the nuclear family—mother, father, and children. For Hispanics, the word most often refers to the extended family which includes grandparents, aunts and uncles, and cousins. It may even be extended to non-blood relatives such as godparents, close relatives of in-laws, those who have married into the family, and relatives of relatives.

Health care professionals who want to really communicate with their non- or limited-English-speaking Hispanic patients must do more than attempt to learn the words and grammar structures of Spanish. They must also learn something about the cultural background of these patients. Health care professionals must remember that people are the products of many different factors: their personal experiences shaped by cultural conditioning; their family experiences; educational attainment; religious practices, beliefs, and values; and socioeconomic status.

Language ability and the right approach to certain complaints are the keys. Potential patients who come for help identifying their disorder as "nervousness" should not be argued with and told that they have some kind of mental disorder. The patient will not stay for treatment. Awareness of cultural nuances will contribute to successful treatment. Comprehensive services offered both in a central facility and elsewhere—such as in churches, parks, libraries, homes, and even broadcast on radio and television—are needed as are programs divided for the benefit of Spanish-speaking and primarily English-speaking Hispanics.

Communication, however, is not only verbal. Much can also be learned from nonverbal cues. When interacting with others, Hispanics tend to prefer being closer to each other than Anglos do. They frequently perceive non-Hispanics who stand at the foot of the bed, for example, as distant and detached.[181] Hispanics tend to be more physical than Anglos. Many expect to shake hands with the health professional when greeting. Female patients may express gratitude by giving gifts or kissing; males often hug to express affection.[182] Another example is how Hispanics express pain. Many are more open in their expression than other cultural groups. Some moan and carry on when in pain, particularly during childbirth. This moaning, however, may be a way of asking others to share their pain. For those who moan and carry on in a rhythmic fashion, their actions may actually reduce pain much like Lamaze breathing.

Nonetheless, for health care professionals to be able to effectively communicate across cultural boundaries, they must have skill, practice, knowledge of the other culture, an ability to be flexible, and a willingness to accept variations. They must also be aware of the fact that Hispanics often have culturally determined values and beliefs, which Anglos may perceive adversely if they are not familiar with the Hispanic culture. Examples of such differences follow.

From earliest childhood, people are taught how to behave in the presence of authority figures. In the Hispanic world, with its sharp social-class distinctions, "place" is determined as much by sex as by the socioeconomic class. The most obvious contrast between Anglo and Hispanic nonverbal communication patterns is that of eye contact and head movement when in the presence of authority figures. For the Anglo, it is important to look into the eye when spoken to. To do otherwise, to look downward, would imply disrespect, dishonesty, or even guilt, especially when the authority figure is a superior. Hispanics are taught the opposite! Hispanic individuals learn from an early age that they must cast their head and eyes downward, especially when being advised by someone in a powerful position. If they look the authority figure directly in the eye, their behavior is considered challenging and disrespectful.

Whereas Anglos tend to value prolonged eye contact as a sign of attention and understanding, even in informal settings with family and friends, Hispanics tend to misinterpret that eye contact as a sign of defiance or anger. In mixed company, Hispanics always avoid staring at members of the opposite sex when they are speaking lest there be any misinterpretation of intent, as prolonged eye contact between the sexes is reserved only for intimate relationships.

Another cultural difference is that the Hispanic world is more formal than the Anglo world, especially concerning the type of behavior that is expected of authority figures by Hispanics. This is particularly true for professionals such as health care workers. Authority figures must look and act as such. Moreover, they must dress appropriately but conservatively. Hispanics would rarely consider addressing authority figures by their first names, for instance. Nonetheless, professionals are expected to show empathy, support, and respect for their clients and patients.

The way Hispanics view family is extended to how they view their communities. For many, the community is the equivalent of the Anglo "extended family." It is used as a support network, which could explain why Hispanics are more likely to turn for advice to family and their community rather than to public hospitals or health agencies. In most Hispanic societies the importance of the family causes them to make their individual needs secondary to the good of the family, including health needs.

The idea of respect (*respeto*) is of utmost importance in the Hispanic world where every living person must have a sense of *dignidad*, or personal worth.[183] Only by respecting oneself first, can Hispanics show others respect. However, showing others respect often takes on certain prescribed physical aspects for Hispanics, which are frequently misinterpreted by some Anglos (and others) as submissiveness, apathy, or acquiescence. When interacting with Anglos, some Hispanics may seem submissive, lacking initiative, or even withdrawn.

There are also many cultural differences toward time.[184] For example, there are differences in the perception of time. In the United States the 24-hour cycle of the day is divided by noon and midnight. These are used to divide the day into A.M. (*ante meridiem* or "before noon") and P.M. (*post meridiem* or "after noon"). In the Hispanic world, however, the 24-hour cycle has four divisions. Hispanics also use noon (*mediodía*) and midnight (*medianoche*), but recognize two additional divisions: *noche* which is used to express the time from sunset to midnight, and *madrugada* which is used for the period between midnight and sunrise. The abbreviation A.M., therefore, is expressed by both *de la mañana* (which covers time from sunrise to noon) and *de la madrugada*, while P.M. is expressed by both *de la tarde* (for the division from noon until sunset) and *de la noche* (for the division from sunset to midnight). Because the time of sunrise and sunset varies from season to season, so, too, does the use of the appropriate form of A.M. or P.M.

Other cultural differences toward time include the following examples. In English, the "clock runs" while in Spanish *el reloj anda* ("the clock walks"). Time in Spanish is never fast or slow, it is *adelantado* (ahead) or *atrasado* (behind), whereas Anglos tend to view time as a commodity to be controlled and utilized. Even socializing in the United States is scheduled much in the same manner as business appointments. Hispanics tend to prefer a slower-paced, flexible lifestyle which places human needs over efficiency and/or productivity. This preference has been viewed in a derogatory way as the *mañana* syndrome. This interpretation incorrectly maintains that Hispanics lack ambition and/or initiative, and their approach to life is fatalistic. Furthermore, it stipulates that Hispanics are disdainful of the modern world of technology and its subsequent efficiency.

Routine medical appointments do not have the same importance for the Spanish-speaking patient. Family needs will often take priority over scheduled appointments. It is important for health care professionals to bear this in mind when they calmly *explain* rather than lecture to the tardy Hispanic patient why it is important to arrive in a timely fashion. It is also important for health care professionals to be as flexible as possible with patients who have arrived late while remembering not to make assumptions about the Hispanic patient's dependability and initiative based solely on that person's punctuality for appointments. Also, when possible, distant appointments should not be scheduled. Moreover, health care professionals would be wise not to take references to *"inmediatamente," "momentico,"* or *"mañana"* literally as "immediately," "in a moment," or "tomorrow," since these expressions could be used to refer to any time in the not too distant future. Finally, when prescribing medications for Spanish-speaking patients, it is better to associate the medicine with specific times such as at mealtime or before going to bed, rather than at arbitrary intervals of every 4 hours. Attitudes toward time will vary from client to client, depending on personal experiences, cultural factors, and the degree of assimilation of the individual into the Anglo society. Those Hispanics who have spent most or all of their lives in the United States will no doubt be more likely to have accepted much of the Anglo's concept of time.

Many Hispanics adhere to the cultural taboo against expressing negative feelings directly, which may manifest itself in many ways. For example, Hispanic patients are usually too respectful to complain about mistreatment or long delays in waiting rooms. When asked if they have already been helped, the reply is usually, *"No me han dicho nada."* ("They haven't told me anything.") Hispanic patients in large urban hospitals regularly suffer from overdoses of lack of attention and insensitivity. In rural areas, they often receive no medical attention at all. In other instances, patients may withhold information, not follow treatment orders, or end medical care entirely.

The American custom of expecting the patient and physician to make important medical decisions often presents problems for some Hispanic communities, when illness involves family or group decisions. Customarily the sick individual consults relatives, both in the United States and in their country of origin, *compadres* (the godparents of their children), friends, and employers before medical consultation.

Long-distance consultations are done with the hope of obtaining advice from both worlds, and especially to fill the gaps that *Hispanos* perceive to exist in treatment that they experience in the United States.

Hispanics express confidence in a physician who diagnoses their complaints through physical examination, X rays, or other lab work. Those who prescribe remedies/treatments without a physical examination or other confirming indicators are criticized by Hispanics.[185] When the health care personnel make recommendations such as, "You need an operation," the Hispanic patient must consult with family members. Such stresses to family functioning may have significant implications to health patterns. When pressed for immediate decisions, the Hispanic often agrees only to be courteous and to avoid dissention. If, upon family consultation, there is disagreement, appointments are broken or cancelled. Surgical procedures in particular are frequently regarded as harmful, dangerous, and unnecessary. Within *familismo* (familism), important decisions are made by the family, not by the individual alone.

STEREOTYPES *ESTEREOTIPOS*

Majority populations view all groups that are different (i.e., minorities) in stereotypical ways. There are several major stereotypes about Hispanics in the United States. One significant stereotype is the belief that Hispanics are "foreign." A corollary to this is the assumption that all Hispanics are also recent immigrants. Neither is correct. The oldest European-influenced settlements in the United States are of Spanish origin. These include St. Augustine, Florida (1565), and Santa Fe, New Mexico (1610). Numerous Hispanic families can trace their antecedents in this country back ten generations or more. Another stereotype is that Hispanics are only found in rural areas. As discussed, an overwhelming number of Hispanics are found in urban areas.[186] This stereotype holds an implicit assumption that Hispanics do not have the skills to work in urban-based occupations. It also implies that they are not consumers for modern products.

Another stereotype has to do with the location of Hispanics in specific regions. As indicated,[186] this stereotype fails to see the Hispanic population as a national presence. Although heavily concentrated in certain parts of the United States, Hispanics have become such a large population that their presence has political, cultural, economic, and health care implications which cannot be ignored.

Despite the media image of illegal aliens and Hispanic poor, they are among the most responsible patients in paying their bills. Another common error is the tendency to lump all immigrants into one group—unskilled, uneducated, and unwanted, which is incorrect. Many migrant workers come to the United States, not just as farm workers, but as professionals.

Early sociological studies completed in the 1950s and 1960s labeled Chicanos "folk oriented" in health care attitudes, superstitious, and living only for the present. This description is not quite accurate in all cases. Assuming that incomes are similar, however, Anglos and Chicanos show very little difference in health attitudes. Economics seem to be the important key—getting an education, getting a job, and then moving up.

Still another stereotype as it applies to Hispanics has to do with race. Americans have attempted to fit people into specific racial categories. Hispanics are not a racial category. They may be Black, White, Native American, American Indian, or a mixture of many racial backgrounds. Hispanics define race with cultural definitions. For example, an individual born in Mexico who speaks Nahuatl—a native language of Mexico—as a first language, is defined as a Native American. However, if that same individual speaks Spanish as a first language, regardless of genes, the individual is no longer considered American Indian. In contrast, in the United States where a genetic, rather than a cultural, standard is used, if an individual has one grandparent who belongs to a different or minority race, the individual is considered to be a member of that ancestor's race, regardless of appearance.

Another stereotype relates to language. Many people wrongly assume that, if a person has an Hispanic surname, he or she either does not speak English or has only learned it recently. A significant percentage of the Hispanic population is monolingual—in English. Obviously, recent Hispanic immigrants reflect more usage of Spanish than Hispanics born in the United States.

CONCLUSION

CONCLUSION

Health care professionals, to effectively meet the needs of the Hispanic communities, must recognize the similarities as well as the differences of this population in comparison with the Anglo society. They must understand the impact of culture and language, develop strong outreach components, and attempt to interact effectively with Hispanic patients. The information provided in this chapter does not imply that all Hispanics believe and interact in the same way. Nevertheless, health care professionals will be more effective if they can appreciate and respond to their patients' values and language needs.

Notes *Notas*

1. The United States has the fifth largest Hispanic population in the world, following Mexico, Spain, Argentina, and Colombia. U.S. Bureau of the Census, *The Hispanic Population in the United States: March 1997* (Update & Current Population Report P20-511); U.S. Bureau of the Census, *U.S. Projection Estimates by Age, Sex, Race, and Hispanic Origin: 1990 to 1996*, April 1997; U.S. Bureau of the Census, *Population Projections of the United States by Age, Sex, Race, and Hispanic Origin: 1995 to 2050*, February 1996.

2. A.C. Novello, P.H. Wise, D.V. Kleinman, "Hispanic Health: Time for Data, Time for Action," *JAMA* 1991, 265: 253–255; M.B. Smith, "Race, Ethnicity, Class, and Culture," *Closing the Gap* March 1998, p. 2.

3. D.E. Hayes-Bautista, J. Chapa, "*Latino* Terminology: Conceptual Bases for Standardized Terminology," *American Journal of Public Health* 1987, 77:61–68.

4. *Diccionario de la Lengua Española*, XXI ed., Madrid: Espasa-Calpe, S.A., 1990.

5. **Assimilation** of one cultural group into another may be evidenced by changes in language preference, adoption of common values and attitudes, and loss of separate ethnic or political identification. **Acculturation** is the process in which members of one cultural group adopt the beliefs and behaviors of another group. Although it is usual for acculturation to go in the direction of the dominant group, it is also possible for the dominant group to adopt patterns typical of the minority group.

6. U.S. citizenship, though limited in scope, entitles Puerto Ricans to move freely from the island to the mainland and it entitles them to fully utilize U.S. social services, among other benefits. Additionally, marriage to a Puerto Rican by an immigrant results in immediate permanent residency for the new spouse and a shortened waiting period of three years rather than five to become a U.S. citizen.

7. U.S. Bureau of the Census, Census of Population & Housing: 1990, STFIA; March 1996.

8. The term *Chicano* derives from the Mexican-American political movement in the 1960s. This term, however, dates back to a much earlier time. Originally it signified someone of a lower socioeconomic status. To some it also implied a certain political radicalism or separatism. The actual origin of the word remains somewhat of a mystery although many have posed suggestions.

9. U.S. Census Bureau definition taken from the *Federal Register*, 1978, p. 19269 which reads, "A person of Mexican, Puerto Rican, Cuban, Central or South American or other Spanish culture or origin, regardless of race."

The U.S. Bureau of the Census refined its definition of *Hispanic* in 1980 and again in 1985 so that Hispanics are now subdivided five ways: Mexican or Mexican American (or Chicano/Chicana); Puerto Rican (or Boricua); Cuban or Cuban American; Central or South American; and "Other" Spanish/Hispanic. It is interesting to note that in some cases people of Portuguese or Brazilian ancestry are considered Hispanic, while in other cases they are not.

10. Racial issues in the Iberian Peninsula theoretically do not exist because all inhabitants are supposedly of Caucasian background. This is not the case in Latin America. Racial problems originated in the sixteenth century when the Conquistadors came to the New World for "gold," "glory," and the "Gospel." Women in the beginning did not come, for the men did not intend to stay permanently. Unions were formed with either native women or with Black slaves who were imported from Africa. New races resulted:

Mestizo—offspring of a European and a Native American
Mulato—offspring of a European and a Black African
Zambo—offspring of a Black African and a Native American

In Latin America the indigenous and Black elements play important roles. As for racial identification, a person is frequently called White if he is not Black. (In the United States a person is classified as African American or Black if he is not completely White.) A number of terms are used when referring to color or racial characteristics: the term *negro* (especially in Puerto Rico) is rarely used. In fact, *negra*, or the diminutive *negrita*, is frequently used as a form of affection for someone who is completely White. The most common term used to designate a Black is *de color*. Problems arise, however, in identifying those people who do not belong to either race solely. Official documents such as marriage and baptismal records use several terms: *pardo, moreno, mulato*. *Trigueño* is perhaps the most commonly used term for the group in-between. *Indio* is used for those with Indian characteristics. *Grifo* designates someone with kinky hair, characteristic of Blacks, but who is of light color. (*Pelo malo*, "bad hair," has the same meaning.) *Trigueño*, which literally means "wheat colored," often is used to describe a person who has dark color but obviously caucasoid features.

Race membership is often more closely linked to socioeconomic status than to physical characteristics. Identification of a person as *White, colored,* or *trigueño* depends in great part on the attitude of the individual making the identification. Two individuals who are both rather dark and similar in physical characteristics, are often judged differently. If socially acceptable, they are considered *trigueños*; if socially unacceptable, they are *de color*. Julian Steward (*People of Puerto Rico*, Champaign: University of Illinois Press, 1946, p. 425) notes that "an individual is 'whiter' in proportion to his wealth." The *Mestizo* inhabits all economic classes, and now occupies many positions which were formerly held by Whites alone. Native Americans are generally country dwellers. The Native American is often poorly educated if not illiterate, poor, and limited in opportunity for future advancement. The *Mulato* and the Black are found along the coastal regions of South America and in the Caribbean. Although poor, and often poorly educated, hope exists for future advancement.

11. Legal and illegal Hispanic immigration to the United States has shown no signs of slackening, nor is immigration expected to make any appreciable declines until such time as Spanish-speaking countries, particularly Mexico, reach relative economic parity with the United States. In 1997, according to *The Foreign-Born Population in the United States: March 1997* (Update), about one in four of the total foreign-born population was born in Mexico (7 million). One of every two foreign-born residents was a native of Central America, South America, or the Caribbean (13.1 million).

12. There are numerous differences between the poorer classes of industrialized Europe who came to the United States as immigrants and those immigrants coming from Latin America. For one thing, industrialization has been slow to reach Latin America, which has historically exported raw materials and agricultural products and imported most of its manufactured goods. The mixed racial heritage of many Hispanics is another factor which has made it difficult for them to "blend in" unlike those Caucasian immigrants of earlier days who came from western Europe. Moreover, today's economy needs workers who are both skilled and technologically educated unlike the economy of earlier times when unskilled laborers willing to work were all that were needed. In fact, the increasing educational minimum makes certain levels of employment somewhat unlikely since the lower classes of Latin America commonly have been given very limited education and/or vocational training. Unlike European immigrants of earlier eras, however, Hispanic immigrants find it relatively easy to return to their homeland or at least keep in close communication with family

and friends back home. They are also encouraged to maintain their cultural mores as ethnic pride has become popular. Finally, a technologically service-oriented society makes it increasingly difficult for most Hispanics to leave the *barrio* and integrate into the mainstream culture.

13. U.S. Bureau of the Census, *The Hispanic Population in the United States: March 1997,* CPR P20-511; U.S. Bureau of the Census, *The Black Population in the United States: March 1997,* CPR P20-508; U.S. Bureau of the Census, *U.S. Projection Estimates by Age, Sex, Race, and Hispanic Origin: 1990 to 1996,* April 1997; U.S. Bureau of the Census, *Population Projections of the United States by Age, Sex, Race, and Hispanic Origin: 1995 to 2050,* February 1996.

14. U.S. Bureau of the Census, *Estimates of the Population of States by Race and Hispanic Origin: July 1, 1994,* August 20, 1996; U.S. Bureau of the Census, *Statistical Tables for the Hispanic Origin Population from March 1994 Current Population Survey;* Robert Aponte and Marcelo Siles, *Latinos in the Heartland: The Browning of the Midwest,* Julian Samora Research Institute, November 1994.

15. It is important to remember that because Hispanics may be of any race, White and Black families may also be Hispanic.

16. U.S. Bureau of the Census,*Current Population Reports,* 1990, Series P-20, Nos. 331, 995, 1045; P.R. Campbell, *Population Projections for States by Age, Sex, Race, and Hispanic Origin: 1995 to 2025,* October 1996, U.S. Bureau of the Census, Population Division, PPL-47.

17. Yankelovich, Skelly & White, *Spanish USA: A Study of the Hispanic Market in the U.S.,* Yankelovich, Skelly and White, Inc., 1984. Only 14% considered themselves primarily American.

18. Yankelovich et al.

19. U.S. Bureau of the Census, *The Foreign-Born Population: 1996,* 1997.

20. Among Central and South Americans, Salvadorans (565,000), Colombians (379,999), Guatemalans (269,000), Nicaraguans (203,000), Ecuadorians (191,000), and Peruvians (175,000) are the largest population groups. Persons of Caribbean origin including a population of 520,000 Dominicans, form the largest component of the "Other" Hispanic subpopulation group. U.S. Bureau of the Census, "Hispanic Americans Today," *Current Population Reports: Population Characteristics,* Series P23-183, June 1993, p. 4.

21. See Chapter 16, note 52.

22. U.S. Bureau of the Census, *Estimates of the Population of States by Race and Hispanic Origin: July 1, 1994,* August 20, 1996. The U.S. Bureau of the Census estimated that there were 7,017,000 people of Mexican origin living here in 1997. *Country of Origin and Year of Entry into the U.S. of the Foreign Born, by Citizenship Status: March 1997.*

23. U.S. Bureau of the Census, *Estimates of the Population of States by Race and Hispanic Origin: July 1, 1994,* August 20, 1996; S. Rodríguez, *Hispanics in the United States: An Insight into Group Characteristics,* Washington, DC: Department of Health & Human Services, July 1995.

24. When reporting statistics and census data on the U.S. Hispanic population, it is customary to exclude data on Puerto Rico, even though persons born on that island are U.S. citizens, too. Census figures indicate that 3.8 million persons lived in Puerto Rico in 1996, a 7.4% increase since 1990. The 1990 census indicated that almost all (90.9%) of these residents were born on the island. Some 2.6 million Puerto Ricans live on the mainland.

25. Florida has a population that is largely Cuban. This population is quite a bit older than other Hispanic subgroups; it also has higher education and income achievement, and is less fecund than the other Hispanic subgroups.

The 1959 exodus of the wealthy and professional class from Cuba to Miami has turned that city today into the "unofficial" Spanish-speaking capital of the United States in terms of services, business, schools, and medical facilities which meet the needs of many of the wealthy members of the upper classes from other Latin American countries as well. (Barbara Lotito, *Entre Nosotros,* New York: Newbury House, 1988)

26. See Chapter 16, page 354, for use of these specific terms of nationality.

27. California's Hispanic population will more than double between 1995 and 2025 (to 21 million and will represent 36% of the total Hispanic population in 2025). While Texas will remain in second place with 17% of the Hispanics in 2025, New York is expected to decline from 9% to 6% and is expected to switch from third to fourth place with Florida. Illinois will remain in fifth place. See P.R. Campbell, *Population Projections for States by Age, Sex, Race, and Hispanic Origin: 1995 to 2025.*

28. The Hispanic population in the United States increased 35.2% between 1980 and 1990 and is projected to increase an additional 43.6% by 2025. (U.S. Bureau of the Census, *U.S. Projection Estimates by Age, Sex, Race, and Hispanic Origin: 1990 to 1996,* April 1997; U.S. Bureau of the Census, *Population Projections of the United States by Age, Sex, Race, and Hispanic Origin: 1995 to 2050,* February 1996, 1025–1130)

In 1995 the Hispanic origin population was the third most populous race/ethnic group in all regions of the United States except the West where it ranks second. The Hispanic population is expected to comprise a substantially larger share of the total population in 2025 than in 1995—up from 21% to 32% in the West, from 9% to 15% in the South and Northeast, and from 3% to 6% in the Midwest. P.R. Campbell, 1996, *Population Projections for States by Age, Sex, Race, and Hispanic Origin: 1995 to 2025,*

29. There is a mistaken perception that Hispanics are a rural phenomenon. About 85% of all Spanish-origin persons live in metropolitan areas compared with 66% of the overall population, compared with 75% of the general U.S. population. (U.S. Bureau of the Census, 1996)

30. U.S. Bureau of the Census, *Population and Housing: 1990 STF4a,* Table PA6; Latino Institute, *Does Chicago's Latino Population Mirror the National Latino Population?* Chicago: Latino Institute, 1993.

31. U.S. Bureau of the Census, *U.S. Population Estimates by Age, Sex, Race , and Hispanic Origin: 1990 to 1996,* April 1997.

It should be noted that these population projections do not include the unknown number of undocumented workers who enter the United States from neighboring Central and South American countries and from Mexico.

32. Between 1990 and 1996 the immigration rate for Hispanics was higher than that of all other groups, having an estimated average of 15.1 immigrants for every 1,000 Hispanic persons per year, compared with 3.1 immigrants for all persons.

33. U.S. Bureau of the Census, *U.S. Projection Estimates by Age, Sex, Race, and Hispanic Origin: 1990 to 1996,* April 1997.

34. National Center for Health Statistics, 1992; U.S. Bureau of the Census, *Fertility of American Women: June 1994,* Current Population Reports, P20-482, 1995.

35. S.J. Ventura, "Births of Hispanic Parentage, 1982." *NCHS, Monthly Vital Statistics Report,* 34(4) Supplement, 1-8. Washington, D.C.: U.S. Government Printing Office, July 23, 1985.

36. Center for Disease Control and Prevention, *Monthly Vital Statistics Report,* June 10, 1997; U.S. Bureau of the Census, *Statistical Tables for the Hispanic Origin Population from March 1994 Current Population Survey,* 1996.

The rate of teen pregnancy among Hispanics is alarmingly high. However, Hispanic teens are more likely to be married when their baby is born than are Black teens, and only slightly less likely than White teens. This varies among Hispanic subgroups: 74.5% of Cuban teen moms, 63.0% Mexican-American teen moms, and 26.4% of Puerto Rican teen moms were married when their baby was born.

The birth rate for Hispanic teen moms is substantially greater than that of the White non-Hispanic teen population. Within the Hispanic population, nonetheless, the rate of teen pregnancy varies widely among subgroups: Mexican-American and Puerto Rican teen moms have a higher birth rate than do Cuban teen moms.

Puerto Rican teen moms are twice as likely as Mexican-American teen moms and three times as likely as Black teen moms to receive prenatal care. (This, of course, could be a factor of their American citizenship.) Pregnant Hispanic teens in 1994 were likely to begin prenatal care at a later stage than non-Hispanics and were more likely to not receive any prenatal care at all. Of Hispanic teen moms, 7.1% received no prenatal care (nationally) in 1994, but 17.5% of New York teens and 10.3% of Texas teens received no prenatal care. It is, nonetheless, unlikely for Hispanic teens in California, Colorado, New Jersey, and Illinois to lack prenatal care. In New York it did not matter which Hispanic subgroup was being studied—few received prenatal care. Early prenatal care rates were the poorest in New York for Mexican-American, Puerto Rican, and Central- and South-American women in general, and teen moms specifically. Early care was most likely to be provided in New Jersey, California, and Illinois.

A low birth weight is considered less than 2,500 grams (or 5 lb 8 oz). In all states, Puerto Ricans had the highest incidence of low-birth-weight babies. Theirs is often a higher rate than that of Blacks. (National Center for Health Statistics, 1996)

37. Women of Mexican ancestry averaged 1.6 children ever born, about 0.5 children higher than non-Hispanic women. Women born in Mexico who were living in the United States had an even higher fertility rate—147 births per 1,000. *Fertility of American Women: June 1994*, CPR P20-482.

38. U.S. Bureau of the Census, 1993.

39. U.S. Bureau of the Census, *The Hispanic Population in the United States: March 1997* (Update) Current Population Report P20-511. In 1997, Hispanics 65 years and older constituted 4.9% of the elderly population of the United States. U.S. Bureau of the Census, *Population Estimates by Age, Sex, Race, and Hispanic Origin*, Appendix A, PPL-57, 1997. Between 1997 and 2030, the number of Hispanic elderly is expected to triple, and in 2030, Hispanics over age 65 are projected to comprise 11.9% of the Hispanic population and 11.2% of the elderly population of the United States. U.S. Bureau of the Census, *Population Projections of the United States by Age, Sex, Race, and Hispanic Origin: 1995–2050*, current Population Reports, P25-1130, February 1996.

40. Many famous people, for somewhat diverse reasons, use only one family name. The great Spanish nineteenth-century author, Benito Pérez Galdós, is known to most as Galdós. Federico García Lorca also retained his maternal name, and is best known as Lorca. However, Jacinto Benavente y Martínez, Miguel de Unamuno y Jugo, and Miguel de Cervantes Saavedra are all known by their paternal surname.

41. E. Gantz McKay, *The Changing Demographics of the Hispanic Family*, Washington, DC: National Council of La Raza, July 1987. In 1996, 67.7% of Hispanic families were headed by married couples, compared with 46.1% of Black families and 81.3% of White families. In 1997, approximately 68.2% of all Hispanic families were comprised of married couple families. *Hispanic Population in the United States: March 1997* (Update) CPR P20-511.

42. Puerto Rican families are more likely to be female headed than other Hispanic families—but this is changing slowly. In 1985, 44.0% of Puerto Rican families were headed by females, compared with 18.6% of Mexican-American families. In 1985, Puerto Ricans had the lowest family income among Hispanics and the highest poverty and unemployment rates. (U.S. Bureau of the Census, *Statistical Tables for the Hispanic Origin Population from the March 1994 Current Population Survey*)

43. Labor force data provided by Jay Meisenheimer, *Employment and Unemployment Statistics*, U.S. Bureau of Labor Statistics, Fall 1997. The unemployment rate for Mexicans was 8.2% that same year, compared with 8.6% for Puerto Ricans and 6.4% for Cubans. U.S. Bureau of the Census, *Selected Characteristics of the Population by Citizenship: March 1997*.

44. U.S. Bureau of Labor Statistics, "Median Weekly Earnings for Full-Time Workers," *Current Population Survey*, 1997. Real per capita income increased more significantly for Hispanics (4.9%) than for Whites (1.8%). In 1996, the median earnings for Hispanic male year-round, full-time workers was $21,056, compared with $32,966 for comparable White workers and $26,404 for comparable Black workers. That same year Hispanic women had lower median earnings than non-Hispanic women. The median earnings of Hispanic women in 1996 was $18,665, compared with $24,160 for comparable White workers and $18,884 for comparable Black workers. In 1996, the real median income of all households was $35,492. The federal government defines a household as a person or group of persons who live in a housing unit. A family is a group of two or more people (one of whom is the householder, the person in whose name the housing unit is owned or rented) living together and related by birth, marriage, or adoption. U.S. Bureau of the Census, *Money Income in the United States: 1996*, CB97-162.

45. U.S. Bureau of the Census, *Dynamics of Economic Well-Being, Poverty 1993–94: Trap Door? Revolving Door? or Both?* Released on 8/10/98, CPS P70-63. The poverty definition used by the federal government for statistical purposes is based on a set of monetary income thresholds which vary by family size and composition.

46. According to the U.S. Bureau of the Census, *Poverty in the United States: March 1997*, CPS P60-198, in 1996, the poverty rate was 11.2% for Whites, 28.4% for Blacks, and 29.4% for persons of Hispanic origin. The poverty rate for all children under 18 years old was 20.5%, higher than that for any other age group. The poverty rate varied across race and ethnic groups for children under 18. About one-third (35.7%) of all Hispanics were under age 18 in 1996. Hispanic children were more likely than non-Hispanic children to be living below the poverty level. In 1996, 40.3% of all Hispanic children lived below poverty, compared with 39.9% of Black children and 16.3% of White children.

U.S. Bureau of the Census, *Poverty in the United States: 1995*, 1996. See page 11, page 31, notes 47 and 48, and page 32, note 49. Single teen moms are likely to become low-income female heads of households. Of Puerto Rican families, 74.4% are headed by females and in 1984 lived below poverty level, as did 43.8% of female-headed Mexican-American families. The 1985 median family income for female-headed Hispanic families was just 39% of the median income for married couple families. In 1985, three-fourths of Hispanic children in female-headed households were poor. The likelihood of poverty increases greatly if the female head of household is young.

47. Among racial and ethnic groups living in poverty, equated to a maximum annual income of $7,995 for one person, $10,233 for two, $12,516 for three, and $16,036 for four, the contrast is even greater: 40.8% of poor Hispanics lacked health insurance coverage compared with 33.3% of poor Whites and 33.5% of poor Blacks. The proportion of poor Hispanic children without health insurance was basically the same as for all Hispanic children. In 1996, 29.9% of poor Hispanic children had no health coverage. The percent of poor White children without health insurance was actually higher than that of poor Black children—25.2% versus 19.7%. (U.S. Bureau of the Census, *Children Without Health Insurance*, CENBR/98-1; U.S. Bureau of the Census, *Health Insurance Coverage: 1995*, September 1996 and U.S. Bureau of the Census, *Health Insurance Coverage: 1996*, September 1997.) This lack of health insurance coverage results in a lack of preventive and supportive services for Hispanic children from the cradle through adolescence.

48. Pregnancy is one of the major reasons cited by Hispanic teen girls for dropping out of school; Hispanic teen moms are considerably less likely to have finished high school than White or Black moms. In 1982, only about 31% of Mexican-American and Puerto Rican teenage moms aged 18 to 19 were high school grads; overall 37.3% of Hispanic teen moms had completed high

school. In that same year only 43.2% of all Hispanic females had completed high school. Data indicate that Cuban teen moms were the only Hispanic subgroup whose educational attainment was generally comparable with that of White graduates.

Hispanics have the lowest educational attainment of any major U.S. population group. About one-fourth of Hispanic youth are unemployed, and changes in the job market are making it very difficult for those with a high school diploma to find work. In 1984, average real annual earnings among males 20 to 24 was $8,072.

The reduced earnings among young men of all population groups increase the likelihood that young families, whether headed by a married couple or a single parent, will live in poverty. In 1985 the Hispanic family received 91% of the Black family income and 71% of the White family income. In 1995, the Hispanic family received 94.6% of the Black family income and 57.6% of the White family income. These numbers reflect the relatively low labor force participation rate of Hispanic women—only half of whom are in workforce—and the fact that both Hispanic male and female workers have lower median weekly earnings than Black or White workers of the same sex. (U.S. Bureau of the Census, *Labor Force Characteristics of Black and Hispanic Workers*, September 1997; U.S. Bureau of the Census, *Poverty in the United States: 1995*, 1996; U.S. Bureau of the Census, *Poverty Status of Families and Persons in Families in 1995*, 1996.

49. The major predictor of poverty among Hispanic families is having a female head of household; 53.1% of Hispanic and 50.5% of Black female-headed households were classified as poor in 1985, compared with 17.0% of Hispanic and 12.2% of Black married couple families.

The Hispanic median family income remains significantly below that of White families. Hispanic median family income was $24,570 in 1995, compared with $42,646 for White families and $25,970 for Black families. Between 1990 and 1995, however, real median family income levels fell 10.1% for Hispanic families and 0.9% for White families, but increased 4.0% for Black families. In 1996, Hispanic families experienced a 5.8% increase in real median family income which offset the drop observed in 1995. The percentage changes in household income of White and Black households were not statistically different from 1995. See page 31, note 48. U.S. Bureau of the Census, *Money Income in the United States: 1995 (With Separate Data on Valuation of Noncash Benefits)*, 1996.

50. The figures do not include the special population target Head Start programs, Migrant Head Start, or Head Start for the Commonwealth of Puerto Rico. Statistical Fact Sheet. Project Head Start, January 1991 and Statistical Fact Sheet. Project Head Start, January 1998.

51. G. A. Mellander, "Tackling Dropouts: New Legislation Proposed," *Hispanic Outlook in Higher Education*, Vol. 8, No. 9, December 26, 1997, p. 4.

52. In 1997, 10% of the Hispanic population ages 25 and over held a bachelor's degree; however, the number of Hispanic young adults completing a bachelor's degree or higher rose to 11% in 1997. U.S. Bureau of the Census, *Educational Attainment in the United States: March 1997*, P20-505.

53. In a number of places in Latin America, despite attempts to eradicate it, the native presence remains strong. This is true in Mexico and most of Central America and the Andean chain. African slaves were introduced to some parts of Latin America, primarily the Caribbean, when the Spaniards eliminated most of the native population.

54. U.S. Bureau of the Census. *Current Population Reports 1990*; series P-60, no. 162; series P-20, no. 431.

55. U.S. Bureau of the Census. *The Hispanic Population in the United States: March 1991. Cur Pop Rep: Pop Characteristics 1993*; series P-20, no. 455.

56. U.S. Bureau of the Census. *Income, Poverty, and Health Insurance, 1992*, September 1993.

57. U.S. Bureau of the Census. *Poverty in the U.S.: 1995*, Current Population Reports 1996.

58. U.S. Bureau of the Census, *Educational Attainment in the United States: March 1997*, P20-505.

59. A U.S.-born Hispanic child is very likely to learn Spanish in the home, which is apt to be in an area populated by other Spanish-speaking families. Upon reaching school age, the Hispanic child begins to develop proficiency in the English language. The Hispanic who immigrates to the United States as an adult usually is drawn to areas with high Hispanic concentrations where language and culture are familiar.

60. M. N. Segal & L. Sosa, "Marketing to the Hispanic Community," *California Management Review*, Vol. XXVI, No. 1, Fall 1983, pp. 120–134.

61. The heaviest users of Spanish language media are recent Hispanic immigrants to the United States and Hispanics with limited English-speaking ability. This group has a lower income than the Spanish origin population, is older, less educated and less integrated into the American mainstream. (A. Guernica, "Consumer Hispanic: A Dual Identity," *Madison Avenue*, July 1983, pp. 35–44)

62. U.S. Bureau of the Census,. *Census of Population and Housing, 1990 and 1980*; U.S. Bureau of the Census. *Language Spoken at Home and Ability to Speak English for United States, Regions and States: 1990*, April 28, 1993.

63. Association of State and Territorial Health Officials, June 1992. Report and recommendations: State health agency strategies to develop linguistically relevant public health systems. *ASTHO Bilingual Health Initiative*.

64. Non-English-speaking patients are more likely to be uninsured or covered by Medicaid, which reimburses for services at a lower rate than private insurance.

65. June 1, 1993, interview with Henri Manasse, vice chancellor at University of Illinois Health Services.

66. See L. Page, "Lost in the Translation," *American Medical News*, Feb. 1, 1993, pp. 37–40; G.A. Galanti, *Caring for Patients from Different Cultures: Case Studies from American Hospitals*, Philadelphia: University of Pennsylvania Press, 1991; R.E. Spector, *Cultural Diversity in Health and Illness*, Connecticut: Appleton & Lange, 1991; J. Shapiro and E. Saltzer, "Cross-Cultural Aspects to Physician-Patient Communication Patterns," *Urban Health*, Dec. 1981, 1–15; Z. Fearon, "Communication and the Medical Care Process," *Consumer Health Perspectives* VII(5):1–7; R. Richman, "Failure to Communicate," *The Chicago Reporter*, XXII (3): 1, 6–9, 11.

67. O.F. Díaz-Duque, "Advice from an Interpreter," *American Journal of Nursing*, 82:1380–1382; R.W. Putsch, III, "Cross-Cultural Communication: The Special Case of Interpreters in Health Care," *Journal of the American Medical Association* 254 (23):3344–3348.

68. Personal interview with Linda Coronado, Director of Volunteer Services, Cook County Hospital, November 27, 1995.

69. "The Culture of Illness," *U.S. News and World Report*, February 15, 1993, p. 76.

70. D. Pinkney, "Where is My Baby?: Immigrants' Health Care Faces Language Barrier," *Chicago Sun Times*, Aug. 16, 1992.

71. C. Prince, "Hablando con el doctor: Communication Problems between Doctors and Their Spanish-speaking Patients," Ph.D. Dissertation, Stanford University, Ann Arbor, MI: University Microfilms International, 1986.

72. U.S. Department of Health and Human Services. *Health US, 1990*. August 1991.

73. Council on Scientific Affairs, "Hispanic Health in the United States," *Journal of the American Medical Association*, 265:248–252; R. Klein, B.E.K. Klein, S.E. Moss, M.D. Davis, D.L. DeMets, "The Wisconsin Epidemiologic Study of Diabetic Retinopathy, III: Prevalence and Risk of Diabetic Retinopathy When Age at Diagnosis is 30 or More Years." *Arch Ophthalmol*. 102:527–242; S.M. Haffner, D. Fong, M.P. Stern et al., "Diabetic Retinopathy in Mexican Americans and non-Hispanic Whites," *Diabetes* 37:878–884; J.A. Pugh,

M.P. Stern, S.M.. Haffner et al., "Excess Incidence of Treatment of End-Stage Renal Disease in Mexican Americans," *American Journal of Epidemiol* 127:135–144.

74. *Diabetes Among Latinos*, National Council of La Raza, 1996.

75. U.S. Department of Health and Human Services. *Health US, 1992*. August 1993.

76. Using the *Hispanic Population in the United States: March 1997* (Update) (*Current Population Report* P20-511 July 1998) figures, Hispanics comprised approximately 11.1% of the total U.S. population.

77. "Cumulative" refers to AIDS cases reported to public health officials since 1981. In 1997, 11.5% of the total male population of the United States was Hispanic, 83.1% and 12.3% was White and Black, respectively. However, Hispanic men accounted for 17.3% of all adolescent and adult male AIDS cases reported to the Centers for Disease Control and Prevention in 1997, while White and Black males accounted for 50.1% and 31.4%, respectively. This makes the AIDS incidence rate (the number of new cases of a disease that occurs during a specific time period) among Hispanics almost four times the rate for Whites and almost half the rate for Blacks. *Impact of HIV/AIDS on Hispanics in the United States*, CDC Update, June 1998.

78. National Commission on AIDS, *The Challenge of HIV/AIDS in Communities of Color: The Hispanic/Latino Community*, 1994.

79. The Chicago Department of Public Health (CDPH) has the only AIDS surveillance program in the United States that as a standard collects AIDS statistics by Hispanic ethnicity. Its data reveal that nine of ten reported Hispanic AIDS cases in that city were adult male cases; that Puerto Ricans accounted for one in every two Hispanic AIDS cases reported in Chicago through December 1996; and that the way HIV is transmitted in Chicago, at least, differs significantly by gender and Hispanic origin. For example, Puerto Rican males were more likely to become infected with HIV through injecting drug use while Mexican and other Hispanic males were more likely to become infected through sex with another male. Chicago's data also indicate that Puerto Ricans, who represent 22.0% of Chicago's Hispanic population, account for 47.4% of all AIDS cases in the city. Mexicans, who represent 64.6% of Chicago's Hispanic population, accounted for 38.5% of all reported Hispanic AIDS cases. Hispanic women were most likely to become infected through heterosexual contact with an infected male partner. (*Census of Population & Housing: 1990*, STFIA; CDPH. *AIDS Chicago: AIDS Surveillance Report*; Fourth Quarter 1996.)

80. The word *pediatric* is used to describe children up to age 13. *Report of Final Mortality Statistics*, 1995, Centers for Disease Control and Prevention, National Center for Health Statistics; *HIV/AIDS Surveillance Report*, 1997, 9 (no. 2), Centers for Disease Control and Prevention, National Center for Health Statistics.

81. Centers for Disease Control and Prevention, *HIV/AIDS Surveillance Report*, December 1993, Table 4.

82. R.M. Díaz, *HIV Risk in Latino Gay/Bisexual Men: A Review of Behavioral Research*. Report prepared for the National Latino/ a Lesbian and Gay Organization, 1995.

83. Puerto Ricans have the highest prevalence of illegal drug use among Hispanics. This may be explained, at least in part, by the fact that 70% of Puerto Ricans living in the United States live in New York City, New Jersey, and Chicago, where rates of poverty are higher and the availability of illegal drugs is higher than in other parts of the country. See M.R. de la Rosa, J.H. Khalsa, and B.A. Rouse, "Hispanics and Illicit Drug Use: A Review of Recent Findings," *International Journal of Addiction* 25:665–691. See also B. Menéndez, E. Drucker, S.H. Vermund et al., "AIDS Mortality among Puerto Ricans and Other Hispanics in New York City, 1981–1987," *Journal of Acquired Immune Deficiency Syndrome* 3:644–648; and R.M. Selik, K.G. Castro, M. Pappaioanou, "Birthplace and the Risk of AIDS among Hispanics in the United States," *American Journal of Public Health* 79:836–839.

84. Dominican-born men living in the United States, unlike those living in the Dominican Republic, have a higher proportion of AIDS cases attributable to injection drug use due to their higher likelihood of exposure to injection drug use in the northeastern United States than in the Dominican Republic. See T. Díaz, J.W. Buehler, K.G. Castro et al., "AIDS Trends among *Hispanos* in the United States," *American Journal of Public Health* 83:504–509.

85. B.V. Marín, *Analysis of AIDS Prevention among African Americans and Latinos in the United States*, Report prepared for the Office of Technology Assessment, 1995. Among men born in Mexico, Cuba, and Central and South America, the predominant exposure category was male–male sex. See T. Díaz, J.W. Buehler, K.G. Castro et al., "AIDS Trends among *Hispanos* in the United States."

86. As of December 1997, a large proportion of Hispanic women were infected through injection drug use (29%) or by having sex with an injection drug user (46%). Centers for Disease Control and Prevention, *HIV/AIDS Surveillance Report*, Vol. 9, No. 2.

87. In a survey, 67% of Hispanic women reported never using condoms with their steady partner. In a traditionally *machista* society, women often do not talk to men about sex because it suggests promiscuity. Frequency and type of sex is most often determined by men. See C.A. Gómez, B.V. Marín, "Gender, Culture, and Power: Barriers to HIV Prevention Strategies for Women," *Journal of Sex Research* 33:355–362. A recent survey found that married Hispanic men were two times (18%) more likely to have multiple partners than non-Hispanic Whites (9%). See B.V. Marín, C.A. Gómez, N. Hearst, "Multiple Heterosexual Partners and Condom Use among Hispanics and non-Hispanic Whites," *Family Planning Perspectives* 25:170–174. A different survey reported that only 20% of Hispanic men with multiple partners report using a condom regularly with their primary partner, and 29% with their secondary partner. F. Sabogal, B. Faigeles, J.A. Catania, "Multiple Sex Partners among Hispanics in the United States: The National AIDS Behavioral Surveys, *Family Planning Perspectives* 25:257–262.

88. R. Díaz, "Latino Gay Men and the Psycho-Cultural Barriers to AIDS Prevention," in M. Levine, J. Gagnon, P. Narde, editors, *A Plague of Our Own: The Impact of the AIDS Epidemic on Gay Men and Lesbians*, Chicago: University of Chicago Press, 1995.

89. It is possible that the information regarding cancer mortality within the Hispanic population is incorrect. This may be the result of late diagnosis associated with misinformation and reluctance to seek out early and adequate medical assistance.

90. *Report of the Secretary's Task Force on Black and Minority Health*, Vol. VIII. *Hispanic Health Issues*. Department of Health and Human Services. Washington, DC: Government Printing Office, 1986.

91. *Secretary's Task Force*, 1986.

92. *Surveillance, Epidemiology, and End Results Program (SEER), 1973–1981*, National Cancer Institute, Annual Cancer Statistics Review by E. Sondik et al., Bethesda, MD: Public Health Service, 1985.

93. National Cancer Institute, *Cancer Rates and Risks*, 3rd ed., Bethesda, MD: DHHS, 1985, 85-91.

94. National Cancer Institute, *Cancer Rates and Risks*.

95. E. Muñoz. "Care for the Hispanic Poor: A Growing Segment of American Society," *Journal of the American Medical Association* 2600:2711–2712.

96. See S.A. Black, K.S. Markides, "Acculturation and Alcohol Consumption in Puerto Rican, Cuban-American, and Mexican-American Women in the United States," *American Journal of Public Health* 83:890–893; E.L. Chavez & R.C. Swaim, "Hispanic Substance Use: Problems in Epidemiology," *Drugs and Society* 6:211–230; L. Susenbury, J.A. Epstein, G.J. Botvin, & T. Díaz, "Social Influence Predictors of Alcohol Use among New York *Latino* Youth," *Addictive Behaviors* 19:363–372; C.Y. Lovato, A.J. Litrownik, J. Elder, & A. Núñez-Liriano, "Cigarette and Alcohol Use among Migrant Hispanic Adolescents," *Family & Community Health* 16:18–31; P. Pérez-Arce, "Substance Use Patterns of Hispanics: Commentary," *International Journal of the Addictions* 29:1189–1199.

97. See also M.P. Stern, S.P. Gaskill, C.R. Allen, J. González, and R.H. Waldrop, "Cardiovascular Risk Factors in Mexican Americans in Laredo, Texas," *American Journal of Epidemiology* 113:5:556–562.

98. *Secretary's Task Force*, 1986.

99. *Secretary's Task Force*, 1986.

100. See S.A. Black & K.S. Markides, "Acculturation and Alcohol Consumption in Puerto Rican, Cuban-American, and Mexican-American Women in the United States," pp. 890–893; J.M. Casas, A. Bimbela, C.V. Corral, I. Yáñez, R.C. Swaim, J.C. Wayman, & S. Bates, "Cigarette and Smokeless Tobacco Use among Migrant and Nonmigrant Mexican American Youth, *Hispanic Journal of Behavioral Sciences* 20, 1, 102–121; J.A. Neff & A.M. Dassori, "Age and Maturing Out of Heavy Drinking Among Anglo and Minority Male Drinkers: A Comparison of Cross-Sectional Data and Retrospective Drinking History Techniques," *Hispanic Journal of Behavioral Sciences* 20, 2, 225–240; J.S. Brook, M. Whiteman, E.B. Balka, & B.A. Hamburg, "African-American and Puerto Rican Drug Use: Personality, Familial, and Other Environmental Risk Factors," *Genetic, Social, and General Psychology Monographs* 118:417–438; A.P. Polednak, "Estimating Smoking Prevalence in Hispanic Adults," *Health Values* 18:32–40; K.W. Smith, S.A. McGraw, & J.E. Carrillo, "Factors Affecting Cigarette Smoking and Intention to Smoke among Puerto Rican–American High School Students," *Hispanic Journal of Behavioral Sciences* 13:401–411; L.B. Szalay, G. Canino, & S.K. Vilov, "Vulnerabilities and Cultural Change: Drug Use among Puerto Rican Adolescents in the United States," *International Journal of the Addictions* 28:327–354; H. Landrine, J.L. Richardson, E.A. Klonoff, & B. Flay, "Cultural Diversity in the Predictors of Adolescent Cigarette Smoking: The Relative Influence of Peers," *Journal of Behavioral Medicine* 17:331–346; G. Marín, E. Pérez-Stable, & B.V. Marín, "Cigarette Smoking among San Francisco Hispanics: The Role of Acculturation and Gender," *American Journal of Public Health* 79:196–198; J. Moor, "The Chola Lifecourse: *Chicana* Heroin Users and the *Barrio* Gang," *International Journal of the Addictions* 29(9):1115–1126.

101. Only 44.3% of all Hispanic and 39.8% of Mexican-American children have been exposed to smoke compared with 50.8% of non-Hispanic White children prenatally according to the National Center for Health Statistics. Postnatally 23.5% of all Hispanic and 24.3% of Mexican-American children 5 years of age and under had been exposed to secondhand smoke compared with 20.9% of non-Hispanic children. ("Children's Exposure to Environmental Cigarette Smoke Before and After Birth," No. 202, June 18, 1991, Table 1.)

102. *1996 National Household Survey on Drug Abuse,* Substance Abuse and Mental Health Services Administration, Department of Health and Human Services.

103. See note 114.

104. National Center for Health Statistics, *Advance Report of Final Natality Statistics, 1991. Monthly Vital Statistics Report* 1993; 42(3; suppl; September), p. 8.

105. The data reflecting infant mortality are gathered from death certificates which the states file and the National Center for Health Statistics compile. This information may not be completely accurate. Infant deaths are likely to be underreported, especially when births occur at home, and among undocumented individuals who fear deportation. Also, there are some states that do not report vital statistics using Hispanic identifiers; additionally, there is not a uniform definition of Hispanic by all states. An earlier study has documented another factor that is commonplace in towns along the border—some families travel to Mexico where they register the deaths. See L.B. Johnson School of Public Affairs, *The Health of Mexican Americans in South Texas,* Policy Research Project, Report No. 32, 1979.

106. See note 114.

107. R.B. Valdez et al., "Insuring Latinos against the Costs of Illness," *Journal of the American Medical Association* 1993:269.

108. Winters Group, *Women of Color Reproductive Health Poll Report,* Table 26. See pages 17–25 for discussion on illness.

109. See page 18.

110. Center for Human Resource Research. *Maternal-Child Health Data from the NLSY. 1991,* Substance Abuse and Mental Health Services Administration. *1992 National Household Survey on Drug Abuse: Final Findings,* 1993; National Center for Health Statistics, *Advance Report of Maternal and Infant Health Data from the Birth Certificate, 1990.* Monthly Vital Statistics 1993; 42(2; July).

111. *Cancer Facts and Figures for Minority Americans,* Atlanta, GA: American Cancer Society, 1991.

112. J.E. Becerra, C.J.R. Hogue, H.K. Atrash, N. Pérez, "Infant Mortality Among Hispanics: A Portrait of Heterogeneity," *Journal of the American Medical Association,* 1991; 265:217–221.

113. Although national data are not available, state and local data indicate that the incidence of measles among Hispanic children is correlated with a lack of immunizations. A 1994 retrospective survey of kindergarten students in California, done by COSSMHO in 1994, showed that in 1991, only 43% of Hispanic children had completed their immunization series at age 2. See *Growing Up Hispanic,* Vol. 1, *Leadership Report.* F.S. Mendoza, S.J. Ventura, R.B. Valdez et al., "Selected Measures of Health Status for Mexican-American, Mainland Puerto Rican, and Cuban-American Children," *Journal of the American Medical Association* 1991: 265:227–232.

114. Hispanic youngsters are twice as likely as non-Hispanic White children to live in communities that do not meet EPA lead air pollutant standards. One survey demonstrated that Mexican-American and Puerto Rican children 4 to 5 years of age are more likely than non-Hispanic White children to have elevated blood lead levels, and Puerto Rican children are three times as likely as non-Hispanic White children to have elevated blood lead levels. This may be correlated to the fact that Hispanics are three times as likely as non-Hispanic Whites (18.5% and 6.0%, respectively) to live in areas designated by the Environmental Protection Agency as not meeting lead air pollutant standards. O. Carter-Pokras, "Blood Lead Levels of 4–11-years-old Mexican American, Puerto Rican, and Cuban Children," *Public Health Reports July–August 1990,* Vol. 105, No. 4, pp. 388–393; *Growing Up Hispanic,* p. 31.

115. While Hispanic children are less likely to contract pneumonia (3.8%) than their Black (4.8%) or White (7.7%) peers, of those with the disease, only 67.5% saw a physician compared with 92.2% of White children. A result of this lower level of care is that Hispanic children with pneumonia are much more likely to miss school days because of the disease (16.3 days) than their Black (5.0 days) and White (5.0 days) peers. Centers for Disease Control and Prevention, "Incidence and Impact of Selected Infectious Diseases in Childhood," *National Center for Health Statistics,* 1991: series 10, no. 180, October.

116. These conditions are widespread among Puerto Rican youngsters where, for example, asthma is twice as high as for other Hispanic groups and they are more than three times as likely as White children to have asthma. Asthma is completely treatable, but requires ongoing monitoring and access to a regular source of health care.

117. National Center for Health Statistics. *Deaths of Hispanic Origin,* Vital Health Stat [20] 1990; no. 18, December.

118. Hispanics represented 22.7% of all drug abuse deaths among young men 10 to 19 years of age. (National Center for Health Statistics, "Advance Report of Final Mortality Statistics, 1991," 42 (2) Supplement, August 31, 1993, p. 8.

119. Hispanic high school students are more likely not to use contraceptives, in particular condoms, than their White peers even though they report about the same level of sexual activity (37.5% and 38.0%, respectively). As a result, they are more likely to contract a sexually transmitted disease. (Centers for Disease Control and Prevention, "Sexual Behavior Among High School Students—United States, 1990.," *Morbidity and Mortality Weekly Report,* Vol. 40, Nos. 51, 52. January 3, 1992. Table 2.)

120. Hispanic adolescents are the racial/ethnic group of adolescents most likely to have attempted suicide. Hispanic high school students are more likely to have made at least one suicide attempt (12%) than their non-Hispanic Black (6.5%) or White (7.9%) peers. They also are more likely to report suicidal thoughts than their non-Hispanic peers. (Centers for Disease Control and Prevention, "Attempted Suicide Among High School Students: United States, 1990," *Morbidity and Mortality Weekly Report*, Youth Risk Behavior Surveillance System, Vol. 40, No. 37, September 21, 1991, Table 1.) See also D. Fraser, J. Piacentini, R. Van Rossem, D. Hien, & M.J. Rotheram-Borus, "Effects of Acculturation and Psychopathology on Sexual Behavior and Substance Use of Suicidal Hispanic Adolescents," *Hispanic Journal of Behavioral Sciences*, 1998, 20(1), 83–101.

121. J.P. Brown, "Dental Health Status and Treatment Needs among Mexican Americans," *Hispanic Health Status Symposium Proceedings*; A.I. Ismail, S.M. Szpunar, "The Prevalence of Total Tooth Loss, Dental Caries, and Periodontal Disease among Mexican Americans, Cuban Americans, and Puerto Ricans: Findings from HHANES 1982-1984," *American Journal of Public Health*, 1990; 80:66–70.

122. G.S. Rust, "Health Status of Migrant Farmworkers: A Literature Review and Commentary," *American Journal of Public Health*, 1990; 9:1218–1224; and Council on Scientific Affairs, "Hispanic Health in the United States," *Journal of the American Medical Association*, 1991; 265:248–252.

123. S. Murphy, R. Castillo et al., "An Evaluation of Food Group Intakes by Mexican American Children," *J Am Diet Assoc*, 1990; 90(3).

124. A.J. Rubel, "Concepts of Disease in Mexican American Culture," *American Anthropologist*, Vol. 62, No. 5 (1960), 795–815.

125. P.A. Poma, "Hispanic Cultural Influences on Medical Practice," *Journal of the National Medical Association*, 1983; 75(10), 941–945.

126. Health care professionals should ask their Hispanic patients which prescription medications, herbs, or over-the-counter medicines they are taking rather than ask if they use folk healers or folk medicine. Most Hispanics do not think of what they do in those terms.

127. J.C. Higginbotham, F.M. Treviño, L.A. Ray, "Utilization of *Curanderos* by Mexican Americans: Prevalence and Predictors, Findings from HHANES 1982-84," *American Journal of Public Health*, 1990; 80(Supplement):32–35.

128. Hispanics broadly define family to include parents, siblings, grandparents, aunts, uncles, cousins, close family friends (considered honorary aunts or uncles), and *padrinos* (godparents). Hispanic families exhibit interdependence, affiliation, and cooperation. (See page 10.) The entire family may be involved in an individual's health and many Hispanics place the responsibility for cure with the entire family. Frequently, Hispanic patients may discuss a physician's diagnosis and treatment recommendations with their families before deciding to follow them. Therefore, including the family is often crucial.

129. Among Hispanics, members of the surrounding community are relied on and interacted with in much the same way as Anglo Americans rely on and interact with their extended families.

130. W. Holland, "Mexican-American Medical Beliefs: Science or Magic? in R. Argüiro Martínez, ed., *Hispanic Culture and Health Care: Fact, Fiction, Folklore*, St. Louis, MO: C.V. Mosby, 1978, pp. 99–119; C. Martínez and H. Martín, "Folk Diseases among Urban Mexican-Americans," *Journal of the American Medical Association*, Vol. 196, No. 2 (April 11, 1966), pp. 161–164.

131. See W. Madsen, "Health and Illness," in J. Burma, ed., *Mexican-Americans in the United States: A Reader*, Cambridge, MA: Schenkman Publishing Co., 1970, pp. 333f.

132. Some common Hispanic sayings include: *Que será, será* (What will be will be); *Esta enfermedad es una prueba de Dios* (This illness is a test of God); and *Que sea lo que Dios quiera* (It's in God's hands now).

133. R. Firth, "Acculturation in Relation to Concepts of Health and Disease," in I. Goldstone, ed., *Medicine and Anthropology*, No. XXI of the New York Academy of Medicine Lectures to the Laity, New York: Books of Libraries Press, 1971, pp. 153–154.

134. H. Fabrega and C.A. Wallace, "Value Identification and Psychiatric Disability: An Analysis involving Americans of Mexican Descent" in C. Hernández, M.J. Haug, and N.N. Wagner, eds., 2nd ed., *Chicanos: Social and Psychological Perspectives*, St. Louis, MO: C.V. Mosby, 1976, pp. 253–261.

135. See L. Saunders, *Cultural Differences and Medical Care*, New York: Russell Sage Foundation, 1954, p. 148.

136. The curandero (curandera) is a person who has a more extensive knowledge of herbs and household remedies than other individuals in the community, and to whom people turn for problems concerning "internal medicine." These individuals are lay practitioners who have no formal training in medicine or allied health fields. See I. V. Octavio Romano, "Charismatic Medicine, Folk-Healing, and Folk-Sainthood," *American Anthropologist*, Vol. 67, pp. 1151–1173.

137. See L. Cohen, *Culture, Disease, and Stress among Latino Immigrants*, Washington, DC: Catholic University of America, 1979, pp. 136–140.

138. See A. Kardec, *El Libro de los espíritus*, Mexico, D.F.: Editorial Diana, 1957.

139. See T. Weaver, "Use of Hypothetical Situations in a Study of Spanish American Illness Referral Systems," *Human Organization*, Vol. 29, No. 2 [1970], pp. 140–154; also J. Kreisman, "The *Curandero's* Apprentice: A Therapeutic Integration of Folk and Medical Healing," *American Journal of Psychiatry*, Vol. 132, No. I [Jan. 1975], pp. 81–83.

140. See M. Kay, "Health and Illness in a Mexican American *Barrio*," in E.H. Spicers, ed., *Ethnic Medicine in the Southwest*, Arizona: University of Arizona Press, 1977," p. 164; W. Gliebe, L. Malley, A. R. Lynn, "Use of the Health Care Delivery System by Urban Mexican-Americans in Ohio," *Public Health Reports*, Vol. 94, No. 3 [May—June, 1979], pp. 226–230.

141. See V.G. de Pineda, *La medicina popular en Colombia*, Bogota: Universidad Nacional de Colombia, Monografías Sociológicas, Vol. 8, pp. 54–55.

142. Pharmacists in the Spanish-speaking world are highly respected and consulted regularly by people suffering from ailments. They receive rigorous training, are current in pharmacology, able to give injections and prescribe medicine, and their advice is taken seriously. See L. Cohen, *Culture, Disease, and Stress*, pp. 171–177.

143. See J. Ramos-MacKay, L. Comas-Díaz, and L. Rivera, "Puerto Ricans," in L. Comas-Díaz and E.H. Griffith, eds., *Clinical Guidelines in Cross-Cultural Mental Health*, New York: John Wiley & Sons, 1988.

144. Thousands of plants are used in Mexico for medicinal purposes. People purchase what they need from *hierberías-yerberías* (herb shops) in open markets. The *hierbero/yerbero / hierbera/yerbera* not only sells dried herbs, but recommends them to alleviate certain ailments. Older generations, especially along the Texas-Mexican border, still shop at *hierberías*.

145. L. Saunders, *Cultural Differences and Medical Care*.

146. M. Clark, *Health in the Mexican-American Culture*, 2nd ed. Berkeley, CA: University of California Press, 1970, pp. 163–183.

147. See also Chapter 8, note 40, page 193 and Chapter 11, note 7, page 249.

148. See G. Foster, "Relationships Between Spanish and Spanish-American Folk Medicine," *Journal of American Folklore*, Vol. 66, No. 261, pp. 201–217; G. Foster & J. Rowe, "Suggestions for Field Recording of Information on the Hippocratic Classification of Diseases and Remedies," in *Kroeber Anthropological Society Papers*, Vol. V, pp. 1–3.

149. See page 23.

150. A. Harwood, "Hot-Cold Theory of Disease" *Journal of the American Medical Association*, 216(7), p. 1154.

151. See M. Kay, "Health and Illness," pp. 162f; C. Martínez and H. Martín, "Folk Diseases among Mexican-Americans," pp. 161–164; N. Galli, "Influence of Cultural Heritage on the Health status of Puerto Ricans," Journal of the School of Health, 45 (1975), pp. 12–13; and I. Murillo-Rohde, "Cultural Sensitivity in the Care of the Hispanic Patient," *Washington State Journal of Nursing*, Special Supplement, 1979, 25–32.

152. See C. Martínez and H. Martín, "Folk Diseases Among Urban Mexican-Americans," p. 148; W. Holland, "Mexican-American Medical Beliefs: Science or Magic?," pp. 99–119.

153. See M. Clark, *Health in the Mexican-American Culture*, pp. 175–176; R. Adams and A. Rubel, "Sickness and Social Relations," *Handbook of Middle American Indians*, Vol. 6, Austin: University of Texas Press, 1967, p. 345.

154. See J. Gillin, "Magical Fright," in *Psychiatry*, 11, 387–400.

155. See A. J. Rubel, "The Epidemiology of Folk Illness: *Susto* in Hispanic America," *Ethnology*, Vol. 3 [1964], pp. 268–283; A. J. Rubel and C. W. O'Nell, "The Meaning of *Susto* (Magical Fright)," paper presented at the XLI International Congress of Americanists, Mexico City, 1974, p. 6.

156. Clark, *Health in the Mexican-American Culture*, p. 177.

157. See Holland, "Mexican-American Medical Beliefs," p. 105.

158. W. Madsen, *Mexican-Americans of South Texas*, 2nd ed. New York: Holt, Rinehart, & Winston, 1973, p. 76.

159. See P. A. Poma, "Hispanos: Impact of Culture on Health Care," *Illinois Medical Journal*, Vol. 156, No. 6, p. 456.

160. This affliction affects Puerto Ricans and Mexicans alike. Some folk healers also use lemons and bay leaves in addition to the raw egg. The *espiritista* calls the treatment a *barrida* (a sweeping) while the *curandero* calls it a *limpia* (cleaning). Whether a *barrida* or a *limpia*, the action is thought to have both diagnostic and treatment value.

161. See D. Werner, *Donde no hay doctor*, 4th ed., México: Editorial Pax-México, 1980, p. 5.

162. See M. Kay, "Health and Illness," p. 140.

163. See A. Kiev, *Curanderismo*, New York: Free Press, 1968, p. 98.

164. See P. A. Poma, "Hispanos," p. 455.

165. See L. Cohen, *Culture, Disease, and Stress among Latino Immigrants*, pp. 162–165.

166. Health workers who deal with nutritional problems should understand theories underlying the diets of their patients; they should recommend the use of different proportions of foods already in the diet of the people rather than encourage complete dietary changes. During times of illness, Hispanics rely greatly on diet modification. (Most of the folk illnesses affect the gastrointestinal tract.)

167. See M. Clark, *Health in the Mexican-American Culture*, pp. 164f; A. J. Rubel, "Concepts of Disease in Mexican-American Culture," *American Anthropologist*, Vol. 62, No. 5 [1960], pp. 795–815.

168. See A. Kiev, *Curanderismo*, p. 95.

169. See P. Poma, "Hispanos," p. 456.

170. See R. Currier, "The Hot-Cold Syndrome and Symbolic Balance in Mexican and Spanish-American Folk Medicine," *Ethnology*, Vol. 5 (1966), pp. 251–263.

171. See Chapter 11, note 7, p. 249. See also D. Werner, *Donde no hay doctor*, p. 23.

172. See M. Clark, *Health in the Mexican-American Culture*, p. 178.

173. R. L. Beals, *Cheran: A Sierra Tarascan Village*, Washington, D.C.: Publications of the Institute of Social Anthropology, 1946.

174. See D. Werner, *Donde no hay doctor*, pp. 26–27.

175. See R. Currier, "The Hot-Cold Syndrome," p. 259; W. Madsen, *Mexican-Americans*, p. 75.

176. See A. Kiev, *Curanderismo*, p. 94.

177. See D. Werner, *Donde no hay doctor*, p. 22.

178. See M. Clark, *Health in the Mexican-American Culture*, p. 180; and D. Werner, *Donde no hay doctor*, p. 28.

179. L.R. Chavez, W.A. Cornelius, & O.W. Jones, "Mexican Immigrants and the Utilization of U.S. Health Services: The Case of San Diego." *Soc.Sci Med.* 21 (1) (1985) 93–102.

180. L.R. Chavez, W.A. Cornelius, & O.W. Jones, "Utilization of Health Services by Mexican Immigrant Women in San Diego." *Women and Health*. Summer 1986; 11(2), 3–20.

181. E.T. Hall, *The Silent Language*, Connecticut: Fawcett Press, 1961.

182. See Chapter 6, p. 118.

183. Hispanic patients can be shown respect, even by health care providers with very limited Spanish, in the following ways: by always using the formal *usted* (you) until the patient suggests the use of the informal *tú*; by addressing patients formally, as *Señor* (Sir) or *Señora* (Mrs./Ma'am), or by using the honorary *Don* or *Doña* and the patient's first name; and by greeting the patients in Spanish with an appropriate *Buenos días* (Good morning) or *Buenas tardes* (Good afternoon). See chapter 6, note 2, page 134. If at all possible, health care providers should not use a curt manner to Hispanics which may be interpreted as not caring about them.

184. See M. Mead, ed., *Cultural Patterns and Technical Change*, Paris: United Nations Educational, Scientific, and Cultural organization, 1953, pp. 179–180.

185. See L. Cohen, *Culture, Disease, and Stress*, pp. 178–179.

186. See page 7.

CHAPTER 2
CAPITULO

Pronunciation
Pronunciación

THE ALPHABET

EL ALFABETO O ABECEDARIO ESPAÑOL

Until March 1994, the Spanish alphabet had thirty letters—five vowels and twenty-five consonants. Since then, it only has twenty-eight—five vowels and twenty-three consonants. With the exception of the consonant *RR*, which never begins a word, each letter has its own separate entry in dictionaries. The two letters that were sacrificed, *CH* and *LL*, traditionally treated by ALL Spanish-speakers as separate letters in their own right, were eliminated in response to calls by the European Union to "'adapt all measures' to aid translation and standardize computer operations." Although the reduction was opposed mainly by Latin Americans and enthusiastically endorsed by the delegates from Spain, the changes adopted at a meeting attended by scholars from all over the Spanish-speaking world do not affect pronunciation, spelling, or syllabication. The main change is found in the way dictionaries are arranged. For example, prior to 1994, the words *Chiapas* and *Chile* were found in dictionaries after *Cuba*. Since 1994, *Chiapas* and *Chile* are found before *Cuba*. Likewise, *lluvia* ("rain") came after *llano* ("plain") and both words followed *lodo* ("mud") in dictionaries published until 1994. Since then, *llano* and *lluvia* are found before *lodo*. Spain did retain the *Ñ*. The letters of the "official" Spanish alphabet are:

Letter	Name	Transliteration	Letter	Name	Transliteration
A	a	ah	Ñ	eñe	eh´-nyay
B	be	bay	O	o	oh
C	ce	say	P	pe	pay
(CH	che	chay/cheh)	Q	cu	coo
D	de	day	R	ere	eh´-ray
E	e	ay/Ā	RR	erre	er´-rray/air rray
F	efe	eh-fay	S	ese	eh-say/essay
G	ge	hay	T	te	tay
H	hache	ah´-chay	U	u	oo
I	i	ee/ē	V	ve/uve	bay or oo-bay
J	jota	hoe´-tah	W	doble ve/	dough̄´-blay bay or
K	ka	kah		doble u/	dough´-blay oo or
L	ele	eh´-lay		ve doble	bay dough´-blay
(LL	elle	ay-yay/L´-yay	X	equis	eh´-keys
M	eme	eh´-may	Y	i griega	ē-grē-ay´-gah
N	ene	eh´-nay	Z	zeta	say´-tah

These letters can also be represented using phonetic transcription:

A	B	C	CH	D	E	F	G	H	I
a	be	θe	ĉe/tʃe	de	e	éfe	xe	áĉe/átʃe	i

J	K	L	LL	M	N	Ñ	O	P	Q
xóta	ka	éle	éʎe	éme	éne	éɲe	o	pe	ku

R	RR	S	T	U	V	W	X	Y	Z
ére	éɾe/érre	ése	te	u	úβe	úβe dóβle	'ekis	iɣriéɣa/i´ɣrjeɣa	θéta

GENERAL REMARKS

OBSERVACIONES GENERALES

Spanish is a language of emotions. This means that when people speak, they use their entire body. Consequently head, hands, and arms are used as auxiliary tools to emphasize the meanings of what is being said. Responses such as "Yes" (*Sí*) or "No" (*No*) are generally repeated since Spanish is an emphatic language as well as a phonetic one.

When learning Spanish, care must be taken to make all pronunciation distinctions. There are no silent letters, except for "h" and "u" in certain limited structures. It is safe to say that if the person learning to speak Spanish does not distinguish between certain sounds and sound contrasts, the learner will be misunderstood when trying to pronounce them. For example, if the distinction is not made between the two types of Spanish *R*, the single tap /r/ and the trilled or multiple tapped /r̄/, the learner will not distinguish between *caro* ("expensive") and *carro* ("automobile") and might erroneously say *Está enterrado*

("He is buried") when intending to say *Está enterado* ("He's informed"). Another example of a mispronunciation which can create a "problem of perception" can occur with the sounds of *P* and *B*. A native English speaker might think he said, «*Déme un peso.*» ("Give me a dollar"), but is heard to say, «*Déme un beso.*» ("Give me a kiss.") by the native Spanish speaker. Sounds that do not exist in English must be pronounced carefully. Distinctions between *sana* ("healthy") and *saña* ("anger") or *unión* ("union") and *uñón* ("big toenail") must be clear. The response to the question, ¿*Cuántos anos tiene usted?* ("How many anuses do you have?") is always "one." The response to the question, ¿*Cuántos años tiene usted?* ("How old are you?") is variable. Failure to pronounce properly can severely impede communication. Spanish-speakers learning English must also learn to make meaningful distinctions of certain English sounds which do not occur in their language. For example, they might say "He went to Yale" when they want to say "He went to jail," or "She is choking" when they mean, "She is joking." Thus, pronunciation is exceptionally important, perhaps, even more important for health care practitioners than grammatical accuracy.

Many Americans mistakenly believe that Spanish is the easiest of all foreign languages to learn. Spanish is considered to be such an "easy" language for Americans primarily because Spanish is relatively easy to pronounce. Also, Spanish is pronounced the way it is written. Spanish letters are treated as feminine nouns, and each has one sound except for *C, D, E, G, N, O, S, X,* and *Y,* which have at least two sounds. The letters *K* and *W* appear only in foreign words. The letter combinations *Ñ, RR* each have one sound and are considered to be one consonant and are alphabetized as such. Because the elimination of the consonants *CH* and *LL* is still considered quite recent, "older" native speakers still use and understand these letters as they have always been. Other native speakers have made the change. This means that non-native speakers may use and hear *che* or *ce hace* ("CH") and *elle* and *doble ele* ("LL") which are used and understood by native speakers. Excluding prefixes and suffixes, *C, R,* and *L* are the only three consonants that may be doubled in Spanish. To help you remember this, think of the word "*CuRL.*"

The Spanish alphabet is divided into vowels (*las vocales*) and consonants (*las consonantes*). The vowels *A, E, I, O,* and *U* are the same as in English. *Y* is a vowel when it is the last letter in a word and a consonant when it begins a word or a syllable. Thus, *Y* serves two functions. An example of *Y*'s use as a vowel is **hoy** ("today"); as a consonant, **inyección** ("injection").[1]

All vowels in Spanish are short, clear, and pure sounds. The position of the mouth remains the same throughout the pronunciation of the vowel. Even in the unstressed position Spanish vowels are pronounced clearly. Also, the time used to produce the Spanish vowel sounds, both in a stressed and unstressed syllable, is the same, unlike English. In a stressed syllable, however, the prominence of the vowel is manifest by its loudness. *A, I,* and *U* each have one sound, although there will be slight variations according to placement within the phrase or word.

RULES OF PRONUNCIATION

REGLAS DE LA PRONUNCIACION

A* sounds like A in "father." Open your mouth wide and pronounce it as a clipped "*ah.*"   /a/

adrenal	ađrənál	*adrenal*	**aparato**	aparáto	*apparatus*
abdomen	abđómēn	*abdomen*	**amígdala**	amígđɐla	*tonsil*

B (**be larga**) is pronounced exactly like *V* (**ve corta** or **uve**). Thus the sounds of *a ver* and *haber, tubo* and *tuvo,* and *las aves* and *la sabes* are the same. Pronunciation of these two letters depends on their position in the word, phrase, or sentence. When *initial,* that is, after a full pause or silence, at the beginning of a sentence, a breath group, or when they follow *M* or *N,* **B** and **V** sound like the English *B* sound of "*boy.*" Lips must be tense.   /b/

hombro	ómbrɔ	*shoulder*	**brazo**	brásɔ/bráθɔ	*arm*
miembro	mjémbrɔ	*limb*	**bazo**	básɔ/báθɔ	*spleen*

Note that in all other positions, especially when the *B* or *V* occurs between two vowels (intervocalic), the sound softens. The *B* or *V* represents a sound that does not exist in English. In order to produce this sound, less lip pressure should be used. Do not quite close the lips, but allow air to escape through the slight opening between them. Lips should be very relaxed.   [ƀ]

cabeza	kaƀésɐ/kaƀéθɐ	*head*	**aborto**	aƀɔ́rtɔ	*abortion*

*Here, and throughout the chapter, the asterisk instructs the reader to see **Dialectal Variations** on pages 44 to 49.

In certain sequences such as /ob-/ and /sub-/ the softened or fricative b [ƀ] disappears, particularly at the beginning of words:

obstáculo [os-tá-ku-lo] *obstruction*   *subjetivo* [su-xe-tíƀo] *subjective*

In many words the alternate spellings reflect the disappearance of the [ƀ] in pronunciation.

C has two sounds.

1. Before *A, O, U,* or a consonant, **C** generally has a hard sound, as in "*cap*" or "*cone,*" but without the slight aspiration (the puff of air) heard in English.* /k/

carne kárnə *flesh*	**cuerpo** kwérpɔ *body*	**clavículas** klaƀíkülas *clavicles*
cadáver kađáƀəɹ *corpse*	**córnea** kɔ́rnəa *cornea*	**cúbito** kúbịto *ulna*

2. **C** before *E* or *I* is pronounced like the **C** in "*city*" throughout most of Latin America and in the southern part of Spain. The sound resembles the English sibilant *s* in the word "*sink.*" In all of Spain except Andalucia, **C** followed by *E* or *I* is pronounced approximately like *TH* in the English word "*thin.*" /s/ or /θ/ Castilian

cintura sịntúrɐ/θịntúrɐ *waist*	**cirujano** sirụxánɔ/θirụxánɔ *surgeon*
cerebro serébrɔ/θerébrɔ *cerebrum*	**contracepción** kọntrasẹƀsjón/kọntraθẹƀθjón *contraception*

CH* is pronounced as the *CH* of "*ch*ild." There is a bit more tension than in the English. /č/

chinelas činélɐs *slippers*	**chicle** číklə *chewing gum*	**gancho** gáṇčɔ *clasp (for a dental bridge)*
chaleco čalékɔ *vest*	**mucho** múčɔ *much, a lot*	**noche** nóčə *night, evening*

D has two different sounds depending on its position.

1. At the beginning of a sentence, after a pause, an *N* or an *L*, it is a hard, strongly dentalized sound. The tip of the tongue presses against the back of the upper front teeth rather than the alveolar ridge [the "bumpy ridge" above the upper front teeth] as in English. Note the difference between English "***day***" and Spanish "***de.***" /d/

   domingo domíŋgɔ *Sunday*
   dolor dolɔ́ɹ *pain*
   dos veces al día dọz ƀéses ạl díɐ/dọz ƀéθes ạl díɐ   *twice a day*

   NOTE: Care must be taken to articulate this Spanish D as a dental sound, and not as an alveolar as it is in English. Intervocalic **D** in English, as in "mu*dd*y," or "la*dd*er," is the equivalent of Spanish **R**.

2. In other positions, such as between vowels, or at the end of a word, Spanish **D** approaches the *TH* of "*the*" or "*they.*" The tongue, however, presses the back of the upper front teeth and should not be as far forward as for the English sound.* [đ]

médicos méđịkọs *physicians*	**codo** kóđɔ *elbow*	**mojado** mọxáᵈɔ *wet*	**radio** ráđjɔ *radius*

E has two sounds.

1. When no other letter follows it in the syllable, it is like the long **A** sound in English "m*a*te," but lacking the "off-glide." It also sounds like this when found in syllables ending in **d, m, n,** or **s.**[2] /e/

higiene ịxjénə *hygiene*	**pelo** pélɔ *hair*	**escayola** eskaŷólɐ *plaster*
teléfono teléfɔnɔ *telephone*	**vena** bénɐ *vein*	**menstruar** menstrụár *to menstruate*
usted ustéđ *you*	**embrión** ẹmbrjón *embryo*	**en el agua** enelágụa *in the water*
entrecano ẹntrəkánɔ *greying*		

2. When followed by a consonant in the same syllable other than **d, m, n, or s,** or in contact with trilled **r** /r̄/ or before /x/, even though final in the syllable, **E** is like the **E** in "m*e*t."* [ɛ]

abertura aƀɛrtúrɐ *opening*	**regla** r̄églɐ *menstrual period*
técnica tégnịka/téknịka *technician*	**oreja** orɛ́xɐ *ear*

F* is pronounced essentially the same as in English, but a bit more tensely. /f/

afeitar afẹịtáɹ *to shave*	**fumar** fümáɹ *to smoke*	**familia** famílȷɐ *family*	**fémur** fémụr *femur*

G has three pronunciations.

Before *A, O, U,* or a consonant it has two sounds.

1. When initial after a full pause or silence or after **N**, the **G** is "hard," like the **G** in "*girls.*" /g/

lengua léŋgwɐ *tongue*	**gotero** gotérɔ *dropper*
garganta gargáṇtɐ *throat*	**glándulas** glánđülas *gland*

2. In all other positions the **G** before *A, O, U,* or a consonant has the weaker **G** of English "su*g*ar." This "softer" version of **G** is very challenging to produce. Raise the back of the tongue toward the soft palate, but do not touch it. Note that a small amount of air should pass through the roof of the mouth and the palate. Proper pronunciation of this sound lessens your English accent.* [g]

su gotero   su gotérɔ   *your dropper*   **hago**   ágɔ   *I am doing. I am making.*
las gafas   laz gafɐs   *the glasses*

The third sound of Spanish **G** is one that does not exist in English. It is a "soft" guttural sound that occurs whenever **G** is before **E** or **I** and is formed in the back of the throat. This sound is similar to the **CH** in the German "A*ch*" or in the Scottish "Lo*ch.*" This is also the same sound of Spanish **J**.   /x/

virgen   bírxən   *virgin*   **ginecólogo**   xinəkólɔgo   *gynecologist*
ingerir   iŋxeríɪ   *to ingest*   **gemelos**   xemélɔs   *twins*

Occasionally a silent **U** will precede the **E** or **I** to indicate that the **G** is "hard" as in English "*gue*st."

pagué   pagé   *I paid*   **guijón**   gixón   *tooth decay*

To keep the **U** sound in the *gue* or *gui* combination, a diæresis (**una diéresis**) (¨) is inserted over the **U** (**Ü**).

vergüenza   bɛrgwénsɐ/bɛrgwénθɐ   *shame*   **ungüento**   uŋgwéŋtɔ   *ointment*
bilingüe   bilíŋgwə   *bilingual*

H   is the only silent Spanish consonant and can best be compared to the *h* of English "*h*onor."

hormonas   ɔrmónɐs   *hormones*   **heroína**   eroínɐ   *heroin*
hematólogo   emɐtólɔgo   *hematologist*   **hígado**   ígeᵈo   *liver*

I   is like the *I* in "mach*i*ne," but without the "off-glide." Contrast the Spanish "*sí*" with the English "*see.*"   /i/

infarto   iɱfártɔ   *infarct*   **interno**   iŋtérnɔ   *intern*   **irritación**   iɾ̯itasɹón/iɾ̯itaθɹón   *irritation*

J   is pronounced just like the soft Spanish **G**. Some feel that it resembles a greatly exaggerated English **H** sound as in English "*h*ouse" or the English **WH** sound in English "*wh*o."   /x/

aguja   agúxɐ   *needle*   **joven**   xóɓən   *young person*
juanete   xwanétɐ   *bunion*   **jeringa**   xeríŋgɐ   *syringe*

K   is pronounced as in English but has no aspiration. It occurs only in **loan words** (i.e., words which Spanish has "borrowed" from other languages).   /k/

kilo   kílɔ   *kilo*   **kilogramo**   kilográmɔ   *kilogram*
kilómetro   kilómətro   *kilometer*   **kiosko**   kɹos´-kɔ   *kiosk*

L*   is pronounced almost the same as in English, but with the tip of the tongue against the upper front teeth, producing a more liquid sound; the Spanish **L** is much more "tense" than the English **L**. Contrast Spanish "*lo*" and English "*low.*"   /l/

líquido   líkɪɖo   *liquid*   **laceración**   laserɐsɹón/laθerɐθɹón   *laceration*
lágrimas   lágrɪmas   *tears*   **exclamar**   es·klɐ-m·ár   *to exclaim*

LL*   is considered to be one consonant in Spanish. In Mexico, many parts of South America, and in some parts of Spain it usually sounds like the **Y** of "*y*es." However, this sound is more closed and tenser in Spanish than in English because the tongue touches the roof of the mouth slightly sounding almost like the **J** in "*j*oke." Contrast the Spanish "*llora*" with the English "*your.*" In most parts of Spain, in Paraguay, most of Peru, and in Bogota, Colombia **LL** approximates the **LLI** in the English word "Wi*lli*am." /y/ or /ḷ/ Castilian

costilla   kɔs̩tíyɐ/kɔs̩tíḷɐ   *rib*   **cuchillada**   kuĉɪyáᵈɐ/kuĉɪḷáᵈɐ   *gash*
espaldilla   espa̩ldíyɐ/espa̩ldíḷɐ   *shoulder blade*   **mellizos**   meyísɔs/meḷíθɔs   *twins*

M   is pronounced essentially the same as in English, but with more tension and is unaspirated. Press your lips together harder and do not allow much air to escape from the lips when the sound is made. Compare the Spanish "*moda*" with the English "*mode.*"   /m/

miope   mɹópə   *myopia*   **mejilla**   məxíyɐ/məxíḷɐ   *cheek*
metabolismo   metaɓolízmɔ   *metabolism*   **menstruar**   mɛnstrwáɹ   *to menstruate*
médula   méɖula   *marrow*   **más suave**   máswáɓə   *softer*

N   has numerous pronunciations.

1.   It is pronounced generally as in English. It is short and clipped; the tip of the tongue touches the alveolar ridge in both languages.   /n/

noche   nóĉə   *night*   **novacaína**   noɓakaínɐ   *novocaine*
nalgas   nálgɐs   *buttocks*   **negro**   négrɔ   *black*
mensual   mɛnwál   *monthly*   **tan gordo**   taŋgórdɔ   *so fat*

The pronunciation of the **N** is influenced by the consonant that follows it. The Spanish **N** takes on characteristics of the consonant. This is called **nasal assimilation.**

2. *N* is pronounced like *M* before *B, F, P, M,* and *V* whether within a word or between words.   [m]

enfermo eɱférmɔ *ill*	**un viejo** ųmbjéxɔ *an old man*
enfermera eɱfɔ̀rmére *nurse*	**un brazo** ųmbrásɔ/ųmbráθɔ *an arm*
un pulmón ųmpųlmǫ́n *a lung*	**un buen día** umbwęŋdía *a good day*
un metatarso ų͈ɱmetɐtársɔ *a metatarsus*	**enviar** embjár *to send*

3. *N* assumes a nasal quality similar to English *N* in "ri*ng*" before *CA, CU, CO, K, G, J, QU,* or *HUE* whether within a word or between words.   [ŋ]

un hueso ųŋwésɔ *a bone*	**un cúbito** ųŋkúbịto *an ulna*
un kilo ųŋkílɔ *one kilo*	**estancado** eṣteŋkáᵈɔ *stagnant*
sangre sáŋgrə *blood*	**estangurria** eṣteŋgúrɟe *catheter*
un jarro ųŋxárɔ *a pitcher*	**estanquidad** eṣteŋkịdáᵈ *watertightness*

4. Before *D* or *T*, Spanish *N* is a **dental** sound, produced by the tip of the tongue touching the upper front teeth.   [ņ]

pantalla paņtáḷa *screen*	**índice** íņdise/íņdiθe *index finger*
un dolor ųņdɔlór *a pain*	**un televisor** ųņtelebisǫ́ɹ *a TV set*

Ñ sounds like the *NI* in English "onion" or the *NY* in "canyon," although in English the *NI* and *NY* have different sounds (glides) and belong to different syllables. Spanish Ñ has one sound and is a single consonant. Ñ always begins a syllable. Contrast Spanish *"com-pa-ÑE-ro"* with English *"com-PAN-ion."*   [ɲ]

riñón r̃iɲ́ón *kidney*	**señor** seɲǫ́ɹ *sir, Mr.*	**niño** níɲɔ *child*

O has two pronunciations.

1. When it ends a syllable, it is comparable to the English *O* in "oak" or in English "no," but without the off-glide. Contrast Spanish *"no"* with English *"no."*   /o/

agotamiento agotamjéņtɔ *exhaustion*	**oreja** oréxɐ *ear*
muslo múzlɔ *thigh*	**emocional** emosjonál/emoθjonál *emotional*
enérgico enérgịko *energetic*	**no** nó *no*

2. When followed by a consonant in the same syllable it sounds like *O* in English "or." Again, it is not diphthongized.   [ǫ]

ombligo ǫmblígɔ *navel*	**hormona** ǫrmóne *hormone*
órgano ǫ́rgeno *organ*	**cónyuge** kǫ́ɲŷ̨xɐ *spouse*

P is pronounced almost as in English but has more tension and is not aspirated. The slight puff of air that is heard after the English *P* is produced is omitted in Spanish. Contrast Spanish *"parte"* with English *"part."*   /p/

pañal paɲál *diaper*	**pecho** péĉɔ *chest, breast*
pijama pịxáme *pajamas*	**pestaña** peṣtáɲe *eyelash*

Although many authorities now omit the initial *P* in the *PS* combination, it is still retained in print.

psicología sikɔlɔxíe *psychology*	**psicoterapia** sikɔterápje *psychotherapy*
psiquíatra sikíetra *psychiatrist*	**psiquiatra** sikjátra *psychiatrist*

Q appears only before *UE* or *UI*. The *U* is always silent and the *Q* has a *K* sound. Nevertheless, care must be taken not to aspirate the *QU* or pronounce it the English way as *KW*. Contrast Spanish *"quieto"* with English *"quiet."*   /k/

quejar kɛxáɹ *to complain*	**bronquios** brǫ́ŋkjɔs *bronchia*
quijada kịxáᵈɐ *jaw*	**química** kímịka *chemistry*

R* has two pronunciations.

1. It is slightly trilled or tapped when not in an initial position. The tip of the tongue is "tapped" against the **alveolar ridge** [the "bumpy ridge" above the upper front teeth]. The sound of Spanish *R* is similar to the English *D* or *T* sounds of mu*dd*y, bu*dd*y, la*dd*er, bu*tt*er, wa*t*er, and le*tt*er. This sound is also called a flap.   /ɾ/

primo hermano prímɔɔrmǻnɔ *first cousin*	**sufrir** sufríɹ *to suffer*

2. It is strongly trilled when initial or after *N, L,* or *S*. This trill or multiple tapping or multiple flap is made by placing the tip of the tongue on the alveolar ridge and letting it vibrate strongly while air passes through the mouth. There is no equivalent in English.   /r̄/

enredar enr̄edáɹ *to implicate*	**roséola** r̄ǫséɔla *roseola*
alrededor ɐlr̄ɛđəđǫ́ɹ *around*	**roncha** r̄ǫ̨ɲĉe *rash; welt*
honrado ǫnr̄áđɔ *honest*	**los ricos** lɔɹr̄íkɔs *the wealthy*
	reumatismo r̄eųmɐtízmɔ *rheumatism*

RR* is very strongly trilled. **RR** is one consonant and always occurs within a word. It has the exact same sound as the **R** which is initial. *RR* often affects the sound of the vowel preceding it. /r̄/

sarro	sár̄ɔ	*tartar of the teeth*	**gonorrea**	gonor̄ɛ́ɐ	*gonorrhea*
diarrea	djar̄ɛ́ɐ	*diarrhea*	**arruga**	ar̄úgɐ	*wrinkle*

Contrast the **r** and the **rr** in the following words. The proper pronunciation of the **r/rr** determines the meaning of the word.

caro	kárɔ	*expensive*	**carro**	kár̄ɔ	*car*	**pero**	péɹɔ	or *but*	**perro**	péɹ̄ɔ or peɹ̄ɔ	*dog*
cero	sérɔ/θérɔ	*zero*	**cerro**	séɹ̄ɔ/θéɹ̄ɔ	*hill*	**para**	páɹɐ	*in order to*	**parra**	páɹ̄ɐ	*vine*
coro	kórɔ or kóɹɔ	*choir/chorus*	**corro**	kóɹ̄ɔ	*circle of people*						

S has two pronunciations.

1. **S** is usually pronounced as *ESS* in English "dre**ss**." /s/

saliva	sạlíβɐ	*saliva*	**toser**	toséɹ	*to cough*	**sudor**	suɖóɹ	*sweat*

2. **S** before *B, D, G, L, M, N,* and *V* has the *Z* sound in English "toy**s**." [z]

asma	ázmɐ	*asthma*	**los dientes**	lọzɖjéṇtəs	*the teeth*	**desgana**	dezgánɐ	*loss of appetite*

T is similar to English, but the tip of the tongue must go directly behind the upper front teeth. There is no aspiration (puff of air) as in the English **T**. **T** is dental in Spanish, but alveolar in English; i.e., the tongue touches slightly above the gums. /t/

tijeras	tịxérɐs	*scissors*	**teléfono**	teléfɔno	*telephone*
asistente de hospital	asịsténtaɖeɔspɪtál	*orderly*			

NOTE: The sound the English *T* sometimes has when it occurs between vowels (wa**t**er, clu**tt**er) is the equivalent of Spanish *R*.

U sounds like the *U* in r**u**le, but without the off-glide. /u/

mujer	mụxéɹ	*woman*	**empujar**	empụxáɹ	*to push*
pulso	púlsɔ	*pulse*	**agudo**	agúɖɔ	*acute*

V* has the same sound as Spanish *B.* /b/ or [b̺]

vaginal	baxɪnál	*vaginal*	**verruga**	beɾ̄úgɐ	*wart*	**la vena**	labénɐ	*the vein*
vacunar	bakünáɹ	*to vaccinate*	**vena**	bénɐ	*vein*	**la vida**	labíɖɐ	*the life*

W occurs only in foreign, loan words and keeps the pronunciation of the original language. /w/

Wáshington	gwásɪŋton	*Washington*	**la wélfer**	lagwélfər	*welfare*	**sándwich**	sáŋwɪche	*sandwich*

X has two pronunciations.

1. Before a consonant, it is usually a hissing *S* as in "**s**it."* /s/

excelente	essəléṇtə/esθəléṇtə	*excellent*	**ambidextro**	ambɪɖéʂtrɔ	*ambidextrous*

   It is also possible to hear the *X* before a consonant pronounced as *KS* by those who wish either to be very careful or emphatic about their pronunciation.

2. Between vowels *X* is generally pronounced like the *X* in English "e**x**amine." [gs]

examen	ẹgsámən/ẹgsámēn	*examination*	**sexual**	sẹgswál	*sexual*	**tóxico**	tógsɪko	*toxic*

   This *X* may also be pronounced as the unvoiced English *KS* sound in "thin**ks**," although this is less common. Repeat the above words using this variation. The *X* of the Spanish words *extra* and *texto* should always be pronounced as fricative *s* or *ks*. It is considered uncultured to pronounce this *X* as an *S*.

extra	ẹgʂtrɐ/ékʂtrɐ	*extra*	**text**	tẹ́gstɔ/tékstɔ	*texto*

   In Mexico the words *México, mexicano, Texas, texano* and other words of Mexican origin are written with an *X*, but pronounced with Spanish *J*. (In Spain these words are written with a *J*.)

Y* has three pronunciations, in part because *Y* is considered both a **semiconsonant** and a **semivowel**. The way that Spanish *Y* is pronounced throughout the Hispanic world varies and no one way is more correct.

1. As a (semi)consonant it is generally pronounced like the *Y* in "**y**es." /y/

yo	yó	*I*	**yeyuno**	yeyúnɔ	*jejunum*	**yerno**	yérnɔ	*son-in-law*
yodo	yóɖɔ	*iodine*	**yeso**	yésɔ	*plaster*			

2. Consonantal *Y* is usually pronounced like the *J* in English "**j**udge" when it follows an *N*. [ŷ]

cónyuge	kọ́ŋ̂ŷuxə	*spouse*	**inyectar**	ịṇŷektáɹ	*to inject*
inyección	ịṇŷeksjón/ịṇŷegθjón	*injection*	**enyesado**	eṇŷəsáɖɔ	*plastering*

3. When it stands alone or after another vowel at the end of a word, *Y* is considered a **(semi)vowel** and is pronounced as the Spanish *I*. /i/

  y i *and*   **estoy** eṣtói̯ *I am*

Z is pronounced the same way as *C* before *E* or *I*. Thus, in Spanish America and in southern Spain it has the *S* sound of English "sit." In central and northern Spain *Z* has the *TH* of English "*th*ink." It is never a voiced sound like the *Z* in English "zoo."   /s/ or /θ/ Castilian

embarazada embaresáᵈɐ/embareθáᵈɐ *pregnant*   **izquierdo** iskjérdɔ/iθkjérdɔ *left*
zurdo súrdɔ/θúrdɔ *left-handed*

DIALECTAL VARIATIONS OF SPANISH

VARIANTES DIALECTALES DE ESPAÑOL

The Iberian Peninsula has four main languages: Castilian, Basque, Catalan, all spoken in Spain, and Portuguese, which is spoken in Portugal. Castilian is the only official language in Spain and is spoken by most people. The term "Spanish" is synonymous with Castilian. However, Castilian has many dialects. Andalusian (*andaluz*), one dialect, is spoken in southern Spain and is closely related to Spanish American Spanish.

As with English, all dialects of Spanish—whether peninsular or Spanish American—are mutually comprehensible, and no speaker of any dialect has any real trouble communicating with speakers of other dialects. Both English and Spanish have many dialectal variations in the pronunciation of some sounds (*phonemes*). A native of Boston, Massachusetts and a native of Atlanta, Georgia rarely sound alike, and neither sounds much like someone from San Antonio, Texas. So too, the Spanish spoken by a Puerto Rican sounds very different from that of a Cuban, and neither sounds much like someone from Mexico or Colombia. With few exceptions, most people can identify a person's place of origin because of certain characteristic features in his speech. Sometimes these features involve phonological differences (that is, differences in sounds such as "*heah*" for *here* or "*cah*" for *car* in English or the pronunciation of such Spanish words as *caza, llave, porque, cielo, perro, mujer,* and *yema*). (In Spanish there are fewer *pronunciation* differences among educated speakers from various parts of the Spanish-speaking world than there are among educated English-speakers from different parts of the United States. A physician from Buenos Aires sounds more like a physician from Mexico City or one from San Juan than he does like a cab driver from Buenos Aires. In the United States, however, a physician from Boston frequently sounds more like a Boston cabdriver than he does a physician from Seattle, at least as far as pronunciation goes.) Sometimes these features may involve lexical differences. This refers to what people call things (i.e., *lift* rather than *elevator, braces* rather than *suspenders*; the use of *guagua* in Cuba, *micro* in Chile, *colectivo* in Argentina, *autobús* in Colombia, *chiva* in Panamá, *camioneta* in Guatemala and El Salvador, and *camión* in Mexico for "*bus.*" Colombians use *saludes* ("healths") rather than *saludos* to send regards. They invite someone to have a cup of coffee, saying *¿Le provoca un tinto?* This same question to a Spaniard might mean, "Does red wine make you fight?") Grammatical differences are usually minor. Thus, any educated Spanish-speaker can easily be understood by any other educated Spanish-speaker. This is due both to unanimity of linguistic standards and to uniformity of education. Dialectal differences are great, however, among the uneducated masses.

In Spanish America the Spanish differs from that of Spain principally in vocabulary and pronunciation and is actually very close in pronunciation to the Spanish spoken in Andalucía/Andalusia, in southern Spain. There are two theories that account for this. One states that the Spanish of America and that of Spain evolved concurrently in similar ways during approximately the same time in history and are therefore quite close today. The other theory is that the majority of the Spanish *conquistadores* and settlers came from southern Spain and obviously brought with them their speech. Evidence indicates that geography has helped to maintain these speech patterns. For the 300 years between 1500, the discovery of the Americas, and 1800, the end of colonization, accessibility to the changes that were occurring in southern Spain seems to have been the main factor in the development of dialectal differences. Thus, the areas of Spanish America which were easily accessible to the Spaniards during the colonial period have been influenced more linguistically than the areas which were landlocked or mountainous. The remote areas of Spanish America did not deviate from the original Spanish spoken at the time of colonization. Areas easily accessible to travelers became influenced linguistically by the changes occurring in Andalusian Castilian. As language evolved in Andalusia, the area from which records indicate nearly all early expeditions originated, the changes reached the accessible regions in America. The development of the interdental /θ/ from an [s] was firmly established in Spain long after the initial colonization of Spanish America and was the norm by 1700. Therefore, it did not affect the Spanish of America. Other factors that also influenced speech patterns were Native American languages, migration from other colonies during the colonial periods, social mobility, and ruralism versus urbanism.

There are now many dialectal variations of the Spanish spoken in America and many subdialects as well. Several scholars have suggested six general dialect areas.[3] Geographically from north to south they are: Southwestern United States (primarily Arizona and New Mexico) and Mexico; Central America (southern Mexico and the Yucatan Peninsula, Guatemala, Honduras, El Salvador, Nicaragua, and Costa Rica); Caribbean (Puerto Rica [and the Puerto Ricans in New York], the Dominican Republic, Cuba [and the Cubans in Florida], Panama, and the northern coast of Colombia and Venezuela); Highlands (the interior of Venezuela, most of Colombia, Ecuador, Peru, and Bolivia); Chile; Southern (Argentina, Uruguay, and Paraguay).

The grammatical aspects of most speakers of Spanish American Spanish is fairly uniform. As with the Spanish of Spain, the principal differences are in vocabulary and pronunciation. The most acceptable dialect of Spanish throughout Spanish America is apparently that spoken in Central America (southern Mexico, the Yucatan Peninsula, Guatemala, Honduras, El Salvador, Nicaragua, Costa Rica) and the Highlands (the interior of Venezuela, Ecuador, most of Colombia, Peru, and Bolivia).[4] The average speaker of a language is perceptive to dialectal variations, and, regardless of how well or poorly educated he or she is and how much linguistic knowledge he or she may have, has certain opinions about different geographical dialects.

Any educated Spanish-speaker can easily understand and be understood by any other educated Spanish-speaker regardless of country of origin. Furthermore, Spanish-speakers are practically forced to use the speech traditions of the community in which they live. Thus, although numerous settlers came to America from northern Spain between 1700 and 1900, they adapted to the American speech pattern of southern Spanish origin through social coercion. In addition, parts of Spanish America were simultaneously settled by Spanish explorers who brought language and culture at the same stages of development to regions far apart. For example, Bolivians use vowel reduction in the unstressed syllable, a speech pattern that is considered typically Mexican, but is also common in highland Ecuador.

As with all languages, Spanish speech is affected by age, sex, social class, profession, education, urban versus rural setting as well as many other factors. Linguists frequently refer to such variations within the area pattern as "attitudinal." Nevertheless, often what is an attitudinal trait in one area may be a general characteristic in another. For example, in the Caribbean the careful articulation of /s/ when it is final in a syllable is considered at best affected and more often effeminate when practiced by men; yet it is the norm in highland Spanish America.

VOWELS *VOCALES*

A In central Mexico and parts of Ecuador, words with an unstressed *A* at the end are occasionally quite relaxed, almost to the *UH* sound in rapid conversation.

E In the Caribbean region Spanish-speakers frequently use the pronunciation of the English *E* as in "b*e*t," even when no other letter follows it in the syllable.

I Has no important dialectal variations.

O In parts of Cuba, Mexico, and Colombia a final unstressed *O* is pronounced as the *U* in English "r*u*le." This usually does not cause confusion.

mucho → muchu

U Has no important dialectal variations.

CONSONANTS *CONSONANTES*

B, V In most of Colombia, El Salvador, Honduras, Nicaragua, and intermittently in the Caribbean and in the Andes these are occlusives after a semivowel or after any consonant.

barba bárbɐ > bárbɐ *chin*   **las vidas** lazbídɐs > lazbídɐs *lives*

BUE, VUE   Many Mexicans and also many uneducated or rural Spanish-speakers will use dialectal variations of **GUE** for **BUE** and **VUE**. This is considered substandard Spanish and is indicated orthographically by the use of **GÜ**:

vuelvo → güelvo   bwélbɔ → gwélbɔ   *I am returning*
abuelo → agüelo   abwélɔ → agwélɔ   *grandfather*
bueno → güeno   bwénɔ → gwénɔ/wénɔ   *okay*

C   In all dialects of Spanish the hard **C** sound at the end of a syllable or at the end of a foreign word is often eliminated when it occurs in rapid speech. This is especially true of Cuban speakers.

coñac   koņák → koņá   *cognac*
doctor → **dotor**   dɔktóɹ → dɔtóɹ   *doctor*
Nueva York → **Nueva Yor**   nwébɐ yórk → nwébɐ yóɹ   *New York*

The final hard **C** in a syllable generally tends to voice to /g/:

doctor → **dogtor**   dɔktóɹ → dɔgtóɹ   *doctor*
técnico → **tégnico**   tékniko → tégniko → tégniko   *technician*

CH   In Cuba, the Dominican Republic, the cities of northern Chile, and Panama a variation of this sound (similar to English "*sh*ell") is freely used in which the tongue assumes almost the same position as for the *CH*, except that the front of the tongue never touches the front palate.   [š]

pecho → péšɔ   *chest*   **chato** → šátɔ   *flat-nosed*   **mucho** → múšo   *much*

In Puerto Rico and on the Colombian coast this sound is often   [ťj].

pecho → péťjɔ   *chest*   **chato** → ťjátɔ   *flat-nosed*   **mucho** → múťjo   *much*

D   Sometimes the intervocalic **D** completely disappears in all dialects of Spanish. This is particularly common for Mexicans and Puerto Ricans.

operado → **operao**   opəráᵈɔ → opəráɔ → opəráɔ → opəráŭ   *operated*

In Colombia other than in Nariño, in El Salvador, Honduras, Nicaragua, and in the Caribbean where -/l/, -/r/ and even -/s/ sound the same, [d] is usual after another consonant or semivowel.

rey de Cuba   r̄ej de kúba   *king of Cuba*   **pardo**   párdo   *dull*

Cubans and Puerto Ricans especially, but even educated Spanish-speakers, will frequently drop it in words ending in -*ado*.

It is usually eliminated when occurring at the end of a word. Mexicans almost always do this and Puerto Ricans eliminate the final d quite frequently. This is also practiced in Guatemala, Ecuador, Peru, and Bolivia, and in Nariño, Colombia.

Madrid → **Madri**   maðríđ → maðríᵈ → maðrí   *Madrid*   **usted** → **uste**   ųstęđ → ųstę̣ᵈ → ųsté   *you (formal, sg)*

The omission of this **D** in any other combination is considered substandard:

nada → **naa** or **na**   náðɐ → náɐ → ná   *nothing*

F   In many parts of Spanish America a rural variant of the *F* sound exists, particularly, after the *M* sound and before the diphthong *UE*. This free variation is a softened *P*:

enfermo → **epermo**   eɱférmɔ → epérmɔ   *ill*   **fuerte** → **puerte**   fwértə → pwértə   *strong*

For many Mexicans when followed by *U* this letter sounds like the English *H*:

fuerte → **huerte**   fwér-te → ẋwér-te   *strong*   **fuera** → **huera**   fwéra → xwéra   *outside*

G   This sometimes disappears at the end of a syllable. In Mexico it is very common to lose the **G** sound in the *GN* combination.

indigno → **indino**   iņdígnɔ → iņdínɔ   *unworthy*

GU   In the speech of uneducated or rural speakers **BU** may be substituted for **GU**. This is considered substandard Spanish.

aguja → **abuja**   agúxa → abúxa   *needle*

GUA   In some dialects of Spanish, but especially in Mexico, this combination sounds like the English *WA*.

agua → **awa**   áwa → áwa   *water*
guagua → **guawa/wawa**   gwágwa → gwáwa wáwa   *bus/baby*

/G/   In most of Colombia, in El Salvador, Honduras, and Nicaragua, this consonant is pronounced as a hard or occlusive after any consonant or semivowel.

la guerra lagéřa *war*
hay guerra aɪgéřa *there is a war*

Many uneducated or rural Spanish-speakers will use dialectal variations of *GU* for *BU*. This is considered substandard Spanish and is indicated orthographically by the use of *GÜ*:

abuela → **agüela** aƀwélɐ → agwélɐ *grandmother*
buenos días → **güenos días** bwénoẓ ðíɐs → gwénoẓ ðíɐs *good morning, good day, hello*

HU   Many educated speakers will pronounce words with these letters as though they were spelled *GU* or *GÜ* or even *BU*:

hueso → **güeso** or **bueso** wésɔ → gwésɔ or ƀwésɔ *bone*   **huele bien** wélebɪɛn → gwélebɪɛn *It smells good.*
un hueso úŋwésɔ → úŋgwésɔ / úmbwésɔ *A bone*   **ahuecar** awekáɪ → agwekáɪ / aƀwekáɪ *to hollow out*

The uneducated speakers make these same sounds stops, instead of fricatives, especially before nasals:

huevo gwéƀɔ → bwéƀɔ *an egg*   **un hueso** úŋ gwésɔ / úm bwésɔ *a bone*

J   In El Salvador this consonant is a weak [h] and tends to drop between vowels especially when the vowel before it is emphasized or stressed.

Méjico méxɪko → méiko *Mexico*

The pronunciation of *J* as [h] rather than [x] is also observed in Guatemala, although in careful speech the sound becomes a voiced palatal fricative.

oreja oréxɐ → ore̞hɐ *ear*

/X/   In southern Spain, the Caribbean, Central America, Panama, and Venezuela, *J*, *GE*, and *GI* are pronounced [h].

girar hirár *to rotate*   **jugar** hugár *to play*

/K/   In Central America, Colombia, Venezuela, and here and there in the Caribbean /K/ is substituted for /P/ in *combinaciones cultas*.

contracepción kontraseksjón *contraception*   **septiembre** sektjémbre *September*

In Nicaragua and El Salvador there is a tendency to use /k/ for /pt/, /bs/, and /ps/.

concepción konseksjón *conception*   **absoluto** aksolúto *absolute*   **acepto** asékto *accept*

L   When *L* occurs at the end of a syllable, it is often replaced by *R* by many uneducated Spanish-speakers in the Caribbean, along the coasts of Colombia and Ecuador, in Puerto Rico, the Dominican Republic, Venezuela, rural Panama and parts of Chile.

papel → paper papél → papéɪ *paper*   **bolsillo** → **borsillo** bolsíyɔ → boɪsıyɔ *pocket*
falta → farta fáltɐ → fáɪtɐ *a lack*

LL   In Uruguay, Argentina, and neighboring countries, *LL* sometimes sounds like *S* in pleasure [ž] and sometimes like *J* in judge [ŷ]. In these countries the consonant *Y* has the *LL* pronunciation.

calle kážə *street*   **hallo** ážɔ/áŷɔ *I find*

In the Río de la Plata region the *LL* is pronounced like *S* in English "pleasure."

calle káʝə → kážə *street*

In Puerto Rico the *LL* sounds like the English *J*.

llegar → **jegar** ʝegár → ŷegár / ĵegár *to arrive*

With the exception of Panama, in all Central American countries intervocalic /ɣ/ is so weak that it usually either disappears or weakens to a semivowel.

silla → sia síʝɐ → síɐ *chair*

N   In Cuba the *N* at the end of a word assumes a nasal quality similar to the *NG* in English "ri*ng*ing" before a pause or a vowel. This is also true in southeastern Mexico, all of Central America, the Dominican Republic, coastal Colombia and Ecuador, most of Venezuela, and the highlands of Ecuador, Peru, and Bolivia. In Panama and Puerto Rico this also occurs but the vowel is nasalized even more sharply.

bien → bieng bjén → bɪɛŋ *well*
ponen → poneng pónən → pónəŋ *they put/give*

But compare: **en aguas**   eɲágwas   in waters with **enaguas**   enágwas   *petticoat*

NS   In the syllables *CONS*, *INS*, and *TRANS*, the *N* is often nasalized or lost in semieducated and uneducated speech.

   constipado   kǫnʂtipáɗɔ → kǫⁿʂtɪpáɗɔ → kõʂtɪ páɗɔ → kǫʂtipáɔ   *head cold*
   transformar   transfǫrmár → traⁿsfǫrmár → trãsfǫrmár → trasfǫrmáɹ   *to transform*

PC   The *P* in the *PC* group of certain learned words is often lost; in ordinary conversation the *P* is often modified to *B*.

   suscripción   sụskrɪpsjón/sụskrɪpθɹón → sụskrɪsjón/sụskrɪθɹón   *subscription*
   concepción   kǫnsępsjón/kǫnθępθɹón → kǫnsębsjón/kǫnθębθɹón   *conception*

PS   In uneducated speech the *P* is suppressed when the *PS* occurs within a word.

   cápsula   kápsüla → káụsüla   *capsule*   **autopsia**   aụtópsja → aụtósja   *autopsy*

In Cuba, Central America, Colombia, and Venezuela *PS* is pronounced *KS*:

   pepsi cola   péksikóle   *Pepsi Cola*

PT is pronounced *KT* and vice versa:

   apto   áptɔ → áktɔ   *apt*

R   Many Spanish-speaking people, even educated speakers, in the Caribbean, the coastal region of Colombia, and parts of Chile, will replace syllables ending with *R* with an *L*.

   carne → calne   kárnə → kálnə   *meat*   **puerta → puelta**   pwérta → pwélta   *port*
   enfermo → enfelmo   ęɱférmɔ → ęɱfélmɔ   *ill*   **izquierdo → izquieldo**   iskjérɗɔ → ihkjéldɔ   *left*
   porque está enfermo   porkęhtáęɱférmɔ → polkęhtáęɱfélmo   *because he is sick*

This is most common in Puerto Rico, and also the northeastern United States.

In Mexico the tendency is to *often* replace the spoken *R* before a consonant or at the end of a word with the sound of *L*.

   hablar → hablal   aƀláɹ→ aƀlál   *to speak*   **pardo → paldo**   párɗɔ→ páḷdɔ   *dull*

In Puerto Rico the *R* is pronounced like an *L* when it precedes a consonant or when it is at the end of a word:

   verdad → veldá   bęrɗáɑ → bęḷdá   *right*   **por favor → pol favol**   pǫr faƀáɹ → pǫl faƀól   *please*

Frequently Puerto Ricans pronounce initial *R* like English *SHR*:

   Puerto Rico → Puelto Shrico   pwértɔríkɔ→ pwéltɔ šríkɔ   *Puerto Rico*

The sound of Spanish *R* is similar to the English *D* or *T* sounds of mu*dd*y, bu*dd*y, butt*er*, or wat*er*. This frequently causes confusion in hearing and speaking for English-speakers of Spanish:

   cata cada cara   **moto modo moro**

The syllable final *R* and the *RR* are strongly assimilated in Guatemala, Costa Rica, Bolivia, Chile, Paraguay and parts of Colombia, Ecuador, and Argentina: [ř][řř]

   mujer   mụxéř   *woman*

RR   Spanish-speakers in Cuba, Puerto Rico, the Dominican Republic, Panama, and coastal Colombia pronounce the *RR* so that the tongue strikes either the uvula or the velum. It resembles the **Jota** of Spain ([x]). This type of sound exists in French (*rouge*) and German (*rot*).

S   The Spanish spoken in Cuba, Puerto Rico, the Dominican Republic, and the coastal regions of Chile, Argentina, and Uruguay substitutes an aspirated *H* sound for both voiced and unvoiced *S*. This pronunciation is common among educated speakers, especially in rapid conversation:

   los codos   loʰ kóɗɔs   *the elbows*   **los chicos**   loʰ ĉíkɔs   *the children*
   esperar   ęʰperáɹ   *to wait*   **Los he visto**   loʰé bíhtɔ   *I have seen them.*
   espero   ęʰpérɔ   *I am waiting*   **¿Quieres más?**   kjéręhmáh   *Do you want more?*

In Costa Rica and Colombia the *S* is often voiced in the middle or at the end of a word, even between vowels:

   presente   prezę́ntə   *present*   **los hijos**   lozíhɔs   *the children*

The lower economic classes in Cuba and the Dominican Republic tend to drop the syllable final /*S*/.

   los dos → lo dó   lǫzdós→ lo ɗó   *the two*

In Ecuador the /s/ is pronounced as a dental [z] when it occurs at the end of a word which precedes a word beginning with a vowel:

más alto   má ẓáltɔ   *higher/louder*   **los animales**   loẓanimáləs   *the animals*

S is pronounced *R* among the uneducated:

exceso   essésɔ /eʂθésɔ → ɛɹsésɔ / ɛɹθésɔ   *excess*   **los dientes**   loẓ đjéɲtes → loɹ đjéɲtəs   *the teeth*

In southern Spain *S* before a voiced consonant drops out, and the voiced consonant becomes unvoiced, shown phonetically by the small circle under the consonant:

mismo   mízmɔ → mímm̥ɔ   *self*   **las botas**   laz bótɐs → laḇóte   *boots*

In Puerto Rico *S* is eliminated when it precedes a consonant.

respirar → repiral   r̄espíráɹ → r̄epˌɪrál   *to breathe*

Often Puerto Ricans eliminate the *S* at the end of a word:

ojos azules → ojo azule   óxɔs asúləs → óxɔ asúlə   *blue eyes*

Frequently Puerto Ricans eliminate the entire syllable containing the *S*.

está → tá   eʂtá → tá   *it is*

V   The occasional use of the *V* sound is not a matter of dialect. Rather, it is a hypercorrection. The *V* sound has never been used consistently in modern Spanish and is best avoided.

X   In Cuba, Puerto Rico, the Dominican Republic, Venezuela, and parts of Argentina and Uruguay, *X* before a consonant has an aspirated *H* sound:

extracción → ehtracción   ekstraksɹón → eʰtraksɹón   *extraction*   **extraño**   eʂtráɲɔ → eʰtráɲɔ   *strange*

In a few words where x is between vowels, many Spanish-speakers use only [s]:

auxilio   au̯sílɹɔ   *help*   **exacto**   esáktɔ   *exact*   **auxiliar**   au̯silɹáɹ   *assistant*

Puerto Ricans often eliminate syllables within words or phrases as well as final syllables of words:

para atrás — > patrá   pára_atráz > patrá   *backwards*
para adelante — > palante   pára ađeláɲtɐ > paláɲtə   *forwards*
nada > na   náđɐ > ná   *nothing*

Y   In eastern Argentina, Uruguay, and central Colombia, *Y* is pronounced like the *S* in English "pleasure."   [ž]

ayer   ayéɹ → ažéɹ   *yesterday*   **mayo**   máyɔ → mážɔ   *May*

In conclusion, dialects tend to be given perhaps too much importance, especially by language students. There is no "best" dialect of Spanish for an English-speaker to learn. The Spanish spoken primarily in southern Mexico, the Yucatan Peninsula, Guatemala, Honduras, El Salvador, Nicaragua, Costa Rica, Ecuador, Bolivia, Peru, most of Colombia, and the interior of Venezuela seems to have the greatest acceptability throughout the Spanish-speaking world of this hemisphere. Nonetheless, any educated speaker of Spanish will have no difficulty being understood by any other educated Spanish-speaker anywhere in the world.

DIPHTHONGS

DIPTONGOS

The vowels are divided into two groups: strong vowels—A, E, O; weak vowels—U, I (Y).

A diphthong is two vowels forming a single syllable. Spanish vowels retain their basic sound when they form part of a diphthong, but they are pronounced more rapidly in succession with a glide and form one syllable. In Spanish a diphthong consists of a strong and a weak vowel, a weak and a strong vowel, or two weak vowels in one syllable.

AU   about like "ow" in "cow." [au̯]

causa   káu̯sɐ   *cause*   **autismo**   au̯tízmɔ   *autism*

UA   about like "wa" in "waffle." [wa]

juanete   xwanétə   *bunion*   **sublingual**   su̯blïŋgwál   *sublingual*
lengua   léŋgwɐ   *tongue*   **su ave**   swáḇe   *his bird*

AI or *AY*   about like "ai" in "aisle," or "y" in "rye."   [aį]

hay áį *there is, there are*   **suprainguinal** supraįŋgınál *suprainguinal*   **aire** áį-r *air*
airoso aįrósɔ *airy*   **ahijado** aįxáɗɔ *godson*

IA   about like "ya" in "yard."   [ja]

arteria artérje *artery*   **tenia** ténje *tapeworm*

EU   an "e" plus "u" *sound.*   [eų]

neurótico neųrótıkɔ *neurotic*   **neurosis** neųrósis *neurosis*
terapéutico terɐpéųtıko *therapeutic*   **leucorrea** leųkọréɐ *leukorrhea*

UE   about like "we" in "wet."   [we]

hueso wésɔ *bone*   **cuerpo** kwérpɔ *body*

EI or *EY*   about like "ei" in "eight" or "ey" in "they."   [eį]

aceite aséįtə/aθéįtə *oil*   **ley** léį *law*   **me imagino** meįmaxínɔ *I imagine.*

IE   about like "ye" in "yes."   [je]

diente djéņtə **tooth**   **tienta** tjéņtɐ *surgical probe*

OI or *OY*   about like the "oy" in "toy."   [ọį]

hoy ọį *today*   **sigmoidoscopio** sigmọįɗɔskópjɔ *sigmoidoscope*

IO   about like "yo" in "yoke."   [jo]

ovario oɓárjɔ *ovary*   **labio** láɓjɔ *lip*   **ilion** í-ljɔn *ilium*   **fisiólogo** fisjólɔgo *physiology*

UO   about like "wo" in "woke" or "uo" in quota   [wo]

duodeno dwoɗénɔ *duodenum*   **sinuoso** sinwósɔ *sinuous*
cuota kwótɐ *payment*   **mutuo** mútwɔ *mutual*

IU   about like "ew" in "chew."   [ju]

diurético djurétıko *diuretic*   **diurno** djúrnɔ *diurnal*

UI or *UY*   like "we."   [wi]

muy mwí *very*   **cuidado** kwiɗáɗɔ *care*

The stress on a diphthong is always on the strong vowel, or on the second of two weak ones.
   The combinations *QUE, QUI, GUE,* or *GUI* are *not* diphthongs: the *U* is silent.

sanguíneo saŋgíneo *blood* (adj)   **inquirir** įŋkırírı *to inquire into*   **aquí** akí *here*
llegué yegé/ʎegé *I arrived*   **querer** kerɛ́ɾı *to want*

Note that an "h" between vowels has no effect on the diphthong combinations or vowels which interact as if they were next to each other.

ahora aọ́ra *now*   **incoherente** įŋkoeréņtə *incoherent*

Two strong vowels never form a diphthong:

íleon íləɔn *ileum*   **coágulo** kɔágulo *clot*   **cráneo** kránəo *skull*

When the weak vowel in a strong and weak vowel combination or when the first vowel of two weak vowels is stressed, a written accent on the weak vowel breaks up the diphthong:

frío frí́ɔ *cold*   **cocaína** kokaínɐ *cocaine*   **había** aɓíɐ *there were/was*

TRIPHTHONGS

TRIPTONGOS

A Spanish triphthong is a combination of three vowels in the same syllable: a weak, a strong, and a weak vowel. The first vowel in this combination functions as a semiconsonant; the last, as a semivowel. The stress falls on the strong vowel. Since the second person plural verb conjugation is not used regularly any more, the number of words which have triphthongs are few. There are only four "true" triphthong combinations in Spanish which can be found within a word: **iei/iey, iai/iay, uei/uey,** and **uai/uay.** Nevertheless, because speakers of Spanish link words together, "pseudo-" triphthongs are common and expand the number of combinations to twelve.

iei/iey Like the English word *yea*.   [jei̯]

    limpiéis lim̦pjéi̯s *that you may clean*   **estudie historia** eștúdjei̯stórja *study history*

ieu [jeu̯]

    estudie usted estúdjeu̯sté̦d *study*

iai/iay Like the *yi* in *yipe*.   [jai̯]

    estudia historia eștúdjəi̯stórja *He studies history*

iau Like "yow" [jau̯]

    Miau Mjau̯ *Meow*

ioi Like "yoe-e" [joi̯]

    Estudió histología eștudjói̯stolɔxíɐ *She studied histology*

iou Like "ē-ow." [jou̯]

    Estudió urología eștudjóu̯rolɔxíɐ *You studied urology*

uei/uey Like *wa* in *wade*.   [wei̯]

    buey bwéi̯ *steer*

ueu Like "way-oo" [weu̯]

    Fue humano fwéu̯mánɔ *It was humane*

uai/uay Like *wi* in *wine*.   [wai̯]

    Paraguay Paragwái̯ *Paraguay*

uau Like "wow" [wau̯]

    Antigua uña an̦tígwau̯ɲɐ *Old fashioned nail*

uoi/uoy [woi̯]

    antiguo y débil an̦tígwoi̯débil *old and weak*

iou [wou̯]

    Antiguo uniforme an̦tígwou̯nifórme *Old fashioned uniform*

A combination of a weak, a strong, and a weak vowel that has a written accent mark on the first weak vowel breaks down into a vowel plus a diphthong: **viviríais** biþi̯ríai̯s *You would live*

When dividing a word into syllables, diphthongs and triphthongs are considered a single vowel and are **NEVER** separated.

REMARKS CONCERNING THE FORMATION OF SOME SPANISH WORDS AND THEIR CORRESPONDING ENGLISH EQUIVALENTS

CORRESPONDENCIA DE PALABRAS

The Spanish ending *ción* corresponds to the English *tion*.

    esterilización sterilization   **obfuscación** obfuscation   **recuperación** recuperation

The Spanish endings *dad* and *tad* correspond to the English *ty*.

    dificultad difficulty   **sexualidad** sexuality   **mortalidad** mortality

The Spanish endings *dad* and *tad* may also correspond to the English *ness*.

    enfermedad illness

The Spanish endings *cia* and *cio* correspond to the English *ce*.

    servicio service   **edificio** edifice   **impotencia** impotence

The Spanish ending *cia* may also correspond to the English *tia*.

    exodoncia exodontia   **demencia** dementia   **ortodoncia** orthodontia

The Spanish endings *ia* and *io* correspond to the English *y*.

    directorio directory   **laboratorio** laboratory   **familia** family

The Spanish ending *ía* also corresponds to the English *y*.

    disentería dysentery   **histerectomía** hysterectomy   **vasectomía** vasectomy

The Spanish ending *oso* (*osa* in the feminine) corresponds to the English *ous*.

cauteloso (cautelosa)   cautious   **nervioso (nerviosa)**   nervous   **generoso (generosa)**   generous

The Spanish ending *ico* (*ica* in the feminine) corresponds to the English *ical* or *ic*.

biológico (biológica)   biological   **físico (física)**   physical   **púbico**   pubic   **música**   music

The Spanish ending *itis* corresponds to the English *itis*.

mastitis   mastitis   **laringitis**   laryngitis

The Spanish ending *scopio* corresponds to the English *scope*.

microscopio   microscope   **estetoscopio**   stethoscope

The Spanish ending *ólogo* (*óloga* in the feminine) corresponds to the English *gist*.

patólogo (patóloga)   pathologist   **oftalmólogo**   ophthalmologist   **neurólogo**   neurologist

The Spanish ending *'tico* (*'tica* in the feminine) corresponds to the English *otic*.

narcótico   narcotic   **neurótico (neurótica)**   neurotic

The Spanish ending *logía* corresponds to the English *logy*.

serología   serology   **biología**   biology

The Spanish ending *ómetro* corresponds to the English *ometer*.

termómetro   thermometer   **esfigmomanómetro**   sphygmomanometer

English words that have **mm** are spelled in Spanish with an **nm**.

la conmoción   commotion

English words that end in *ist* end in *ista* in Spanish and are both masculine and feminine.

dentista   dentist   **especialista**   specialist

Many English words that begin with *s* and a consonant, insert *e* before the *s* for the corresponding Spanish word.

esfigmomanómetro   sphygmomanometer   **escroto**   scrotum   **esquizofrénico**   schizophrenic

English words that have the *ph* sound are spelled in Spanish with an *f*.

físico   physical   **fósforo**   phosphorus   **flebitis**   phlebitis

The **th** of many English words becomes **t** in their Spanish equivalents.

la catedral   cathedral

The English -**que** or **qua**- is often expressed with **cue, ca** or **cua** in Spanish.

frecuente   frequent   **la calidad/la cualidad**   quality   **cuarto**   quarter

The English vowel *y* is replaced in Spanish by the *i*.

esfigmomanómetro   sphygmomanometer   **hímen**   hymen

Many English words ending in silent *e*, drop the *e* and add *o* or *a* in Spanish.

medicina   medicine   **caso**   case   **intenso (intensa)**   intense   **dentífrico**   dentifrice

Many English words that end in a consonant add *o, a,* or *e* in Spanish.

accidente   accident   **mucho**   much   **víctima**   victim

The endings *ar, er,* and *ir* are added to some English infinitives that end in a consonant to form the corresponding verbs in Spanish.

permitir   permit   **comprender**   comprehend   **inyectar**   inject

Many English infinitives ending in silent *e*, drop the *e* and add *ar* or *ir* to form the Spanish equivalent.

terminar   terminate   **revivir**   revive   **cauterizar**   cauterize

ACCENTUATION

ACENTUACION

Stress is the prominence given to certain syllables: *HOS-pi-tal.* Spanish has only two degrees of stress—strong and weak:

docTOR   weak + strong   **enFERmo**   weak + strong + weak

In English, stress is occasionally used to differentiate between words:

    wind (n)   wind (v)   object (n)   object (v)   live (adj)   live (v)

In Spanish the same use of stress occurs:

pracTIco	(I practice)	**conTInuo**	(prolonged, continuous)
practiCÓ	(he practiced)	**contiNÚo**	(I continue.)
PRÁctico	(practical, medical practitioner)	**contiNUÓ**	(he continued)
LIbro	(book)	**liBRÓ**	(She expelled the placenta.)

Spanish words do not usually bear a written accent ('). Rules for determining the stressed syllable are clear:

1. Words ending in a vowel, an *-N*, or *-S*, stress the next to the last syllable:

    a-ci-DO-sis acidosis   **BUS-can** they are looking for   **me-di-CI-na** medicine

2. Words ending in a consonant other than *-N* or *-S*, are stressed on the last syllable:

    pe-OR worst   **es-pa-ÑOL** Spanish

    NOTE: Final *Y*, although pronounced as a vowel, is considered a consonant for the purpose of written accentuation.

3. Words that do not follow rules 1 and 2 must have a written accent mark (') on the syllable stressed.

    Á-ci-do acid   **ac-NÉ** acne   **MÉ-du-la** marrow   **tam-PÓN** tampon   **MÉ-di-co** physician

    NOTE: Spanish has only one written accent, which always indicates that the syllable bearing it is *stressed*.

- Interrogative words are always accented:

    ¿qué? what?   **¿cuánto?** how much?   **¿cuándo?** when?

- A written accent differentiates similarly spelled words, usually monosyllabic, with different meanings:

él	he	**el**	the	**sí**	yes	**si**	if
dé	give (command)	**de**	of, from	**solo**	alone *adj*	**sólo**	only (adv)
se	himself, etc.	**sé**	I know				

The accent mark may be omitted over capital letters: **PRONUNCIACION DE CONVERSACION MEDICA.**

DIVISION OF WORDS INTO SYLLABLES

SEPARACION POR SILABAS

Spanish words are syllabified according to simple but rigid rules:

1. A word has as many syllables as it has vowels, diphthongs, and triphthongs.
2. A single consonant, including *CH, LL, RR*, goes with the following vowel:

    sa-rro tartar   **ni-ño** little boy   **mu-cha-cha** girl   **ma-no** hand

3. Two consonants are usually separated:

    som-no-len-cia sleepiness   **a-del-ga-zar** to lose weight   **bar-bi-lla** chin

    (*a*) A combination of a consonant and an *L* or an *R* (which can begin a word in English) goes with the following vowel in Spanish:

        re-tra-í-do withdrawn   **pla-no** plain   **sa-cro** sacrum   **a-fli-gi-do** suffering

    (*c*) There is one expression: *-S* plus a consonant. Since this combination cannot begin a syllable, the *-S* goes with the preceding syllable:

        as-cen-sor elevator   **es-to-ca-da** stab

4. Three consonants are usually divided after the first one, unless the second is an *S*:

in-gle groin	**abs-ten-ción** withdrawal	**ins-tan-te** instant
tem-blar to tremble	**hom-bre** man	**trans-por-te** transport

5. Four consonants between vowels are a very rare Spanish combination. They are always divided after the second:

    obs-truc-ción blockage   **trans-plan-te** transplant   **re-cons-truc-ti-vo** reconstructive

DICTATION   DICTADO

In pairs ask each other to spell the following words. The person who is writing should have the book closed. Each person should spell five words:

1. especialista	4. accidente	7. diagnóstico	9. nitroglicerina
2. urgencia	5. físico	8. alcohol	10. mejilla
3. horrible	6. deshidratación		

PRACTICE   *PRACTICA*

Pronounce each word aloud and indicate which syllable (vowel) is stressed:

1.	medicamento	4.	palillo	7.	epilepsia	9.	quimioterapia
2.	inmediatamente	5	agua	8.	período	10.	diabetes
3.	colesterol	6.	indigestión				

Say each word, then say how it is spelled using spanish pronunciation for the names of the letters.

1.	torniquete	3.	historial	5.	jeringa	7.	antibiótico
2.	enfermera	4.	sangre	6.	muestra	8.	farmacia

Indicate the correct number of syllables in each word. It may help to divide the words into syllables first.

1.	epilepsia	4.	muñeca	7.	agarra	9.	conduzca
2.	asma	5.	cierre	8.	farmacéutico	10.	neumonía
3.	obesidad	6.	examinar				

Rewrite the following words. Divide them into syllables and indicate the stressed syllable.

therapist **terapeuta** _____	diaphragm **diafragma** _____
to rinse **enjuagar** _____	enema **lavativa** _____
vulva **vulva** _____	dressing **vendaje** _____
umbilicus **ombligo** _____	drainage **drenaje** _____
jaw **mandíbula** _____	crutch **muleta** _____
mirror **espejo** _____	infarct **infarto** _____
chemistry **química** _____	hoarseness **carraspera** _____
shoulder **hombro** _____	lump **borujo** _____
anatomic **anatómico** _____	measles **sarampión** _____
red-haired **pelirrojo** _____	nit **liendre** _____
X-ray therapy **radioterapia** _____	tongue **lengua** _____
ammonia **amoníaco** _____	German measles **rubéola** _____
vaccination **inoculación** _____	

PRONUNCIATION PRACTICE   *PRACTICA DE LA PRONUNCIACION*

Contrast the two sounds.

Practice the contrasting *b* sounds.

		/b/	/b̶/
vagina	the vagina	**vagina**	la **v**agina
beard	the beard	**barba**	la **barb**a
mouth	the mouth	**boca**	la **b**oca
I drink	I drink	**bebo**	yo **bebo**
he came	he came	**vino**	él **v**ino
bladder	the bladder	**vejiga**	la **v**ejiga

Practice the contrasting *d* sounds.

		/d/	/đ/
finger	my finger	**dedo**	mi **dedo**
weakness	the weakness	**debilidad**	la **debilidad**
pain	a little pain	**dolor**	poco **dolor**
doubt	the doubt	**duda**	la **duda**

Practice the contrasting *g* sounds.

		(g)	/g/
it pleases	I like	**gusta**	me **gusta**
drop	a drop	**gota**	una **gota**
expenses	your expenses	**gastos**	sus **gastos**

Practice the contrasting *r* sounds.

		/r̄/	/r/
knee	the knee	**rodilla**	la **rodilla**
cold		**resfriado**	
diarrhea		**diarrea**	
	uterus		**útero**

radius	my radius	radio	mi radio
	urethra		uretra
rectum	his rectum	recto	su recto
	relative		pariente
kidney	another kidney	riñón	etro riñón
	ear		oreja
gonorrhea		gonorrea	
	nose		nariz

READING EXERCISE *EJERCICIO DE LECTURA*

Read the following aloud for pronunciation practice.

Un doctor me dijo que no podía quedarme en este lugar y que tendría que dormir más, hacer más ejercicios y comer menos.

—Pero, doctor, ¿adónde iré para vivir de este modo? No puedo dormir tanto si me despiertan temprano todos los días. Y no me gusta divertirme con deportes.

El perro de San Roque no tiene rabo porque Ramón Ramírez se lo ha cortado.

LINKING

ENCADENAMIENTO

In spoken Spanish words are uttered in breath groups rather than in isolation. This is one reason that Spanish seems to be spoken very rapidly. This combining is called **linking**. Sometimes the final vowel of one word is pronounced with the initial vowel of the next word. It is important to try to link words together when speaking Spanish.

Opero a las siete.   I operate at 7 o'clock.

If both vowels in this case are identical or if two identical vowels occur within a word, they are pronounced slightly longer than one vowel would be.

Beba ahora.   *Be-ba-ho-ra.*   Drink now.

Often a diphthong or triphthong is formed by joining the final vowel of one word and the initial vowel of the next. When there is a combination of three vowels, a triphthong is formed.

mi oftalmólogo   *miof-tal-mó-lo-go* My ophthalmologist   **ocio inútil** *o-cioi-nú-til* useless leisure time

Sometimes the final consonant of a word is pronounced together with the initial vowel of the next word.

El enfermo no quiere tomar esta medicina.   *E-len-fer-mo-no-quie-re-to-ma-res-ta-me-di-ci-na.*
The sick man doesn't want to take this medicine.

When the final consonant of one word is the same as the initial consonant of the following word, only one sound is made, but it is of slightly longer duration.

Carlos sufre *Car-lo-su-fre* Carlos is suffering.

INTONATION

ENTONACION

Intonation is the way the voice rises and falls in delivering a phrase or sentence, or its tone or pitch. Like stress, tone can change the meaning of a sentence. Spanish sometimes appears to be less emphatic than English because pitch in Spanish tends to be more constant than in English which often has great variations.

Spanish intonation for statements known as declarative sentences starts in a low pitch, raises to a higher one on the first stressed syllable, maintains that pitch until the last stressed syllable, and then goes back to the initial low pitch, dropping even lower at the very end.

El doctor Godoy es oncólogo.   **La clínica está lejos de aquí.**
Dr. Godoy is an oncologist.   The clinic is far from here.

In general, the speech pattern is different in Spanish for interrogative statements which are also known as questions. There are basic types of questions, each with its own pattern of intonation: information questions, which use question or interrogative words and need more than a yes or no answer; yes/no questions; and tag questions.

Information questions, like declarative sentences, end with a falling tone. Because they begin with an interrogative word, they are never confused with statements. (The pattern is similar to English.)

¿De dónde es la paciente?↘   **¿Quién tiene mis píldoras?**↘
Where is the patient from?   Who has my pills?

In Spanish yes/no questions end with rising intonation, which expresses the speaker's uncertainty as to the correct response.

¿Hace mucho tiempo que usted está enfermo?↗   **¿Tiene mucho dolor?**↗
Have you been sick for a long time?   Do you have a lot of pain?

However, these yes/no questions can be asked using falling tones. To do so either means that the interrogator knows the answer or is trying to direct it.

¿Tiene mucho dolor?↘   **¿La señora Gómez es su paciente?**↘
Is Mrs. Gómez your patient?

Tag questions, which are statements followed by a short "tag," usually end with a rising tone.

Vd. tiene fiebre, ¿verdad?↗
You have a fever, don't you?

PUNCTUATION

PUNTUACION

Spanish punctuation is the same as English punctuation with the following exceptions:

1. A question has an inverted question mark (¿) at the beginning of the question as well as the regular question mark (?) at the end.

    ¿Dónde está el médico?   Where is the physician?

2. An inverted exclamation point (¡) precedes exclamations and a regular exclamation mark (!) concludes them.

    ¡Qué magnífica enfermera es!   What a magnificent nurse she is!

3. In quotations a dash (—) is generally used to indicate a change of speaker instead of quotation marks. Quoted speech and dialogue may also be indicated by « ».

    El doctor dijo:—¿Qué es lo que Vd. padece?—   The doctor said: "What is the matter with you?"
    Siento mucha opresión en el pecho.—   "I feel a lot of congestion in my chest,"
    respondió Pablo.   responded Paul.
    «No sufro de nada.»   "I'm not suffering from anything."

Common Punctuation Symbols		*Frecuentes símbolos de puntuación*
apostrophe	'	**apóstrofo**
asterisk	*	**asterisco**
braces	{ }	**corchetes**
brackets	[ ]	**paréntesis cuadrados**
colon	:	**dos puntos**
comma	,	**coma**
dash	—	**raya**
diaeresis	ü	**crema / diéresis**
exclamation point	¡ !	**principio de exclamación (¡); fin de exclamación (!)**
hyphen	-	**guión**
parentheses	( )	**paréntesis**
period	.	**punto**
question mark	¿ ?	**principio de interrogación (¿); fin de interrogación (?)**
quotation marks	«/»	**comillas**
semicolon	;	**punto y coma**
suspension points	. . .	**puntos suspensivos**

The conjunction *o* ("or") is accented between numbers to avoid confusion with zero.

Tengo 7 ó 8.   I have 7 or 8.

CAPITALIZATION

USO DE MAYUSCULAS

Capital letters are not used as frequently in Spanish as in English. Only proper nouns and topographic nouns are capitalized.

The pronoun **yo** ("I") is not capitalized, except at the beginning of a sentence.

The days of the week and the months of the year are not capitalized except at the beginning of a sentence. Names of political parties, languages, and titles are not capitalized except at the beginning of a sentence.

Hoy es miércoles   Today is Wednesday.
Es el veinte de agosto.   It is the twentieth of August.
El es republicano, no demócrata.   He is a Republican, not a Democrat.

An adjective of nationality is not capitalized. Some authors capitalize adjectives of nationality used as nouns while others do not.

Dígalo Vd. en inglés.   Say it in English.
Hablo con un español.
Le hablo a un Español.   } I am speaking to a Spaniard.

The following words are capitalized when they are abbreviated:

usted–Vd. (Ud.)   ustedes–Vds. (Uds.) you
señor–Sr.   señora–Sra.   señorita–Srta. Mr. Mrs. Miss
doctor—Dr.   doctora—Dra. Dr.

The following nouns are also capitalized:

1. Divine attributes
   Creador Creator   **Redentor** Redeemer
2. Titles and nicknames which designate specific people
   el Duque de Windsor the Duke of Windsor
3. Names of important positions and public powers when they are equivalent to proper names
   el Rey the King   **el Presidente** the President
4. Certain collective nouns
   la Nación the Nation   **el Reino** the Kingdom

EXERCISES EJERCICIOS

A. Rewrite the following passages, inserting proper punctuation and capitals.
   1. **qué causa la alta presión arterial el 90–95% de la todos los casos de alta presión arterial es debido a una causa desconocida**
      what causes high blood pressure 90–95% of all cases of high blood pressure is due to an unknown cause
   2. **el tiempo en la sala de recuperación varía de una hora a 3 o 4 horas o más**
      the time in the recovery room varies from an hour to 3 or 4 or more
   3. **la siguiente información es exigida por la administración de alimentos y drogas de los estados unidos**
      the following information is required by the food and drug administration of the united states
   4. **la píldora es el más eficaz de todos los anticonceptivos si sigue completamente las instrucciones sobre su uso.**
      the pill is the most effective of all the contraceptives if you are completely following the instructions about its use
   5. **por favor vaya a llamar al dr. garcía del departamento de psiquiatría a ver si puede continuar con el examen**
      please go call dr garcia from the psych department to see if you can continue the exam
   6. **inglaterra tiene un sistema de la medicina socializada en que el gobierno paga los gastos médicos**
      england has a system of socialized medicine in which the government pays for medical expenses

B. Examine the following sentences. Note the differences between the Spanish writing system and the English writing system. Draw circles around examples of such differences.
   1. **—¡Hola, Carlos! ¿Qué tal? ¿Cómo estás?**
   2. **—Muy bien, gracias, ¿y tú?**
   3. **—¿Cómo está usted, doctor?**[5]
   4. **—Estoy bien, gracias. ¿Y Vd., señor?**[5]

Notes *Notas*

1. *Vowel:* found in the center of a syllable and the most prominent sound in a syllable; it is formed without any constriction of the oral cavity. Vowels are *a, e, i, o, u.*
Semivowel: very brief and always in the same syllable with a true vowel. *U, i,* and final *y* are semivowels.
2. To remember these four letters more easily, think of the word *DeMoNS* (***DeMoNioS***).
3. D. Lincoln Canfield, *La pronunciación del español en América: Ensayo histórico-descriptivo.* Bogotá: Institute Caro y Cuervo, 1962 and Pedro Henríquez Ureña, "Observaciones sobre el español de América," *Revista de filología española* VIII (1921): 357–390.
4. Henríquez Ureña, "Observaciones sobre el español de América."
5. Note that the titles **doctor** (Dr.) and **señor** (Mr.) are not capitalized as they would be in English. Spanish uses a capital with these titles only when they are abbreviated. See page 57.

CHAPTER 3

Anatomic and Physiological Vocabulary
Vocabulario anatómico y fisiológico

PARTS OF THE BODY

LAS PARTES DEL CUERPO

MISCELLANY   MISCELÁNEA

albumin   **albúmina** *f*
aorta   **aorta** *f*
artery   **arteria** *f*
  brachial artery   **arteria humeral**
  carotid artery   **arteria carótida**
  coronary artery   **arteria coronaria**
  facial artery   **arteria facial**
  pulmonary artery   **arteria pulmonar**
  subclavian artery   **arteria subclavia**
  temporal artery   **arteria temporal**
articulation   **articulación** *f;*
  coyuntura *f*
blood   **sangre** *f*
body   **cuerpo** *m*
  ciliary body   **cuerpo ciliar**
bone   **hueso** *m*
breath   **aliento** *m*
capillary   **capilar** *m*
cardiovascular system   **aparato**
  cardiovascular *m;* **sistema**
  cardiovascular *m*
cartilage   **cartílago** *m*
cavity   **cavidad** *f*
cholesterol   **colesterol** *m;* **grasa en las**
  venas *f, fam*
circulation   **circulación** *f*
circulatory (or hematologic) system
  aparato circulatorio (o
  hematológico) *m;* **sistema**
  circulatorio (o hematológico) *m*
crow's feet   **patas de gallo** *f*
diastole   **diástole** *f*
digestive system   **aparato digestivo** *m;*
  sistema digestivo *m*
enrocrine system   **aparato endócrino** *m;*
  sistema endócrino *m*
endometrium   **endometrio** *m*
enzyme   **enzima** *f;* **jugo digestivo** *m*
epidermis   **epidermis** *f*
excretion   **excreción** *f;* **excremento** *m*
extrasystole   **extrasístole** *f*
fibroid   **fibroideo** *adj*
flesh   **carne** *f*
follicule   **folículo** *m*

freckles   **pecas** *f*
gastrointestinal system   **aparato**
  gastrointestinal *m;* **sistema**
  gastrointestinal *m*
genitourinary system   **aparato**
  genitourinario *m;* **sistema**
  genitourinario *m*
hairy   **peludo** *adj;* **tarántula** *adj,*
  Chicano
hormone   **hormona** *f;* **hormón** *m*
joint   **articulación** *f;* **coyuntura** *f*
ligament   **ligamento** *m*
limb   **miembro** *m;* **extremidad** *f*
lingual   **lingual** *adj*
lymph node   **nódulo linfático** *m;* **nudo**
  linfático *m, fam*
marrow   **médula** *f*
membrane   **membrana** *f*
mole, birthmark   **lunar** *m*
muscle   **músculo** *m*
  involuntary muscle   **músculo**
    involuntario
  smooth muscle   **músculo liso**
  striated muscle   **músculo estriado**
  voluntary muscle   **músculo**
    voluntario
myometrium   **miometrio** *m*
nerve   **nervio** *m*
  cranial nerve   **nervio craneal**
  motor nerve   **nervio motor**
  parasympathetic nerve   **nervio**
    parasimpático
  sensory nerve   **nervio sensorial**
  sympathetic nerve   **nervio simpático**
nervous system, autonomic
  aparato nervioso autónomo *m;*
  sistema nervioso autónomo *m*
nervous system, central   **aparato**
  nervioso central *m;* **sistema nervioso**
  central *m*
olfactory   **olfatorio** *adj*
organ   **órgano** *m*
perimetrium   **perimetrio** *m*
periosteum   **periostio** *m*

perspiration   **transpiración,** *f*
pore   **poro** *m*
pulse   **pulso** *m*
reflex   **reflejo** *m*
reproductive system   **aparato**
  reproductivo *m;* **sistema reproductivo**
  m
respiratory system   **aparato respiratorio**
  m; **sistema respiratorio** *m*
sense   **sentido** *m*
  sense of feel (tactile)   **sentido del**
    tacto
  sense of hearing (auditory)
    sentido del oído
  sense of pain   **sentido del dolor**
  sense of sight (visual)   **sentido de la**
    vista
  sense of smell (olfactory)   **sentido**
    del olfato
  sense of taste (gustatory)   **sentido del**
    gusto; sentido gustatorio
sensorial   **sensorial** *adj*
skeleton   **esqueleto** *m;* **armazón** *m*
skin   **piel** *f*
  flap of skin   **colgajo** *m*
sphincter   **esfínter** *m*
systole   **sístole** *f*
tactile   **táctil** *adj*
tendon   **tendón** *m*
tissue   **tejido** *m*
urine   **orina** *f;* **orines** *m*
valve   **válvula** *f*
vein   **vena** *f*
  brachial vein   **vena humeral**
  deep vein   **vena profunda**
  facial vein   **vena facial**
  great cardiac vein   **vena coronaria**
    mayor
  inferior vena cava vein   **vena cava**
    inferior
  jugular vein   **vena yugular**
  pulmonary vein   **vena pulmonar**
  small cardiac vein   **vena coronaria**
    menor

The Human Body—Rear View *El cuerpo humano—vista posterior*

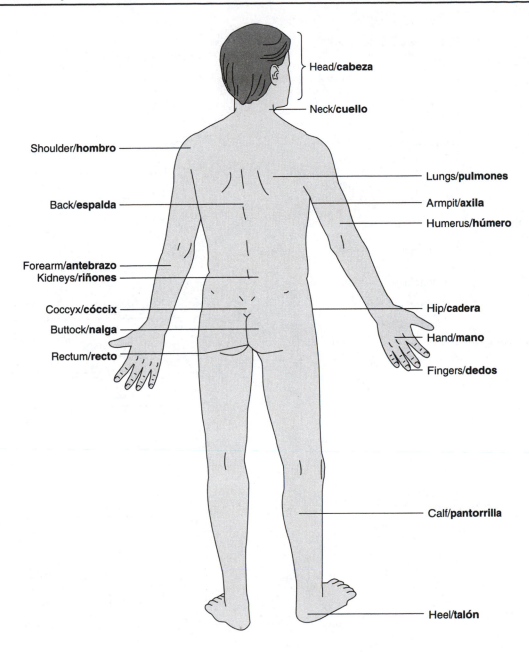

Head/**cabeza**

Neck/**cuello**

Shoulder/**hombro**

Lungs/**pulmones**

Back/**espalda**

Armpit/**axila**

Humerus/**húmero**

Forearm/**antebrazo**

Kidneys/**riñones**

Coccyx/**cóccix**

Hip/**cadera**

Buttock/**nalga**

Hand/**mano**

Rectum/**recto**

Fingers/**dedos**

Calf/**pantorrilla**

Heel/**talón**

The Human Body—Front View *El cuerpo humano—vista anterior*

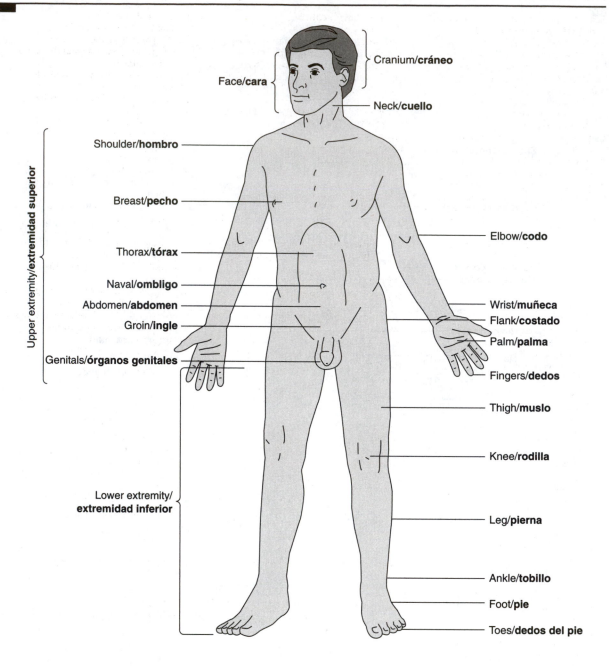

Cranium/**cráneo**

Face/**cara**

Neck/**cuello**

Shoulder/**hombro**

Breast/**pecho**

Thorax/**tórax**

Naval/**ombligo**

Abdomen/**abdomen**

Groin/**ingle**

Genitals/**órganos genitales**

Upper extremity/**extremidad superior**

Lower extremity/ **extremidad inferior**

Elbow/**codo**

Wrist/**muñeca**

Flank/**costado**

Palm/**palma**

Fingers/**dedos**

Thigh/**muslo**

Knee/**rodilla**

Leg/**pierna**

Ankle/**tobillo**

Foot/**pie**

Toes/**dedos del pie**

THE HEAD *LA CABEZA*

Adam's apple **nuez de Adán** *f*; **bocado de Adán** *m*; **manzana** *f, Mex.*
adenoids **adenoides** *m, pl*
beard **barba** *f*
blood vessel **vaso sanguíneo** *m*
brains **sesos** *m*
cell **célula** *f*
  ciliated cell **célula ciliada**
cerebral cortex **corteza cerebral** *f*; **materia gris** *f, fam*
cerebral hemisphere **hemisferio cerebral** *m*
cerebrum **cerebro** *m*
  anterior chamber of cerebrum **cámara anterior del cerebro** *f*
  posterior chamber of cerebrum **cámara posterior del cerebro** *f*
cheek **mejilla** *f*; **carrillos** *m*; **cachete** *m*
  cheekbone **pómulo** *m*
chin **barbilla** *f*; **mentón** *m*; **barba** *f*
cranium **cráneo** *m*
  base of the cranium **base del cráneo** *f*
crown of the head **mollera** *f*
ear **oreja** *f*
  auditory **auditivo** *adj*
  ear (organ of hearing) **oído** *m*
  earwax **cerumen** *m*; **cera de los oídos** *f*; **cerilla** *f*
  Eustachian tube **trompa de Eustaquio** *f*
  external ear **oído externo** *m*; **pabellón externo de la oreja** *m*; **aurícola** *f*
    external ear canal **conducto**[1] **auditivo externo** *m*
  lobe of the ear **pulpejo** *m*; **lóbulo** *m*
  eardrum (tympanic membrane) **tímpano** *m*
  inner ear **oído interno** *m*
    cochlea **cóclea** *f*; **caracol** *m*
    semicircular canal **conducto semicircular** *m*
  middle ear **oído medio** *m*
    anvil (incus) **yunque** *m*
    hammer (malleus) **martillo** *m*
    stirrup (stapes) **estribo** *m*
  saccule **sáculo** *m*
eye **ojo** *m*
  aqueous humor **humor acuoso** *m*
  chorioid **corioide** *f*; **coroides,** *f, inv*
  cone **cono** *m*
  conjunctiva **conjuntiva** *f*
  cornea **córnea** *f*
  eyeball **globo del ojo** *m*; **globo ocular** *m*; **tomate** *m, slang, Chicano*
  eyebrow **ceja** *f*
  eyelash **pestaña** *f*
  eyelid **párpado** *m*
  eye socket **cuenca de los ojos** *f*
  fovea centralis **fóvea central** *f*
  iris **iris** *f*
  lachrymal **lacrimal** *adj*; **lagrimal** *adj*
  lens (of eye), crystalline **cristalino** *m*
  optic nerve **nervio óptico** *m*
  pupil **pupila** *f*; **niña del ojo** *f*
  retina **retina** *f*
  rod **bastoncillo** *m*
  sclera **esclerótica** *f*
  tear duct **conducto lagrimal** *m*
  tear sac **bolsa de lágrimas** *f*
  vitreous humor **humor vítreo** *m*
face **cara** *f*; **rostro** *m*; **carátula** *f, slang, Chicano*
features **facciones** *f*
fontanelle **fontanela** *f*; **mollera** *f*
forehead **frente** *f*
fossa **fosa** *f*
frontal **frontal** *adj*
ganglion **ganglio** *m*
hair **cabello** *m*; **pelo** *m*; **chimpa** *f, Chicano*
  curl of hair **rizo** *m*; **tirabuzón** *m*; **chino** *m, Chicano*
  curly hair **pelo crespo**; **pelo rizado**
  kinky hair **pelo grifo** (Chicano); **pelo pasudo**
  (premature) gray hair **canas (verdes)** *f, pl*
  straight hair **pelo liso**
  wavy hair **pelo quebrado**; **pelo ondulado**
jaw **mandíbula** *f*; **quijada** *f*
jawbone **mandíbula** *f*
larynx **laringe** *f*
lip **labio** *m*
lymph glands **glándulas linfáticas** *f*
maxillar **maxilar** *adj*
moustache **bigote** *m*; **mostacho** *m*
mouth **boca** *f*
mucus **moco** *m*
nape (of neck) **nuca** *f*
neck **cuello** *m*
nose **nariz** *f*; **nayotas** *f, pl, slang, Chicano*
  bridge of the nose **caballete de la nariz** *m*
nostril **fosa nasal** *f*; **ventana de la nariz** *f*; **ventanilla de la nariz** *f*
occipital **occipital** *adj*
palate **paladar** *m*
  hard palate **paladar duro** *m*; **bóveda ósea del paladar** *f*
  soft palate **paladar blando** *m*; **velo del paladar** *m*
parotid gland **glándula parótida** *f*
pharynx **faringe** *f*
pituitary gland **glándula pituitaria** *f*
saliva **saliva** *f*
salivary gland **glándula salival** *f*
scalp **cuero cabelludo** *m*; **pericráneo** *m*
septum **tabique** *m*
sinus **seno** *m*
skin (of the face) **cutis** *m*
  light skinned/complexioned **de tez blanca**
  olive skinned/complexioned **trigueño** *adj*
  very dark skinned, but lacking Negroid features **pinto** *adj*; **retinto** *adj*
skull **cráneo** *m*; **calavera** *f, Chicano*
  top of the skull **tapa de los sesos** *f, fam*
sputum **esputo** *m*; **saliva** *f*; **desgarro** *m, Sp. Am.*; **pollo** *m, Chicano*
sublingual gland **glándula sublingual** *f*
submaxillary gland **glándula submaxilar** *f*
suture **sutura** *f*; **comisura** *f*
tear **lágrima** *f*
tear gland **glándula lagrimal** *f*
temple **sien** *f*
throat **garganta** *f*
tongue **lengua** *f*
tonsils **amígdalas** *f*; **anginas** *f, Mex., Ven.*; **tonsils** *m, Chicano*
tooth **diente** *m*
trachea **tráquea** *f*; **gaznate** *m*
uvula **úvula** *f*; **campanilla** *f, fam*; **galillo** *m, fam*
vocal cord **cuerda vocal** *f*
wrinkle **arruga** *f*

The Head *La cabeza*

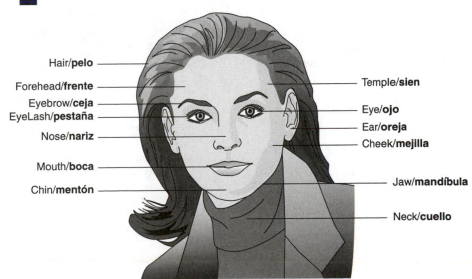

Hair/**pelo**
Forehead/**frente**
Eyebrow/**ceja**
EyeLash/**pestaña**
Nose/**nariz**
Mouth/**boca**
Chin/**mentón**
Temple/**sien**
Eye/**ojo**
Ear/**oreja**
Cheek/**mejilla**
Jaw/**mandíbula**
Neck/**cuello**

Principal Speech Organs   *Organos principales del habla*

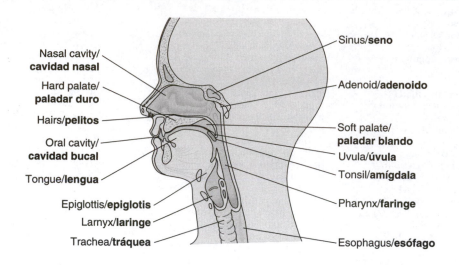

Nasal cavity/**cavidad nasal**

Hard palate/**paladar duro**

Hairs/**pelitos**

Oral cavity/**cavidad bucal**

Tongue/**lengua**

Epiglottis/**epiglotis**

Larnyx/**laringe**

Trachea/**tráquea**

Sinus/**seno**

Adenoid/**adenoido**

Soft palate/**paladar blando**

Uvula/**úvula**

Tonsil/**amígdala**

Pharynx/**faringe**

Esophagus/**esófago**

Structures of the Ear   *Estructuras del oído*

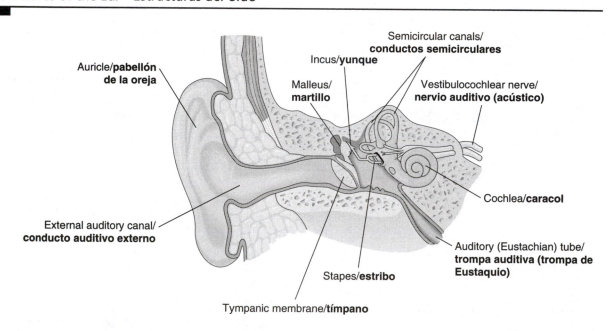

Auricle/**pabellón de la oreja**

Malleus/**martillo**

Incus/**yunque**

Semicircular canals/**conductos semicirculares**

Vestibulocochlear nerve/**nervio auditivo (acústico)**

Cochlea/**caracol**

External auditory canal/**conducto auditivo externo**

Stapes/**estribo**

Tympanic membrane/**tímpano**

Auditory (Eustachian) tube/**trompa auditiva (trompa de Eustaquio)**

Structures of the Eye   *Estructuras del ojo*

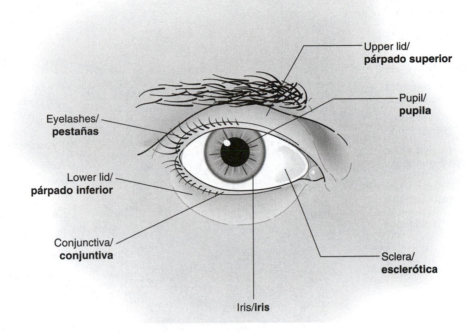

Upper lid/
párpado superior

Pupil/
pupila

Eyelashes/
pestañas

Lower lid/
párpado inferior

Conjunctiva/
conjuntiva

Sclera/
esclerótica

Iris/**iris**

Lateral View of the Eyeball Interior   *Vista lateral del globo del ojo interior*

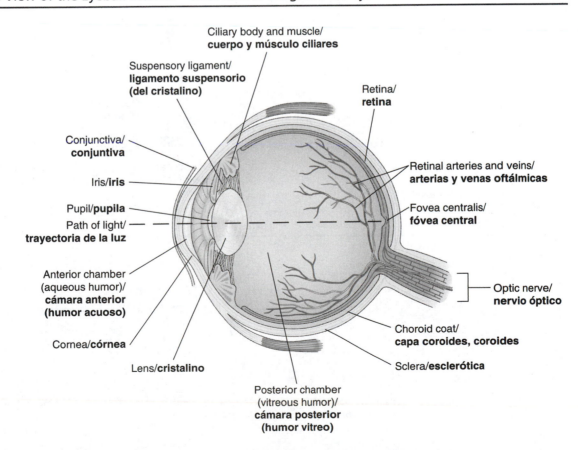

Ciliary body and muscle/
cuerpo y músculo ciliares

Suspensory ligament/
**ligamento suspensorio
(del cristalino)**

Retina/
retina

Conjunctiva/
conjuntiva

Iris/**iris**

Retinal arteries and veins/
arterias y venas oftálmicas

Pupil/**pupila**

Fovea centralis/
fóvea central

Path of light/
trayectoria de la luz

Anterior chamber
(aqueous humor)/
**cámara anterior
(humor acuoso)**

Optic nerve/
nervio óptico

Cornea/**córnea**

Choroid coat/
capa coroides, coroides

Lens/**cristalino**

Sclera/**esclerótica**

Posterior chamber
(vitreous humor)/
**cámara posterior
(humor vitreo)**

Structures of the Mouth   *Estructuras de la boca*

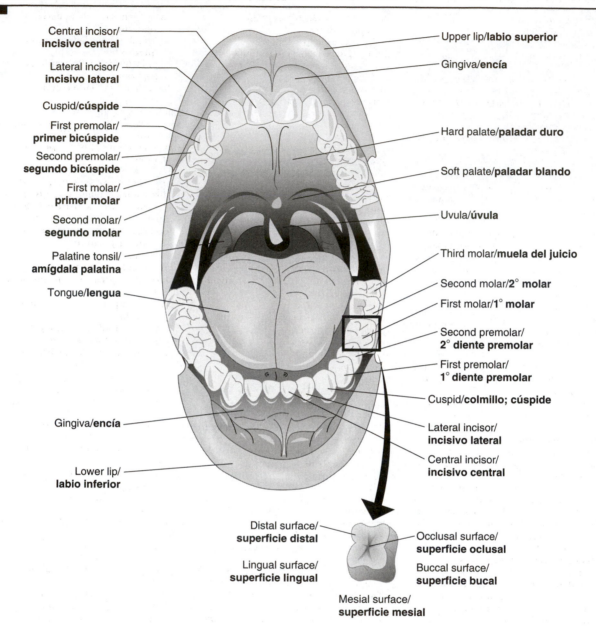

Central incisor/**incisivo central**

Lateral incisor/**incisivo lateral**

Cuspid/**cúspide**

First premolar/**primer bicúspide**

Second premolar/**segundo bicúspide**

First molar/**primer molar**

Second molar/**segundo molar**

Palatine tonsil/**amígdala palatina**

Tongue/**lengua**

Gingiva/**encía**

Lower lip/**labio inferior**

Upper lip/**labio superior**

Gingiva/**encía**

Hard palate/**paladar duro**

Soft palate/**paladar blando**

Uvula/**úvula**

Third molar/**muela del juicio**

Second molar/**2° molar**

First molar/**1° molar**

Second premolar/**2° diente premolar**

First premolar/**1° diente premolar**

Cuspid/**colmillo; cúspide**

Lateral incisor/**incisivo lateral**

Central incisor/**incisivo central**

Distal surface/**superficie distal**

Lingual surface/**superficie lingual**

Occlusal surface/**superficie oclusal**

Buccal surface/**superficie bucal**

Mesial surface/**superficie mesial**

Buccal and Proximal Views   *Vistas bucales y proximales*

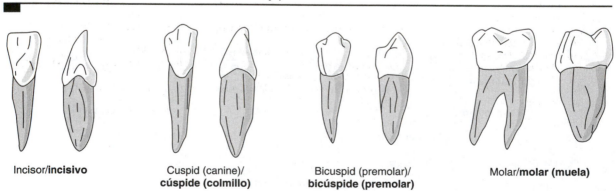

Incisor/**incisivo**

Cuspid (canine)/**cúspide (colmillo)**

Bicuspid (premolar)/**bicúspide (premolar)**

Molar/**molar (muela)**

DENTAL VOCABULARY   *VOCABULARIO DENTAL*

abscess   **absceso** *m*
acrylic   **acrílico** *adj*
amalgam   **amalgama** *f*
apex   **vértice** *m*
arch   **arco**
artificial, false teeth   **dientes postizos** *m*
base   **base** *f*
block the nerve, to   **obstruir el nervio**
bite, to   **morder (ue)**
border   **borde** *m*
braces   **aparato ortodóntico** *m*; **frenos**
   m, Mex., Arg.
bridge (dental)   **puente** *m*
   fixed dental bridge   **puente fijo** *m*
   removable bridge   **puente movible** *m*
brush one's teeth, to   **cepillarse los**
   dientes
burr   **fresa** *f*
canker sore   **ulceración** *f*; **postemilla** *f*
capillaries   **capilares** *m*; **vaso capilar** *m*
caries   **caries** *f inv.*
cavity   **caries** *f inv*; **diente picado** *m*;
   diente cariado *m*; **cavidad** *f*; **picadura**
   f; **guijón** *m*
cementum   **cemento** *m*
chew, to   **mascar; masticar**
clasp   **gancho** *m*
cleaning   **limpieza** *f*
crown   **corona** *f*
   acrylic jacket crown   **corona acrílica**
   porcelain jacket crown   **corona de**
      procelana
cut teeth, to   **dentar (ie); endentecer**
deaden the nerve, to   **adormecer el**
   nervio
dental   **dental** *adj*
dental drill   **taladro** *m*
dental floss   **hilo dental** *m*; **seda**
   encerada *f*
dental forceps   **pinzas** *f, pl*; **tenazas de**
   extracción *f, pl*; **gatillo** *m*
dental hygienist   **higienista dental** *m/f*
dental office   **clínica dental** *f*
dentine   **dentina** *f*
dentition   **dentición** *f*
denture   **dentadura (postiza)** *f*;
   placa *f*
   full denture   **dentadura completa**
   partial denture   **dentadura parcial**
diet, liquid   **dieta de líquidos** *f*
drill   **taladro** *m*; **torno** *m*; **trépano** *m*
drill, to   **perforar; taladrar**
emesis basin   **riñonera** *f*
enamel   **esmalte** *m*
   end   **extremo**
   end, distal   **extremo distal**
   end, lower   **extremo inferior**
   end, proximal   **extremo proximal**
   end, upper   **extremo superior**
extraction   **extracción** *f*
fauces   **fauces** *f, pl*
feel nothing, to   **no sentir (ie) nada**
file down, to   **limar**

fill, to   **empastar; tapar; calzar;**
   emplomar *Arg.*
   fill with gold, to   **orificar**
filling   **empaste** *m*; **empastadura** *f*;
   relleno *m*; **tapadura** *f*; **emplomadura**
   f, Arg.
frenum of the tongue   **frenillo** *m*
gargle (liquid)   **gargarismo** *m*
gargle, to   **hacer gárgaras; hacer buches**
   (de sal) *fam*; **gargarizar**
gold   **oro** *m*
groove   **canal** *m*
gums   **encías** *f*
headrest   **apoyo para la cabeza** *m*
impression   **impresión** *f*
immobilization   **inmovilización** *f*
impaction   **impacción** *f*
inlay   **incrustación** *f*; **orificación** *f*
jaw   **quijada** *f*; **mandíbula** *f*
   broken jaw   **quijada rota** *f*;
      mandíbula rota *f*
margin   **borde** *m*
neck of the tooth   **cuello del diente** *m*
nerve   **nervio** *m*
novocaine   **novocaína** *f*
numb   **entumecido** *adj*; **adormecido**
   adj; **entumido** *adj*
occlusion   **oclusión** *f*
palate   **paladar** *m*
plaque   **placa** *f*
plate, dental   **placa** *f*
polish (up), to   **limar**
porcelain   **porcelana** *f*
pressure   **presión** *f*
   exert pressure on, to   **ejercer presión**
      sobre
   sensations, pressure   **sensaciones de**
      ser apretado
pull out, to   **extraer**
pulp   **pulpa** *f*
pulpotomy   **pulpotomía** *f*
put to sleep, to   **adormecer por**
   anestesia
pyorrhea   **piorrea** *f*
reimplantation   **reimplantación** *f*;
   reinjertación *f*
remove the nerve, to   **sacarle el nervio a**
   alguien; matarle el nervio a alguien
ridge   **elevación** *f*; **reborde** *m*
rinse, to   **enjuagarse**
roof of the mouth   **cielo de la boca** *m*;
   paladar *m*
root   **raíz** *f*
root canal   **canal radicular** *m*
root canal work   **extracción del nervio** *f*;
   curación del nervio *f*
saliva   **esputo** *m*; **saliva** *f*; **expectoración**
   f
set a fracture, to   **reducir una fractura;**
   componer una fractura
show one's teeth, to   **enseñar los**
   dientes *fam*; **mostrar (ue) los dientes**
side   **lado** *m*

upper right side   **lado derecho**
   superior
lower right side   **lado derecho**
   inferior
upper left side   **lado izquierdo**
   superior
lower left side   **lado izquierdo**
   inferior
smooth (over), to   **limar**
sodium pentothal   **pentotal de sodio** *m*
spit in the bowl, to   **escupir en la taza**
straighten the teeth, to   **enderezar los**
   dientes
surface   **superficie** *f*
   buccal surface   **superficie bucal**
   distal surface   **superficie distal**
   lingual surface   **superficie lingual**
   mesial surface   **superficie mesial**
   occlusal surface   **superficie oclusal**
suture (dental)   **sutura** *f*
tartar   **sarro** *m*
teeth   **dientes** *m*; **mazorca** *f, slang*
   bicuspids   **bicúspides** *m*; **premolares**
      m
   canine, cuspid, eyetooth   **canino** *m*;
      colmillo *m*
   deciduous teeth   **dientes de leche**
   even teeth   **dientes parejos**
   incisors, front teeth   **incisivos** *m*
   lacking teeth   **chimuelo** *adj, Chicano*
   molars   **molares** *m*
      third molar   **tercer molar**
   stained teeth   **dientes manchados**
   white teeth   **dientes blancos**
   wisdom teeth   **muelas del juicio** *f*;
      muelas cordales *f*
teething   **dentición** *f*; **salida de los**
   dientes *f*
temporary filling   **empaste provisional**
   m; **empaque** *m, Chicano*
tingling   **hormigueo** *m*
tooth   **diente** *m*
   baby tooth   **diente mamón; diente**
      de leche; diente temporal
   back tooth   **muela** *f*; **molar** *m*
   impacted tooth   **diente impactado**
   large, misshapen tooth   **diente de ajo**
      fam
   lower tooth   **diente inferior**
   toothache   **dolor de muelas** *m*; **dolor**
      de dientes *m*; **odontalgia** *f*
   toothbrush   **cepillo de dientes** *m*
   toothpaste   **pasta de dientes** *f*; **pasta**
      dentífrica *f*
   toothpick   **palillo de dientes** *m*;
      mondadientes *m, inv*
   tooth socket   **alvéolo** *m*
   upper tooth   **diente superior**
wall   **pared** *f*
waterpick   **limpiador de agua a presión**
   m
wire, to   **atar con alambre**

Parts of a Tooth   *Partes de un diente*

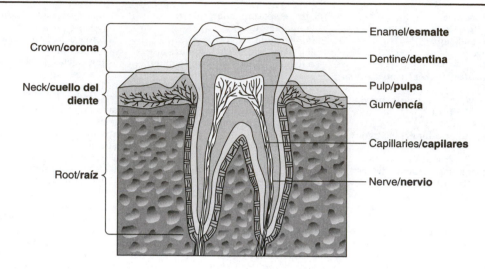

Crown/**corona**

Neck/**cuello del diente**

Root/**raíz**

Enamel/**esmalte**

Dentine/**dentina**

Pulp/**pulpa**

Gum/**encía**

Capillaries/**capilares**

Nerve/**nervio**

Adult Dentition   *Dentición adulta*

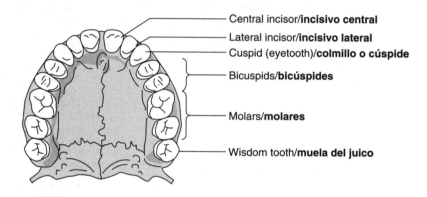

Central incisor/**incisivo central**

Lateral incisor/**incisivo lateral**

Cuspid (eyetooth)/**colmillo o cúspide**

Bicuspids/**bicúspides**

Molars/**molares**

Wisdom tooth/**muela del juico**

Deciduous Teeth   *Los dientes de leche*

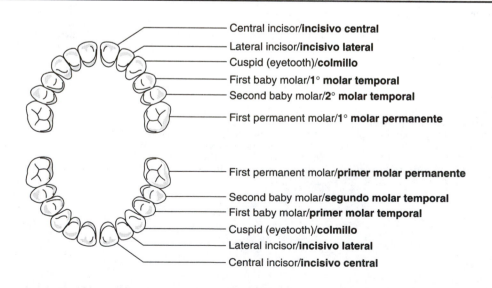

Central incisor/**incisivo central**

Lateral incisor/**incisivo lateral**

Cuspid (eyetooth)/**colmillo**

First baby molar/**1° molar temporal**

Second baby molar/**2° molar temporal**

First permanent molar/**1° molar permanente**

First permanent molar/**primer molar permanente**

Second baby molar/**segundo molar temporal**

First baby molar/**primer molar temporal**

Cuspid (eyetooth)/**colmillo**

Lateral incisor/**incisivo lateral**

Central incisor/**incisivo central**

THE TRUNK *EL TRONCO*

abdomen **abdomen** *m*; **vientre** *m*; **panza** *f, fam*

alveolus **alvéolo** *m*

anus **ano** *m*; **agujero** *m, vulgar, Chicano*; **chicloso** *m, vulgar, Chicano*; **chiquito** *m, vulgar; Chicano*; **fundillo** *m, Mex.* **istantino** *m, fam*

appendix **apéndice** *m*; **apendix** *f*; **tripita** *f, fam*

back **espalda** *f*; **dorso** *m*

backbone **columna vertebral** *f*

belly **barriga** *f*; **panza** *f, fam*

bile **bilis** *f*; **hiel** *f*

bladder **vejiga** *f*; **vesícula**

bosom **senos** *m, pl*

bowel **intestino inferior** *m*

bowels **entrañas** *f*; **tripa** *f, fam*

breast **pecho** *m*; **busto** *m*; **agarraderas** *f, Chicano*; **chichas** *f, pl, C.R.*; **chichi** *f, Mex.*; **teta** *f, slang*; **tele** *f*

breastbone **esternón** *m*

bronchia **bronquios** *m*

buttock **nalga**[2] *f*; **sentadera** *f*; **anca** *f*; **aparato** *m, Chicano*; **pellín** *m, Chicano*; **común** *m, Mex.*; **fondillo** *m, Cuba*; **fundillo** *m, Mex.*; **olla** *f, slang, Chicano*; **fondongo** *m, slang*; **buche** *m, vulgar, Chicano*

cervix **cervix** *f*; **cerviz** *f*; **cuello de la matriz** *m*

chest **pecho** *m*; **tórax** *m*

clitoris **clítoris** *m*; **bolita** *f, slang*; **pelotita** *f, slang*; **pepa** *f, slang*

coccyx **cóccix** *m*; **cócciz** *m, Chicano*; **colita** *f*; **coxis** *m*

collar bone/clavicle **clavícula** *f*; **cuena** *f, Chicano*

colon **colon** *m*

sigmoid colon **colon sigmoide**

coronary **coronario** *adj*

cortex **corteza**

crotch **entrepiernas** *f, pl*

diaphragm **diafragma** *m*

disc **disco** *m*

duodenum **duodeno** *m*

epididymis **epidídimo** *m*

esophagus **esófago** *m*; **tragante** *m, Chicano*

Fallopian tubes **trompas de Falopio** *f*; **tubos** *m*

flank **costado** *m*

foreskin **prepucio** *m*

fundus **fondo** *m*

gallbladder **vesícula biliar** *f*; **vejiga de la bilis** *f*

gastric juice **jugo gástrico** *m*

genitals **órganos genitales** *m*; **partes** *f, slang*; **partes ocultas** *f, slang*

gland **glándula** *f*

adrenal gland **glándula suprarrenal**

carotid gland **glándula carótida**

Cowper's gland **glándula de Cowper**

endocrine gland **glándula endocrina**

lymph gland **glándula linfática**

mammary gland **glándula mamaria**

parathyroid gland **glándula paratiroides**

pineal gland **glándula pineal**

pituitary gland **glándula pituitaria**

prostrate gland **próstata** *f*; **glándula de la próstata**; **glándula prostática**

sebaceous gland **glándula sebácea**

sweat gland **glándula sudoripara**

thyroid gland **glándula tiroides**

glans (penis) **glande** *m*; **bálano** *m*; **cabeza** *f, slang*

gluteal region **región glutea** *f*; **gluteo** *m*

heart **corazón** *m*

apex of the heart **punta del corazón** *f*

auricle **aurícula** *f*

heart valve **válvula del corazón** *f*

ventricle **ventrículo** *m*

hip **cadera** *f*; **cuadril** *m, Mex., Chicano*

ileum **íleon** *m*

ilium **ilion** *m*

intestines **intestinos** *m*; **tripas** *f*

large intestine **intestino grueso**

small intestine **intestino delgado**

Islets of Langerhans **islotes de Langerhans** *m*

jejunum **yeyuno** *m*

kidney **riñón** *m*

lap **regazo** *m*

liver **hígado** *m*

loin **lomo** *m*

lung **pulmón** *m*; **bofe** *m, Chicano, Sp. Am.*

marrow **médula** *f*

myocardium **miocardio** *adj*

navel **ombligo** *m*

neck **cuello** *m*

back of neck **nuca** *f*; **cerviz** *f*

nipple (female) **pezón** *m*; **chichi** *f, slang*

nipple (male) **tetilla** *f*

ovary **ovario** *m*

pancreas **páncreas** *m*

pelvis **pelvis** *f*

penis **pene** *m*; **miembro** *m*; **pito** *m, slang*; **verga** *f, slang*; **balone** *m, Chicano*; **chale** *m, vulgar, Chicano*; **chalito** *m, vulgar, Chicano*; **chicote** *m, slang*; **chile** *m, slang*; **chorizo** *m, vulgar*; **güine** *m, vulgar*; **palo** *m, slang*; **picha** *f, vulgar*; **pichón** *m, vulgar*; **pilinga** *f, vulgar*; **pilonga** *f, slang, vulgar*; **pinga** *f, vulgar*; **reata/riata** *f, vulgar*

pubic hair **vello púbico pelitos** *m, pl, Chicano*

pubis **pubis** *m*

rectum **recto** *m*

rib **costilla** *f*

false/floating rib **costilla falsa o flotante** *f*

true rib **costilla verdadera** *f*

sacroiliac **sacroilíaco** *adj*

sacrum **sacro** *m*

sciatic **ciático** *adj*

scrotum **escroto** *m*; **bolsa de los testículos** *f*

semen **semen** *m*; **esperma** *f*

seminal vesicle **vesículo seminal** *m*

shoulder blade (scapula) **espaldilla** *f*; **omóplato** *m*; **escápula** *f*; **paletilla** *f*

side **costado** *m*; **lado** *m*

skin **piel** *f*

spermatic cord **cordón espermático** *m*

spinal column **columna vertebral** *f*; **espina dorsal** *f*

spinal cord **médula espinal** *f*

spleen **bazo** *m*; **esplín** *m*

stomach **estómago** *m*; **vientre** *m*

stomach (pit of) **boca del estómago** *f*

testis **testículo** *m*; **testis** *m*

testicle **testículo** *m*; **huevos** *m, pl, vulgar, slang*; *Mex.* **compañones** *m, pl, slang*, **cuates** *m, pl, slang, Chicano*; **blanquillo** *m, slang, Chicano*; **bola** *f, pl, slang*

thoracic cavity **caja torácica** *f*

thorax **tórax** *m*

thymus **timo** *m*

thyroid **tiroides** *m*

umbilical cord **cordón umbilical** *m*

umbilicus **ombligo** *m*

ureter **uréter** *m*

urethra **uretra** *f*, **canal urinario** *m*; **caño urinario** *m*

urinary bladder **vejiga de la orina** *f*

urinary tract **vías urinarias** *f*

uterus **útero** *m*; **matriz** *f*

vagina **vagina** *f*; **panocho** (*m, slang*); **pan** *m, slang, vulgar*; **cueva** *f, slang, vulgar, Chicano*; **linda** *f, slang*; **partida** *f, vulgar*; **agujero** *m, vulgar, Chicano*; **concha** *f, vulgar, Arg., Chile, Ur.*

vas deferens **conducto deferente** *m*

vertebra **vértebra** *f*

vulva **vulva** *f*; **panocha** *f, slang*; **rajada** *f, vulgar*

waist **cintura** *f*

womb **matriz** *f*; **útero** *m*

Anterior View of Skeleton *Vista anterior del esqueleto*

Posterior View of Skeleton *Vista posterior del esqueleto*

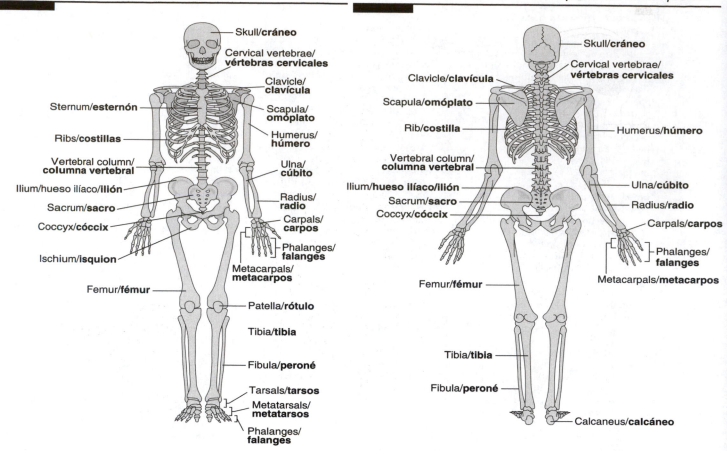

Anterior view labels:
- Skull/**cráneo**
- Cervical vertebrae/**vértebras cervicales**
- Clavicle/**clavícula**
- Sternum/**esternón**
- Scapula/**omóplato**
- Ribs/**costillas**
- Humerus/**húmero**
- Vertebral column/**columna vertebral**
- Ulna/**cúbito**
- Ilium/hueso ilíaco/**ilión**
- Radius/**radio**
- Sacrum/**sacro**
- Coccyx/**cóccix**
- Carpals/**carpos**
- Phalanges/**falanges**
- Ischium/**isquion**
- Metacarpals/**metacarpos**
- Femur/**fémur**
- Patella/**rótula**
- Tibia/**tibia**
- Fibula/**peroné**
- Tarsals/**tarsos**
- Metatarsals/**metatarsos**
- Phalanges/**falanges**

Posterior view labels:
- Skull/**cráneo**
- Cervical vertebrae/**vértebras cervicales**
- Clavicle/**clavícula**
- Scapula/**omóplato**
- Rib/**costilla**
- Humerus/**húmero**
- Vertebral column/**columna vertebral**
- Ilium/**hueso ilíaco/ilión**
- Ulna/**cúbito**
- Sacrum/**sacro**
- Radius/**radio**
- Coccyx/**cóccix**
- Carpals/**carpos**
- Phalanges/**falanges**
- Femur/**fémur**
- Metacarpals/**metacarpos**
- Tibia/**tibia**
- Fibula/**peroné**
- Calcaneus/**calcáneo**

Fractures *Fracturas*

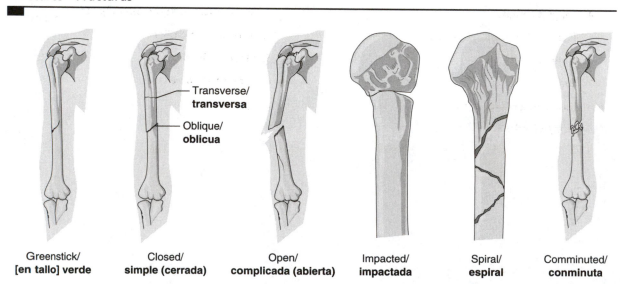

- Greenstick/**[en tallo] verde**
- Closed/**simple (cerrada)**
- Open/**complicada (abierta)**
- Impacted/**impactada**
- Spiral/**espiral**
- Comminuted/**conminuta**
- Transverse/**transversa**
- Oblique/**oblicua**

Internal Organs *Los órganos internos*

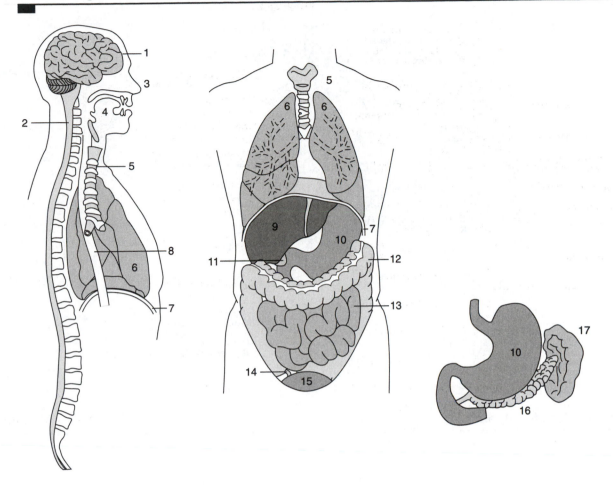

1. Brain/**Cerebro**

2. Spinal Cord/**Médula espinal**

3. Nose/**Nariz**

4. Tongue/**Lengua**

5. Trachea (Windpipe)/**Tráquea**

6. Lungs/**Pulmones**

7. Diaphragm/**Diafragma**

8. Esophagus/**Esófago**

9. Liver/**Hígado**

10. Stomach/**Estómago**

11. Gallbladder/**Vesícula biliar**

12. Large Intestine/**Intestino grueso**

13. Small Intestine/**Intestino delgado**

14. Appendix/**Apéndice**

15. Bladder/**Vejiga**

16. Pancreas/**Páncreas**

17. Spleen/**Bazo**

General or Systemic Circulation   *Circulación general o sistemática*

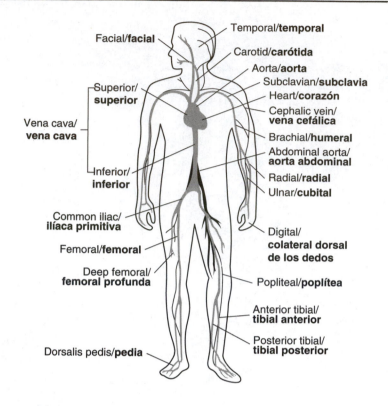

Facial/**facial**
Temporal/**temporal**
Carotid/**carótida**
Aorta/**aorta**
Subclavian/**subclavia**
Superior/**superior**
Heart/**corazón**
Cephalic vein/**vena cefálica**
Vena cava/**vena cava**
Brachial/**humeral**
Abdominal aorta/**aorta abdominal**
Inferior/**inferior**
Radial/**radial**
Ulnar/**cubital**
Common iliac/**ilíaca primitiva**
Digital/**colateral dorsal de los dedos**
Femoral/**femoral**
Deep femoral/**femoral profunda**
Popliteal/**poplítea**
Anterior tibial/**tibial anterior**
Posterior tibial/**tibial posterior**
Dorsalis pedis/**pedia**

Digestive System   *Aparato o sistema digestivo*

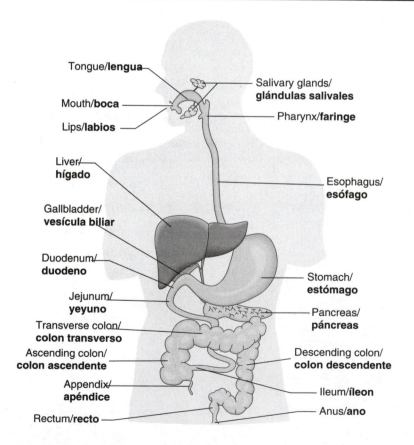

Tongue/**lengua**
Salivary glands/**glándulas salivales**
Mouth/**boca**
Pharynx/**faringe**
Lips/**labios**
Liver/**hígado**
Esophagus/**esófago**
Gallbladder/**vesícula biliar**
Duodenum/**duodeno**
Stomach/**estómago**
Jejunum/**yeyuno**
Pancreas/**páncreas**
Transverse colon/**colon transverso**
Ascending colon/**colon ascendente**
Descending colon/**colon descendente**
Appendix/**apéndice**
Ileum/**íleon**
Rectum/**recto**
Anus/**ano**

The Endocrine System   *Aparato o sistema endocrino*

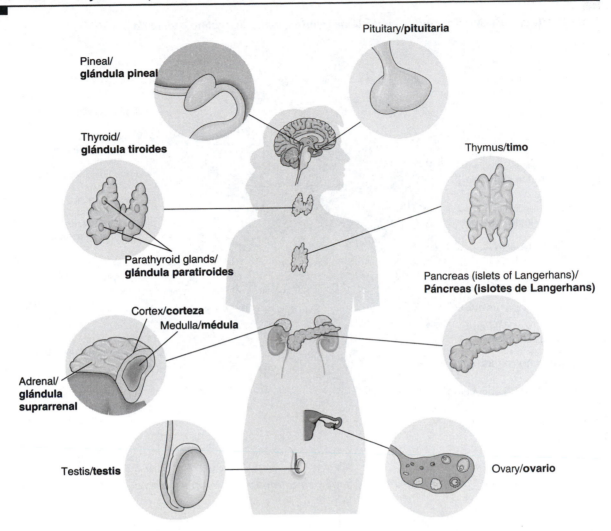

Pineal/
glándula pineal

Pituitary/**pituitaria**

Thyroid/
glándula tiroides

Thymus/**timo**

Parathyroid glands/
glándula paratiroides

Pancreas (islets of Langerhans)/
Páncreas (islotes de Langerhans)

Cortex/**corteza**
Medulla/**médula**

Adrenal/
glándula
suprarrenal

Testis/**testis**

Ovary/**ovario**

Posterior view/Vista posterior

Reproductive Organs *Organos reproductivos*

*Male Genitourinary System—Side View/***Sistema genitourinario masculino—vista de perfil**

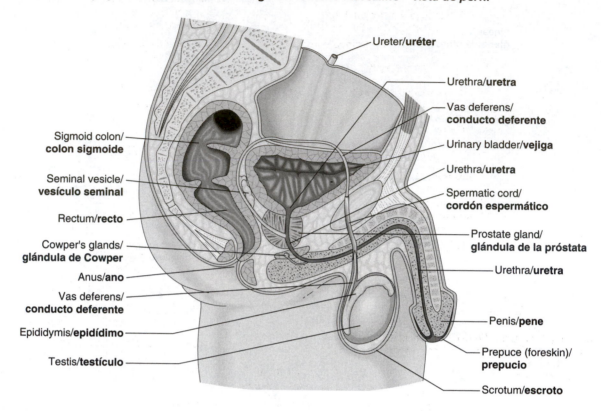

Ureter/**uréter**

Urethra/**uretra**

Vas deferens/
conducto deferente

Sigmoid colon/
colon sigmoide

Urinary bladder/**vejiga**

Urethra/**uretra**

Seminal vesicle/
vesículo seminal

Spermatic cord/
cordón espermático

Rectum/**recto**

Cowper's glands/
glándula de Cowper

Prostate gland/
glándula de la próstata

Urethra/**uretra**

Anus/**ano**

Vas deferens/
conducto deferente

Penis/**pene**

Epididymis/**epidídimo**

Testis/**testículo**

Prepuce (foreskin)/
prepucio

Scrotum/**escroto**

*Female Genitourinary System—Side View/***Sistema genitourinario femenino—vista de perfil**

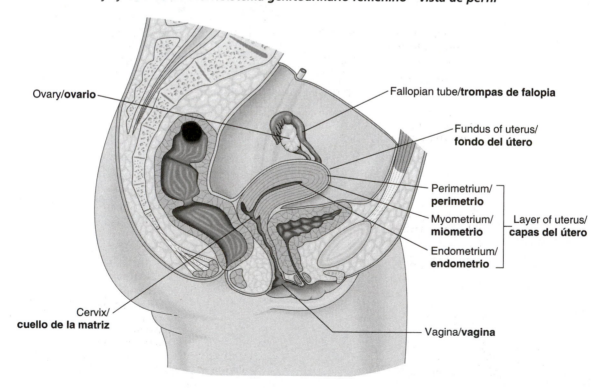

Ovary/**ovario**

Fallopian tube/**trompas de falopia**

Fundus of uterus/
fondo del útero

Perimetrium/
perimetrio

Myometrium/
miometrio

Layer of uterus/
capas del útero

Endometrium/
endometrio

Cervix/
cuello de la matriz

Vagina/**vagina**

Respiratory System   *Aparato o Sistema respiratorio*

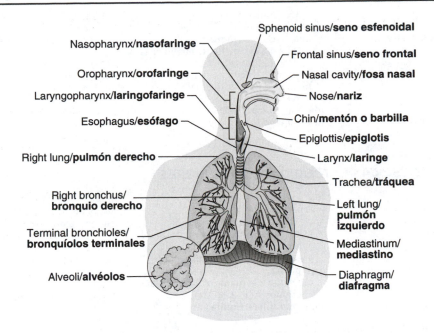

Nasopharynx/**nasofaringe**

Oropharynx/**orofaringe**

Laryngopharynx/**laringofaringe**

Esophagus/**esófago**

Right lung/**pulmón derecho**

Right bronchus/**bronquio derecho**

Terminal bronchioles/**bronquíolos terminales**

Alveoli/**alvéolos**

Sphenoid sinus/**seno esfenoidal**

Frontal sinus/**seno frontal**

Nasal cavity/**fosa nasal**

Nose/**nariz**

Chin/**mentón o barbilla**

Epiglottis/**epiglotis**

Larynx/**laringe**

Trachea/**tráquea**

Left lung/**pulmón izquierdo**

Mediastinum/**mediastino**

Diaphragm/**diafragma**

Urinary System   *Sistema urinario o Aparato urinario*

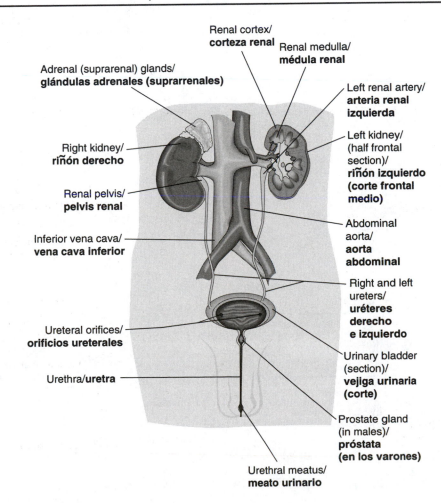

Renal cortex/**corteza renal**

Renal medulla/**médula renal**

Adrenal (suprarenal) glands/**glándulas adrenales (suprarrenales)**

Left renal artery/**arteria renal izquierda**

Right kidney/**riñón derecho**

Left kidney/ (half frontal section)/**riñón izquierdo (corte frontal medio)**

Renal pelvis/**pelvis renal**

Abdominal aorta/**aorta abdominal**

Inferior vena cava/**vena cava inferior**

Right and left ureters/**uréteres derecho e izquierdo**

Ureteral orifices/**orificios ureterales**

Urinary bladder (section)/**vejiga urinaria (corte)**

Urethra/**uretra**

Prostate gland (in males)/**próstata (en los varones)**

Urethral meatus/**meato urinario**

UPPER EXTREMITIES   *LAS EXTREMIDADES SUPERIORES*

arm   **brazo** *m*
  bend of the arm   **flexura del brazo** *f*
armpit   **sobaco** *m*; **axila** *f*; **arca**
  (*f*, Mex.)
biceps   **biceps** *m*; **conejo** (*m*, sg.
  Chicano); **mollero** (*m*, Cuba, Sp., *fam*
cuticle   **cutícula** *f*
elbow   **codo** *m*
finger   **dedo** *m*
  ball of thumb   **pulpejo** *m*
  fleshy tip of the finger   **yema** *f*

index   **índice** *m*
knuckle   **nudillo** *m*
little finger   **meñique** *m*
middle finger   **dedo del medio** *m*;
  dedo del corazón *m*
ring finger   **dedo anular** *m*
thumb   **pulgar** *m*; **dedo gordo** *m*
fist   **puño** *m*
forearm   **antebrazo** *m*
hand   **mano** *f*

back of the hand   **dorso de la mano**
  m
palm of the hand   **palma de la mano**
  f
humerus   **húmero** *m*
nail   **uña** *f*
phalanx   **falange** *f*
radius   **radio** *m*
ulna   **cúbito** *m*
wrist   **muñeca** *f*

LOWER EXTREMITIES   *LAS EXTREMIDADES INFERIORES*

ankle   **tobillo** *m*
big toe   **dedo grueso o gordo** *m*
bunion   **juanete** *m*
calcaneus   **calcáneo** *m*
callus   **callo** *m*
femur   **fémur** *m*
fibula   **peroné** *m*
foot   **pie** *m*
groin   **ingle** *f*; **empeine**[3] *m*
heel   **talón** *m*; **calcañar** *m*

hip   **cadera** *f*
instep   **empeine**[3] *m*
knee   **rodilla** *f*
  knee (back of the)   **corva** *f*; **flexura de
    la pierna** *f*
  kneecap   **rótula** *f*; **choquezuela** *f*
leg   **pierna** *f*
  calf of the leg   **pantorrilla** *f*; **canilla** *f*;
    chamorro (*m*, Chicano)
shin   **espinilla** *f*; **canilla** *f*

shinbone   **tibia** *f*
sole of the foot   **planta del pie** *f*
tendon   **tendón** *m*
thigh   **muslo** *m*
tibia   **tibia**
toe   **dedo (del pie)** *m*

Lateral View of the Adult Human Skeleton
Vista lateral del esqueleto humano adulto

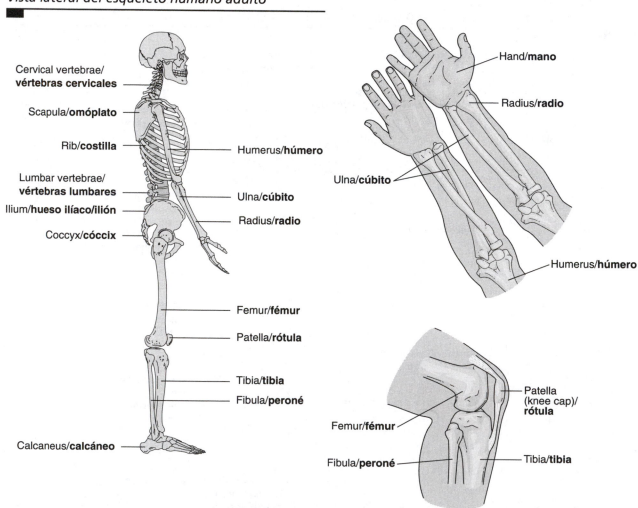

Cervical vertebrae/**vértebras cervicales**
Scapula/**omóplato**
Rib/**costilla**
Lumbar vertebrae/**vértebras lumbares**
Ilium/**hueso ilíaco/ilión**
Coccyx/**cóccix**
Calcaneus/**calcáneo**

Humerus/**húmero**
Ulna/**cúbito**
Radius/**radio**
Femur/**fémur**
Patella/**rótula**
Tibia/**tibia**
Fibula/**peroné**

Hand/**mano**
Radius/**radio**
Ulna/**cúbito**
Humerus/**húmero**

Femur/**fémur**
Fibula/**peroné**
Patella (knee cap)/**rótula**
Tibia/**tibia**

El cuerpo humano   *Vista posterior*

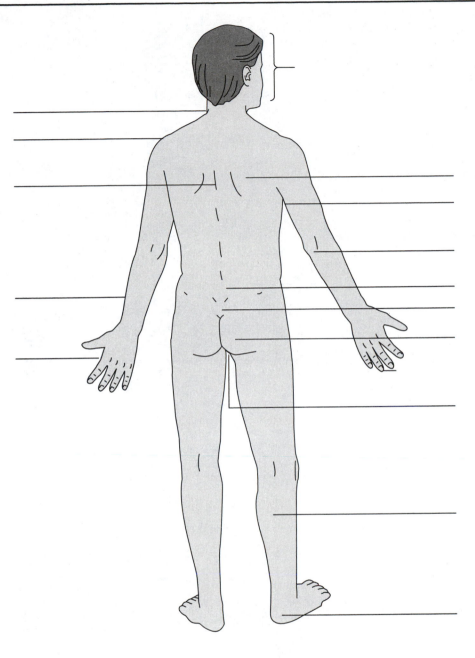

El cuerpo humano   *Vista anterior*

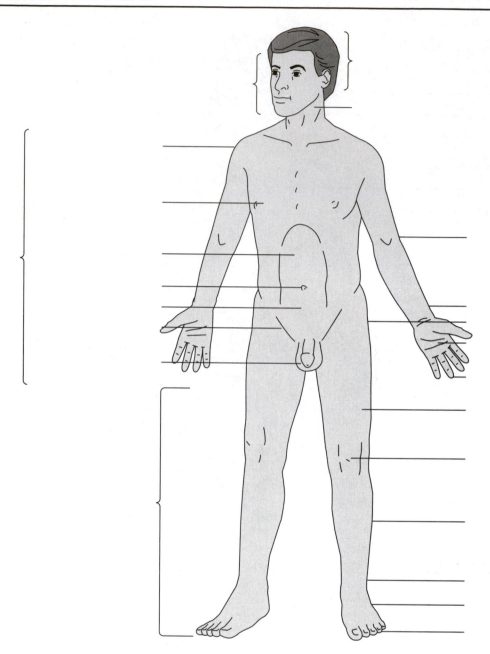

Identify the items on these diagrams.   **Ponga letreros en este esquema.**

A. _____   G. _____   M. _____   R. _____

B. _____   H. _____   N. _____   S. _____

C. _____   I. _____   O. _____   T. _____

D. _____   J. _____   P. _____   U. _____

E. _____   K. _____   Q. _____   V. _____

F. _____   L. _____

Partes de un ojo

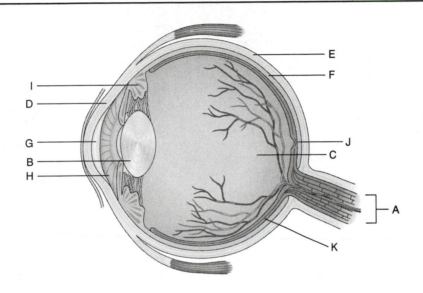

Partes de un oído

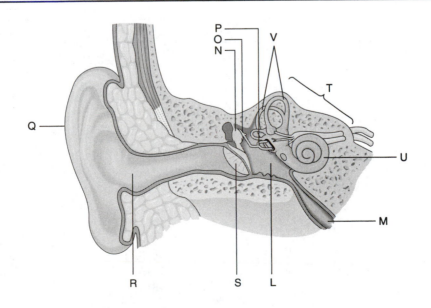

Los órganos internos

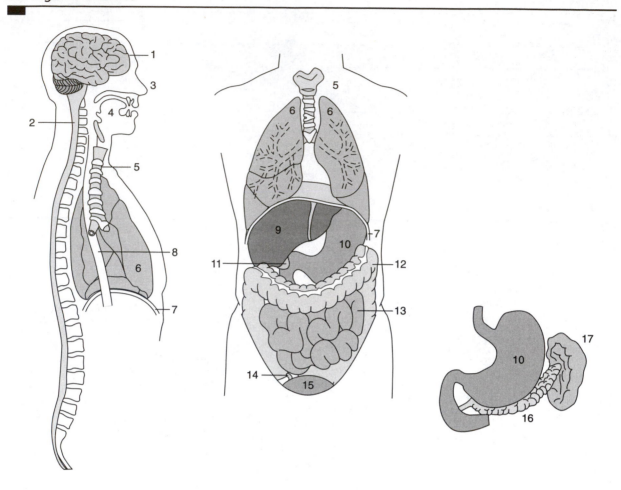

Identify the items on this diagram. **Ponga letreros en este esquema.**

1. _____   7. _____   13. _____

2. _____   8. _____   14. _____

3. _____   9. _____   15. _____

4. _____   10. _____   16._____

5. _____   11. _____   17. _____

6. _____   12. _____

Sistema digestivo

Identify the items on this diagram.   **Ponga letreros en este esquema**

A. _____

B. _____

C. _____

D. _____

E. _____

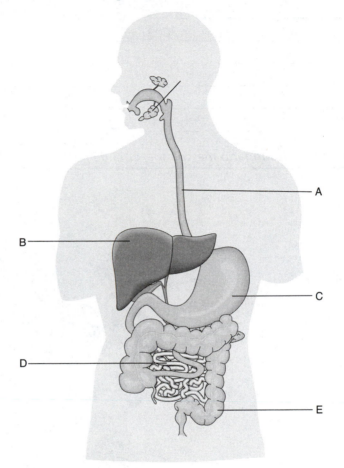

Organos reproductivos

Identify the items on this diagram.   **Ponga leteros en este esquema**

A. _____   G. _____   L. _____

B. _____   H. _____   M. _____

C. _____   I. _____   N. _____

D. _____   J. _____   O. _____

E. _____   K. _____   P. _____

F. _____

Sistema genitourinario masculino—vista de perfil

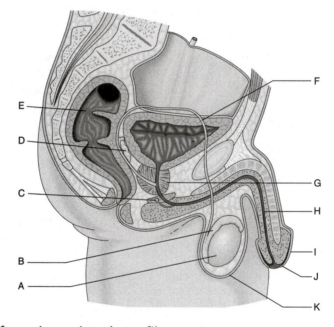

Sistema genitourinario femenino—vista de perfil

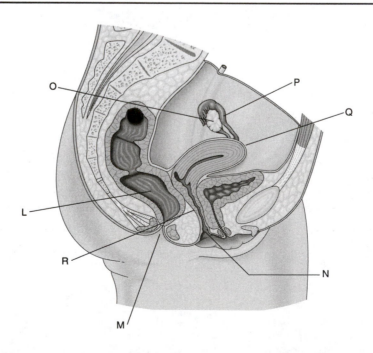

Estructuras de la boca

**Identify the Items on this Diagram/
Ponga letreros en este esquema**

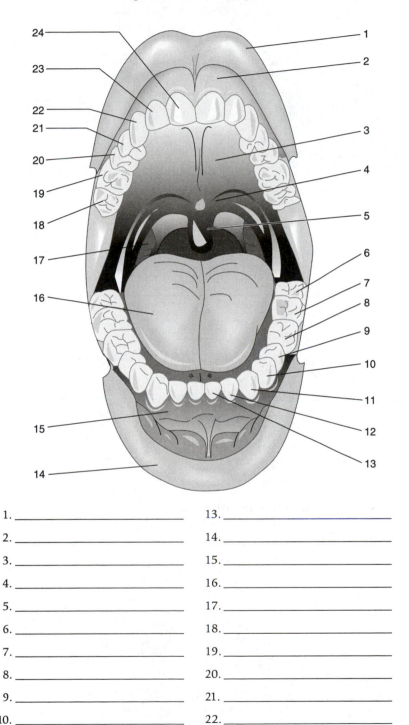

1. _____   13. _____

2. _____   14. _____

3. _____   15. _____

4. _____   16. _____

5. _____   17. _____

6. _____   18. _____

7. _____   19. _____

8. _____   20. _____

9. _____   21. _____

10. _____   22. _____

11. _____   23. _____

12. _____   24. _____

Partes de un diente

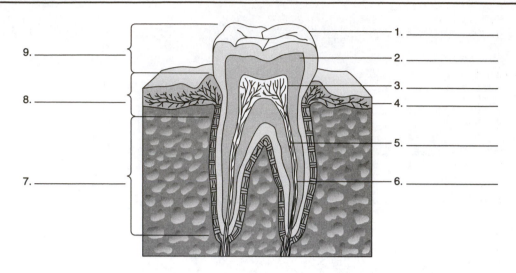

9. _____
8. _____
7. _____

1. _____
2. _____
3. _____
4. _____
5. _____
6. _____

La dentadura del adulto

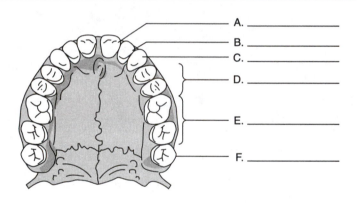

A. _____
B. _____
C. _____
D. _____
E. _____
F. _____

Los dientes de leche

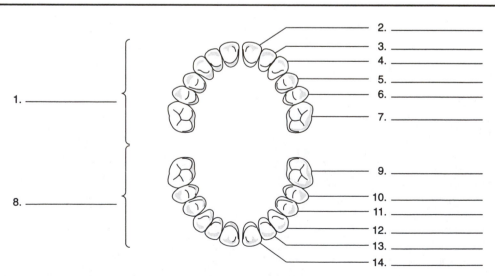

1. _____
8. _____

2. _____
3. _____
4. _____
5. _____
6. _____
7. _____
9. _____
10. _____
11. _____
12. _____
13. _____
14. _____

Spanish, like all languages of the world, has a wealth of *dichos, proverbios, y refranes* ("sayings, proverbs, and refrains"). These sayings and proverbs are one way that ethnic groups are able to maintain their heritage. These expressions are used almost exclusively in informal situations and are commonly heard. A small sampling of those that use anatomical vocabulary along with their comparative English version include:

De *la mano* a *la boca*, se pierde la sopa.
There's many a slip 'twixt the cup and the lip.

¡Ojo!
Careful! or Watch out!

Tengo la palabra en *la punta de la lengua*.
I have the word on the tip of my tongue.

Habla hasta por *los codos*.
(S)He runs off at the mouth.

Notes   *Notas*

1. In Spanish **canal** is an open duct, **conducto** is closed.
2. The plural of **nalga** is less polite.
3. Multiple meanings of **empeine** *m* include these and ringworm.

CHAPTER 4
CAPITULO

Numerical Expressions

Expresiones numéricas

NUMBERS
NUMEROS

CARDINALS *CARDINALES*

0	cero[1]	31	treinta y uno (un, una)
1	uno, un, una	32	treinta y dos, etc.
2	dos	40	cuarenta
3	tres	50	cincuenta
4	cuatro	60	sesenta
5	cinco	70	setenta
6	seis	80	ochenta
7	siete	90	noventa
8	ocho	100	ciento, cien
9	nueve	105	ciento cinco
10	diez	200	doscientos, -as
11	once	300	trescientos, -as
12	doce	400	cuatrocientos, -as
13	trece	500	quinientos, -as
14	catorce	600	seiscientos, -as
15	quince	700	setecientos, -as
16	dieciséis, diez y seis	800	ochocientos, -as
17	diecisiete, diez y siete	900	novecientos, -as
18	dieciocho, diez y ocho	999	novecientos noventa y nueve
19	diecinueve, diez y nueve	1.000[2]	mil
20	veinte	1.009	mil nueve
21	veintiuno, veintiún, veintiuna, veinte y uno, veinte y un, veinte y una	2.000	dos mil
		7.555	siete mil quinientos cincuenta y cinco
22	veintidós, veinte y dos	27.777	veintisiete mil setecientos setenta y siete
23	veintitrés, veinte y tres		
24	veinticuatro, veinte y cuatro		
25	veinticinco, etc.	100.000	cien mil
26	veintiséis	1.000.000	un millón
27	veintisiete	2.000.000	dos millones
28	veintiocho	4.196.234	cuatro millones ciento noventa y seis mil doscientos treinta y cuatro
29	veintinueve		
30	treinta	1.000.000.000	mil millones

In Spanish **un billón** is a million **millones**. To express 1.000.000.000 **mil millones** is used.

Cien is used in counting or before a noun. **Ciento** is used in compound numbers between 100 and 200. **Ciento** is *never* followed by the conjunction **y**

noventa y ocho, noventa y nueve, cien, ciento uno, etc.   No hay cien médicas aquí.

With the exception of *primero* (first), cardinal numbers and not ordinals are used in Spanish to express the days of the month.

el primero de diciembre December 1st *but:* **el dos de octubre** October 2nd **el diez de mayo** May 10th

Years are also expressed with cardinal numbers. Years in this century are expressed differently in Spanish than in English. They are *never* expressed as "nineteen ninety eight." In Spanish years are expressed as **mil** + **novecientos** + two-digit number.

1998 mil novecientos noventa y ocho Years in the next century will be expressed as **dos mil** + appropriate numbers.

2.005 **dos mil cinco**   2050 **dos mil cincuenta**

ORDINALS *ORDINALES[3]*

1st	primer(o), -a (1er, 1°, 1ª)	5th	quinto, -a (5°, 5ª)	8th	octavo, -a (8°, 8ª)
2nd	segundo, -a (2°, 2ª)	6th	sexto, -a (6°, 6ª)	9th	noveno, -a (9°, 9ª)
3rd	tercer(o), -a (3er, 3°, 3ª)	7th	séptimo, -a (7°, 7ª)	10th	décimo, -a (10°, 10ª)
4th	cuarto, -a (4°, 4ª)				

Ordinals above ten are rarely used; they are replaced by cardinals. When a cardinal is used for an ordinal, it is placed after the noun it modifies.

    segunda lección   second lesson   **lección doce**   twelfth lesson

In Spanish ordinal numbers do not occur with the same frequency as in English. Ordinal numbers when used as adjectives agree with the nouns they modify in gender. The formation of the feminine and the plural of ordinals is regular in Spanish.

    el segundo quirófano   the second operating room   **las segundas copias**   the second copies
    la segunda cirugía plástica   the second plastic surgery

Primero and **tercero** drop the **o** when they precede a masculine singular noun.

    el primer paciente }
    la primera paciente }   the first patient   **los primeros pacientes** }
                                                   las primeras pacientes }   the first patients

Primero and not a cardinal number is always used to express the first day of the month.

    May 1st   **el primero de mayo**

Spanish does not use ordinal numbers to designate centuries, unlike English.

    el siglo veinte   the twentieth century

Ordinal numbers are used to designate monarchs up to only ten.

    Alfonso sexto   Alfonso VI   **Isabel segunda**   Isabel II   *but:* **Alfonso trece**   Alfonso XIII

Aniversario is one noun, however, that always calls for an ordinal number.

    en el primer aniversario   on the first anniversary   **el octogésimo segundo aniversario**   the 82nd anniversary

POSITION OF NUMBERS   *POSICION DE LOS NUMEROS*

Cardinal numbers usually precede the noun. If they are used to substitute for ordinals, they follow.

    Operó quince horas.   He operated for 15 hours.
    Estuvo en la Unidad de Cuidado Intensivo tres días.   She was in ICU for three days.
    El quirófano está en el piso veintiuno del hospital.   The OR is on the twenty-first floor of the hospital.

Ordinal numbers may precede or follow the noun that they modify. Generally they follow when they indicate a member of a recognized series. Cardinal numbers may precede or follow ordinal numbers.

    Las tres primeras suturas }
    las primeras tres suturas }   the first three sutures

EXERCISES *EJERCICIOS*

A. Write the cardinal numbers in Spanish.

1. 1 _____ espéculo
2. 31 _____ baños de asiento
3. 16 _____ píldoras
4. 64 _____ cápsulas
5. 14 _____ aspirinas para niños
6. 3 _____ tobilleras
7. 50 _____ transfusiones de sangre
8. 21 _____ radiografías
9. 36 _____ onzas
10. 72 _____ vendas

B. Say the following in Spanish.

1. 2,000,000
2. 17,592
3. 8,653
4. 706
5. 911
6. 1492
7. 875
8. 1,812
9. $25
10. 2598
11. 1124
12. 100,400
13. 3,247
14. 449

C. Practice saying the following years in Spanish:

1. 1492
2. 1776
3. 1910
4. 1942
5. 1936
6. 1971
7. 1928
8. 1953
9. 1512
10. 2001

Países de mayor población hispana

1.	Méjico	85.950.000	6. Perú	23.450.000
2.	España	43.522.000	7. Venezuela	19.800.000
3.	Argentina	36.321.000	8. Chile	12.820.000
4.	Colombia	33.800.000	9. Cuba	11.950.000
5.	Estados Unidos	29.700.000	10. Ecuador	10.230.000

Using the information above, answer the following questions. Remember to put the numbers into Spanish.

1. ¿Cuántos habitantes (*inhabitants*) tiene Colombia?
2. ¿Cuál es la población de Méjico?
3. ¿Cuántos habitantes hispanos tienen los Estados Unidos?
4. ¿Cuántos millones de habitantes tiene Cuba?
5. ¿Cuántos habitantes tiene Venezuela?

Countries with greatest Hispanic population
Países de mayor población hispana

1.	Méjico	85.950.000		6.	Perú	23.450.000
2.	España	43.522.000		7.	Venezuela	19.800.000
3.	Argentina	36.321.000		8.	Chile	12.820.000
4.	Colombia	33.800.000		9.	Cuba	11.950.000
5.	Estados Unidos	28.300.000		10.	Ecuador	10.230.000

1. Read the population figures out loud until you are comfortable pronouncing the numbers.
2. Answer in Spanish:
   a. ¿Cuántos habitantes más tiene Argentina que Colombia?
   b. ¿Cuántos habitantes menos tiene Cuba que España?
   c. ¿Cuántos habitantes hispanos hay en los Estados Unidos?

Top Ten U.S. States by Hispanic Population (7.1996)
Los diez estados principales con población hispana

California	9.630.000	Florida	2.022.000
Texas	5.503.000	Illinois	1.136.000
New York	2.538.000		

1. Read these population numbers until you are comfortable.
2. Conteste:
   a. ¿Cuántos habitantes hispanos hay en Texas, Florida, e Illinois?
   b. ¿Cuántos habitantes hispanos tienen Illinois y Nueva York?
   c. ¿Cuántos habitantes hispanos hay en Nueva York y California?

AGE *LA EDAD*

To ask someone's age Spanish generally uses **¿Cuántos años tiene Vd.?** (literally, How many years do you have?) An alternative is to ask **¿Qué edad tiene Vd?** (What age do you have). Responses may be **Tengo veintiún años** or **Voy a cumplir veintiún.** (I'm going to be 21.)

How old is she? ¿Cuántos años tiene ella?   She is thirty years old.   **Ella tiene treinta años.**

Oral Practice

Answer the questions using the numbers as cues.

Model: ¿Cuántos años tiene él?   51
[El tiene] cincuenta y un años.

1. ¿Cuántos años tiene la enfermera? 27
2. ¿Cuántos años tiene el médico? 55
3. ¿Cuántos años tiene la paciente? 33
4. ¿Cuántos años tiene su dentista? 61
5. ¿Cuántos años tiene su esposa? 45
6. ¿Cuántos años tiene mi padre? 87
7. ¿Cuántos años tiene el paciente? 75
8. ¿Cuántos años tiene el especialista? 39
9. ¿Cuántos años tiene la higienista? 19
10. ¿Cuántos años tiene el camillero? 25

FRACTIONS *FRACCIONES*

½	**un medio (la mitad)**	⅔	**dos tercios**
⅓	**un tercio (la tercera parte)**	¾	**tres cuartos**
¼	**un cuarto (la cuarta parte)**	⅘	**cúatro quintos**

NOTE: The numerator of a fraction is a cardinal number. The denominators from ¼ to ¹⁄₁₀ are the corresponding ordinals. From ¹⁄₁₁ to ¹⁄₉₉, the denominators end in the suffix **-avo**, which is added to the cardinal after the final **e** or **a** has been dropped. There are two exceptions to the apocopation of the final **e**—**siete** and **nueve**.

²⁄₇ **dos siete*avo*s**   ¹⁄₁₉ **un diecinueve*avo***

The word **parte(s)** may be used to express all fractions higher than, and including, one-third.

⁴/₇ **las cuatro séptimas partes**

SYMBOLS *SIMBOLOS*

The equal symbol (=) is pronounced **es igual a.** The plus symbol (+) is pronounced **más.**

1/4 tablet = one quarter of a tablet/
1/4 pastilla = un cuarto o la cuarta
      parte de una pastilla

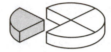
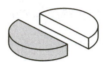

1 1/2 tablet = one and a half tablets/
1 1/2 pastilla = una pastilla y media

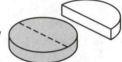

1/2 tablet = one half of a tablet/
1/2 pastilla = media pastilla

1/8 tablet = one eighth of a tablet/
1/8 pastilla = un octavo de una pastilla

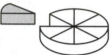

ARITHMETICAL SIGNS *OPERACIONES ARITMETICAS*

The signs +, ×, −, ÷, = are read respectively **más, por, menos, dividido por, igual a**

To Read	Para leer
2 + 2 = 4	dos **más** dos es igual a cuatro.
6 − 2 = 4	seis **menos** dos es igual a cuatro.
4 × 4 = 16	cuatro **por** cuatro es igual a dieciséis.
10 ÷ 2 = 5	diez **dividido por** dos es igual a cinco.

A. *Exercise:* Calculate the cost of the following.

   a. 4 bottles of cough syrup/15 pesos/bottle   c.   100 grams of aspirin/12 pesos/kilo
   b. ½ kilo of ointment/8¼ pesos/kilo   d.   200 grams of eyedrops/27 pesos/kilo

B. *Lea estas operaciones aritméticas*

   5 + 7 = 12   40 − 15 = 25   24 ÷ 8 = 3   12 × 12 = 144

DECIMALS *NUMEROS DECIMALES*

Fractions in the form of so many tenths (**décimas**) or hundredths (**centésimas**) or thousandths (**milésimas**) are called decimal fractions (**quebrados decimales**), from the Latin word for *ten.* The decimal point (**punto decimal**) marks off integers (units [**unidades**], tens [**decenas**], hundreds [**centenas**], etc.) from fractions (**fracciones decimales**).

   Additional decimal equivalents are:

ten thousandths **diezmilésimas**	ten millionths **diezmillonésimas**
hundred thousandths **cienmilésimas**	hundred millionths **cienmillonésimas**
millionths **millonésimas**	

   Spanish decimals are read in several ways. The number 12.435,678 can be expressed

12 unidades, 4 décimas, 3 centésimas, 5 milésimas, etc. or
12 unidades, 435,678 millonésimas or
12 unidades, 435 milésimas, 678 millonésimas

SOCIAL SECURITY NUMBERS *NUMEROS DEL SEGURO SOCIAL*

The nine digits in the social security numbers are expressed in Spanish according to the following breakdown:

   123-45-6789   **123-45-67-89** or   **ciento veintitrés, cuarenta y cinco, sesenta y siete, ochenta y nueve**

Some Spanish-speakers will express their social security number as: **1-2-3-45-6-7-8-9** or **uno, dos, tres, cuarenta y cinco, seis, siete, ocho, nueve.**

   Others prefer to use: **1-23-45-67-89** or **uno, veintitrés, cuarenta y cinco, sesenta y siete, ochenta y nueve.**

All ways are acceptable. Many speakers will insert **el** in front of the social security number.

Mi número de seguro social es *el* **tres treinta y dos dieciocho cero cero setenta.**

STREET ADDRESSES *SEÑAS DEL DOMICILIO*

Addresses in Spanish are given with the street number following the name of the street. Street direction is the last item mentioned:

651 West Main Avenue   **Avenida Main, número seiscientos cincuenta y uno, oeste**
street   **calle** *f*   boulevard   **paseo** *m*   lane   **callejuela** *f*

It is not uncommon, however, to hear the anglicism *la _____ Street.*

Trabajo en la Court Street.

When Spanish speakers give their apartment or office address, they always include the floor number and exact location of the apartment or office, i.e., fifth floor, apartment 12. Frequently the location is given with a direction such as *derecho* (*der.*) or *izquierdo* (*izq.*).

Office addresses are often given with the name of the building preceded by the Spanish word for building (*edificio* / *Edif.*) Floors of a building generally begin in Spanish-speaking countries with the *planta baja* or ground floor, so that the first floor above the street level is considered *el primer piso* / *1°*. Nonetheless, the floors of a house are numbered as in the U.S. which means that the ground floor in Spanish is *el primer piso* and the second floor is *el segundo piso.*

Zip codes are expressed by giving the first number separately and pairing the others. In a complete sentence the *el* is usually inserted before the number:

La zona postal es el 48503 (cuatro ochenta y cinco cero tres).

NOTE: When expressing either addresses, zip codes, telephone numbers, or area codes in Spanish, it is customary to group them in sets of twos after the initial number. (See example immediately above.) If a zero occurs at the beginning of any group of two numbers, Spanish-speakers will pronounce both numbers individually, using the written word *cero* for the zero.

TELEPHONE NUMBERS *NUMEROS DE TELEFONO*

Spanish-speakers living in the U.S. express their 7 digit telephone number in a variety of ways.
The first number is usually given separately, and the other numbers are grouped in twos:

762-3445 → 7-62-34-45

Some will insert the definite article before the number in a complete sentence:

Todavía es el 7-62-34-45 (siete sesenta y dos treinta y cuatro cuarenta y cinco).

Others have adopted the U.S. custom of expressing all digits as units numbers:

7-6-2-3-4-4-5   **(siete seis dos tres cuatro cuatro cinco)**

Area codes are generally expressed as a single number and a group of two:

847   **ocho cuarenta y siete**   212   **dos doce**

EXERCISES *EJERCICIOS*

Practice reading the following sentences aloud until you can express the numbers without hesitation:

1. **Mi número de seguro social es el 316-09-1167.**
2. **Su número de fax es el 732 3938.**
3. **Cambiaron** (they changed) **el código del área de 810 a 248.**
4. **Su número de seguro social es el 041 289116.**
5. **La zona postal es 60521.**

DIMENSIONS *LAS DIMENSIONES*

Dimension is expressed with **ser** or with **tener.** The nouns and adjectives needed to express dimension are:

Nouns		*Adjectives*	
la altura	height	**alto**	tall, high
la anchura	width	**ancho**	wide
la longitud	length	**largo**	long
la profundidad	depth	**profundo**	deep
el espesor	thickness	**grueso**	thick

How deep is the wound?	¿Cómo es de profunda la llaga?
How wide is the cyst?	¿De qué ancho es el lobanillo?

How long is the baby?

The baby is 50 centimeters long. ⎰ El nene tiene una longitud de cincuenta centímetros. El nene tiene cincuenta centímetros de largo.

CONVERSION

CONVERSION

FAHRENHEIT/CENTIGRADE   *FAHRENHEIT/CENTIGRADO*

32 degrees (**grados**) Fahrenheit (**Fahrenheit**) (F) = 0° centigrade (**centígrado**)
Each centigrade degree is equal to 1.8 Fahrenheit degrees.

To change degrees F to degrees C, subtract 32 and multiply by ⅝.

$(F - 32) \times ⅝ = C$

To change degrees C to degrees F, multiply by ⅘ and add 32.

$(C \times ⅘) + 32 = F$

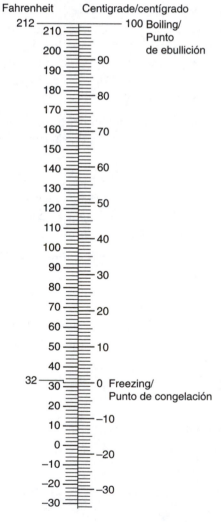

Fahrenheit	96°	97°	98°	98.6°	99°	100°	101°	102°	103°	104°	105°
Centigrade	35.6°	36.1°	36.7°	37°	37.2°	37.8°	38.3°	38.9°	39.4°	40°	40.6°

To Read   Para leer
20°   **Estamos a veinte grados.**
−5°   **Estamos a cinco grados bajo cero.**
2°   { **Estamos a dos grados sobre cero.**
         { **Estamos a dos grados por encima de cero.**
0°   **Estamos a cero grados.**

DECIMAL/METRIC   *DECIMAL/METRICO*

1 centimeter (**centímetro**) = .393 inches (**pulgadas**)   1 foot = .304 meters
1 inch = 2.54 centimeters   1 yard = .914 meters

$$1 \text{ meter (\textbf{metro})} = \begin{cases} 39.37 \text{ inches} \\ 3.28 \text{ feet (\textbf{pies})} \\ 1.903 \text{ yards (\textbf{yardas})} \end{cases}$$

1 kilometer (**kilómetro**) = .621 miles
1 mile (**milla**) = 1.609 kilometers
1 gram (**gramo**) = .035 ounces (**onzas**)

Centimeters/   Inches/
centímetros   Pulgadas

```
 0 ———— 0.0
 1 ————
        0.5
 2 ————
        1.0
 3 ————
 4 ———— 1.5
 5 ————
        2.0
 6 ————
        2.5
 7 ————
        3.0
 8 ————
 9 ———— 3.5
10 ————
        4.0
```

1 hectogram (**hectogramo**) = 3.53 ounces   1 pint = .473 liters
1 ounce = 28.35 grams   1 quart = .946 liters
                                                 1 gallon = 3.785 liters

$$1 \text{ kilogram (\textbf{kilo})} = \begin{cases} 2.204 \text{ pounds (\textbf{libras})} \\ 35.273 \text{ ounces} \end{cases}$$

1 pound = .453 kilograms (**kilogramos**)

$$1 \text{ liter (\textbf{litro})} = \begin{cases} 2.113 \text{ pints (\textbf{pintas})} \\ 1.056 \text{ quarts (\textbf{cuartos})} \\ .264 \text{ gallons (\textbf{galones})} \end{cases}$$

To Read   Para leer
½ l   **medio litro**
¼ kg   **cuarto kilo**
            un cuarto de kilo
¾ l   **tres cuartos de litro**
1½ kg   **un kilo y medio**

El niño enfermo mide 1.5 (**uno cincuenta/un metro cincuenta centímetros**)

de altura / estatura

El quirófano mide 7 × 4 m (**siete metros de largo por cuatro de ancho**).

El chófer de la ambulancia iba conduciendo a 90 km. (noventa kilómetros por hora)

EXERCISES *EJERCICIOS*

In the United States we are used to using a measuring system that is not used in other parts of the world. The metric system is the universally accepted system of measurement.

Length is perhaps the most familiar measure. The ruler is used to measure something. For Americans the yard is the most commonly used measure. The yard measurement does not exist in the metric system, nor do the foot or inch. The basic unit of measure in the metric system is the meter. It is called the basic unit because the metric systems of weight and volume are derived from the meter.

The meter can easily be divided into 100 or 1,000 equal parts: centimeters or millimeters. Since one part of 1,000 is called a millimeter (mm), then a metric ruler consists of 1,000 mm. Ten millimeters make up a centimeter. There are 100 centimeters (cm) in a meter (m).

1 m = 1,000 mm = 100 cm   10 mm = 1 cm

In the metric system volume is measured in liters. There is a similarity between the liter and the meter. The liter can also be divided into 1,000 equal parts (milliliter). Therefore, 1 liter = 1,000 ml.

Volume means the quantity of material that a cube can hold. The volume of a cube is measured by dividing the length, width, and height. If a 10 cm cube holds one liter in quantity (10 cm × 10 cm × 10 cm = 1,000 cc [cc = cubic centimeter]), 1 liter = 1,000 cc.

Just as a metric system of length and volume exists, so too there is one for weights. The kilo is the measure used to weigh materials in this system. It also can be divided into 1,000 equal parts, which are called grams (g).

The metric system is easier than the English system. It can easily be divided into hundreds or thousands, which can be reduced to decimals. Moreover, length, volume, and weight are related.

En los Estados Unidos nos hemos acostumbrado a usar un sistema de medidas que no se usa en otras partes del mundo. El sistema métrico es el sistema de medidas aceptado universalmente.

El largo es tal vez la medida más conocida. La regla se usa para medir algo. La medida más comúnmente usada es la yarda para los estadounidenses. La yarda no existe en el sistema métrico, tampoco el pie ni la pulgada. La unidad fundamental de medida en el sistema métrico es el metro. Se llama la unidad fundamental porque es del metro que se derivan los sistemas métricos de peso y volumen.

El metro se puede dividir fácilmente en 100 o 1000 partes iguales: centímetros o milímetros. Puesto que una parte de 1000 se denomina milímetro (mm), entonces una regla métrica consta de 1000 mm. Diez milímetros se agrupan en un centímetro. Hay 100 centímetros (cm) en un metro (m).

1 m = 1000 mm = 100 cm   10 mm = 1 cm

En el sistema métrico, el volumen se mide en litros. Existe una afinidad entre el litro y el metro. El litro también puede dividirse en 1000 partes iguales (mililitro). Por lo tanto, 1 litro = 1000 ml.

Volumen quiere decir la cantidad de material que un cubo puede contener. El volumen de un cubo se mide multiplicando la longitud y el ancho y el alto. Si un cubo de 10 cm contiene un litro en cantidad (10 cm × 10 cm × 10 cm = 1000 cc [cc = centímetro cúbico]), 1 litro = 1000 cc.

Así como existe un sistema métrico de longitud y volumen, de la misma manera existe uno para los pesos. El kilo es la medida que se usa para pesar materiales en este sistema. También se puede dividir en 1000 partes iguales llamadas gramos (g).

El sistema métrico es más fácil que el sistema inglés. Se puede dividir con facilidad en cientos o miles, los cuales se pueden reducir a décimos. Además, longitud, volumen y peso están relacionados entre sí.

A. Convert the following.

   1.   50 mm = _____ cm   2.   50 cm = _____ m   3.   75 mm = _____ cm   4.   500 mm = _____ m

B. Answer the following in Spanish.

   1.   **¿Cuántos cm hay en un pie?**   4.   **¿Cuál es la unidad básica de medida en la yarda?**
   2.   **¿Cuántos mm hay en un pie?**   5.   **¿Cuál es la unidad básica de medida en el metro?**
   3.   **¿Cuál es su altura en pies, metros, centímetros?**   6.   **¿Cuántas pulgadas hay en una yarda? ¿en un metro?**

C. Solve the following problems.

1. A man tells you that he is 185 centimeters tall (**ciento ochenta y cinco centímetros**). How tall is he in feet and inches? (conversion: 1 cm = .4 [.393] in.)
2. A woman says that her baby weighs 5 kilos (**cinco kilos**) now. How much does the baby weigh in pounds? (conversion: 1 k = 2 lb [2.204])
3. A man arrives at the hospital with a gash made by a knife that was about 8 centimeters long by 2 centimeters wide. How long and how wide was the knife? (conversion: 1 cm = .4 in.)
4. A woman says that she cannot walk more than 30 meters before she begins to have trouble breathing. How many feet can she walk? (conversion: 1 m = 3 ft [3.28])

Medicines are packaged by weight—in grams (**gramos[g]**) and milligrams (**miligramos[mg]**). 1,000 mg = 1 g (**mil miligramos es igual a un gramo**). 1 mg = .001 g = 1/1,000 g (**un miligramo es una milésima de un gramo**). In some countries medicines are still weighed in grains (**grano[gn]**). 1 gn = 65 mg.

EXERCISES *EJERCICIOS*

1. Convert the following according to the model.
   How many mg does a 5 gn aspirin contain? (conversion: 1 gn = 65 mg)
   How many mg = 0.5 g? (conversion: 1 g = 1,000 mg)
2. Terramycin comes in capsules (**cápsulas**) of 50 mg, 100 mg, and 250 mg doses. Convert to 50 mg and 100 mg doses an R$_x$ that reads: **Tome Terramicina, 4 cápsulas de 250 mg diarias.**

TELLING TIME

LA HORA

For medical purposes it is often necessary to record a precise time. Depending on their country of origin, Spanish-speakers will write the actual hour in one of the following ways:
10.25 / 10,25 / 10'25 / 10:25.

NOTES ON TELLING TIME *OBSERVACIONES ACERCA DE LA HORA*

The verb **ser** is always used in telling time. The singular verb **es** is used to express one o'clock; from two o'clock on, the plural verb **son** is used.

> It's one o'clock.   Es la una.   It's three o'clock.   Son las tres.

Note that the definite article **la** stands for **la hora**, and **las** stands for **las horas**. These definite articles are loosely translated as *o'clock*.

Spanish **y** loosely expresses the English of *past* or *after*. **Menos** approximates *to* or *till*. **El mediodía** is the equivalent of *noon*; **la medianoche** is the equivalent of *midnight*.

To express time from the hour to the half hour, minutes are added to the hour by **y**. When the number of minutes past the hour is greater than thirty, minutes are subtracted from the next hour, using the word **menos**. Thus, "six thirty-eight" becomes "seven minus twenty-two."

It's four ten.		It's five fifty five.	
It's ten past four.	**Son las cuatro y diez.**	It's five to six.	**Son las seis menos cinco.**
It's ten after four.		It's five till six.	

Remember that from 12:31 to 1:30 singular verb **es** and the article **la** are used.

The Spanish **cuarto** and **media** approximate the English quarter and half. **Media** (½) is a feminine adjective that agrees with the understood **hora**; **cuarto** (¼) is a masculine noun and therefore does not have to agree in gender with **hora**.

> It's half past four.   **Son las cuatro y media.**
> It's a quarter after four.   **Son las cuatro y cuarto.**
> It's a quarter to four.   **Son las cuatro menos cuarto.**

Numbers can be substituted for the expressions **cuarto** and **media**.

> It's a quarter after four.   **Son las cuatro y quince.**
> It's four fifteen.
> It's four thirty.   **Son las cuatro y media.**

Colloquially it is acceptable to say **"Faltan diez para las diez"** instead of **"Son las diez menos diez."**
Asking the time in Spanish closely resembles English except that the word *hour* is substituted for the word *time*. The question always uses a singular verb.

What time is it?   **¿Qué hora es?**

To ask at what time an event occurs, use **¿A qué hora . . . ?** To answer use **a** + **la(s)** + time.

I leave at one o'clock.   **Salgo a la una.**

When making appointments, it is polite to ask if a specific time is convenient. Use **¿ Le conviene + a + time?** (literally "Is it good for you at + *time?*) In order to respond only the indirect object pronoun needs to be changed since the subject, the appointment at a specific hour, has not changed.

Is 10:15 convenient?   **¿Le conviene a las diez y cuarto?**
Ten fifteen is good for me.   **Me conviene a las diez y cuarto.**

The Spanish "day" is divided into **mañana** (from sunrise to noon), **tarde** (from noon to sunset), **noche** (from sunset to midnight), **madrugada** (from midnight to sunrise). When the hour is specified, **de** must be used to translate *in* and *at* in the expressions **de la mañana,** and so on. When there is no definite hour specified, **por** is used for *in* or *at:* **por la mañana** (in the morning), **por la tarde** (in the afternoon, evening), and **por la noche** (in the evening, at night).

He is operating at 6:30 A.M.   **Opera a las seis de la madrugada.**
He operates in the (early) morning.   **Opera por la madrugada.**

Official time in Spain and other Spanish-speaking countries is expressed on a 24-hour basis. This applies to radio, television, train, and airline schedules among other things. To figure out the equivalent time after 12 noon and before midnight (P.M.) you would need to subtract 12 hours. Thus, **las diecinueve** is 7:00 P.M., **las veintitrés** is 11:00 P.M.

One o'clock is good for me.   **Me conviene a las trece de la tarde.**
22:45 = **las once menos cuarto**

FURTHER EXAMPLES   *EJEMPLOS ADICIONALES*

1. What time is it?
   ¿Qué hora es?
   ¿Qué horas son? (Sp. Am.)

2. Do you know what time it is?
   ¿Sabe usted la hora?

3. I cannot say because I haven't any watch.
   No puedo decir porque no tengo reloj.

4. It is one o'clock.
   Es la una.

5. It is two o'clock.
   Son las dos.

6. It is three o'clock.
   Son las tres.

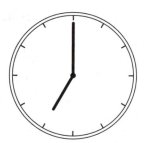

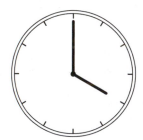

7. **Son las cuatro.**
8. It is five o'clock.
   Son las cinco.
9. It is six o'clock.
   Son las seis.

10. **Son las siete.**
11. It is eight o'clock.
    Son las ocho.
12. It is nine o'clock.
    Son las nueve.
13. It is ten o'clock.
    Son las diez.
14. It is eleven o'clock.
    Son las once.

15. **Son las doce.**

16. It is one thirty.
    Es la una y media.

17. It is 4:30.
    Son las cuatro y media.

18. It is 11:30.
    Son las once y media.

19. It is 1:15.
    Es la una y cuarto.

20. It is 2:15.
    Son las dos y cuarto.

21. It is 2:10.
    Son las dos y diez.

22. It is 11:10.
    Son las once y diez.

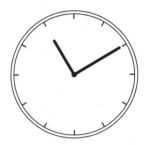

23. It is 10:10 P.M.
    Son las veintidós y diez.

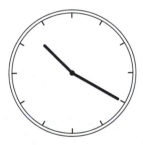

24. **Son las diez y veinte.**
25. It is 12:05.
    Son las doce y cinco.

26. It is 2:45.
    Son las tres menos cuarto.

27. **Son las ocho menos cuarto.**

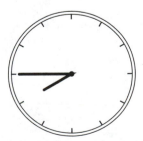

28. **Son las diez menos cuarto.**

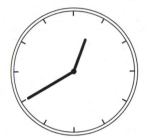

29. It is 6:55. (It is five to seven.)
    Son las siete menos cinco.

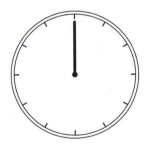

30. **Es la una menos veinte.**
31. It is 6 A.M.
    Son las seis de la mañana.

32. It is 5 P.M. (in the afternoon).
    Son las cinco de la tarde.

33. It is 8 P.M. (in the evening).
    Son las ocho de la noche.

34. It is exactly three o'clock.
    Son las tres en punto.

35. It is approximately nine.
    Son las nueve, más o menos.

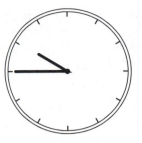

36. It is noon.
    Es mediodía.

37. It is midnight.
    Es medianoche.

38. At 3:00.
    A las tres.

39. At 5:05.
    A las cinco y cinco.

40. At 12:50 (at ten to one).
    A la una menos diez.

41. My watch is slow.
    Mi reloj se atrasa.

42. My watch is fast.
   Mi reloj se adelanta.

43. My watch has stopped.
   Mi reloj se ha parado.

44. My watch is 8 minutes slow.
   Mi reloj se atrasa 8 minutos.

45. My watch is 5 minutes fast.
   Mi reloj se adelanta cinco minutos.

PRACTICE   *PRACTICA*

¿Qué hora es?

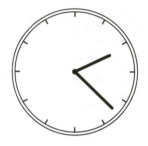

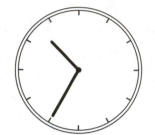

_____

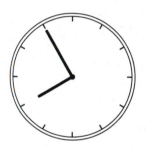

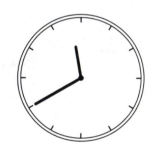

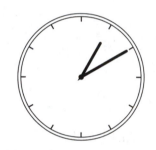

_____

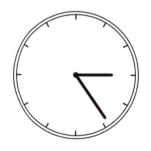

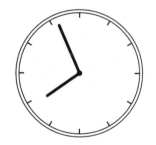

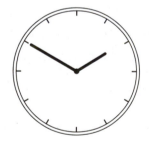

_____

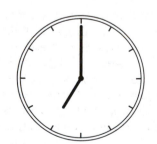

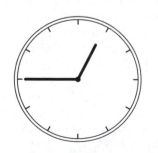

_____

Write out these times in Spanish.

1. 2:15 P.M.	5. 6:17 P.M.	9. 4:27 A.M.	13. 5:38 P.M.
2. 7:42 A.M.	6. 8:18 A.M.	10. 7:55 P.M.	14. 12:20 P.M.
3. 1:19 P.M.	7. 10:30 P.M.	11. 3:14 A.M.	15. 11:39 A.M.
4. 12:48 A.M.	8. Midnight	12. 9:50 A.M.	

ADDITIONAL EXPRESSIONS OF TIME   *MAS EXPRESIONES HORARIAS*

a short while ago   **hace poco**
a week from today   **de hoy en ocho**
after meals   **después de comer**
as of now   **por ahora**
at bedtime   **al acostarse**
at the same time   **a la vez**
before meals   **antes de comer**
by that date   **para esa fecha**
by then   **para entonces**
constantly   **constantemente**
daily   **diario**
during the day   **durante el día**
early   **temprano**
every hour   **(a) cada hora**
every other day   **cada dos días**
every hour   **(a) cada hora**
first time   **primera vez**
for how long?   **¿por cuánto tiempo?**
for many years   **por muchos años**
for the time being   **por ahora**
four a day   **cuatro veces al día**
from time to time   **de vez en cuando**
how many times?   **¿cuántas veces?**

how often?   **¿cada cuánto (tiempo)?,
¿con qué frecuencia?**
immediately, at once   **en seguida**
in a few minutes, shortly   **dentro de
poco**
last time   **última vez**
late   **tarde**
lately   **últimamente**
minute   **minuto**
moment   **momento**
month   **mes**
monthly   **mensual, mensualmente**
next month   **el mes que viene**
next week   **la semana que viene**
next year   **el año que viene**
now   **ahora**
occasionally   **a veces**
often   **a menudo, seguido** *Mex.*
on time   **a tiempo**
once   **una vez**
once a day   **una vez al día**
per day   **al (por) día**
per month   **al (por) mes**

per week   **a (por) la semana**
second   **segundo**
since when?   **¿desde cuándo?**
the day after tomorrow   **pasado
mañana**
the day before yesterday   **anteayer,
antier** *Mex.*
three a day   **tres veces al día**
today   **hoy**
tomorrow   **mañana**
tonight   **esta noche**
twice a day   **dos veces al día**
two weeks from today   **de hoy en
quince**
upon getting up   **al levantarse**
upon waking up   **al despertarse**
week   **semana**
weekly   **semanal**
year   **año**
year round   **todo el año**
yearly   **anual, anualmente**
yesterday   **ayer**

THE CALENDAR

EL CALENDARIO

In Spanish calendars begin the week with Monday rather than Sunday.

DAYS OF THE WEEK   *LOS DIAS DE LA SEMANA*

Monday   **el lunes**
Tuesday   **el martes**
Wednesday   **el miércoles**

Thursday   **el jueves**
Friday   **el viernes**

Saturday   **el sábado**
Sunday   **el domingo**

SEASONS   *LAS ESTACIONES*

spring   **la primavera**   summer   **el verano**   autumn   **el otoño**   winter   **el invierno**

In much of Hispanic America, from Guatemala through Peru, there are no seasons of hot and cold since summer and winter depend on altitude. Countries that are located close to the equator do not have the variation of seasons that countries farther away from the equator have. The equator passes through northern Ecuador, giving that country its name, southern Colombia, and northern Brazil. In the countries closest to the equator there are typically two seasons. In those countries each season lasts about six months. The dry season, often referred to as "summer" or *verano*, is called *la época seca*; the rainy season, also called *invierno*, "winter," is *la época de lluvia*. Peru, Bolivia, Paraguay, Chile, Argentina, Uruguay, and most of Brazil, all located south of the equator, have four distinct seasons as does the United States, but in a pattern that is the opposite of the seasons in the United States. In Puerto Rico, for example, there are only two seasons—rainy and dry—and the weather (hurricanes, storms, drought, or rain) is responsible for the major climatic changes.

MONTHS OF THE YEAR   *LOS MESES DEL AÑO*

January **enero**	May **mayo**	September **septiembre**
February **febrero**	June **junio**	October **octubre**
March **marzo**	July **julio**	November **noviembre**
April **abril**	August **agosto**	December **diciembre**

Observe that in Spanish the months, seasons, and days of the week are not capitalized. The masculine definite article is used with the days of the week except when the days of the week are preceded by the adjectives **cada, muchos, pocos,** by any number, or by the verb **ser.** When the English *on* is expressed or implied before a day of the week or month, the definite article **el** (or **los**) is used.

on Saturday   **el sábado**   on Wednesdays   **los miércoles**   on April 23   **el veintitrés de abril**

In expressing dates, **primero** is used for the first day of the month. All other days of the month are counted in Spanish by the cardinal numbers, preceded by the definite article. The month and year, when expressed, are connected with the date by the preposition **de:**

on April 1   **el primero de abril**
January 7, 1970   **el siete de enero de mil novecientos setenta**
December 29, 1999   **el veintinueve de diciembre de mil novecientos noventa y nueve**
July 4, 2000   **el cuatro de julio de dos mil**

When the month is omitted, it is common to place the word **día,** day, before the number.

Today is the 23rd.   **Hoy es el día veintitrés.**

There are several ways to ask the day of the month. All are acceptable. When answering, the response should use the same terms as the question.

	¿A cuánto(s) estamos?
	¿Cuál es la fecha?
	¿Qué fecha tenemos?
What day of the month is it?	**¿Qué día del mes tenemos?**
	¿Qué día del mes es hoy?
	¿A qué fecha estamos?
	¿A qué día del mes estamos?
	Hoy es el veintitrés de abril.
(Today) It is the 23rd of April.	**Tenemos el veintitrés de abril.**
	Estamos a veintitrés de abril.

MORE CALENDAR VOCABULARY   *MAS VOCABULARIO DEL CALENDARIO*

birthday **cumpleaños** *m, inv*
calendar **calendario** *m*
century **siglo** *m*
date **fecha** *f*
day **día** *m*
daylight **luz del día** *f*
eve **víspera** *f*
fortnight **quincena** *f*
holiday **fiesta** *f;* **día de fiesta** *m;* **día festivo** *m*
April Fools Day **el día de los Inocentes**[5]
Christmas **Navidad** *f*
Christmas Eve **Nochebuena** *f*
Columbus Day **el día de la Raza**
Easter **pascua de resurrección** *f,* **pascua florida** *f,* **pascua de flores** *f;*

día de la coneja (*m,* Chicano)
Friday the 13th **martes el trece**[6]
Independence Day (USA) **día de la independencia** *m*
Labor Day (USA) **día del trabajo** *m*
Memorial Day (USA) **día (de recordación) de los caídos** *m*
New Year's Eve **Nochevieja, víspera de año nuevo** *f*
Pentecost **pascua del espíritu santo** *f,* **pascua de Pentecostés** *f*
hour, time **hora** *f*
daylight saving time **hora de verano** *f*
standard time **hora legal** *f,* **hora normal** *f*

minute **minuto** *m*
midnight **medianoche** *f*
month **mes** *m*
noon **mediodía** *m*
week **semana** *f*
weekend **fin de semana** *m*
workday **día de trabajo** *m,* **día laborable** *m*
saint's day **(día del) santo** *m*
year **año** *m*
fiscal year **año económico** *m*
leap year **año bisiesto** *m*
school year **año escolar** *m,* **año lectivo** *m*

It is interesting to note that Spanish-speakers, when using numerals to express the date, will generally use one of the following styles:

20/VII/99
20 de julio de 1999
20/7/99

Care must be taken to always remember that the middle number, whether expressed in Roman numerals or cardinal numbers, always refers to the month of the year, not the day.

SPANISH ADAGE *UN REFRAN ESPAÑOL*

Treinta días tiene noviembre,
con abril, junio y septiembre;
veintiocho tiene uno,
y los demás treinta y uno.

EXERCISES *EJERCICIOS*

A. Translate the following into Spanish.

1. Conchita was born February 17, 1973.
2. The operation is going to cost $985.
3. At what time does the technician arrive here?
4. It is 3:45 P.M., November 29, 1982.
5. Two hundred children are sick today.
6. They operate at 6:30 A.M.
7. We do not work on Wednesdays.
8. She goes to the laboratory every Saturday.
9. The baby always has a cold in the winter.
10. I have an appointment with my doctor every Tuesday morning at the clinic during the summer.

B. Answer in Spanish.

1. ¿Qué día es hoy? (Hoy es lunes, etc. . . .)
2. ¿Qué día es mañana?
3. ¿Qué día fue (was) ayer?
4. Si hoy es lunes, ¿qué día es mañana? (Si hoy es lunes, mañana es . . .)
5. Si hoy es lunes, ¿qué día fue ayer?
6. Si hoy es jueves, ¿qué día es mañana?
7. Si hoy es miércoles, ¿qué día fue ayer?
8. Si hoy es martes, ¿qué día es pasado mañana?
9. Si hoy es martes, ¿qué día fue anteayer?
10. Si hoy es domingo, ¿qué día es pasado mañana?
11. ¿Cuáles son (Which are) los meses de la primavera? ¿del verano? ¿del otoño? ¿del invierno?
12. ¿En qué mes estamos ahora?
13. ¿Cuál es la fecha de hoy?
14. ¿En qué mes celebramos (do we celebrate) la Navidad? ¿La independencia de los Estados Unidos (United States)?
15. ¿En qué mes tiene Vd. su cumpleaños (do you have your birthday)? (Tengo mi cumpleaños en . . .)

C. With a partner ask and answer the following questions in Spanish.

1. ¿Qué mes tiene 28 días?
2. ¿Cuáles son los meses que tienen 30 días?
3. ¿Cuáles son los meses que tienen 31 días?
4. ¿Cuáles son dos meses del verano?
5. ¿Cuál es un mes de la primavera?
6. ¿Cuál es un mes del invierno que tiene 31 días?
7. ¿Cuál es un mes del otoño que tiene 30 días.
8. ¿En qué mes es su cumpleaños?

D. Item substitution:

1. **La farmacia está cerrada los sábados.** (The pharmacy is closed on Saturdays.)
2. _____ domingos.
3. _____ días de fiesta.
4. _____ abierta (open) _____ .
5. _____ todos los días.
6. **La clínica** _____ .

E. Fill in the grid with the name of the season that occurs in the countries listed during the months indicated. You may find it helpful to refer to the map of the Americas on page 358.

		Primavera Verano Otoño Invierno
País	**Mes**	**Estación**
Argentina	julio	
Bolivia	agosto	
Illinois	diciembre	
Paraguay	abril	
Chile	febrero	
Uruguay	septiembre	
Ecuador	junio	
Venezuela	marzo	
Honduras	enero	
Colombia	octubre	
Perú	mayo	
Nueva York	noviembre	

Notes *Notas*

1. To avoid confusion with *cero,* the conjunction **o** ("or") has a written accent mark on it when the conjunction occurs between two numbers: i.e., **7 ó 9 siete ó nueve**

2. Note that in Spanish a period is used to punctuate thousands; a comma is used as a decimal point.

3. Ordinal numbers do exist for *11th* to *100th.* These are for reference use only. (11th   **undécimo, -a;** 12th   **duodécimo, -a;** 13th **décimo tercero, -a;** 14th   **décimo cuarto, -a;** 15th   **décimo quinto, -a;** 20th   **vigésimo, -a;** 30th   **trigésimo, -a;** 40th **cuadragésimo, -a;** 50th **quincuagésimo, -a;** 60th   **sexagésimo, -a;** 70th   **septuagésimo, -a;** 80th   **octogésimo, -a;** 90th **nonagésimo, -a;** 100th   **centésimo, -a).**

4. In Spain this is December 28th.

5. In the U.S. Friday the 13th is often considered a day when bad luck may happen. In Hispanic countries, however, the bad luck is associated with Tuesday the 13th. Hence, the expression *"Martes, ni te cases, ni te embarques, ni de la casa te apartes."* (On Tuesdays, don't get married, don't take a trip, and don't leave your home.)

CHAPTER 5

Conversations for Administrative Personnel

Conversaciones para personal administrativo

GENERAL QUESTIONS

PREGUNTAS GENERALES

1. Hello. May I help you?
   Hola. ¿En qué puedo servirle (servirla)?*

2. What is your name?
   ¿Cómo se llama usted?

3. Do you speak any English?
   ¿Habla usted algo en inglés?

4. Can you understand what I am saying?
   ¿Puede usted comprender lo que digo?

5. My Spanish is not very good yet.
   Mi español no es perfecto todavía.

6. I can say some words in Spanish.
   Puedo decir algunas palabras en español.

7. Please try to speak slowly when you answer me.
   Favor de tratar de responder despacio al contestarme.
   Por favor, trate de responder despacio cuando me conteste.

8. I probably will not understand what you are saying.
   Probablemente no voy a comprender lo que usted dice.

9. Tell me more slowly, please.
   Dígamelo más despacio, por favor.

10. May I practice speaking Spanish with you?
    Puedo practicar mi español con usted?

11. Are you in good health?
    ¿Tiene usted buena salud?

12. Are you having any problems with your general health?
    ¿Tiene usted algún problema con su salud en general?

13. Do you feel okay generally?
    ¿Se siente bien en general?

14. Are you under any doctor's care?
    ¿Está usted en tratamiento con algún médico/alguna médica?
    ¿Recibe usted tratamiento de cualquier médico (médica)?

15. I'm sorry. I don't understand you.
    Lo siento. No le comprendo.

16. Would you repeat that slowly, please?
    ¿Puede usted repetirlo despacio?

17. Thank you.
    Gracias.

18. What is your doctor's name?
    ¿Cómo se llama su médico (médica)?

19. Do you have any heart problems?
    ¿Padece usted de problemas cardíacos?
    ¿Sufre usted de problemas cardíacos?

20. Do you have . . .?
    ¿Padece usted de . . .?   ¿Sufre usted de . . .?
    asthma?   diabetes?   epilepsy?
    ¿asma?   ¿diabetes?   ¿epilepsia?

In Spanish, the direct object pronoun for the English words "him" or "you" *m* may be either **le,** which is preferred in Spain, or **lo,** which is more common in Spanish America. The English plural, "them," when it is masculine, may be either **les,** preferred in Spain, or **los,** more common in Spanish America. These forms are all correct and understood by all. Although not as common in the United States, **le** and **les** will be used throughout this work as the masculine direct object pronouns referring to people.

---

*Feminine alternatives are listed in parenthesis throughout the book.

21. Are you allergic to any medications?
     ¿Es usted alérgico (alérgica) a algún medicamento?
     | Aspirin? | Codeine? | Penicillin? | Sulfa? |
     | **¿Aspirina?** | **¿Codeína?** | **¿Penicilina?** | **¿Sulfa?** |

22. Have you ever had an unusual or allergic reaction to any medicine or drug?
     ¿Ha tenido alguna vez una reacción extraordinaria o alérgica a alguna medicina o droga?

23. I want you to fill out this health form questionnaire.
     Necesito que usted llene este cuestionario de salud.

24. Do you have someone who can drive you home?
     ¿Le acompaña alguien que le lleve a casa?

25. Come with me.
     Venga conmigo.

PAYMENT AND INSURANCE

PAGOS Y SEGUROS

1. I have to ask you some questions.
    Tengo que hacerle algunas preguntas.

2. Please answer only "yes," "no," or "I don't know" to the questions if possible.
    Por favor, conteste a las preguntas solo con <<si,>> <<no,>> o <<no sé>> si es posible.

3. Do you have any dental insurance?
    ¿Tiene usted algún tipo de seguro dental?

4. May I see the card?
    ¿Puedo ver la tarjeta?

5. Do you have a Medicare Card?
    ¿Tiene usted la tarjeta de Medicare?

6. May I see it?
    ¿Puedo verla?

7. Will you pay for this yourself?
    ¿Pagará esto usted mismo?

8. What is your profession / occupation?
    ¿Cuál es su profesión / trabajo / (ocupación)?

9. Where do you work?
    ¿Dónde trabaja usted?

10. This will cost _____ dollars.
    Esto le costará _____ dólares.

    | 20 twenty | **veinte** | 300 three hundred | **trescientos** |
    | 30 thirty | **treinta** | 400 four hundred | **cuatrocientos** |
    | 40 forty | **cuarenta** | 500 five hundred | **quinientos** |
    | 50 fifty | **cincuenta** | 600 six hundred | **seiscientos** |
    | 60 sixty | **sesenta** | 700 seven hundred | **setecientos** |
    | 70 seventy | **setenta** | 800 eight hundred | **ochocientos** |
    | 80 eighty | **ochenta** | 900 nine hundred | **novecientos** |
    | 90 ninety | **noventa** | 1,000 one thousand | **mil** |
    | 100 one hundred | **cien** | 2,000 two thousand | **dos mil** |
    | 200 two hundred | **doscientos** | 3,000[1] three thousand | **tres mil** |

11. We can make a payment plan.
    Podemos arreglar un plan de pago.

12. You have to pay half before we start.
    Usted tiene que pagar la mitad por anticipado.

13. You have to pay _____ before we start.
    Usted tiene que pagar _____ antes de que podamos empezar.
    | 1/3 one third | **la tercera parte / un tercio** |
    | 1/4[2] one fourth | **la cuarta parte / un cuarto** |

REPORT FOR BLUE CROSS/BLUE SHIELD

1. Admitting Date _____

2. Patient's Complete Name _____

3. Blue Cross Certificate Number _____

The following questions must be answered for all claims which may be "work related" in order for Blue Cross to determine eligible benefits. Thank you for cooperating.

4. Was the condition which required hospital care caused by your employment? If yes, answer only questions 5 through 9.

5. Are you entitled to Workmen's Compensation benefits for the disability?

6. Give reason:_____

7. Briefly explain in what way condition was caused by employment.

8. If you are employed, give the following information:
    What is the name of your employer?_____
    What is his address?_____
    In what city and state is he?_____
    What is the zip code?_____
    What is the telephone number where you work? _____

9. Signature of informant_____
    Date_____ Informant's telephone number _____
    If the response to Question 4 is no, answer only what follows, Skip questions 5–9.

10. Signature of informant. _____
    Date _____ Informant's telephone number _____

Note carefully: If subsequent investigation reveals your condition is "work related," benefits paid for you by Blue Cross must be returned.

INFORME PARA BLUE CROSS/BLUE SHIELD

1. Fecha de admisión _____

2. Nombre completo del paciente _____

3. Número del certificado de Blue Cross _____

Hay que contestar a las preguntas que siguen para todas las reclamaciones que estén "relacionadas al trabajo" para que Blue Cross determine los beneficios admisibles. Gracias por su colaboración.

4. ¿Fue la condición por la que necesitó hospitalización causada por su empleo? Si la respuesta es afirmativa, conteste a las preguntas 5 a 9 solamente.

5. ¿Tiene derecho a recibir beneficios de la compensación obrera por esta incapacidad?

6. Explique. _____

7. Con brevedad explique la manera en que su empleo causó esta incapacidad.

8. Si tiene trabajo, dé la información siguiente:

    ¿Cómo se llama su patrón? _____

    ¿Cuál es su dirección? _____

    ¿En qué ciudad y estado está? _____

    ¿Cuál es el número de teléfono del lugar donde trabaja? _____

9. Firma del informante _____

    Fecha _____ Número de teléfono del informante _____

    Si la respuesta es negativa, solamente conteste a lo que sigue y omita las preguntas 5 a 9.

10. Firma del informante. _____

    Fecha _____ Número de teléfono del informante _____

Nota importante: Si investigación subsecuente revela que su estado de salud está <<relacionado al trabajo,>> será preciso devolver todos los beneficios pagados por Blue Cross.

INFORMATION FOR ADMISSION

INFORMACION PARA ADMISION

1. What is the patient's complete and correct name?[3]
   Dígame el nombre completo y correcto del (de la) paciente.
   ¿Cómo se llama el (la) paciente?

2. What is the address and zip code of the patient?
   ¿Cuál es la dirección y la zona postal del (de la) paciente?

3. What is your former address?
   ¿Donde vivía antes?

4. Is there a telephone?
   ¿Hay teléfono?

5. What is the patient's telephone number?[4]
   ¿Cuál es el número de teléfono del (de la) paciente?

6. What is the sex of the patient?
   ¿Cuál es el sexo del paciente?

7. To what race does the patient belong?[5]
   ¿A qué raza pertenece el (la) paciente?

8. How old is the patient?[6]
   ¿Qué edad tiene el (la) paciente?
   ¿Cuántos años tiene el (la) paciente?

9. On what day, month, and year was the patient born?[7]
   ¿En qué día, mes y año nació el (la) paciente?

10. Where was the patient born?
    ¿Dónde nació el (la) paciente?

11. Tell me the name of the town, the state, and the country.
    Dígame el nombre del pueblo, del estado, y del país.

12. How long have you been in the United States?
    ¿Desde cuándo está Vd.* en los Estados Unidos?

13. What is the patient's religion?[8]
    ¿Cuál es la religión del (de la) paciente?

14. What is the patient's marital status?
    ¿Qué es su estado civil?

15. If married, what is the spouse's name?
    Si es casado (casada), ¿cómo se llama la esposa (el esposo)?

16. What kind of work does the patient do?[9]
    ¿Qué clase de trabajo hace el (la) paciente?
    ¿Cuál es su ocupación?

17. What is the name of the patient's employer or responsible party?
    ¿Cómo se llama el patrón (la patrona) del (de la) paciente o la persona responsable?

18. What is the address of that employer?
    ¿Cuál es la dirección de ese patrón (esa patrona)?

19. What is the telephone number there?
    ¿Cuál es el número de teléfono allí?

20. Of what country is the patient a citizen?
    ¿De qué país es ciudadano (ciudadana) el (la) paciente?

21. What is the name of the patient's nearest relative?
    ¿Cómo se llama el pariente más cercano del (de la) paciente?

22. What is his/her address?[10]
    ¿Cuál es su dirección?

---

*The pronoun **usted** and its plural, **ustedes** may be abbreviated as **Vd.** or **Ud.** and **Vds.** or **Uds.** This book will employ the abbreviations **Vd.** and **Vds.** for "you."

23. What is his/her telephone number?[4]
    ¿Cuál es su número de teléfono?

24. What is the relationship with the patient?
    ¿Qué parentesco tiene con el (la) paciente?
    ¿Cuál es la relación entre ellos?

25. What is the patient's social security number?[11]
    ¿Cuál es el número de la tarjeta de seguro social del (de la) paciente?

26. To whom shall the bill be sent?
    ¿A quién debemos mandar la cuenta?

27. What is the address and zip code of this person?[10]
    ¿Cuál es la dirección y zona postal de esta persona?

28. When was the patient admitted to the hospital?
    ¿Cuándo fue admitido el paciente (admitida la paciente) al hospital?
    ¿Cuándo ingresó el (la) paciente al hospital?

29. What was the time?[12]
    ¿Qué hora era?

30. When was the patient discharged?
    ¿A qué hora le dieron de alta al (a la) paciente?

31. Is this his/her first time in the hospital?
    ¿Es ésta la primera vez en el hospital?

32. Was the patient admitted to the hospital within the last six months?
    ¿Tuvo el (la) paciente admisión previa al hospital durante los últimos seis meses?
    ¿Fue admitido el paciente (admitida la paciente) al hospital durante de los últimos seis meses?

33. Does the patient have Blue Cross/Blue Shield?
    ¿Tiene el (la) paciente Blue Cross o Blue Shield?

34. What is the certificate and group number of the patient's Blue Cross?
    ¿Cuál es el número del certificado y del grupo de la Blue Cross del (de la) paciente?

35. What is the name of the policyholder?
    ¿Cómo se llama el tenedor de la póliza?

36. What is the sex of the policyholder?
    ¿Cuál es el sexo del poseedor de la póliza?

37. What is the patient's relation to the policyholder?
    ¿Cuál es la relación entre el (la) paciente y el asegurado (la asegurada)?

38. What is the social security number of the policyholder?
    ¿Cuál es el número de la tarjeta de seguro social del tenedor de la póliza?

39. Does the patient have other medical, hospitalization, or health insurance?
    ¿Tiene el (la) paciente algún otro seguro médico, de hospital, o de enfermedad?

40. What is the name(s) of his/her insurance company (companies)?
    ¿Cuál es el nombre (los nombres) de su(s) aseguranza(s)?
    ¿Cómo se llama(n) la(s) empresa(s) con que está asegurado (asegurada)?

41. What is the insurance policy number?
    ¿Cuál es el número de su póliza de seguros?

42. What is the name of the policyholder?
    ¿Cómo se llama el tenedor de esta póliza?

43. What is the name of the policyholder's employer?
    ¿Cómo se llama el patrón (la patrona) del tenedor de esta póliza?

44. What is the employer's address?[10]
    ¿Cuál es la dirección del patrón (la patrona)?

45. Was the patient admitted because of an accident?
    ¿Se le admitió al (a la) paciente a causa de un accidente?

46. When did the accident happen?
    ¿Cuándo ocurrió el accidente?

47. Where did the accident happen?
    ¿Dónde ocurrió el accidente?

48. Was the patient admitted from a general hospital?
    ¿Ingresó el (la) paciente de un hospital general?

49. From home?
    ¿De casa?

50. From an extended-care facility?
    ¿De una institución de cuidado prolongado?

51. What was the admission diagnosis?
    ¿Cuál fue el diagnóstico al ingresar?

52. Is the condition due to injury or sickness arising from the patient's employment?
    ¿Se debe este estado a una herida o enfermedad que proviene del empleo del (de la) paciente?

53. If "Yes," what is the name and address of the employer?
    Si lo es, dígame el nombre y la dirección del patrón (de la patrona).
    Si lo es, ¿cuál es el nombre y la dirección del patrón (de la patrona)?

54. Does the patient want a private room?
    ¿Desea el (la) paciente un cuarto privado (individual)?

55. A semiprivate room?
    ¿Un cuarto semiprivado (doble)?

56. A ward?
    ¿Una crujía (una sala de los enfermos) (un pabellón)?

57. What is the name and address of the patient's physician?[10]
    Dígame el nombre y la dirección del médico (de la médica) del (de la) paciente.

58. Whom shall we notify in case of emergency?
    ¿A quién se notifica en caso de emergencia?
    ¿A quién podemos notificar en caso de emergencia?

59. Is this person a relative? a friend? a neighbor?
    ¿Es un pariente? ¿amigo? ¿vecino?

60. Where does this person live?
    ¿Dónde vive esta persona?

61. What is his telephone number?[4]
    ¿Cuál es su número de teléfono?

62. Does the patient authorize release of information requested on this form by the above- named hospital?[13]
    ¿Autoriza el (la) paciente una communicación de la información pedida en este informe por el hospital ya nombrado?

63. Does the patient authorize payment directly to the above named hospital of any benefits payable in this case, realizing that the patient shall be responsible for the charges not covered?
    ¿Autoriza el (la) paciente el pago de todos los beneficios aplicables en este caso directamente al susodicho hospital, dándose cuenta de que tendrá que pagar lo que no pague el seguro?

64. Does the patient consent to and authorize all treatments, surgical procedures, and administration of all anesthetics that in the judgment of his/her physician may be considered necessary for the diagnosis or treatment of this case while a patient in _____ hospital?
    ¿Da el (la) paciente su consentimiento y autorización para todos los tratamientos, procedimientos quirúrgicos y administración de todas las anestesias que crea necesarios su médico (médica) para el diagnóstico o tratamiento de este caso mientras que sea paciente en el hospital de_____?

THE ADMISSIONS OFFICE

Receptionist: Who is the patient?
Patient: I am the patient. This is my husband.
Receptionist: Very well. What is your complete and correct name, please?
Patient: María Angel Ramírez de Fernández.
5 Receptionist: Oh, yes. I have your name on the list. Do you want a private room or a semi-private one?
Patient: A semi-private room, please.
Receptionist: Do you have medical insurance or other hospitalization insurance?
Patient: Yes, Miss. Here is all the information.
10 Receptionist: Please fill in the admission form.
[Several minutes pass.]

	Patient:	I have filled it out now.
	Receptionist:	Okay. Your room will be 682B, on the sixth floor.
	Patient:	Can my husband go with me?
15	Receptionist:	Yes, Ma'am. The bed is ready. The elevator is on your left.
	Patient:	What are the visiting hours?
	Receptionist:	From noon until 8:30 at night.
	Patient:	How many visitors are allowed at a time?
	Receptionist:	Only two visitors.
20	Patient:	Thank you.
	Receptionist:	You are welcome.

Situation   *Situación*

You are the admitting clerk. Greet the patient, ask about insurance, and have him/her fill out the admitting form.

LA OFICINA DE INGRESOS

	Recepcionista:	¿Quién es el paciente?
	Paciente:	Yo soy la paciente. Este es mi esposo.
	Recepcionista:	Muy bien. ¿Cuál es su nombre completo y correcto, por favor?
	Paciente:	María Angel Ramírez de Fernández.
5	Recepcionista:	Ah, sí. Aquí tengo su nombre en la lista. ¿Quiere Vd. un cuarto individual o un cuarto semi-privado?
	Paciente:	Un cuarto semi-privado, por favor.
	Recepcionista:	¿Tiene Vd. seguro médico u otro seguro de hospital?
	Paciente:	Sí, señorita. Aquí tiene Vd. toda la información.
10	Recepcionista:	Favor de llenar el formulario de entrada.
		[Unos minutos pasan.]
	Paciente:	Ya lo he llenado.
	Recepcionista:	Muy bien. Su cuarto será 682B [seiscientos ochenta y dos Be], en el sexto piso.
	Paciente:	¿Puede acompañarme mi esposo?
15	Recepcionista:	Sí, señora. La cama está lista. A la izquierda tienen Vds. el ascensor.
	Paciente:	¿Cuáles son las horas de visita?
	Recepcionista:	Desde las doce de la tarde hasta las ocho y media de la noche.
	Paciente:	¿Cuántos visitantes se permiten a la vez?
	Recepcionista:	Sólo dos visitantes.
20	Paciente:	Gracias.
	Recepcionista:	De nada.

Questions   *Preguntas*

1. ¿Quién acompaña a la Sra. Fernández a la oficina de ingresos?
2. ¿Qué tiene que llenar?
3. ¿Cuándo puede visitarla su esposo?

EMERGENCY ROOM REPORT

INFORME DE LA SALA DE EMERGENCIA

1. Are you the patient?[14]
   ¿Es Vd. el (la) paciente?

2. What is your name?
   ¿Cómo se llama Vd.?
   Dígame su nombre completo y correcto.

3. What is your last (surname) name?[15]
   ¿Cuál es su apellido?

4. How is it spelled?
   ¿Cómo se deletrea (escribe)?

5.   What is your first name?
¿Cuál es su nombre?
¿Cuál es su nombre de bautismo?

6.   What is your middle initial?
¿Cuál es su segunda inicial?

7.   What is your maiden name?
¿Cuál es su nombre de soltera?

8.   What is your home telephone number?[4]
¿Cuál es el número de teléfono de su casa?

9.   What is your address?[10]
¿Cuál es su dirección?
¿Dónde vive Vd.?

10.   What is your zip code?[10]
¿Cuál es su zona postal?

11.   What is the name of your nearest relative?
¿Cómo se llama su pariente más cercano (cercana)?

12.   What is the relationship with you?
¿Qué parentesco tiene con Vd.?
¿Cuál es la relación entre Vds.?

13.   How is she/he related to you?
¿Qué es de Vd.?

14.   Where does she/he live?
¿Dónde vive?

15.   What is the zip code there?[10]
¿Cuál es la zona postal allí?

16.   What is her/his telephone number?[4]
¿Cuál es su número de teléfono?

17.   How old are you?[6]
¿Qué edad tiene Vd.?
¿Cuántos años tiene Vd.?

18.   On what day, month, and year were you born?[7]
¿En qué día, mes y año nació Vd.?

19.   Where were you born?
¿Dónde nació Vd.?

20.   What is your race?[5]
¿A qué raza pertenece Vd.?

21.   What is your marital status?
¿Cuál es su estado civil?

22.   Are you married?
¿Es. Vd. casado (casada)?

23.   Are you divorced?
¿Es Vd. divorciado (divorciada)?

24.   Are you single?
¿Es Vd. soltero (soltera)?

25.   Are you a widow(er)?
¿Es Vd. viudo (viuda)?

26.   Are you separated?
¿Está Vd. separado (separada)?

27.   When were you hurt?
¿Cuándo se lastimó?

28.   What was the time?[12]
¿A qué hora?

29.   When did the accident happen?
¿Cuándo ocurrió el accidente?

30. What kind of work do you do?[9]
   ¿Qué clase de trabajo hace Vd.?
   ¿Cuál es su ocupación?

31. What is the complete name of your employer?
   Dígame el nombre completo del lugar donde trabaja.

32. What is the address of the place where you work?[10]
   ¿Cuál es la dirección del lugar donde trabaja?

33. What is the zip code?[10]
   ¿Cuál es la zona postal?

34. What is the telephone number where you work?[4]
   ¿Cuál es el número del teléfono donde trabaja?

35. Do you have Blue Cross and/or Blue Shield?
   ¿Tiene Vd. Blue Cross y/o Blue Shield?

36. What is the number of your Blue Cross policy? of your Blue Shield policy?
   ¿Cuál es el número de su certificado de Blue Cross? ¿de Blue Shield?

37. What is the name of the group policyholder?
   ¿Cómo se llama el tenedor de la póliza del grupo?
   Dígame el nombre del asegurado (de la asegurada) del grupo.

38. Do you have a Medicare card?
   ¿Tiene Vd. tarjeta de Medicare?

39. What is the number of your card? (You must include all the letters, also.)
   ¿Cuál es el número de su tarjeta? (Vd. debe incluir todas las letras también.)

40. Do you receive public assistance?
   ¿Recibe Vd. asistencia pública?

41. What is the number of your green card?[16]
   ¿Cuál es el número de su tarjeta verde?

42. When does the card expire?
   ¿Cuándo expira la tarjeta?

43. Do you have medical insurance?
   ¿Tiene Vd. seguro médico?

44. Do you have hospitalization?
   ¿Tiene Vd. seguro de hospital?

45. What type of insurance do you have?
   ¿Qué tipo de seguros tiene Vd.?

46. What is the name of your insurance company?
   ¿Cuál es el nombre de su compañía de seguros?
   ¿Cuál es el nombre de la empresa con que está asegurado (asegurada)?

47. Where did the injury occur?
   ¿En qué lugar ocurrió la herida?

48. Where was the onset of the illness?
   ¿En qué lugar empezó la enfermedad?

49. Were the police notified?
   ¿Fue notificada la policía?

50. What was the police district number?
   ¿De qué barrio era la policía?

51. Does it hurt a lot?
   ¿Le duele mucho?

52. You will be OK.
   Vd. va a estar bien.

53. You will (won't) need stitches (sutures).
   Vd. (no) va a necesitar suturas/puntos.

54. When was your last tetanus shot?
   ¿Cuándo fue su última inyección (vacuna) contra el tétano?

55.   How did you burn yourself?
      ¿Cómo se quemó Vd.?

56.   Hot water, grease, fire, acid, the stove?
      ¿Agua caliente, grasa, fuego,[17] ácido, la estufa/el horno?

57.   Tell me if this hurts.
      Dígame si le duele esto.

58.   You must keep it clean at all times.
      Vd. tiene que mantenerla limpia todo el tiempo.

59.   I want to check it again in a week.
      Quiero examinarla otra vez de hoy en ocho (días).

60.   The above instruction(s) have been explained to me as continued care following treatment in the emergency room at _____ Hospital.
      Se me han explicado las antedichas instrucciones como cuidado continuo siguiendo el tratamiento en la sala de emergencia en el Hospital _____.

INFORMATION FOR THE CERTIFICATE OF LIVE BIRTH

INFORMACION PARA LA PARTIDA DE NACIMIENTO VIVO

CHILD   *NIÑO*

1.   Tell me the complete and correct name of the child.[3]
     Dígame el nombre completo y correcto del niño.

2.   On what day, month, and year was he/she born?[7]
     ¿En qué día, mes y año nació?

3.   At what time was the child born?[12]
     ¿A qué hora exacta nació?

4.   What is the sex?
     ¿De qué sexo es?

5.   Was this a single birth, twin, triplet, etc.?
     ¿Fue un parto único, doble, triple, etc.?

6.   If this was not a single birth, was this child born first, second, third, etc.? (Specify)
     Si éste no fue un parto único, ¿nació este hijo primero, segundo, tercero, etc.? (Especifique.)

7.   In what county was the child born?
     ¿En qué condado nació el niño?

8.   Tell me the name of the city, town, township.
     Dígame el nombre de la ciudad, del pueblo, del municipio.

9.   Was the child born inside the city?
     ¿Nació el niño dentro de la ciudad?

10. What is the name of the hospital? If the birth did not occur in the hospital, tell me the street and number.
     ¿Cómo se llama el hospital? Si el parto no ocurrió en hospital, dígame el nombre de la calle y el número.[10]

MOTHER   *MADRE*

11. What is your complete and correct maiden name?
     Dígame su nombre completo y correcto de soltera.[3]

12. How old are you at the time of this birth?[6]
     ¿Cuántos años tiene al parir?

13. Where were you born? Tell me the state or foreign country.
     ¿Cuál es su lugar de nacimiento? Dígame el nombre del estado o del país extranjero.

14. In what state is your permanent address?
     ¿En qué estado es su dirección permanente?

15. In what county is your permanent address?
     ¿En qué condado es su dirección permanente?

16. In what city, town, or township do you live?
    ¿En qué ciudad, pueblo, o municipio vive Vd.?

17. Do you live inside the city?
    ¿Vive Vd. dentro de la ciudad?

18. What is your exact address?[10]
    ¿Cuál es su dirección exacta?

19. What is your complete mailing address?[10]
    ¿Cuál es su dirección completa del correo?

20. Is this your first pregnancy?
    ¿Es su primer embarazo?

21. How many living children have you had?
    ¿Cuántos hijos vivos ha tenido?

22. How many miscarriages or abortions have you had?
    ¿Cuántos malpartos o abortos ha tenido?

23. How many still births have you had?
    ¿Cuántos nati-muertos ha tenido?

24. What is your blood type?
    ¿Qué tipo de sangre tiene?

25. Are you going to nurse the baby?
    ¿Piensa darle el pecho al bebé?

FATHER *PADRE*

26. Tell me the complete and correct name of the father.[3]
    Dígame el nombre completo y correcto del padre.

27. How old is the father at the time of this birth?[6]
    ¿Qué edad tiene el padre al nacer su bebé?

28. Where was the father born? Tell me the state or foreign country.
    ¿Dónde nació el padre? Dígame el nombre del estado o del país extranjero.

29. Signature of the informant.
    Firma del (de la) informante.

30. What is the relation to the child?[18]
    ¿Cuál es la relación entre Vd. y el niño?

Notes *Notas*

1. For additional information about numbers, refer to Chapter 4.
2. For additional information on Fractions *Fracciones*, see Chapter 4, pages 89–90.
3. See Chapter 1, pages 9–10.
4. See Chapter 4, page 91, and Chapter 6, note 12.
5. See Chapter 1, page 28, and note 10, page 29, for a more complete discussion on race.
6. Chapter 4, page 89.
7. See Chapter 4, page 99.
8. See Chapter 16, pages 353–354.
9. See Chapter 16, pages 354–355.
10. See Chapter 4, page 91.
11. See Chapter 4, pages 90–91.
12. See Chapter 4, page 95.
13. See sample form in Chapter 14, pages 302–303.
14. Because several family members usually accompany the Hispanic patient about to be hospitalized, this question eliminates unnecessary confusion and delay for the person in charge of admitting. See Chapter 6, note 23, page 135.
15. Refer to Chapter 1 for the discussion on Hispanic nomenclature.
16. Mexicans and others often confuse this "green card" with another one, the **mica**, or *migration card*.
17. **Lumbre** (fire) is used in the southwestern part of the United States.
18. In many Latin American countries the term *illegitimate* is never used. A child born to a married couple is called *legitimate* and is a "legal" child. All other children are often termed "natural." A third term, **hijo reconocido** (recognized child) is coming into use. Some countries, such as Puerto Rico, require the father of such a child, whether he is living with the mother or not, to recognize the child, thus giving the offspring the right to use the father's name, the right to support, and some rights of inheritance.

CHAPTER 6

Conversations for Health Professionals: Basic Preliminary Communication

Conversaciones para personal médico y paramédico: Comunicación básica preliminar

TITLES
TITULOS

1. Doctor
   doctor (Dr.)[1] (*masculine*)
   doctora (Dra.)[1] (*feminine*)

2. Mr. / Sir
   señor (Sr.)[2]

3. Mrs. / Ma'am
   señora (Sra.)[2]

4. Miss
   señorita (Srta.)[2]

GREETINGS AND RESPONSES
SALUDOS Y RESPUESTAS

1. Good morning (good day).
   Buenos días.

2. And to you.
   Muy buenos.

3. Good afternoon (*used from noon until sunset*).[3]
   Buenas tardes.

4. Good afternoon (*response*).
   Muy buenas.

5. Good evening (*used from sundown until the end of the evening; also used to say "good-bye" at night*).[3]
   Buenas noches.

6. Good evening (*response*).
   Muy buenas.

INTRODUCTION
PRESENTACION

1. Hello. (Hi.)
   Hola.

2. Let me introduce myself.
   Déjeme presentarme.
   Permita usted (Vd.) que me presente.

3. Let me introduce you to_____.
   Déjeme presentarle a_____.

4. My name is_____.
   Me llamo_____, a sus órdenes.[4]

5. I am_____.
   Soy_____, a sus órdenes.[4]
   Dr. Burton (*male physician*)
   el doctor Burton.
   Dr. Burton (*female physician*)
   la doctora Burton
   Jaime Burton (*no title*)
   Jaime Burton

6. What is your name?
   ¿Cómo se llama usted?

7. I am glad to meet you.
   Me alegro de conocerle (conocerla).

8. I am glad to see you.
   Me alegro de verle (verla).

9. It's a real pleasure (to meet / see you).
   Mucho gusto.
   Tanto gusto.

10. I'm delighted (to meet you).
    Encantado (Encantada).

11. I am pleased to meet you.
    Estoy encantado (encantada) de conocerle (conocerla).

12. The pleasure is mine.
    El gusto es mío.

13. Same here.
    Igualmente.

> #### NONVERBAL COMMUNICATION: INTRODUCTIONS AND GREETINGS
>
> Cultural differences exist for English-speaking Americans—Anglos—and the Spanish-speaking-Hispanics—when they meet. Anglos tend to be less physical than Hispanics when meeting people they are acquainted with in social or business settings. However, when meeting for the first time, Hispanics tend to be less animated than Anglos. There are certain nonverbal gestures that the majority of Hispanics use when interacting with each other. Hispanics tend to use a polite handshake with limited animation **both** when meeting and saying good-bye. This can be seen through the Spanish expression *dar la mano* (*to give one's hand*), very different than the English expression *to shake hands.* Until very recently in Hispanic cultures, members of the opposite sex rarely touched each other when being introduced. Care is taken to ensure that the handshake is neither held too tightly, too long, nor too vigorous, especially on the part of a woman. When introducing yourself in a formal setting, it is customary to give your full name as you extend your hand (*dar la mano*.) This may be followed by the phrase *a sus órdenes* (*at your service*).
>
> With family and friends, however, most Hispanics are usually much more physically demonstrative. Men generally greet each other with a firm hug, *un abrazo,* a strong handshake, and pats on the back. Women tend to be just slightly less energetic than men when they hug, and usually greet each other and their male friends by lightly kissing each other's cheek. (Sometimes this kiss is given to the "space" close to the side of the face of the other party.)

COURTESY

CORTESIA

1. Please.
   Por favor.

2. Excuse me. (*I must leave. I'd like to get through, etc.*)
   Con permiso.[5]

3. Yes, of course.
   Sí, cómo no.

4. Pardon (me). (*for interrupting, but . . .*)
   Perdón.[5, 6]
   Perdóneme usted.[5]
   Dispense usted.[5]

5. Don't worry (about it).
   No se preocupe.

6. May I come in?
   ¿Se puede?

7. Yes, come in. (*literally, come forward*).
   Sí, adelante.
   Sí, pase.

8. Thank you (very much).
   (Muchas) gracias.

9. Thanks a million.
   Mil gracias.

10. You're welcome.
    De nada.

11. I appreciate it a lot.
    Se lo agradezco mucho.

12. Don't mention it.
    No hay de qué.

13. Gladly. / I'd be glad to. / With much pleasure.
    Con mucho gusto.

14. Don't trouble yourself.
    No se moleste.

15. It's no bother at all.
    No es ninguna molestia.

16. I'm sorry.
    Lo siento.

17. My deepest sympathy.
    Mi sentido pésame.

EXERCISES EJERCICIOS

A. It's your first day in the hospital. Greet and introduce yourself to at least three other people and ask their names.

B. Enter the room and greet the people there, your "friends," the Hispanic way. Do not use words. Then, say good-bye without using words.

C. Using the Hispanic tradition, exchange greetings with a patient of the same sex whom you have just met without using any words. Do the same thing with a patient of the opposite sex. Repeat this exercise in the Anglo tradition still non-verbally.

D. You are working as a receptionist at a local clinic. How would you greet the following people in Spanish?

MODELO: 8:00 am *Buenos días, doctor.*

1. Mrs. García 6:30am
2. Sr. Gómez 3:45pm
3. Dra. Navas 8:00pm
4. María Paz 5:00pm
5. Srta. Villarreal 12:30pm
6. Dr. Brown 10:00am

COMMUNICATION
COMUNICACION

1. Do you speak English?
   ¿Habla usted inglés?

2. Do you understand English?
   ¿Entiende usted (el) inglés?[7]

3. Do you speak Spanish?
   ¿Habla usted español?

4. Do you understand Spanish?
   ¿Entiende usted (el) español?[7]

5. What other languages do you speak?
   ¿Qué otras lenguas habla usted?
   ¿Qué otros idiomas habla usted?

6. Really?
   ¿Verdad?
   ¿De veras?

7. What is your name?
   ¿Cómo se llama?

8. Repeat, please.
   Repita, por favor.

9. Please speak slowly.
   Hable usted despacio, por favor.
   Favor de hablar despacio.

10. I can say some words in Spanish
    Puedo decir algunas palabras en español.

11. I do not understand Spanish very well.
    No entiendo el español muy bien.[7]

12. I am. . . .
    Soy. . .
    nurse Abrams (*female*).
    la enfermera Abrams.
    nurse Abrams (*male*).
    el enfermero Abrams
    Sandy Abrams (*no title*)
    Sandy Abrams.

13. Do you understand?
    ¿Comprende?[7]

14. Can you understand me?
    ¿Puede entenderme?[7]

15. Am I speaking clearly?
    ¿Hablo claramente?

16. Please answer my questions slowly.
    Por favor, conteste Vd. a mis preguntas despacio.

17. Nod your head for "yes."
    Mueva la cabeza para arriba y para abajo cuando quiera decir "sí."
    Favor de mover la cabeza para arriba y para abajo cuando quiera decir "sí."

18. Shake it for "no."
    Muévala de un lado a otro cuando quiera decir "no."
    Favor de moverla de un lado a otro cuando quiera decir "no."

19. Answer as briefly as possible, please.
    Conteste Vd. lo más breve posible, por favor.

20. Answer in a different way, please.
    Conteste de otra manera, por favor.

21. Don't talk so fast.
    No hable Vd. tan de prisa.

22. Please answer my questions more slowly.
    Por favor, conteste Vd. a mis preguntas más despacio.

23. Please speak louder.
    Hable usted en voz más alta, por favor.
    Favor de hablar en voz más alta.

24. Please speak softer.
    Hable usted en voz más baja, por favor.
    Favor de hablar en voz más baja.

25. Be calm, please.
    Cálmese Vd., por favor.

26. Don't be frightened.
    No se asuste Vd.
    No tenga Vd. miedo.

27. What's the matter?
    ¿Qué pasa?

28. Tell me, please.
    Dígame, por favor.
    Favor de decirme.

29. How can I help you?
    ¿En qué puedo servirle (servirla)?

30. Do you need something?
    ¿Necesita usted algo?

31. Do you want something?
    ¿Desea usted algo?

32. What does _____ mean?
    ¿Qué significa _____?
    ¿Qué quiere decir _____?

33. It means _____.
    Significa _____.
    Quiere decir _____.

34. How do you say _____?
    ¿Cómo se dice _____?

35. You say _____.
    Se dice _____.

36. Did I say that right?
    ¿Lo dije correctamente?

37. How do you spell it?
    ¿Cómo se escribe?
    ¿Cómo se deletrea?

38. It is spelled _____.
    Se escribe _____.
    Se deletrea _____.

39. Write it here, please.
    Escríbalo aquí, por favor.
    Favor de escribirlo aquí.

CONVERSATION FOR ROUNDS

CONVERSACION PARA VISITAS DE RUTINA

1. How are you?
   ¿Cómo está usted?[8]

2. How's it going? / What's up?
   ¿Qué tal?

3. How are things? / How's it going?
   ¿Cómo le va?[8]

4. Fine, thank you.
   Bien, gracias.

5. Very well, thanks.
   Muy bien, gracias.

6. How do you feel today?
   ¿Cómo se siente hoy?[8, 9]

7. Marvelous, thanks.
   Maravilloso (Maravillosa), gracias.

8. I'm feeling great!
   Estoy de lo más bien. *PR*

9. So, so. / Fair.
   Más o menos.
   Así, así.
   Regular.
   Pasándolo.
   Pasándola. *Mex.*
   Así no más. *SpAm*

10. Same as always.
    Igual que siempre.

11. And (how are) you?
    ¿Y usted?

12. What's wrong?
    ¿Qué tiene?[8]

13. I'm okay.
    Me siento bien.

14. I feel bad.
    Me siento mal.

15. I feel better.
    Me siento mejor.

16. Better than yesterday.
    Mejor que ayer.

17. Better than before.
    Mejor que antes.

18. Pretty well.
    Bastante bien.

19. I feel worse.
    Me siento peor.

20. Worse than yesterday.
    Peor que ayer.

21. Worse than before.
    Peor que antes.

22. I'm a bit / slightly ill.
    Estoy un poco enfermo (enferma).
    Estoy un poco malo (mala).

23. I feel blue.
    Tengo murria.

24. I have a cold.
    Tengo (un) catarro.
    Tengo un resfriado.
    Tengo resfrío.

25. Please sit up.
    Haga Vd. el favor de sentarse recto.

26. Breathe slowly.
    Respire Vd. despacio.

27. Breathe deeply.
    Respire Vd. profundo.

28. Cough, please.
    Tosa Vd., por favor.

29. Please be quiet for a moment.
    Haga el favor de callarse un momento.

30. Please lie down.
    Haga el favor de acostarse.

31. You cannot eat yet.
    Vd. no puede comer todavía.

32. You have to eat (more).
    Vd. tiene que comer (más).

33. You cannot drink yet.
    Vd. no puede beber todavía.

34. You have to drink (more).
    Vd. tiene que beber (más).

35. You have to stay in bed (today)(this week).
    Vd. tiene que quedarse en cama (hoy)(esta semana).

36. You may walk around (tomorrow)(today).
    Vd. puede caminar (mañana)(hoy).

37. You are doing very well.
    Vd. va muy bien.

FAREWELLS

DESPEDIDAS

1. I will talk with you later.
   Le hablaré más tarde.

2. I will explain it to your family when they come.
   Se lo explicaré a su familia cuando venga.

3. Good-bye.
   Adiós.
   ¡Que le vaya bien!
   Chao. Chau.

4. Well, good-bye.
   Pues, adiós.

5. So long. / See you later.
   Hasta luego.
   Hasta lueguito. *Chile Arg.*

6. See you soon.
   Hasta pronto.

7. Until we meet again.
   Hasta la vista.

8. See you tomorrow. / Until tomorrow.
   Hasta mañana.

9. Until next time.
   Hasta la próxima vez.

10. I'll see you.
    Nos veremos.
    Nos vemos. *Mex.*

11. God willing. / If God wills.
    Si Dios quiere.[10]

12. Come again.
    Vuelva otra vez.

13. Regards to . . .
    Recuerdos . . .
    the family.
    a la familia.
    your parents.
    a sus padres.
    your wife.
    a la esposa.
    your husband.
    al esposo.

14. Say hello to . . .
    Saludos . . .
    the family.
    a la familia.
    your parents.
    a sus padres.
    your wife.
    a la esposa.
    your husband.
    al esposo.

EXERCISES *EJERCICIOS*

A. With another person, assume the roles of doctor and patient. Greet each other and ask how things are.

B. Greet someone, ask how he/she is feeling, and then say good-bye.

C. The following is a conversation between a nurse and a patient in the hospital. Take the part of the nurse, filling in her comments and reactions. Use the new vocabulary that you have just learned.

NURSE: Good morning. I am Mary, your nurse.

ENFERMERA:_____

PATIENT: Good morning, I am Mrs. García.

PACIENTE: **Muy buenos. Soy la señora García.**

NURSE: I am glad to meet you.

ENFERMERA:_____

PATIENT: The pleasure is mine.

PACIENTE: **El gusto es mío.**

NURSE: How do you feel today?

ENFERMERA:_____

AMBULANCE[11]

AMBULANCIA

1. I am . . .
   Soy . . .
   a doctor.
   médico (médica).
   doctor (doctora).
   an EMT / emergency medical technician.
   especialista en emergencia médica.
   a nurse.
   enfermero (enfermera).
   a paramedic.
   paramédico (paramédica).
   a fireman.
   bombero (bombera).
   a policeman / policewoman.
   policía.

2. Stay calm.
   Quédese tranquilo (tranquila).

3. Don't move.
   No se mueva.

4. Don't move . . .
   No mueva . . .
   your head.
   la cabeza.
   your legs.
   las piernas.
   your arms.
   los brazos.

5. Are you hurt?
   ¿Está herido? (herida?)
   ¿Está lastimado? (lastimada?)

6. Show me where.
   Muéstreme dónde.
   Enséñeme dónde.

7. Where does it hurt?
   ¿Dónde le duele?

8. Can you talk?
   ¿Puede hablar?

9. Do not speak now.
   No hable ahora.

10. Do you have a doctor?
    ¿Tiene médico (médica)?

11. Who is your doctor?
    ¿Cómo se llama su médico (médica)?

12. What is his/her phone number?[12]
    ¿Cuál es su número de teléfono?

13. I cannot help the patient here.
    No puedo ayudar al (a la) paciente aquí.

14. You must go to the hospital.[13]
    Tiene que ir al hospital.

15. You do not need to go to the hospital by ambulance.
    Usted no necesita ir al hospital por ambulancia.

16. You may go on your own.
    Puede ir por su cuenta.

17. I am going to call an ambulance.
    Voy a llamar una ambulancia.

18. We must take the patient to the hospital (to the clinic[14]).[15]
    Debemos llevar al (a la) paciente al hospital (a la clínica).

19. We have to take you to the hospital (to the clinic).
    Tenemos que llevarlo (llevarla) al hospital (a la clínica).

20. We are going to take you to the hospital.
    Vamos a llevarlo (llevarla) al hospital.

21. Which hospital do you prefer?
    ¿A qué hospital prefiere ir?

22. You have to go to the nearest trauma center.
    Tiene que ir al centro de trauma más cercano.

23. We are going to take the patient to a trauma center.
    Vamos a llevar al (a la) paciente a un centro de trauma.

24. We are going to move the patient to a stretcher.
    Vamos a pasar al (a la) paciente a una camilla.

25. Don't be afraid.
    No tenga Vd. miedo.

26. Someone ought to accompany the patient in the ambulance.
    Alguien debe acompañar al (a la) paciente en la ambulancia.

27. Is the patient comfortable?
    ¿Se siente cómodo (cómoda) el (la) paciente?

28. We will be at the hospital (clinic) soon.
    Estaremos en el hospital (la clínica) dentro de pronto.

29. We are here.
    Ya llegamos.

30. We are going to move you onto a bed.
    Vamos a transportarle a una cama.

31. We are going to pull the sheet at the count of three.
    Vamos a jalar la sábana al contar tres.

32. Don't worry, but don't move either.
    No se preocupe, pero no se mueva tampoco.

ADMISSION OF THE PATIENT TO THE ROOM[16]

ADMISION DEL (DE LA) PACIENTE AL CUARTO

1. I am _____ .
   Soy _____ .

2. I am the day nurse, night nurse, nurse on duty, nurse's aide, head nurse.
   Soy la enfermera de día, la enfermera de noche, la enfermera de guardia, la ayudante de enfermera, la jefa de enfermeras.

3. I am the public health nurse, visiting nurse.
   Soy la enfermera de salud pública, la enfermera ambulante.

4. Do you need a wheelchair?
   ¿Necesita Vd. una silla de ruedas?

5. Your family may accompany you to the room.
   Su familia puede acompañarle al cuarto.

6. You can accompany your wife (husband) to her (his) room.
   Vd. puede acompañar a su esposa (esposo) hasta el cuarto.

7. When is your family coming? I want to talk to them.[17]
   ¿Cuándo viene su familia? Quiero hablarles.

8. I want to introduce you to ____ (other patient in the room).
   Quiero presentarle a ____. (otro/otra paciente en el cuarto)

9. Here is a hospital gown; please put it on. Do you need help?
   Aquí tiene una bata del hospital; favor de ponérsela. ¿Necesita ayuda?

10. Ask your family (or a friend) to take your suitcase home.
Pida Vd. que su familia (un amigo) lleve su maleta a casa.

11. Your clothes go in the closet.
Su ropa va en el armario.

12. Put your clothes in the closet.
Ponga su ropa en el ropero.

13. Your family (friend) can bring you your clothes tomorrow.
Su familia (amigo / amiga) puede traerle su ropa mañana.

14. I need a urine specimen.
Necesito una muestra de orina de Vd.

15. When you urinate, fill up this bottle and give it to the nurse on duty.
Cuando Vd. orine, llene este frasco y déselo a la enfermera de guardia.

16. Here is a booklet that deals with the rules of the hospital.
Aquí tiene un folleto que trata de las reglas del hospital.

17. This is the buzzer (bell).
Este es el timbre.

18. This is the call light.
Esta es la luz para llamar a la enfermera.

19. If you need anything, press the button.
Si Vd. necesita algo, apriete el botón.

20. The light over your door will stay on until a member of the nursing staff answers your call.
La luz que está sobre la puerta se mantendrá prendida hasta que un miembro del personal de enfermeras conteste a su llamada.

21. This button raises the headboard.
Este botón levanta la cabecera de la cama.

22. This button lowers the headboard.
Este botón baja la cabecera de la cama.

23. This button raises (lowers) the bed.
Este botón levanta (baja) la cama.

24. This button raises the foot of the bed.
Este botón levanta el pie de la cama.

25. This button lowers the foot of the bed.
Este botón baja el pie de la cama.

26. Call someone to help you.
Llame a alguien para que le (la) ayude.

27. Do not turn without calling the nurse.
No se voltee sin llamar a la enfermera.
No se dé vuelta sin llamar a la enfermera.

28. Do you want me to raise your headboard?
¿Quisiera la cabecera de la cama más alta?
¿Quiere Vd. que le levante un poco la cabecera de la cama?

29. Do you want me to lower your headboard?
¿Quiere Vd. que le baje un poco la cabecera de la cama?

30. Do you want me to raise the knee rest (your knees)?
¿Quiere Vd. que le levante (suba) un poco las rodillas?

31. Do you want me to lower your knees?
¿Quiere Vd. que le baje un poco las rodillas?

32. The side rails on your bed are for your protection.
Los rieles del costado están para su protección.
Las barandas protectoras de la cama están para su protección.

33. Please do not try to lower or climb over the side rail.
No pretenda bajarlos (bajarlas) o treparse sobre ellos (ellas).

34. Please wear slippers or shoes and a robe at all times when you are out of bed.
Por favor, use Vd. pantuflas o zapatos y una bata siempre que no esté en la cama.

35. Don't walk barefoot.
No camine descalzo (descalza).

36. Your bathroom is behind this door.
Su baño está detrás de esta puerta.
Su servicio (*Spain*) está detrás de esta puerta.

37. You (do not) have a private bathroom.
Vd. (no) tiene un baño privado.

38. The bathtub is along the hall to the right (to the left).
La bañera (la bañadera *Amer.*) está por el pasillo (corredor) a la derecha (a la izquierda).

39. There are bathrooms in the hall for visitors.
Hay baños en el pasillo para las visitas/los visitantes.
Hay servicios (*Spain*) en el pasillo para las visitas/los visitantes.

40. This is a special denture cup to store your dentures in when you are not wearing them.
Este es un recipiente especial para guardar su dentadura postiza cuando no la use.

41. You must remove your dentures or any partial dentures before surgery or any procedure involving a general anesthetic.
Vd. debe quitarse la dentadura postiza o cualquier diente postizo antes de la cirugía, o si Vd. está en la lista para algún tratamiento que requiera anestesia general.

42. You can (not) tape cards to the wall.
Vd. (no) puede pegar tarjetas en la pared.

43. You can put your things on the shelf.
Vd. puede poner sus pertenencias (cosas) en el estante.

44. You cannot hang anything from the door.
Vd. no puede colgar nada de la puerta.

45. You may use the telephone to make local calls.
Vd. puede usar el teléfono para hacer llamadas locales.

46. To place a local telephone call, dial 9 (nine), wait for the dial tone, then dial the number you wish.
Para hacer una llamada local, marque 9 (nueve), espere el tono, luego marque el número que Vd. desee.

47. For long distance or suburban calls, dial 0 (zero) and the operator will help you.
Para llamadas de larga distancia o a las afueras, marque 0 (cero) y la operadora lo (la) asistirá.

48. You can call collect or use a credit card.
Vd. puede llamar por cobrar o usar una tarjeta de crédito.

49. Telephone calls can (not) be added to your hospital bill.
Las llamadas telefónicas (no) pueden ser agregadas a su cuenta del hospital.

50. Newspapers are sold each morning and evening throughout the hospital and are also available in the lobby.
Se venden los periódicos todas las mañanas y todas las noches por todo el hospital y también están a disposición en el salón de entrada.

51. Television sets can be rented here in the hospital at a nominal cost.
Se puede alquilar televisores (aparatos de televisión) aquí en el hospital por un pago nominal.

52. The television has _____ channels.
El televisor tiene _____ canales.

53. You may view religious services on channel _____ on Sundays.
Puede observar los servicios religiosos en el canal _____ los domingos.

54. There is also a medical educational channel.
También hay un canal educativo médico.

55. I will call the dietician to discuss your menu.[18]
Llamaré al (a la) dietista para que hablen de su menú.

56. You will be given a choice of foods for your meals according to the diet prescribed by your doctor.
Se le darán a elegir los alimentos para sus comidas según la dieta que su médico (médica) le prescriba.

57. You have to choose three meals a day.
Vd. tiene que escoger tres comidas por día.

58. You can order double portions if you wish.
Vd. puede pedir porciones dobles si desea.

59. Breakfast is served at 8:00 A.M.[19]
Se sirve el desayuno a las ocho de la mañana.

60. Lunch is served at 11:30.[19]
Se sirve el almuerzo a las once y media.

61. Dinner is at 5:00 P.M.[19]
Se sirve la cena a las cinco de la tarde.

62. A snack is served at 8:45 P.M.[19]
Se sirve una merienda (una colación) a las nueve menos cuarto de la noche.

63. We need to send your menu choices to the kitchen.
Necesitamos enviar su selección del menú a la cocina.

64. You can eat in your room or in the visitors' room.
Vd. puede comer o en su cuarto o en el cuarto para visitas.

65. The patients' chapel is located on the main floor and is open to members of all faiths.
La capilla de los pacientes se halla en la planta baja (el piso principal) y está a disposición de los miembros de todos los credos.

66. There are brief services there every Sunday at 10:30 A.M.[19]
Hay breves servicios allí todos los domingos a las diez y media de la mañana.

67. If you wish, your own priest, minister, or rabbi can come to visit you.
Si Vd. desea, su propio sacerdote, ministro, o rabino (rabí) puede venir a visitarle.

68. Do you want to see the chaplain?
¿Desea ver al capellán?

69. The head nurse is _____.
La jefa de enfermeras es _____.

70. Your doctor usually visits at _____.[19]
Su médico (médica) suele visitar a las _____.

71. You may not smoke in the room.
No se puede fumar en el cuarto.

72. You cannot smoke here.
Vd. no puede fumar aquí.

73. You can smoke _____.
Vd. puede fumar _____.
   in the lobby.
   en el vestíbulo.
   outside.
   afuera.

74. Is the room too hot?
¿Hace demasiado calor en el cuarto?

75. You cannot open the windows.
Vd. no puede abrir las ventanas.

76. Do you want me to open (close) the window?
¿Quiere que yo abra (cierre) la ventana?

77. Do you want me to turn on (turn off) the lights?
¿Quiere Vd. que encienda (apague) la luz?

78. Do you need more blankets or another pillow?
¿Necesita Vd. más frazadas (cobijas) u otra almohada?

79. Are you allergic to any medication?
    ¿Padece Vd. de alguna alergia?
    ¿Es Vd. alérgico (alérgica) a alguna medicina?

80. Are you on a special diet?[20]
    ¿Sigue dieta especial?

81. Are you on a restricted diet?
    ¿Sigue Vd. dieta limitada (restringida/ rigurosa)?

82. Do you need to speak with a dietitian?
    ¿Necesita hablar con un(a) dietista?

83. Are you hungry?
    ¿Tiene Vd. hambre?

84. Have you eaten today?
    ¿Ha comido hoy?
    breakfast?
    ¿Se desayunó?[21]
    lunch
    ¿Almorzó?
    dinner?
    ¿Cenó?

85. Are you thirsty?
    ¿Tiene Vd. sed?

86. Do you want water?
    ¿Quiere agua?

87. Do you want a glass of water?
    ¿Quiere un vaso con agua?

88. Do you want a drink?
    ¿Quiere beber?

89. There is ice water in the pitcher.
    Hay agua con hielo en la jarra.

90. I am the technician.
    Soy el (la) laboratorista (técnico/técnica).

91. I am here to draw your blood.[22]
    Estoy aquí para tomarle una muestra de sangre.

92. I am the orderly.
    Soy el ayudante.

93. I have come to take you for your tests.
    He venido para llevarle a que le hagan sus análisis.

94. Please move over to the stretcher.
    Acuéstese en la camilla, por favor.
    Por favor, pásese a la camilla.

95. Can you move over to the stretcher?
    ¿Puede Vd. acostarse en la camilla?
    ¿Puede Vd. pasarse a la camilla?

96. I am going to help you lie down on the stretcher.
    Voy a ayudarlo (ayudarla) a acostarse en la camilla.

97. I am going to cover you with a blanket (sheet).
    Voy a cubrirlo (cubrirla) con una frazada (una sábana).

98. Please sit down in the wheelchair.
    Siéntese Vd. en la silla de ruedas, por favor.

99. Wait here until you hear your name.
    Espere aquí hasta oír su nombre.
    que oiga su nombre.
    que escuche su nombre.

100. You will have to wait your turn.
    Vd. tendrá que esperar su turno.

101. Transportation will take you for tests and will take you back to your room when you are finished.
    El transporte lo (la) llevará para las pruebas y lo (la) regresará a su cuarto cuando termine.

102. You may be here a long time.
    Estará aquí mucho tiempo.

EXERCISES *EJERCICIOS*

A. Answer the questions using the cue given in parenthesis.

1. **¿Quién es Vd.?** (el cirujano)
   _____

2. **¿Quién es Vd.?** (la enfermera de guardia)
   _____

3. **¿Quién es Vd.?** (la jefa de enfermeras)
   _____

4. **¿Quién es Vd.?** (la enfermera diplomada)
   _____

5. **¿Quién es Vd.?** (la ayudante de enfermera)
   _____

6. **¿Quién es Vd.?** (el ayudante de hospital)
   _____

7. **¿Quién es Vd.?** (el enfermero de guardia)
   _____

8. **¿Quién es Vd.?** (la enfermera ambulante)
   _____

9. **¿Quién es Vd.?** (el enfermero de salud pública)
   _____

10. **¿Quién es Vd.?** (el camillero)
   _____

B. Make the appropriate substitutions.

1. **Este botón levanta la cabecera de la cama.**
   (baja) _____

2. **Este botón baja la cabecera de la cama.**
   (la cama) _____

3. **Este botón baja la cama.**
   (apaga la luz) _____

4. **Este botón apaga la luz.**
   (el televisor) _____

5. **Este botón apaga el televisor.**

VISITING HOURS

LAS HORAS DE VISITAS

1. Visitors are allowed unless you or your physician request "no visitors."
   Se permiten visitas a no ser que Vd. o su médico (médica) dispongan lo contrario.

2. Visitors are only allowed during visiting hours.
   Se admiten visitantes solamente durante las horas de visita.

3. The visiting hours are from _____ to _____.[19]
   Las horas de visita son desde la(s) _____ hasta las _____ de la tarde.

4. Visitors must obtain a pass from the information desk in the lobby.
   Los visitantes deben obtener un pase en la mesa de información del salón de entrada.

5. No more than two visitors at a time.[23]
   No más de dos visitas (visitantes) al mismo tiempo.

6. Only two visitors per patient are allowed.[23]
   Solamente se permiten dos visitantes por paciente.

7. Please return the passes when you leave.
   Por favor, no se olviden de devolver los pases cuando Vds. salgan.

8. There are too many visitors in the room.[23]
   Hay demasiados visitantes en el cuarto.

9. Please do not smoke in the patients' room.
   Le(s) pedimos que siga(n) las reglas de no fumar en el cuarto de los pacientes.

10. Smoking is allowed in the waiting room of each floor.
    Se permite fumar solamente en la sala de espera que está en cada piso.

11. Children under 14 are not able to visit the patients.
    Los niños menores de catorce años no pueden visitar a los pacientes.

12. Children under 12 are not allowed to visit the patients.
    A los niños menores de doce años no se les permite visitar a los pacientes.

13. Children between 12 to 16 must be accompanied by an adult.
    Los visitantes entre la edad de doce a dieciséis años tienen que ser acompañados por un adulto.

14. Children accompanying visitors should not be left unattended in the lobby.
    No se debe dejar solos en el salón de entrada a los niños que acompañan a los visitantes.

15. Visiting hours for the Intensive Care Unit are:[19]
    Las horas de visita para la Unidad de Cuidados Intensivos son:

16. Visiting hours for the Cardiac Care Unit are:[19]
    Las horas de visita para la Unidad de Cuidados Coronarios son:

17. One (two) visitors for 5 minutes every hour on the hour beginning at _____ and ending with _____.[19, 23]
    Un (dos) visitante(s) por cinco minutos cada hora en la hora que comienza a la(s) _____ y termina con _____.

18. One visitor for 5 minutes every hour on the half hour beginning at _____ and ending with _____.[19, 23]
    Un visitante por cinco minutos cada hora en la media hora que comienza a la(s) _____ y termina con _____.

Visiting Policy For All Maternity and Gynecology Patients

Fathers and/or husbands are permitted to visit from 2 P.M. to 8 P.M. The father of the baby visiting during feeding hours must wash his hands and be gowned.

Other visitors to Maternity and Gynecology are permitted from 2 P.M. to 3 P.M. and 7 P.M. to 8 P.M.

Maternity and Gynecological patients are permitted two visitors per day, exclusive of the father and/or husband.

No persons under 16 years of age are permitted to visit a maternity or gynecological patient other than the father of the baby or husband of the patient.

Horas de visita para pacientes del piso de maternidad y del piso ginecológico

Se permiten visitas de los padres y/o los esposos desde las dos de la tarde hasta las ocho de la noche. Durante las horas de alimentación, el padre del recién nacido debe lavarse las manos y ponerse la bata de hospital si está presente.

Se permiten otros visitantes al piso de maternidad y al piso ginecológico desde las dos hasta las tres de la tarde y desde las siete hasta las ocho de la noche.

Además del padre y/o esposo, se permiten dos visitantes a cada paciente de maternidad o de ginecología por día.

Nadie menor de dieciséis años está permitido visitar a ninguna paciente de maternidad o de ginecología a menos que sea el padre del recién nacido o el esposo de la paciente.

CONVERSATION WITH THE PATIENT
CONVERSACION CON EL PACIENTE

NURSING CARE *CUIDADOS AUXILIARES*

1. May I help you?
   ¿En qué puedo servirle (servirla)?

2. Did you call?
   ¿Me llamó Vd.?
   ¿Me ha llamado Vd.?

3. Did you sleep well?
   ¿Durmió Vd. bien?

4. Do you feel better today?
   ¿Se siente mejor hoy?

5. Do you still feel (very) weak?
   ¿Todavía se siente (muy) débil?

6. Are you sleepy?
   ¿Tiene Vd. sueño?

7. It is necessary to rest more.
   Es necesario descansar más.

8. Try to sleep.
   Trate de dormir.

9. Do you want to sit up?
   ¿Quiere Vd. sentarse?

10. Do you want to lie down?
    ¿Quiere Vd. acostarse?

11. Do you want me to call the nurse?
    ¿Quiere que llame a la enfermera?

12. Can I help you?
    ¿Puedo ayudarle (ayudarla) en algo?

13. Can you help me?
    ¿Puede ayudarme?

AMBULATION *TRATAMIENTO AMBULATORIO*

1. You are not well enough yet to get out of bed.
   Todavía Vd. no está bastante fuerte para levantarse.

2. You are to remain in bed today.
   Vd. debe guardar cama hoy.
   Vd. debe permanecer en cama hoy.

3. You may get out of bed, but not by yourself.
   Vd. puede salir de la cama, pero no sin ayuda.

4. You may be able to get (up) out of bed tomorrow.
   Vd. podrá levantarse de la cama mañana.

5. You may get up for about 15 minutes this afternoon.
   Vd. puede levantarse por unos quince minutos esta tarde.

6. You will not be able to walk for ten days.
   No podrá caminar por diez días.

7. You must lie flat in bed until tomorrow.
   Vd. debe permanecer acostado (acostada) hasta mañana.

8. You have to get out of bed.
   Vd. tiene que salir de la cama.
   Vd. tiene que levantarse de la cama.

9. You may walk around today.
   Vd. puede caminar hoy.

HYGIENE *HIGIENE*

1. You may take a bath.[24]
   Vd. puede bañarse.

2. You may take a shower.[24]
   Vd. puede ducharse.
   Vd. puede darse una ducha.
   Vd. puede darse un regaderazo. *Mex.*

3. You may take a sitz bath.[24]
   Vd. puede darse un baño de asiento (un semicupio).

4. Take a hot sitz bath every four hours.[24]
   Tome Vd. un baño de asiento (un semicupio) caliente cada cuatro horas.

5. Do not lock the door, please.
   No cierre Vd. la puerta con llave, por favor.

6. Call if you feel faint or in need of help.
   Llame si Vd. se siente débil, o si necesita ayuda.

7. Can you wash yourself or do you need help?
   ¿Puede Vd. lavarse, o necesita ayuda?

8. Do you want me to wash you?
   ¿Quiere Vd. que yo le (la) bañe?
   ¿Quiere Vd. que yo le (la) lave?

9. We are going to give you a (sponge) bath.
   Nosotros vamos a darle un baño (de esponja).

10. You may use the wash basin.
    Vd. puede usar la jofaina.
                               palangana.
                               ponchera. *C.A.*
                               palangana. *Mex.*
                               vasija (basija).

11. Wash your genitals.
    Lávese los privados (los [órganos] genitales).

12. Can you comb your hair without help?
    ¿Puede peinarse sin ayuda?

13. Can you shave yourself or do you want me to shave you?
    ¿Puede afeitarse a sí mismo, o quiere que yo le afeite?

14. Try to do it yourself.
    Trate de hacerlo por sí mismo (misma).

15. Call when you have to go to the toilet.
    Llame cuando tenga que ir al inodoro.
                               a los servicios.
                               al [cuarto de] baño.

16. Do you need the bed pan, or do you want to go to the bathroom?
    Necesita Vd.   la cuña o quiere ir al inodoro?
                    la silleta o quiere ir al inodoro?
                    el cómodo *Mex.* **o quiere ir al inodoro?**

17. I am going to put the bed pan on the table.
    Voy a dejar la cuña (el cómodo *Mex.* **sobre la mesa.**

18. Flex your knees and raise your buttocks off the bed.
    Flexione Vd. las rodillas y levante las nalgas de la cama.

19. Use the signal cord to call as soon as you have urinated.
    Use Vd. el botón para llamar tan pronto como Vd. haya orinado.

20. Do you need tissues or toilet paper?
    ¿Necesita Vd. kleenex (pañuelo de papel) o papel higiénico (papel de baño)?

21. Are you constipated?
    ¿Está Vd. estreñido (estreñida)?

22. I will give you an enema.
    Le pondré una enema.

23. Turn on your left (right) side.
    Acuéstese Vd. sobre el lado izquierdo (derecho).

24. Turn over.
    Dése vuelta, por favor.
    Voltéese del otro lado, por favor.
    Vírese Vd. del otro lado.
    Vuélvase del otro lado, por favor.

DIAGNOSIS   *DIAGNOSIS*

1. I still don't know exactly what is wrong with you.
   Todavía no sé exactamente lo que Vd. tiene.

2. I think that we have found the cause of your illness.
   Pienso que hemos descubierto la causa de su enfermedad.

3. We are still trying to find the cause of your illness.
   Todavía estamos tratando de saber la causa de su enfermedad.

4. I (do not) know why you are sick.
   (No) sé por qué está enfermo (enferma).

5. What do you think is the matter with you?
   En su parecer, ¿de qué padece?[25]

6. Have you visited a *curandero* or *santero* or a *botánica*[26] recently?[25]
   ¿Ha visitado un curandero o santero o botánica recientemente?

7. It seems that you have heart disease.[27]
   Parece que Vd. tiene enfermedad cardíaca.

PROHIBITIONS   *PROHIBICIONES*

1. It is very harmful for you to smoke so much.
   Le hace mucho daño fumar tanto.

2. You have to stop smoking.
   Vd. tiene que dejar de fumar.

3. Don't drink any alcohol.
   No tome Vd. ninguna bebida alcohólica.

4. Don't have any sexual relations until . . .
   No tenga relaciones sexuales hasta que . . .
       you are treated.
       se cure.
       you finish this medicine.
       termine este medicamento.

5. Avoid physical exercise.
   Evite Vd. los ejercicios físicos.

6. Don't do any heavy work.
   No haga Vd. ningún trabajo pesado.

7. Don't drive a car.
   No conduzca Vd. el coche.

8. Don't lose weight.
   No pierda Vd. peso.

9. Don't gain weight.
   No aumente Vd. peso.

10. Avoid salt.
    Evite Vd. la sal.

11. Avoid tobacco.
    Evite Vd. el tabaco.

12. Don't swim for the next few weeks.
    No debe nadar durante las semanas que vienen.

13. Don't use this hand for the next few days.
    No debe usar esta mano durante los próximos días.

14. Don't lift anything that weighs more than _____ pounds.[28]
    No levante nada que pese más de _____ libras.

APPOINTMENTS *CITAS*

1. The doctor wants to see that prescription.
   El médico (La médica) quiere ver esa receta.

2. The doctor will examine you now.
   El doctor (La doctora) le (la) examinará ahora.

3. The doctor wants to see how you are getting along.
   El doctor (La doctora) quiere ver cómo (le) va.

4. What day and time can you make an appointment?
   ¿Cuándo puede venir para una cita / un turno?
   ¿Qué día? ¿A qué hora?

5. Do you have directions to our office?
   ¿Sabe Vd. dónde está nuestro consultorio?

6. Make an appointment to come back to the clinic to see me in two weeks.[29]
   Haga Vd. una cita en la clínica para verme de hoy en quince días.

7. I will make an appointment for you to see Dr. Ortiz on Tuesday, February 17 at 11:30 A.M.
   Le haré una cita a Vd. para ver a la doctora Ortiz el martes, el diecisiete de febrero, a las once y media de la mañana.[19, 29]

8. Here is an appointment card.
   Aquí tiene Vd. una tarjeta con la información escrita.

9. Don't fail to return on the 17th (of February).[19, 29]
   No deje de volver el diecisiete (de febrero).

10. Don't forget.
    No se olvide.

11. The appointment is important.
    La cita es importante.

12. I'll need to take a message and have the doctor call you.
    Necesito apuntar un recado / mensaje. El médico / La médica le llamará más tarde.

DISCHARGE *EL ALTA*

1. I think that you should not return home just yet.
   Creo que Vd. no debe volver a su casa todavía.

2. I think that you will be much better soon.
   Creo que Vd. se sentirá mucho mejor dentro de poco.

3. I think that it may take you quite a while to recuperate.
   Creo que tardará mucho en recobrar la salud.

4. You are going to be discharged (released) today.
   A Vd. le van a dar de alta hoy.
   A Vd. van a darle de alta hoy.

5. The patient was discharged this morning.
   A la (Al) paciente le dieron de alta esta mañana.

6. If you have any questions, ask your doctor (ask for me).
   Si Vd. quiere saber algo, pregunte por su doctor(a) (por mí).

SUPPLIES *MATERIALES*

1. Do you need supplies?
   ¿Le faltan artículos (materiales)?

2. Do you need a sleeping pill?
   ¿Necesita Vd. una pastilla para dormir?
   una píldora somnífera?
   un somnífero?
   algo para ayudarle a dormir?

3. Do you need a stool softener?
   ¿Necesita Vd. una cápsula para ablandar sus evacuaciones?

Notes *Notas*

1. When people are not on a first name basis, it is far more common for them to address someone using just that person's title rather than the title and last name. Note that titles are not capitalized unless they are abbreviated.

2. When interacting with "older" people, instead of addressing them by their first names only, as is often the case with Anglo health care practitioners, it is more respectful to precede their name with the untranslateable *don* (for men) or *doña* (for women). i.e., *doña Carmen* rather than Carmen when speaking with 80 year old Carmen Sánchez De Llama.

3. In Spanish-speaking countries, people tend to use the words *tarde* (afternoon) and *noche* (evening) differently than people in the United States. For most people who live in the United States, the afternoon is considered to be the time between noon and 5 or 6 P.M.—the end of the work day—at which time the evening begins and extends until bedtime. In the Spanish-speaking world, however, the afternoon extends far beyond 5 or 6 P.M.; people work until 7 or 8 in the "afternoon." The evening meal may be served between 9 and 10 P.M. They tend to go to bed much later as well. See Chapter 4, page 95.

4. It is customary to give your entire name.

5. *Con permiso* asks for permission *before* an action that inconveniences someone happens; *perdón* and its derivatives are used *after* an offensive or disturbing action occurs.

6. Many Hispanics will say ¡*Perdón*¡ when they sneeze. People around them are likely to reply, ¡*Salud*¡ or ¡*Jesús!* In some areas of Mexico and in parts of Central America, it is common to hear ¡*Salud!* when a person sneezes once, ¡*Dinero!* (Money!) after the second sneeze, and ¡*Amor!* (Love!) in response to the third sneeze in a row.

7. Although often used interchangeably as synonyms, *comprender* generally refers to understanding an idea or a concept; *entender* refers to understanding linguistically or conceptually.

8. ¿*Cómo se siente?* and ¿*Qué tiene Vd.?* are used to inquire about physical health and appearance. ¿*Cómo está Vd.?*, although it literally asks "How are you?," is considered more of a greeting. Responses are not meant to include comments about physical health. ¿*Qué le pasa?* usually refers to emotional conditions or situations.

9. The verb *sentirse* (ie) is used when discussing one's health or mental state. i.e., *Me siento tan mal.* could mean I feel so sick, meaning that I am unwell; it could also mean that I am extremely upset. Context clues will give hints. The non-reflexive form of the verb, *sentir*, also has the meaning of "to feel." It is used with nouns to refer to the physical senses. *No siento una brisa.* I don't feel a breeze. "To be sorry" or "to regret" are additional meanings. *Lo siento (mucho).* I'm very sorry.

10. Many Hispanics tack on this response to someone else's arrangement of a future occurrence. It is illustrative of their faith and the important role that religion plays in their lives. It is also common to hear people say,¡*Jesús!* when someone sneezes or invoke either the name of God or Jesus in conversation. This is not considered disrespectful or blasphemous. On the contrary, many Spanish expressions of surprise or excitement have a religious source. Commonly heard are ¡*Virgen santa!*, ¡*Por Dios!* ("For God's sake") ¡*Dios mio!* ("My God"), *Con la ayuda de Dios* ("With God's help"), ¡*Sabe Dios!* ("Goodness/God knows") *Dios mediante* ("God willing") *Que Dios te acompañe* ("God go with you"), or ¡*Ave María purísima!*. These can best be likened to "My goodness" or "God Help Me" in English.

11. Students may find it helpful to review Spanish Verbs.

12. Local telephone numbers in many Spanish-speaking countries are composed of between two and seven digits: Costa Rica: 6 digits; El Salvador: 6 digits; Guatemala: 2-6 digits; Philippines: 4-7 digits; Spain 6-7 digits; Venezuela: 4-6 digits.

Inhabitants tend to express their telephone numbers in groups of twos. Thus, 230695 becomes: 23-06-95. If the telephone number contains an odd number of digits, the first number is given separately whereas the remaining digits are grouped in twos: 7123445 becomes: 7-12-34-45.

Some Spanish-speakers adopt the U.S. custom of expressing all digits as units numbers: 525-4123 becomes: 5-2-5-4-1-2-3.

13. Many foreign-born Hispanics are familiar with the special centers of their countries known as *Casa de Primeros Auxilios* (House of First Aid) or *Casa de Socorro* (House of Help). They are taken there when a medical emergency arises rather than going directly to a hospital. The health care practitioners there either take care of the problem entirely, or, in serious cases, refer the patients to a hospital for more extensive treatment. Consequently, some individuals might be fearful of being taken directly to the hospital for fear of a more serious problem than is the case.

14. The terms *hospital, clínica,* and *consultorio* ("doctor's office") do not necessarily mean the same thing to foreign-born Hispanics as to others. In many Spanish-speaking countries individuals in search of medical assistance will go to any of the above, or they will receive the necessary treatment at home.

Hospitales in many countries, including Mexico, are government-subsidized public health facilities that offer free or nominally priced medical care. The intention is to provide some type of health care treatment to everyone, regardless of the ability to pay. These facilities vary greatly in what resources they can provide, and in some areas segments of population consider them places where people go to die.

Popular among the wealthier individuals are the *clínicas* which are not State owned. Rather, they are usually owned privately by a group of physicians. Although these facilities are generally not nearly as large as the *hospitales,* they frequently have better, more modern equipment and better educated, often in the United States, physicians. Health care in the *clínicas* is never subsidized by the government. Consequently, it is expensive, which results in fewer people using the facilities and hence, more attention and better care. Many *clínicas* have their own surgeries, and most provide in-patient care.

Consultorios are exclusively for out-patient treatment. They resemble many U.S. physicians' offices. Doctors attempt to serve their patients as best they can in the office. In the event that more is needed, patients are sent either to the *hospital* or to a *clínica.*

15. The Hispanic family is usually reluctant to give up its responsibility for sick family members and may be very resistant to hospitalization. There are many underlying causes. Despite rapid urbanization, many Hispanics still live in areas where medical facilities are not readily available; the Spanish-speaking as a group tend to be poor, and Anglo medical care is very expensive. Fear of separation from the family is another important factor (see footnote 23). The formality and impersonality of the Anglo health care personnel, the hospital schedule, and unfamiliar foods may be distasteful to Hispanics. Finally, there is the fear of the hospital itself, for it is viewed as the place where people go to die. (See John H. Burma, ed., *Mexican-Americans in the United States: A Reader,* Cambridge: Schenkman Publishing Co., 1970, page 329; Pedro Poma, "Hispanos: Impact of Culture on Health Care," *Illinois Medical Journal,* Vol. 156, No. 6, page 457).

16. See Chapter 1, page 25.

17. Health care practitioners should always remember the strong influence of the Hispanic family. Consequently, when speaking with Hispanic patients, they are often speaking with the entire family even if not every one is actually present. It is common for Hispanic patients to discuss the physician's diagnosis and plan of treatment with the family although this response is not limited solely to Hispanics. See Chapter 1, page 25.

18. See Chapter 11, page 247, **Diet** *Dieta.*
19. See Chapter 4, "Numerical Expressions," pages 95–99.
20. See Chapter 16, page 356.
21. The verb "to eat breakfast" is expressed in some Spanish-speaking countries as *desayunar.* Consequently, both are acceptable.
22. See Chapter 12, pages 252–253 for more extensive blood tests.
23. This standard American policy of hospitalization often presents problems for the Hispanic community. Hospitalization often means a separation from family and the temporary loss of the emotional support of kinship. Consequently, family members and close friends may go to the hospital in large numbers to visit the sick individual, thus creating disruptions to hospital regulations. (See P. Poma, "Hispanos: Impact of Culture on Health Care," *Illinois Medical Journal*, Vol. 156, page 457.)
24. Some Hispanic women who have just given birth may choose to follow the rules of *la cuarentena* and may object to bathing or showering. For a more complete discussion about this, see Chapter 8, note 40, Chapter 11, note 7, and M. Kay, "Health and Illness in a Mexican American Barrio," in Spicers, ed., *Ethnic Medicine in the Southwest*, Arizona: University of Arizona, 1977, pages 155f.
25. It is not always necessary to ask this question; nonetheless, many less acculturated Hispanics, especially those foreign-born individuals with little or no formal education, have definite ideas about the etiology of their health problem. Some believe that illness is related to sins they may have accidentally committed, or to "spells" that have been cast on them. It is not uncommon for someone with very limited formal education to describe his illness in terms of his cultural understanding. Such individuals may easily confuse neurological problems with nervous problems and use the expression *problemas de los nervios* ("nervous problems") even when speaking in Spanish to refer to mental health.

   Although it is not clear how many Hispanics make use of these alternative medical options, it is possible that a patient may have also sought help from a *curandero* and that the *curandero* may have prescribed some type of medication or herbs. Consequently, it might prove helpful to ask these questions.
26. *Botánicas* are stores where different types of powders, herbs, and roots can be purchased. Because of the effectiveness of many herbal treatments, there is wide-spread confidence in the use of such *remedios*. These stores are especially popular in the Caribbean region; they are also located in any area of the United States where there is a significant Hispanic population.
27. See Chapter 16, **Key Diseases,** pages 333–338.
28. Remember that all Spanish-speaking countries use the metric system, which may cause some misunderstanding or confusion when discussing weights and measures with a Hispanic patient.
29. For important cultural differences in orientation to time, see Chapter 1, pages 25–28.

CHAPTER 7

Conversations for Health
Professionals: Present Illness
and Past Medical History

*Conversaciones para personal médico y
paramédico: Enfermedad actual
y previa historia médica*

PRESENT ILLNESS[1]

ENFERMEDAD ACTUAL

1. What is wrong with you?[2]
   ¿De qué se queja Vd.?
   ¿Qué le pasa a Vd.?
   ¿Qué le sucede a Vd.?

2. What's wrong with the child?
   ¿De qué se queja la niña / el niño?
   ¿Qué le pasa a la niña / al niño?
   ¿Qué le sucede a la niña / al niño?

THE PEDIATRICIAN

(It is 8pm. Mrs. Reyes is telephoning Dr. Poma, her daughter's pediatrician.)

	Service:	Hello.
	Mrs. Reyes:	Hello. This is Helen Reyes speaking. I need to speak with Dr. Poma.
	Service:	What is the problem, Ma'am?
5	Mrs. Reyes:	My daughter Marcelina has a cold. Moreover, she is suffering from a horrible earache in her right ear and bad chest pains. Her temperature has risen to 102.2°F [39°C].
	Service:	I will get in touch with the doctor. What is your telephone number?
	Mrs. Reyes:	It is 932-67-84.
10	Service:	Doctor will call you as soon as possible.
	Mrs. Reyes:	Thank you. Good-bye.
		(A short while later the telephone rings in the Reyes' home.)
	Mrs. Reyes:	Hello.
	Doctor:	Hello. Dr. Poma speaking. Is this Mrs. Reyes?[3]
15	Mrs. Reyes:	Speaking.
	Doctor:	My service tells me that Marcelina has a serious problem. I am not far from you. I can make a house call and be there within fifteen minutes.
	Mrs. Reyes:	Oh, Doctor. That would be so nice.

(The doctor arrives within 15 minutes. After having a cup of tea in the Reyes' kitchen and chatting pleasantly,
20 Mrs. Reyes suggests that the doctor examine the irritable child.)

	Doctor:	Good evening, Marcelina. How are you feeling?
	Marcelina:	Horrible.
	Doctor:	I am going to take your temperature and examine your ears and chest.
	Mrs. Reyes:	The poor thing is all worn out.
25	Doctor:	How old are you now, Marcelina?
	Marcelina:	Five.
	Mrs. Reyes:	Marcelina has a dry cough and a problem bringing up phlegm sometimes. She has lost her color.
	Doctor:	What hurts you, Marcelina?
30	Marcelina:	It hurts me here [indicating the sternum area] and here [indicating her throat] when I swallow, and here [pointing to her right ear].
	Doctor:	It seems that she has an ear infection, tonsillitis, and bronchitis. I am going to prescribe some drops for her ear and an antibiotic for the infections. If it is possible, she can gargle either with salt water or with Listerine.
35		While her temperature is high, it is necessary for Marcelina to stay in bed. For her ear, besides the drops every four hours, a hot water bottle, warm enough so that she may rest her head on it, can help.
		Now, I want to give her a penicillin injection. Is the child allergic to penicillin?
	Mrs. Reyes:	No, Doctor.
40	Doctor:	Okay. Give her warm (hot) drinks like tea made from "dock herb." She should drink lots of liquids. When the cough is very severe, use the vaporizer to add humidity to the room. As a general rule, the vaporizer helps to soothe a dry, non-productive cough. I am going to prescribe
45		an expectorant (cough syrup). How much does Marcelina weigh?
	Mrs. Reyes:	About 50 lbs. [22.65 kilos].

Doctor:	Give the medicine like this: One teaspoonful every four hours, following my orders exactly. The sore throat will disappear when the cold is cured.
50	Marcelina, open your mouth. I am going to tickle your throat with this swab. Mother, I have to do a throat culture (take a small sample of the secretions of her pharynx). She should take three baby tylenols after every meal and upon going to bed. Here are the prescriptions that you will need. It is necessary to keep on taking the antibiotic until it is finished in order to be sure
55	of the cure. If the fever is still not down in the morning, I want to see the child tomorrow afternoon. If the temperature comes down, I will see her next week.
Mrs. Reyes:	Thank you very much, Doctor. Good night.
Doctor:	Good night.

Situation

You are the pediatrician. A mother calls about her three year old who shows early signs of dehydration, severe diarrhea, and high fever. Tell her what to do. Suggest lots of fluids, tylenol, cool baths or alcohol rubs, and 1–2 tablespoonsful of Kaopectate after every bowel movement.

LA PEDIATRA

(Son las ocho de la noche. La señora Reyes llama por teléfono a la pediatra de su hija, la doctora Poma.)

	Servicio:	Diga.[4]
	Sra. Reyes:	Oiga. Habla Elena Reyes. Necesito hablar con la doctora Poma.
	Servicio:	¿Cuál es el problema, señora?
5	Sra. Reyes:	Mi hija Marcelina está resfriada. Además, padece de un tremendo dolor del oído derecho y de dolor torácico. Su temperatura sube a los 102.2°F [39°C].
	Servicio:	Voy a notificar a la doctora. ¿Cuál es su número de teléfono?
	Sra. Reyes:	Es 932-67-84.
10	Servicio:	La doctora le llamará tan pronto como sea posible.
	Sra. Reyes:	Gracias. Adios.

(Al rato suena el teléfono en casa de los Reyes.)

	Sra. Reyes:	Diga.
15	Dra. Poma:	Oiga. Habla la doctora Poma. ¿Tengo el gusto de hablar con la señora Reyes?[3]
	Sra. Reyes:	Servidora de Vd.[3]
	Dra. Poma:	Mi servicio me dice que Marcelina tiene un problema grave. No estoy muy lejos de Vds. Puedo hacer una visita facultativa y estar allí dentro de quince minutos.
20	Sra. Reyes:	Oh, doctora. Nos gustaría muchísimo.

(La doctora llega dentro de 15 minutos. Después de tomar una taza de té en la cocina con los Reyes y de charlar amablemente, la señora sugiere que la doctora vea a la irritable niña.[5])

	Dra. Poma:	Buenas noches, Marcelina. ¿Cómo te sientes?[6]
	Marcelina:	Malísima.
25	Dra. Poma:	Voy a tomarte la temperatura y examinarte los oídos y el pecho.
	Sra. Reyes:	Está agotada la pobrecita.
	Dra. Poma:	¿Cuántos años tienes ahora, Marcelina?
	Marcelina:	Cinco.
	Sra. Reyes:	Marcelina tiene una tos seca y tiene dificultad para expectorar tragando flemas a veces.
30		Ha perdido el color.
	Dra. Poma:	¿Qué te duele, Marcelina?
	Marcelina:	Me duele aquí (indicando la región del esternón) y aquí (indicando la garganta) al tragar, y aquí (señalando el oído derecho).
	Dra. Poma:	Parece que tiene una infección del oído y de las amígdalas y bronquitis. Voy a recetar unas
35		gotas para el oído y un antibiótico para las infecciones. Si es posible, ella puede hacer gárgaras antisépticas o con agua salada o con Listerine.
		Mientras la temperatura sea alta, Vd. debe mantener a Marcelina en cama. Para el oído, además de las gotas cada cuatro horas, puede ayudar una bolsa de agua caliente, bastante
40		templada para que la pequeña recline encima su cabeza.
		Ahora, quiero darle una inyección de penicilina. ¿Es la niña alérgica a penicilina?
	Sra. Reyes:	No, doctora.
45	Dra. Poma:	Bueno. Déle bebidas calientes como té hecho de hierba colorada[7]. Debe tomar muchos líquidos, señora. Cuando la tos sea muy molesta, utilice el vapor de agua para humedecer el ambi-

50   Sra. Reyes: ente. Por regla general, el vapor de agua ayuda a suavizar una tos seca y no productiva. Voy a recetar un (jarabe) expectorante. ¿Cuánto pesa Marcelina?

           Sra. Reyes: Unas cincuenta libras [22.65 kilos].

           Dra. Poma: Administre la medicina así: Una cucharadita cada cuatro horas, siguiendo exactamente la prescripción facultativa. El dolor de garganta suele desaparecer cuando se cura el resfriado.

              Marcelina, abre la boca. Voy a cosquillear la garganta con este tapón. Señora, tengo que tomarle una pequeña muestra de la garganta (de la secreción faríngea). Ella debe tomar tres tylenol para niños después de cada comida y al acostarse. Aquí están las recetas que necesitarán. Hay que seguir tomando el antibiótico hasta terminarlo para estar segura de la cura. Si mañana la fiebre no baja todavía, quiero ver a la niña mañana por la tarde. Si la temperatura

60   baja, la veré la semana que viene.

           Sra. Reyes: Muchas gracias, doctora. Buenas noches.

           Dra. Poma: Muy buenas.

Preguntas

1. **¿Cuál es el problema de Marcelina?**
2. **¿Necesita alguna medicina?**
3. **¿Qué debe hacer la familia si la fiebre no baja?**

3. Did you have an accident?
   ¿Tuvo Vd. un accidente?
   ¿Sufrió Vd. un accidente?

4. When did it occur?
   ¿Cuándo ocurrió?

5. Where did it happen?
   ¿Dónde ocurrió?

6. Were you hurt at work?
   ¿Fue lastimado (lastimada) en el trabajo?
   ¿Se lastimó en el trabajo?
   ¿Se hizo daño en el trabajo?

7. What is the name of your employer?
   ¿Para qué compañía trabaja Vd.?
   ¿Dónde trabaja Vd.?
   ¿Quién le emplea?

8. What is the address of your employer?[8]
   ¿Cuál es la dirección de su trabajo?
   ¿Dónde está Vd. empleado (empleada)?

9. Did you faint before the accident?
   ¿Se desmayó Vd. antes del accidente?

10. Did you faint after the accident?
    ¿Se desmayó Vd. después del accidente?

11. Did you have a dizzy spell before the accident?
    ¿Tuvo Vd. mareos antes del accidente?
    Se sintió Vd. mareado (mareada) antes del accidente?

12. Did you lose consciousness after the accident?
    ¿Perdió Vd. el conocimiento después del accidente?

13. How long?
    ¿Por cuánto tiempo?

14. How did this illness begin?[9]
    ¿Cómo empezó esta enfermedad?
    ¿Cómo ha empezado esta enfermedad?

15. When were you first taken sick?
    ¿Cuándo ha empezado esta enfermedad?

16. Please try to remember (the) dates and times accurately.
    Por favor, trate de recordarse de las fechas y la hora exactas.

17.   Have you taken any medicine for this?
¿Ha tomado Vd. alguna medicina para esto?

18.   What have you taken?
¿Qué ha tomado Vd.?

A MEDICAL PROBLEM

	Mr. Gómez:	What is today's date?
	Mrs. Gómez:	Today is August 18. But, what's the matter? You don't look well.
	Mr. Gómez:	I don't feel well. I have lost my appetite, and I think I need to see a doctor. How much does Dr. Ortiz charge for a house call?
5	Mrs. Gómez:	It doesn't matter. You are ill and you need medical attention, but he no longer makes house calls. Let's call his office (clinic) and make an appointment for this afternoon if possible.
		[An hour later.]
10	Mrs. Gómez:	We will take a taxi and go to the clinic. Here comes a taxi. Driver, is your car for hire?
	Driver:	Yes. Where do you want to go?
	Mrs. Gómez:	Take us to #2 La Brea Avenue, as fast as possible. Hurry and you will have a big tip. Stop here; this is the building. We will get out here.
	Mr. Gómez:	Ring the doorbell.
15	Mrs. Gómez:	Is the doctor in?
	Receptionist:	Yes. Who are you?
	Mrs. Gómez:	This is Ernesto Gómez; he has an appointment with Dr. Ortiz for two o'clock.
	Receptionist:	Ma'am, you can wait here; go right in, Mr. Gómez.
	Dr. Ortiz:	How long have you been feeling indisposed?
20	Mr. Gómez:	Since last night; I was sweating when I left my office, and I caught a bad cold.
	Dr. Ortiz:	Let me take your pulse. Stick out your tongue.
	Mr. Gómez:	Doctor, do you think that the symptoms are serious?
	Dr. Ortiz:	No, Sir. Now I am going to take your temperature.
		[Two minutes later]
25		The thermometer shows that you only have slight fever.
	Mr. Gómez:	I have a **BAD** headache and I feel dizzy.
	Dr. Ortiz:	Take these pills (aspirins) and the pain will pass.
		[After several minutes]
		Don't you feel better now?
	Mr. Gómez:	On the contrary, I feel worse.
30	Dr. Ortiz:	In that case, perhaps you need something stronger. Fill this prescription at the pharmacy, and take a tablespoonful of the medicine every four hours. If you don't feel better, return in three days.
	Mr. Gómez:	Thank you very much, Doctor.

Situation

1.   You are the patient. You have a high fever, chills, sore throat and persistent cough. You need medical attention. Call the doctor's office and set up an appointment as soon as possible.
2.   You are the receptionist. The doctor that you work for is away on vacation. Try to schedule an appointment for a routine check-up for the week after the doctor returns.

UN PROBLEMA MEDICO

	Señor Gómez:	¿Cuál es la fecha de hoy?
	Señora Gómez:	Hoy es el dieciocho de agosto. Pero, ¿qué tienes? No luces muy bien.
	Sr. Gómez:	No me siento bien. He perdido el apetito, y creo que necesito ver a un médico. ¿Cuánto co-
5		bra el doctor Ortiz por hacer una visita facultativa?
	Sra. Gómez:	No importa. Estás enfermo y necesitas ayuda médica, pero ya no hace visitas facultativas. Vamos a llamar a su clínica y pedir turno (hora) para esta tarde si es posible.
		[Una hora después]
10	Sra. Gómez:	Tomaremos un taxi e iremos a la clínica. Aquí viene un taxi. Chófer, ¿está su auto desalquilado?

	Chófer:	Sí, señores, ¿adónde desean Vds. ir?
15	Sra. Gómez:	Llévenos Vd. a la avenida La Brea, número dos, lo más aprisa posible. Dése prisa y tendrá una buena propina. Pare Vd. aquí; éste es el edificio. Vamos a bajar.
	Sr. Gómez:	Toca el timbre de la puerta.
	Sra. Gómez:	¿Está en casa el doctor?
	Recepcionista:	Sí. ¿Quiénes son Vds.?
	Sra. Gómez:	Este es Ernesto Gómez; tiene un turno con el doctor Ortiz para las dos.
20	Recepcionista:	Señora, Vd. puede esperar aquí; pase Vd. adelante, Sr. Gómez.
	Dr. Ortiz:	¿Desde cuándo se siente Vd. indispuesto?
	Sr. Gómez:	Desde anoche; estaba sudando al salir de mi oficina, y cogí un fuerte resfriado.
	Dr. Ortiz:	Déjeme tomarle el pulso. Saque la lengua.
25	Sr. Gómez:	¿Cree Vd., doctor, que los síntomas son serios?
	Dr. Ortiz:	No, señor. Ahora voy a tomarle la temperatura.
		[Dos minutos más tarde.]
		El termómetro indica que Vd. tiene sólo una pequeña [leve] fiebre.
	Sr. Gómez:	Siento un GRAN dolor de cabeza y mareo.
30	Dr. Ortiz:	Tome Vd. estas píldoras (aspirinas) y se le pasará el dolor. [Después de unos minutos.] ¿No se siente Vd. mejor ahora?
	Sr. Gómez:	Al contrario, me siento peor.
	Dr. Ortiz:	En ese caso, tal vez le falta a Vd. algo más fuerte. Envíe esta receta a la farmacia y tome una cucharada de la medicina cada cuatro horas. Si no se siente mejor, vuelva (hágame el favor de volver) dentro de tres días.
35	Sr. Gómez:	Muchas gracias, doctor.

Preguntas

1. ¿Cómo se siente el Sr. Gómez?
2. ¿Qué tiene?
3. ¿Tiene otros síntomas?
4. ¿Cuánto tiempo hace que se siente mal?
5. ¿Cómo llega al consultorio del Dr. Ortiz?
6. ¿Entra en la sala de reconocimientos la señora Gómez?
7. Después de ver al médico, ¿cuál es el diagnóstico?
8. ¿Cuándo tiene que volver?

PAIN *DOLOR*

18. Is the pain better after the medicine?
    ¿Siente Vd. alivio después de tomar la medicina?

19. Does it make it worse?
    ¿Lo hace sentir peor?

20. Are you in pain?
    ¿Siente Vd. dolor?

21. When did your pains begin?
    ¿Cuándo empezaron sus dolores?

22. Where is the pain?
    ¿Qué le duele?
    ¿Dónde le duele?
    ¿Dónde siente Vd. el dolor?

23. In the head?
    ¿En la cabeza?[10]

24. In the abdomen?
    ¿En el abdomen?

25. In the chest?
    ¿En el pecho?

26. In the side?
    ¿En el lado?
    ¿En su costado?

27. Which one?
    ¿En qué lado?

28. In the shoulder blades?
    ¿En los hombros?

29. In the back?[11]
    ¿En la espalda?

30. In the lower back?
    ¿En los riñones?[12]
    ¿En la cintura?[13]
    ¿En el cinturón?[14]

31. In the legs?
    ¿En las piernas?

32. In the bones?
    ¿En los huesos?

33. Here?
    ¿Aquí?

34. Are you in pain now?
    ¿Tiene Vd. dolores ahora?
    ¿Siente Vd. dolores ahora?
    ¿Sufre Vd. de dolor ahora?

35. Does the pain radiate?
    ¿Se corre el dolor?

36. From where to where?
    ¿Hacia dónde?

37. Is it a constant pain, or does it come and go?
    ¿Es un dolor constante, o va y vuelve?

38. Is it dull, sharp, steady pain, or a feeling of pressure?
    ¿Es un dolor sordo, agudo, continuo, o una sensación de presión?

39. Do you have pain here?
    ¿Siente Vd. dolor aquí?
    ¿Le duele aquí?

Practice *Práctica*

Conteste Vd. a las preguntas que siguen según el modelo:

¿Dónde le duele a la abuela? (las rodillas)
Le duelen las rodillas.

¿Dónde le duele a Vd.? (la cabeza)
Me duele la cabeza.

1. **¿Dónde le duele a su tío? (el codo izquierdo)**
2. **¿Dónde le duele al niño? (los oídos)**
3. **¿Dónde le duele al paciente? (el corazón)**
4. **¿Dónde le duele a Miguel? (el tobillo)**
5. **¿Dónde le duele a su madre? (el estómago)**

40. Has the pain eased a great deal?
    ¿Ha disminuido mucho el dolor?

41. How long have you had the pain?
    ¿Desde cuándo tiene Vd. el dolor?

42. Is there anything that makes the pain better?
    ¿Hay algo que lo alivie?

43. Is there anything that makes the pain worse?
    ¿Hay algo que lo haga sentir peor?

44. What is it?
    ¿Qué es?

45. Is there anything else that accompanies the pain?
    ¿Hay otras molestias que acompañan el dolor?

46. Does the pain go away when you rest?
    Al descansar, ¿se alivia el dolor?

47. Does the pain awaken you at night?
    ¿Le (La) despierta el dolor durante la noche?

48. Is the pain very strong at night?
    ¿Es mayor el dolor durante la noche?
    ¿Aumenta el dolor en la noche?

49. More during the daytime?
    ¿Mayor durante el día?

50. All the time?
    ¿Todo el tiempo?

51. Before eating?
    ¿Antes de comer?

52. After eating?
    ¿Después de comer?

53. While eating?
    ¿Al comer?

54. When it is (was) cold?
    ¿Cuando hace (hacía) frío?

55. When it is (was) hot?
    ¿Cuando hace (hacía) calor?

56. When it is (was) humid?
    ¿Cuando está (estaba) húmedo?

57. When you are (were) upset?
    ¿Cuando está (estaba) molesto (molesta)?

58. When you are worried?
    ¿Cuando está (estaba) preocupado (preocupada)?

59. When you exercise(d)?
    ¿Cuando hace (hacía) ejercicios?

60. When you urinate(d)?
    ¿Cuando orina (orinaba)?

61. When you defecate(d)?
    ¿Cuando defeca (defecaba)?

62. When you have (had) sexual relations?
    ¿Cuando tiene (tenía) relaciones sexuales?

63. When you swallow(ed) liquids, solids, or both?
    ¿Cuando traga (tragaba) líquidos, sólidos o ambos?

64. When you stand (stood)?
    ¿Cuando está (estaba) de pie?

65. When you sit (sat) down?
    ¿Cuando está (estaba) sentado (sentada)?

66. When you lie (lay) down?
    ¿Cuando está (estaba) acostado (acostada)?

67. When you walk (walked)?
    ¿Cuando camina (caminaba)?

68. When you climb(ed) stairs?
    ¿Cuando sube (subía) escaleras?

69. When you bend (bent) over?
    ¿Cuando se agacha (agachaba)?

70. Do you have a lot of pain in your left (right) leg?
    ¿Le duele mucho la pierna izquierda (derecha)?

71. Does it hurt more when I press, or when I stop pressing suddenly?
    ¿Le duele más cuando le aprieto o cuando dejo de apretar de repente?

72. Does it hurt only where I am pressing, or somewhere else?
    ¿Le duele solamente donde aprieto, o en otros lugares más?

73. Can you sleep with the pain?
    ¿Lo (La) deja dormir el dolor?

74. I will not hurt you.
    No voy a hacerle daño.

75. It is not painful.
    No le va a doler.
    No va a dolerle.

76. Tell me when you feel pain.
    Avíseme cuando sienta dolor.

Practice   *Práctica*

Conteste Vd. a las preguntas que siguen según el modelo:

    ¿Cuándo le duele a la abuela? (subir las escaleras)
    Le duele a la abuela cuando sube las escaleras.

    ¿Cuándo le duele a Vd.? (toser mucho)
    Me duele cuando toso mucho.

1. **¿Cuándo le duele la garganta a la niña? (comer)**
2. **¿Cuándo le duelen los pies? (andar demasiado)**
3. **¿Cuándo le duele a Vd.? (hacer ejercicios físicos)**
4. **¿Cuándo le duele al viejecito? (orinar)**
5. **¿Cuándo le duele el tobillo? (correr)**

77. Have you had a heart attack?
    ¿Sufrió Vd. un ataque cardíaco?

78. When did you have your first attack?
    ¿Cuándo sufrió Vd. su primer ataque?

79. Have you or another person in your family or neighborhood suffered from this same illness previously?
    ¿Ha padecido Vd. u otra persona de la familia o vecindad antes de esta misma dolencia?

80. What is bothering you most right now?
    ¿Qué es lo que más le molesta en este momento (ahora mismo)?

81. Do you have or have you had . . .
    ¿Tiene o ha tenido Vd. . . . .
        stiffness here?
        rigidez aquí?
        swelling here?
        hinchazón aquí?
        redness here?
        enrojecimiento aquí?
        sensation of warmth here?
        una sensación de calor aquí?
        tenderness here?
        sensibilidad aquí?
        limited movement here?
        movimiento limitado aquí?

82. Does the wound have any pus?
    ¿Tiene pus la herida?

83. Has pus drained from the wound?
    ¿Ha salido pus de la herida?

A WOUND

Doctor: Let's see that wound. Does it hurt you a lot?
Patient: So, so. My whole leg hurts a little.
Doctor: That is normal. Such a deep wound takes a long time to heal.
Patient: Is there any infection or gangrene?
5 Doctor: There is nothing to worry about. There is neither infection nor gangrene. Let's see this bandage. It will be necessary to change the dressing now and then again every two days.
Patient: Who will change my bandage at home?
Doctor: Your daughter can do it for you. The nurse will show her how to do the best dressing for your
10 (type of) wound. When she comes to visit you, tell her to check with the nurse on duty.
Patient: Thank you, doctor. I am going to telephone her right now.

Questions

1. What is the matter with the patient?
2. Who will do his bandage when he returns home?
3. When will he have to change it?

UNA HERIDA

Médico:	A ver esa herida. ¿Le duele mucho?
Paciente:	Así, así. Me duele un poquito toda la pierna.
Médico:	Es normal. Una herida tan profunda tarda mucho tiempo en curarse.
Paciente:	¿Hay infección o gangrena?
5 Médico:	No hay que preocuparse. No hay ni infección ni gangrena. A ver este vendaje. Será preciso cambiar la venda ahora y después cada dos días.
Paciente:	¿Quién me hará el vendaje en casa?
Médico:	Su hija puede hacérselo. La enfermera le enseñará cómo hacer la mejor venda para su
10	herida. Cuando ella venga a visitarle, dígale que consulte con la enfermera de guardia.
Paciente:	Gracias, doctor. Voy a telefonearle ahorita.

Preguntas

1. ¿De qué sufre el paciente?
2. ¿Quién le hará el vendaje al volver a casa?
3. ¿Cuándo tiene que cambiarlo?

84. Do you know where you are?
    ¿Sabe Vd. dónde está?

85. You are in the hospital.
    Vd. está en el hospital.

86. What day is today?
    ¿Qué día es hoy?

87. What month is it?
    ¿Cuál es el mes?

88. You will be OK.
    Vd. va a estar bien.

89. You will need an operation.
    Vd. va a necesitar una operación.

90. I am calling a specialist to see you.
    Voy a llamar a un(a) especialista que le (la) vea.

REVIEW *REPASO*

Learn the following dialogue.

Aprenda el diálogo que sigue.

DOCTOR: Good morning. What is wrong with you?

DOCTOR: **Buenos días. ¿De qué se queja Vd.?**

PATIENT: I don't feel very well.

PACIENTE: **No me siento muy bien.**

DOCTOR: What happened?

DOCTOR: **¿Qué le pasó?**

PATIENT: I had an accident. A huge box fell on my head.

PACIENTE: **Sufrí un accidente. Una caja enorme se me cayó en la cabeza.**

DOCTOR: When did it occur?

DOCTOR: **¿Cuándo ocurrió?**

PATIENT: It happened during my shift at the plant about 9:30.

PACIENTE: **Ocurrió durante mi turno en la fábrica más o menos a las nueve y media.**

DOCTOR: For whom do you work?

DOCTOR: **¿Quién le emplea?**

PATIENT: Delphi West.

PACIENTE: **Delphi West.**

DOCTOR: What is the address of your employer?

DOCTOR: **¿Cuál es la dirección de su trabajo?**

PATIENT: 4800 South Saginaw, Flint.

PACIENTE: **Calle Saginaw cuarenta y ocho cero cero Sur, Flint.**

DOCTOR: Did you faint after the accident?

DOCTOR: **¿Se desmayó Vd. después del accidente?**

PATIENT: I suddenly lost consciousness.

PACIENTE: **De repente perdí el conocimiento.**

DOCTOR: For how long?

PATIENT: A minute.

DOCTOR: Are you in pain now?

PATIENT: Yes, and I feel dizzy.

DOCTOR: Where is the pain? Show me.

PATIENT: My head and neck hurt me.

DOCTOR: Is it a constant pain or does it come and go?

PATIENT: It is a constant pain.

DOCTOR: Is it dull, sharp, steady, or a feeling of pressure?

PATIENT: It is a sharp pain in my head and a feeling of pressure on my neck.

DOCTOR: Has the pain eased a lot?

PATIENT: It is better.

DOCTOR: We must have more information. Please give the nurse the information she requests. You will also need some tests before we can make a diagnosis.

DOCTOR: ¿Por cuánto tiempo?

PACIENTE: Un minuto.

DOCTOR: ¿Siente Vd. dolor ahora?

PACIENTE: Sí, y me siento mareada.

DOCTOR: ¿Qué le duele? Muéstreme.

PACIENTE: Me duelen la cabeza y el cuello.

DOCTOR: ¿Es un dolor constante, o va y vuelve?

PACIENTE: Es un dolor constante.

DOCTOR: ¿Es un dolor sordo, agudo, continuo, o una sensación de presión?

PACIENTE: En la cabeza es un dolor agudo, y en el cuello, una sensación de presión.

DOCTOR: ¿Ha disminuido mucho el dolor?

PACIENTE: Me siento mejor.

DOCTOR: Debemos tener más información. Tenga la bondad de contestar a las preguntas de la enfermera. Además, Vd. necesitará algunos análisis antes de que podamos hacer un diagnóstico.

PAST MEDICAL HISTORY[15]

PREVIA HISTORIA MEDICA

1. Have you ever had . . . ?
   ¿Ha sufrido Vd. alguna vez de . . . ?
   ¿Ha padecido Vd. alguna vez de . . . ?

rheumatic fever
fiebre reumática
measles
sarampión
German measles
rubéola; sarampión alemán; alfombría
Chicano; **fiebre de tres días**
scarlet fever
fiebre escarlatina
mumps
paperas; farfoyota *PR;* **bolas** *slang*
typhoid fever
fiebre tifoidea
polio
polio
chicken pox
varicela; viruelas locas *slang*
cholera
cólera
diphtheria
difteria
small pox
viruela
whooping cough
tos ferina; tos convulsiva; coqueluche
chronic tonsilitis
amigdalitis crónica

chronic laryngitis
laringitis crónica
tuberculosis[16]
tuberculosis
amebic dysentery
disentería amebiana
high blood pressure
hipertensión arterial; presión arterial alta
low blood pressure
hipotensión arterial; presión arterial baja
diabetes[17]
diabetes
goiter
bocio; buche *slang*
anemia
anemia (un número bajo de los glóbulos rojos)
venereal disease
enfermedades venéreas; la secreta *slang*
gonorrhea
gonorrea; purgación *slang*
syphilis
sífilis; sangre mala *slang*
heart disease
enfermedades cardíacas; enfermedad del corazón; cardiopatías

any kidney ailment
cualquier enfermedad del riñón
kidney stones
cálculos en el riñón
allergies
alergias
hay fever
fiebre del heno
sinusitis
sinusitis
arthritis
artritis
cystitis
cistitis (infección de la vejiga)
spastic colon
colon espástico; colitis mucosa
pneumonia
neumonía; pulmonía
emphysema
enfisema
varicose veins
**várices; venas varicosas; venas infla-
madas**
brain stroke
**derrame cerebral; embolia cerebral;
parálisis; hemorragia vascular**
blurred vision
vista borrosa
Parkinson's disease
**la parálisis agitante; la enfermedad de
Parkinson**
chorea (any spastic paralysis)
**corea; el mal o la danza o el baile de San
Vito o de San Guido**

tetanus
tétanos; el mal de arco *slang*
pancreatitis
pancreatitis
cirrhosis
cirrosis del hígado
epileptic attacks
ataques epilépticos; convulsiones
ulcers (stomach or duodenal)
úlceras (de estómago o duodeno)
mononucleosis
mononucleosis infecciosa
gall bladder attack
**ataque de la vesícula; derrame de bilis;
ataque vesicular**
gall stones
cálculos en la vejiga
appendicitis
apendicitis
jaundice
derrame biliar; ictericia; piel amarilla *fam*
hepatitis
hepatitis
pleurisy
pleuresía
large boils
furúnculos grandes
cancer
cáncer[18]
tropical diseases
enfermedades tropicales
diverticulitis
diverticulitis; colitis ulcerosa
any previous surgery
cualquier cirugía anterior; cirugía previa

2. Do you have problems with your thyroid gland?
   ¿Tiene Vd. problemas con la glándula tiroides?
   ¿Tiene Vd. problema de tiroides?

3. What immunizations have you had?[19]
   ¿Qué clase de inmunizaciones ha tenido Vd.?
   cholera
   cólera
   yellow fever
   fiebre amarilla
   tetanus
   tétanos
   polio (myelitis)
   polio (mielitis)—(la vacuna oral)
   polio (mielitis)—(en forma de inyección)

   measles
   sarampión
   measles, mumps, rubella
   la triple
   Hib vaccine (meningitis)
   la vacuna contra meningitis
   BCG
   BCG para tuberculosis

4. Were you vaccinated against smallpox?
   ¿Le vacunaron contra la viruela?

5. Did you get an inoculation for typhoid?
   ¿Le pusieron una inoculación contra el tifus?

6. Were there many people in your town with that disease?
   ¿Había mucha gente en su pueblo con esa enfermedad?

7. Do you have asthma?
   ¿Sufre Vd. de asma?
   ¿Ha padecido Vd. de asma?
   ¿Sufre Vd. de fatiga? *fam*

8. Are you allergic to . . . ?
   ¿Tiene Vd. alergias a . . . ?
   ¿Es Vd. alérgico (alérgica) a . . . ?
   ¿Padece Vd. de alergias a . . . ?

any food	sleeping pills
alguna comida	**píldoras para dormir**
ice cream	dust or pollen or mold
helado[20]	**polvo o polen o moho**
penicillin	animals
penicilina	**animales**
aspirin	insect bites
aspirina	**picaduras de insectos**
sulfa	
sulfas	

9. Have you ever had welts/rashes, itching, swelling or asthma after getting penicillin?
   ¿Ha tenido Vd. alguna vez ronchas, comezón, hinchazones o asma después de recibir penicilina?

10. Do you have any drug reactions?[21]
    ¿Tiene Vd. alguna sensibilidad a productos químicos?

11. Have you been hospitalized within the last five years?
    ¿Ha estado Vd. internado (internada) por cualquier razón durante los últimos cinco años?

12. Why?
    ¿Por qué?

13. When did you come here (to the hospital) for the first time?
    ¿Cuándo vino Vd. aquí (al hospital) por primera vez?

14. How long had you been in the hospital?
    ¿Cuánto tiempo hacía que Vd. estaba en el hospital?

15. Which hospital was it?
    ¿En qué hospital?

16. What is the address?
    ¿Cuál es la dirección?

17. How long have you been in the hospital?
    ¿Cuánto tiempo lleva Vd. internado (internada)?

18. Do you have your own doctor?
    ¿Tiene Vd. su propio médico (propia médica)?

19. What is his (her) name?
    ¿Cómo se llama?

20. Where is his (her) office?
    ¿Dónde está su consultorio?

21. What is the telephone?[4]
    ¿Cuál es su número de teléfono?

22. When was the last time you saw a doctor?[22]
    ¿Cuándo fue la última vez que visitó a su médico (médica)?
    ¿Cuándo fue la última vez que ha visitado a un médico (una médica)?
    ¿Cuándo fue la última vez que ha visto a un médico (una médica)?

23. What was the visit for?
    ¿Para qué consultó Vd. a su médico (médica)?

24. Have you seen another doctor or native healer for this problem?[2]
    ¿Ha visto Vd. a otro médico o curandero tocante a este problema (por este problema)?

25. Why did you go to the doctor at that time?
    ¿Por qué fue Vd. a ver al médico entonces?

26. How long had you been sick?
    ¿Cuánto tiempo hacía que estaba enfermo (enferma)?
    ¿Cuánto tiempo llevaba Vd. enfermo (enferma)?

27. What was the name of the medicine that the doctor gave you?
    ¿Cómo se llama la medicina que el médico le recetó?
    ¿Cuál era el nombre de la medicina que le recetó el médico?

28. Are you taking any medicine, or are you undergoing any medical treatment at present?[23]
    ¿Toma Vd. alguna medicina o está siguiendo algún tratamiento médico actualmente?

29. What are the names of the medicines?
    ¿Cuáles son los nombres de las medicinas?

30. What are the medicines for?
    ¿Para qué son las medicinas?

31. How many pills do you have at home?
    ¿Cuántas píldoras tiene Vd. en casa?

32. Have you ever had surgery?
    ¿Ha sido operado (operada) jamás?

33. How many times?
    ¿Cuántas veces?

34. Where were you operated on?
    ¿En qué parte fue operado (operada)?

35. Please show me.
    Muéstremela, por favor.

36. When was your last operation?
    ¿Cuándo fue la última operación?

37. Did you have much bleeding during or after the operation?
    ¿Sangró Vd. mucho durante la operación o después?

38. Did you receive blood transfusions?
    ¿Tuvieron que darle una transfusión de sangre?

39. Do you travel much abroad?
    ¿Viaja Vd. mucho al extranjero?

40. Were you sick?
    ¿Se enfermó?

41. Did you see a physician?
    ¿Vio Vd. a un(a) médico (médica)?

42. What did he (she) diagnose?
    ¿Qué diagnosticó?

43. What was the treatment?
    ¿Cuál fue el tratamiento?

44. How do you travel? By plane, train, boat, or car?
    ¿Por qué medio viaja Vd.? ¿Por avión, por tren, por barco o en auto?

45. How long do you spend away from the USA?
    ¿Cuánto tiempo pasa Vd. fuera de los Estados Unidos?

46. Where do you stay?
    ¿Dónde se queda Vd.?

47. Were you wounded while in the military service?
    ¿Fue Vd. herido (herida) mientras (que) estuvo en el servicio militar?

48. Have you ever been wounded by a gun?
    ¿Jamás le dieron un balazo?
    ¿Ha tenido jamás escopetazo?

49. Were you ever cut with a knife?
    ¿Le cortaron jamás con un cuchillo (una daga, un puñal, una navaja)?

50. Were you hit with a stick, stone, fist?
    Le pegaron con un palo, una piedra, el puño (la mano)?

51. Please show me where you were wounded.
    Muéstreme, por favor, dónde fue herido (herida).

52. Have you ever been badly hurt in an automobile accident?
    ¿Ha sido gravemente herido (herida) en un accidente de automóvil?

53. In any other kind of accident?
    ¿En otra clase de accidente?

Although the drills that follow are designed to be done actively in class by the instructor and the students, they are arranged so that the student may do them individually outside the class. The student must cover the drill with a card, move the card down the page until the first question or response is visible, make the appropriate answer aloud, and then move the card down until the correct answer appears. This procedure is followed until the end of the drill, when the student may repeat the drill (for additional practice) or go on to the next one.

EXERCISES *EJERCICIOS*

A. Ask the following questions using the cues in parenthesis:

1. ¿Ha padecido Vd. alguna vez de tuberculosis?
   (reumatismo)
2. ¿Ha padecido Vd. alguna vez de reumatismo?
   (furúnculos grandes)
3. ¿Ha padecido Vd. alguna vez de furúnculos grandes?
   (enfermedades tropicales)
4. ¿Ha padecido Vd. alguna vez de enfermedades tropicales?
   (cálculos en la vejiga)
5. ¿Ha padecido Vd. alguna vez de cálculos en la vejiga?
   (piel amarilla)
6. ¿Ha padecido Vd. alguna vez de piel amarilla?
   (alergias)
7. ¿Ha sufrido Vd. alguna vez de alergias?
   (artritis)
8. ¿Ha sufrido Vd. alguna vez de artritis?
   (vista borrosa)
9. ¿Ha sufrido Vd. alguna vez de vista borrosa?
   (viruelas locas)
10. ¿Ha sufrido Vd. alguna vez de viruelas locas?
    (paperas)
11. ¿Ha sufrido Vd. alguna vez de paperas?

B. Ask the hypothetical patients about immunizations, using the cues in parenthesis:

1. ¿Fue inmunizada María contra la difteria?
   (la viruela)
2. ¿Fue inmunizada María contra la viruela?
   (Roberto y Pablo)
3. ¿Fueron inmunizados Roberto y Pablo contra la viruela?
   (fiebre amarilla)
4. ¿Fueron inmunizados Roberto y Pablo contra la fiebre amarilla?
   (Carmen)
5. ¿Fue inmunizada Carmen contra la fiebre amarilla?
   (Carlos)
6. ¿Fue inmunizado Carlos contra la fiebre amarilla?
   (sarampión)
7. ¿Fue inmunizado Carlos contra el sarampión?
   (los niños)
8. ¿Fueron inmunizados los niños contra el sarampión?
   (Marta)
9. ¿Fue inmunizada Marta contra el sarampión?
   (las chicas)
10. ¿Fueron inmunizadas las chicas contra el sarampión?
    (el tifus)
11. ¿Fueron inmunizadas las chicas contra el tifus?

Notes *Notas*

1. See Chapter 1, page 14.
2. See Chapter 6, note 25.
3. The English translations in some instances are a bit free. Contemporary English frowns upon the sometimes flowery way of speaking still in use in Spanish.

4. See Chapter 6, note 12, page 134.

5. See Chapter 1, p. 25.

6. Notice that in conversation with the child, the doctor uses the *tú* forms. She is *tuteando*. It is not customary to address a youngster using the polite *Vd.* The child, on the other hand, never addresses adults using *tú*.

7. *Hierba colorada* or dock herb [*Rumex crispus*] is used by many Hispanic individuals to treat tonsillitis.

8. See Chapter 4, "Numerical Expressions," page 91.

9. Depending on the degree of acculturation, the typical Hispano uses a variety of curing patterns. Whether rural or urban, many Hispanos work at low-level, low-income jobs, requiring a minimum of specialized skills or education. There are many Hispanic doctors, dentists, and attorneys, but they usually assume the general social class characteristics of the dominant Anglo society. See Chapter 1, pages 13, 17–18, and 28.

10. Some Spanish-speaking patients will use the word *el cerebro*, which literally means "brain," to describe a headache localized in the occipital area of the head and even radiating down the posterior neck, or *el cuello*.

11. Many Spanish-speaking patients will use the *el pulmón*, which literally means "the lung" when referring to upper paraspinal musculoskeletal pain.

12. Many Spanish-speaking patients complain literally of "kidney" pain when they really mean lower back pain. Physical examination usually clarifies this, however.

13. Although this literally means "waist," it is not uncommon for some Spanish-speakers to use this when referring to lower back pain.

14. This literally means "belt," but is commonly used by many Spanish-speakers when referring to lower back pain.

15. See Chapter 16 for a fuller list of Key Diseases. In order to elicit the best responses and build patient trust, before beginning either the medical history or the physical, it is often helpful to request the Hispanic patient's permission to ask personal questions and to examine him/her. This display of courtesy requires professionals to use the phrases *Con su permiso* [**With your permission**] and *sin querer ser indiscreto* (*indiscreta*) . . . [**without wanting to be indiscreet . . .**].

16. Hispanics have a higher incidence of tuberculosis than other ethnic groups. (Hispanic Health and Nutrition Examination Survey, 1982–1984)

17. Diabetes and obesity are health issues of some importance in the Hispanic population. The HHANES reported that 26.1% of Puerto Ricans, 23.9% of Mexican Americans, and 15.8% of Cubans in the 45–74 age bracket have diabetes. The HHANES elaborates on this, saying that Mexican Americans are at higher risk for complications because their type of diabetes is of greater metabolic severity. Mexican Americans have a significantly higher incidence of diabetic retinopathy and diabetes-related end-stage renal disease. For further information about diabetes, see Chapter 15, pp. 316–324.

18. In rural areas Hispanics often use the word *cáncer* to refer to any serious skin infection, especially infected wounds or gangrene. The term *lepra* refers to any sore that spreads on the skin. This frequently causes confusion for health care personnel. Among the diseases that are called *lepra* are impetigo, boils, allergic skin reactions, scabies, insect bites, skin ulcers, chronic sores, skin cancer, and even skin TB or leprosy.

19. Significant numbers of children in some Hispanic countries have not been vaccinated, primarily because of the family's inability to pay. Nonetheless, there are some Hispanic families (and some from other ethnic groups) who do not understand that the "traditional" childhood diseases such as whooping cough and diphtheria, have not been eradicated as the result of vaccinations. Other families have put off vaccinating their children until they are of school age. Migrant (Hispanic) workers often have difficulty with their children's vaccination schedules because they move around so much. Health care practitioners must encourage parents to update their children's vaccinations and to keep written records in a place where they won't be lost. See E. R. Zell *et al.*, "Low Vaccination Levels of US Preschool and School-age Children: Retrospective Assessments of Vaccination Coverage, 1991–1992," *Journal of the American Medical Association*, 1994; 271:833–839 and T. A. Lieu *et al*, "Risk Factors for Delayed Immunization among Children in an HMO," *American Journal Public Health*, 1994; 84:1624–1625.

20. Patients from South America might substitute *la nieve*, which means "snow" for ice cream.

21. It is important to recognize that the word "drug" is NOT translated into Spanish by *droga*. The latter is used by Hispanics to refer to narcotics and other illegal drugs.

22. As indicated in Chapter 1, the use of health care services by Hispanics greatly depends on whether or not their employment provides them with health care insurance; it also depends on socioeconomic conditions. Data from HHANES indicates that uninsured Hispanics are less likely to have visited a physician within the past year, less likely to have had a routine physical exam, and less likely to have a regular source of health care than Hispanics with private health insurance.

In many Spanish-speaking countries, people go to their local pharmacists to consult about their health problems. In the Hispanic world pharmacists receive demanding training and make an effort to stay current in pharmacology. It is not uncommon for pharmacists to give shots and even prescribe medicines since the government does not regulate the sale of medication. Therefore, it is also possible that they may have consulted with the local pharmacist in the U.S., or with a *curandero* or other alternative practitioner. See Chapter 1, pages 10–11 and 17, and 6, notes 25 & 26, page 135.

23. See Chapter 6, note 25., page 135

24. See Chapter 1, page 20 for discussion about the Hispanic custom of borrowing and lending medication.

CHAPTER 8

Conversations for Health Professionals: Review of Systems

Conversaciones para personal médico y paramédico: Repaso de sistemas

REVIEW OF SYSTEMS

REPASO DE SISTEMAS

GENERAL *GENERAL*

1. How much do you normally weigh?[1]
   ¿Cuánto pesa Vd. por lo regular?

GROWTH PROGRESS

	Visiting Nurse:	Good afternoon, Mrs. Félix. How are you and your new infant?
	Mrs. Félix:	Good afternoon. I am very well, thank you, and my son is well, too.
	V. Nurse:	Today we ought to prepare a growth chart card for your son. We will need it to write down the most important facts that will occur related to his health. I will explain it to you later.
5		With your permission, I will ask you some questions about the baby.
	Mrs. Félix:	Gladly.
	V. Nurse:	What is the baby's name?
	Mrs. Félix:	His name is Maximiliano.
10	V. Nurse:	And what is your full and correct name?
	Mrs. Félix:	It is María Angela Hernández de Félix.[2]
	V. Nurse:	What is your husband's full name?
	Mrs. Félix:	His name is Jorge Luis Félix y Gómez.
	V. Nurse:	What is your address?
	Mrs. Félix:	We live on Alvarado Street. The houses there do not have numbers, but we live near the catholic church.
	V. Nurse:	What was the date of Maximiliano's birth?
	Mrs. Félix:	He was born on October 29th.
20	V. Nurse:	How many brothers and sisters does Maximiliano have?
	Mrs. Félix:	Only one sister. Her name is Teresita.
	V. Nurse:	Do you have a growth chart card for Teresita?
	Mrs. Félix:	No.
	V. Nurse:	On what date was she born?
25	Mrs. Félix:	On August 27th, more than three years ago. Teresita has always enjoyed good health.
	V. Nurse:	I'm glad, but it is advisable to immunize her so that she doesn't become ill. With your permission, I can vaccinate her today against TB. But now, I should like to weight Maxi. [She does it.] He weighs five and a half kilos. I want you to look at what I write down on the
30		card. I wrote the names of the months on this card, in the boxes which are on the bottom part. I began with October—the month in which Maximiliano was born. I will make a big dot on top of this month, which is December, at the height which corresponds to 5.5 kilos.
35	Mrs. Félix:	Is his weight okay?
	V. Nurse:	Yes, it is good for a baby almost two months old. From here on, we will weigh Maximiliano monthly in order to be certain that he is gaining weight. In this way we will know if he is growing well.

CRECIMIENTO

	Enfermera visitante:	**Buenas tardes, Sra. Félix. ¿Cómo están usted y su nuevo bebé?**
	Sra. Félix:	**Muy buenas. Estoy muy bien, gracias, y mi hijo está bien, también.**
	Enf. visi.:	**Hoy debemos preparar una ficha de crecimiento para su hijo. La**
5		**necesitaremos para anotar lo más importante que ocurra relacionado con su salud. Se lo explicaré más tarde. Con su permiso, le haré algunas preguntas acerca del bebé.**
	Sra. Félix:	**Con mucho gusto.**
	Enf. visi.:	**¿Cómo se llama el bebé?**
10	**Sra. Félix:**	**Se llama Maximiliano.**
	Enf. visi.:	**Y, ¿cuál es el nombre completo y correcto de usted?**
	Sra. Félix:	**Es María Angela Hernández de Félix.**
	Enf. visi.:	**¿Cuál es el nombre completo de su esposo?**
	Sra. Félix:	**Se llama Jorge Luis Félix y Gómez.**

15	Enf. visi.:	¿Cuál es su dirección?
	Sra. Félix:	Vivimos en la calle Alvarado. Las casas allá no tienen números, pero vivimos cerca de la iglesia católica.
	Enf. visi.:	¿En qué fecha nació Maximiliano?
	Sra. Félix:	Nació el 29 de octubre.
20	Enf. visi.:	¿Cuántos hermanos tiene Maximiliano?
	Sra. Félix:	Una sola. Se llama Teresita.
	Enf. visi.:	¿Tiene usted una ficha de crecimiento para Teresita?
	Sra. Félix:	No.
	Enf. visi.:	¿En qué fecha nació ella?
25	Sra. Félix:	El 27 de agosto, hace más de tres años. Teresita siempre ha gozado de buena salud.
	Enf. visi.:	Me alegro, pero conviene ponerle unas vacunas para que no se enferme. Con su permiso, puedo vacunarla hoy contra la tuberculosis. Pero ahora, quisiera pesar a Maxi. [Lo hace.] Pesa 5 kilos y medio. Quiero que usted
30		mire lo que anoto en la ficha. Escribí los nombres de los meses en esta ficha, en las casillas que hay en la parte baja. Comencé con octubre—el mes en que nació Maximiliano. Haré un punto grueso a la altura que corresponde a 5,5 kg, encima de este mes, que es diciembre.
	Sra. Félix:	¿Su peso está bien?
35	Enf. visi.:	Sí, es bueno para un bebé de casi dos meses. De aquí en adelante le pesaremos a Maximiliano mensualmente para estar seguras de que aumenta de peso. De esta manera sabremos si crece bien.

2. Do you have chills?
   ¿Tiene Vd. escalofríos?

3. Do the chills come every day?
   ¿Siente Vd. los escalofríos todos los días?
   every other day?
   cada dos días?
   every three days?
   cada tres días?

4. Are you hot or cold frequently?
   ¿Tiene Vd. calor o frío con frecuencia?[3]

5. Are you nervous?
   ¿Está Vd. nervioso (nerviosa)?

6. Are you depressed?
   ¿Está Vd. deprimido (deprimida)?
   ¿Sufre Vd. de depresiones severas?

PRACTICE   *PRACTICA*

With a friend practice the following dialogue until you have mastered it.

DOCTOR: Good afternoon, Mr. Gómez. I would like you to answer my questions to the best of your ability

DOCTOR: Buenas tardes, señor Gómez. Quiero que Vd. conteste a mis preguntas lo mejor que pueda.

MR. GÓMEZ: Okay, Doctor.

SR. GÓMEZ: Muy bien, doctor.

DOCTOR: How much do you normally weigh?

DOCTOR: Por lo regular, ¿cuánto pesa?

MR. GÓMEZ: 140 pounds.

SR. GÓMEZ: Ciento cuarenta libras.

DOCTOR: What was your minimum body weight, and when was it?

DOCTOR: ¿Cuál fue su peso mínimo, y cuándo fue?

MR. GÓMEZ: When I was in the army, I weighed only 130 pounds.

SR. GÓMEZ: Cuando estaba en el ejército, pesaba solamente ciento treinta libras.

DOCTOR: When were you in the army?

DOCTOR: ¿Cuándo estuvo en el ejército?

MR. GÓMEZ: I was in the army from 1990 to 1994. I was in the Gulf War for 3 months.

SR. GÓMEZ: Estuve en el ejército desde mil novecientos noventa hasta el noventa y cuatro. Estuve en la Guerra del Golfo por tres meses.

DOCTOR: What was your maximum body weight, and when was that?

DOCTOR: ¿Cuál fue su peso máximo, y cuándo pesaba eso?

MR. GÓMEZ: A year ago I weighed 175 pounds.

SR. GÓMEZ: Hace un año (que) pesaba ciento setenta y cinco libras.

DOCTOR: Then you have lost a lot of weight?

DOCTOR: Entonces, ¿ha perdido mucho peso últimamente?

MR. GÓMEZ: Yes, I have lost thirty-five pounds.

SR. GÓMEZ: Sí, he perdido treinta y cinco libras.

DOCTOR: Were you ever ill while in the army?

DOCTOR: ¿Sufrió Vd. enfermedades mientras estaba en el ejército?

MR. GÓMEZ: Never.

SR. GÓMEZ: Nunca.

DOCTOR: Do you sweat much?

DOCTOR: ¿Suda Vd. mucho?

MR. GÓMEZ: No, I sweat very little.

SR. GÓMEZ: No, sudo muy poco.

DOCTOR: Do you have chills?

DOCTOR: ¿Tiene escalofríos?

MR. GÓMEZ: Yes, I often have the chills.

SR. GÓMEZ: Sí, a menudo tengo escalofríos.

DOCTOR: Do the chills come every day?

DOCTOR: ¿Siente los escalofríos todos los días?

MR. GÓMEZ: I have the chills every other day, usually in the evening.

SR. GÓMEZ: Siento los escalofríos cada dos días, generalmente por la noche.

DOCTOR: Are you nervous?

DOCTOR: ¿Está Vd. nervioso?

MR. GÓMEZ: Yes, I am very nervous, and I eat little.

SR. GÓMEZ: Sí, estoy nervioso, y como poco.

DOCTOR: Very well, let's find out more about the problem.

DOCTOR: Muy bien. Vamos a averiguar cuál es el verdadero carácter de su problema.

SKIN, HAIR   *LA PIEL, EL PELO*

1. Do you have any bleeding problems if you cut yourself?
   ¿Tiene Vd. problemas de sangrar si se corta?

2. How long does it last?
   ¿Cuánto tiempo le dura?

3. Does this happen frequently?
   ¿Ocurre con frecuencia?

4. When you cut yourself, do you bleed more than most people, or about the same?
   Cuando Vd. se corta, ¿sangra más que la mayoría de las personas o igual que ellas?

5. Do you have any rash on your *face?*[4]
   ¿Tiene Vd. alguna erupción en *la cara?*

6. Where else do you have the rash?[4]
   ¿En qué otra parte tiene Vd. la erupción (el salpullido)?

7. How long have you had this rash?
   ¿Desde cuándo tiene Vd. esta erupción?

8. Have you had this before?
   ¿Ha tenido Vd. esto antes?

9. Has an insect bitten you?
   ¿Le (La) ha picado un insecto?

10. Have you eaten anything different lately?
    ¿Ha comido Vd. algo diferente últimamente (recientemente)?

11. Have you used a new soap lately, either for yourself or in the wash?
    ¿Ha usado Vd. un jabón nuevo últimamente, ya sea para usted mismo (misma) o cuando lava la ropa?

12. Does it irritate much?
    ¿Le (La) irrita mucho?

13. Is it itchy?
    ¿Le da comezón?

14. Does it hurt?
    ¿A Vd. le duele?

15. Did you take anything for it?
    ¿Ha tomado Vd. algo para curarlo?

16. Do you have chronic skin diseases, like psoriasis or seborhea?
    ¿Sufre Vd. de enfermedades crónicas de la piel, como psoriasis (la sarna *slang*) o seborrea?

17. Do you have any black or dark red moles that have changed in size?
    ¿Tiene Vd. lunares negros o colorados que hayan sufrido cambios?

18. Do you have any moles that bleed?
    ¿Tiene Vd. lunares que sangren?

19. Do you break out in hives?
    ¿Brota Vd. de urticarias severas en la piel?

20. Are you losing your hair?
    ¿Está Vd. perdiendo el pelo?

21. Does your scalp itch?
    ¿Le pica la cabeza?

HEAD[5] *LA CABEZA*

1. Do you get headaches?
   ¿Tiene Vd. dolores de cabeza?[6]
   ¿Tiene Vd. jaquecas?
   ¿Le duele la cabeza?[6]
   ¿Le dan dolores de cabeza?[6]

2. Do you get migraines?
   ¿Tiene Vd. migrañas?
   ¿Tiene Vd. jaquecas?

3. What part of your head hurts?
   ¿Qué parte de la cabeza le duele?

4. Show me where.
   Enséñeme dónde.

5. Does it hurt you here?
   ¿Le duele aquí?

6. Is it the first time that you have had a headache as strong as this?
   ¿Es la primera vez que tiene dolor de cabeza tan fuerte como éste?

7. When did it begin?
   ¿Cuándo empezó?

Ten minutes ago?	Today?
¿Hace diez minutos?	**¿Hoy?**
An hour ago?	Yesterday?
¿Hace una hora?	**¿Ayer?**

8. When did it begin for the first time?
   ¿Cuándo empezó por primera vez?
   Last week?
   ¿La semana pasada?
   Last month?
   ¿El mes pasado?
   Last year?
   ¿El año pasado?

9. Do you ever feel dizzy?
   ¿Tiene Vd. vértigo alguna vez?
   ¿Suele Vd. tener mareos? *fam*

10. How long do you feel dizzy?
    ¿Cuánto tiempo le duran los mareos?

11. How long have you had the headache?
    ¿Cuánto tiempo hace que Vd. tiene el dolor de cabeza?

12. Show me where it hurts you.
    Enséñeme Vd. dónde le duele.

13. How did the pain begin?
    ¿Cómo empezó el dolor?

14. Gradually?
    ¿Poco a poco?

15. Suddenly?
    ¿De repente?

16. What is the pain like?
    ¿Cómo es el dolor?

17. Is it strong?
    ¿Es fuerte?

18. Is it mild?
    ¿Es leve?

19. Is it throbbing, or is it a constant pain?
    ¿Le palpita, o es un dolor constante?

20. Is it aching?
    ¿Es dolorido?
    ¿Es adolorido?

21. Is it dull?
    ¿Es sordo?

22. Is it like shooting pain?
    ¿Es como punzada?

23. Do you have nausea with the pain?
    ¿Tiene náuseas con el dolor?

24. Have you vomited?
    ¿Ha vomitado Vd.?

25. Do you have dizziness with the pain?
    ¿Tiene mareos con el dolor?

26. Is something else hurting you?
    ¿Le duele algo más?

27. Where?
    ¿Dónde?

28. Does your neck hurt?
    ¿Le duele el cuello?

29. How often do you have pain?
    ¿Cada cuánto tiempo tiene dolor?

30. Every _____ minutes?[7]
    ¿Cada _____ minutos?

31. How did the pain begin?
    ¿Cómo empezó el dolor?

32. Gradually?
    ¿Poco a poco?

33. Suddenly?
    ¿De repente?

34. What is the pain like?[8]
    ¿Cómo es el dolor?

35. Is the pain the same each time?
    ¿Es el dolor igual cada vez?
    ¿Es el dolor lo mismo cada vez?

36. Is the pain in the same place each time?
    ¿Es el dolor en el mismo sitio cada vez?

37. Have you been feeling depressed?
    ¿Ha estado Vd. deprimido (deprimida)?

38. Did you get hit in the head?
    ¿Recibió un golpe en la cabeza?

39. Have you ever been hit in the head? face?
    neck? eyes? nose?
    ¿Se ha golpeado jamás la cabeza? ¿la cara?
    ¿el cuello? ¿los ojos? ¿la nariz?

40. Have you ever lost consciousness?
    ¿Ha perdido jamás el conocimiento?

41. For how long?
    ¿Por cuánto tiempo?

42. When?
    ¿Cuándo?

43. What happened?
    ¿Qué le pasó?

44. Is this the strongest headache you have ever had?
    ¿Es éste el dolor de cabeza más fuerte de su vida?

45. Are you running a fever now?
    ¿Tiene fiebre ahora?

46. Do you have a stiff neck?
    ¿Tiene el cuello tieso?

47. Does light bother you?
    ¿Le molesta la luz?

48. Do you have numbness anywhere?
    ¿Tiene entumecida alguna parte?

49. Do you have weakness anywhere?
    ¿Tiene débil alguna parte?

50. How old are you?[9]
    ¿Cuántos años tiene?

51. Do your temples hurt?
    ¿Le duelen las sienes?

52. Are you having problems with your vision?
    ¿Tiene problemas con la vista?

53. Do you lose vision? Suddenly?
    ¿Pierde la vista? ¿De repente?

54. Have you lost weight?
    ¿Perdió peso?

55. Does your head hurt more at night?
    ¿Le duele la cabeza más por la noche?

56. Do your hips or shoulders hurt?
    ¿Le duelen las caderas o los hombros?

57. Does it hurt more at night than during the day?
    ¿Le duele más por la noche que por el día?

58. Are you taking any medication? What?
    ¿Toma alguna medicina? ¿Qué?

59. Do your teeth hurt?
    ¿Le duelen los dientes?

60. Does any tooth hurt with ice?
    ¿Le duele algún diente con hielo?

61. Which tooth?
    ¿Qué diente?

62. Are your gums swollen?
    ¿Se le hinchan las encías?

63. Do you have or have you had frequent headaches?
    ¿Tiene Vd. o ha tenido dolores de cabeza frecuentemente?

64. Is your headache worse when you cough?
    ¿Es peor el dolor de cabeza cuando tose?

65. Is it worse when you move?
    ¿Es peor cuando se mueve?

66. Does it awaken you at night?
    ¿Le despierta por la noche?

67. Did you get hit in the head?
    ¿Recibió un golpe en la cabeza?

68. Did you lose consciousness?
    ¿Perdió conocimiento?

69. Are you allergic to any food or medicine?
    ¿Tiene alergia a alguna comida o medicina?

70. Do you get a headache from ice cream?
    ¿Sufre de dolores de cabeza al comer helado?[10]

71. Do you have diabetes?[11]
    ¿Sufre de diabetes?
    ¿Tiene diabetes?

72. Do you take insulin?
    ¿Toma insulina?

THE NEW DIABETIC

Nurse:	Good afternoon, Mr. Fernández. My name is Juan Mendoza, and I am the public health nurse. I see that you are going to be discharged from the hospital soon and that you will be able to return home in a few days. They have already confirmed that you are a diagnosed diabetic. Your doctor and the hospital dietician already spoke with you about your diet and the state of your health so that the transition from the hospital to home would not cause problems. I want to show you how to give yourself insulin.
Patient:	Thank you, Sir. I appreciate your interest.
Nurse:	Before I begin, do you have any questions about what has happened to you, and why you have to follow a special diet and exercise regularly?
Patient:	Well, I know that I suffered a diabetic coma and that foods which have refined sugar and starch poison me. Am I going to have another attack?
Nurse:	Nobody knows that. If you follow the diet, exercise, and take your insulin, it is unlikely that you will have another coma. In your case it is very important for you to lose weight. When you lose it, we hope that your glucose tolerance improves. Until you lose about 20 lbs., you will have to follow a salt-free diet.
Patient:	Why should I follow a salt-free diet if I have diabetes?
Nurse:	Salt retains fluids in the tissues and causes edema or swelling. When you eliminate salt from your diet, it helps the tissues to not retain fluids. These excessive fluids enter the blood system and are eliminated by the kidneys. There is better control of the blood sugar and the serum lipids when weight is not excessive.
Patient:	How can I remember what I ought to eat when I return home?
Nurse:	I am going to give you an Exchange List.
Patient:	Thank you. Are there any diabetic cookbooks?
Nurse:	Of course! Bookstores have them, libraries, too. And the Diabetes Association offers some. Why don't you write to the American Diabetes Association of Greater Chicago and Northern Illinois, 620 N. Michigan Avenue, Chicago, Illinois 60611?
Patient:	Thank you for the address.
Nurse:	If you don't have any other questions, I am going to teach you how to give yourself a shot of insulin. I suggest that you use disposable syringes. If you use a glass syringe, remember that the syringe and needle should be sterilized before each injection. You will be using slow-acting insulin, which is a cloudy preparation. Mix it thoroughly by rotating the bottle, not shaking it, so that there is no foam. Remove the cover and clean the stopper with an alcohol-soaked cotton ball. Take into the syringe an amount of air equal to the dosage of insulin that you are going to take out of the flask. Insert the needle into the center of the rubber stopper and let out the air. Turn the syringe and flask upside down. Take in the specified dosage. Clean the injection site with a cotton ball soaked in alcohol. Pinch the skin of the injection site together and then rapidly insert the needle. Inject the insulin dosage. Soak the injection area with alcohol as you withdraw the needle. Rub the area with alcohol.
Patient:	Can I use the same area every day?
Nurse:	No. You have to change the place every time, or you will develop insulin resistance or brittle diabetes. Use the rule of 48. Divide both arms, both thighs, and both sides of your abdomen (mentally) into rectangles of eight squares each. Six times eight squares make up 48 different places into which to take your injections. I want you to try injecting now. Don't be discouraged. Try it again. That's better. I'll see you again tomorrow.
Patient:	Good-bye.

EL NUEVO DIABETICO

Enfermero:	Buenas tardes, señor Fernández. Me llamo Juan Mendoza, y soy el enfermero de salud pública. Veo que le darán de alta del hospital pronto, y que Vd. podrá volver a casa dentro de unos días. Ya han confirmado que Vd. es un diabético diagnosticado [confirmado]. Su médico y la dietista del hospital ya hablaron con Vd. acerca de su dieta y el estado de su salud para que la transición del hospital a casa no causase problemas. Quiero mostrarle cómo debe inyectarse con insulina.
Paciente:	Gracias, señor. Le agradezco mucho el interés suyo.
Enfermero:	Antes de que empiece yo, ¿tiene Vd. algunas preguntas sobre lo que le ha ocurrido y el por qué tiene que seguir una dieta especial y hacer ejercicios regularmente?

Paciente:	Pues, sé que he sufrido un coma diabético y que las comidas que contienen azúcar refinado y almidón me envenenan. ¿Sufriré otro ataque?
Enfermero:	Eso no se sabe. Si Vd. sigue la dieta, hace los ejercicios, y toma su insulina, es difícil que Vd. sufra otro coma. En el caso de Vd., es muy importante que pierda peso. Al perderlo esperamos que su tolerancia a la glucosa mejore. Tendrá que seguir una dieta sin sal hasta que pierda unas veinte libras.
Paciente:	¿Por qué debo seguir una dieta sin sal si tengo diabetes?
Enfermero:	La sal retiene los líquidos en los tejidos, y causa edema o hinchazón. El eliminar la sal de su dieta ayuda a los tejidos a no retener los flúidos. Estos flúidos excesivos entran en el sistema circulatorio y son eliminados por los riñones. Hay mejor control de la glucosa sanguínea y de los lípidos del suero cuando el peso no es excesivo.
Paciente:	¿Cómo puedo recordar lo que debo comer cuando regrese a casa?
Enfermero:	Voy a darle una lista de intercambios.
Paciente:	Gracias. ¿Hay libros de cocina para diabéticos?
Enfermero:	¡Cómo no! Las librerías los tienen, las bibliotecas, también. Y la Asociación para diabetes ofrece algunos. ¿Por qué no le escriba Vd. a la American Diabetes Association of Greater Chicago and Northern Illinois, Avenida de Michigan, Número 620, norte, Chicago, Illinois, 60611 [seis cero seis once] para más información?
Paciente:	Gracias por la dirección.
Enfermero:	Si Vd. no tiene otras preguntas, voy a enseñarle cómo inyectarse con insulina. Sugiero que use una jeringuilla desechable. Si Vd. usa una jeringuilla de cristal, recuerde que la jeringuilla y la aguja deben ser esterilizadas antes de cada inyección. Vd. va a usar insulina con reacción lenta, que es una solución que luce turbia. Mezcle Vd. el medicamento completamente moviendo el frasco en rotación, no agitándolo, para evitar que se forme espuma. Quítele la tapa protectora y limpie el tapón de caucho del frasco con una mota de algodón empapada en alcohol. Con la jeringuilla tome una cantidad de aire igual a la de la dosis de insulina que va a extraer del frasco. Inserte la aguja a través del centro del tapón de caucho y expulse el aire dentro. Invierta el frasco y la jeringuilla. Extraiga con la jeringuilla la dosis especificada. Limpie el área de la inyección con otra mota de algodón empapada en alcohol. Pliegue la piel y rápidamente introduzca toda la aguja. Inyecte la dosis de insulina. Moje el área de inyección con alcohol mientras que retrae la aguja.
Paciente:	¿Puedo usar el mismo área cada día?
Enfermero:	No, hay que cambiar el área cada vez que se inyecte o sufrirá de resistencia a insulina o de diabetes quebradiza. Emplee Vd. la regla de cuarenta y ocho. Mentalmente divida los dos brazos, los dos muslos, los dos lados del abdomen en rectángulos, cada uno de ocho cuadrados. Seis por ocho cuadrados consituyen cuarenta y ocho áreas diferentes donde puede inyectarse. Quiero que Vd. trate de inyectarse ahora. No se desaliente. Hágalo otra vez. Eso es mejor. Le veré de nuevo mañana.
Paciente:	Adiós.

73. Do you have high blood pressure?
    ¿Tiene la presión alta?

74. Do you take medication for it? What?
    ¿Toma medicina para ella? ¿Qué?

75. Do you have a cold? frequent colds?
    ¿Tiene catarro? ¿Sufre de catarros frecuentemente?

76. Do you have a (frequent) stuffed-up nose?
    ¿Tiene la nariz tapada (frecuentemente)?

77. Do you have pain in your forehead?
    ¿Tiene dolor en la frente?
    ¿Le duele la frente?

78. Does your cheek hurt?
    ¿Le duele el pómulo?

79. Do you have any pain under your eyes?
    ¿Tiene algún dolor debajo de los ojos?

80. Do you have trouble breathing through your nose?
    ¿Tiene dificultad al respirar por la nariz?

81. Do you have sinusitis?
    ¿Sufre de sinusitis?

82. What is the pain like?
    ¿Cómos es el dolor?

83. Is it on one side or on both?
    ¿Es de un lado o los dos?

84. Is it constant or does it come and go?
    ¿Es constante o va y vuelve (viene)?

85. Are you nauseous with the pain?
    ¿Tiene náuseas con el dolor?

86. Does dizziness accompany the pain?
    ¿Tiene mareos con el dolor?

87. Are you vomiting?
    ¿Vomita?

88. Is there someone in the family who has migraines?
    ¿Hay alguien en la familia que tiene migrañas?

89. Who?
    ¿Quién? ¿Quiénes?[12]

90. Does the headache begin suddenly?
    ¿Empieza de repente el dolor de cabeza?

91. Do you know when you are going to have a headache?
    ¿Sabe cuándo le dolerá la cabeza?

92. Do you have tingling . . .
    ¿Tiene hormigueo . . .
    before the pain?
    antes del dolor?
    during the pain?
    durante el dolor?
    after the pain?
    después del dolor?

93. Do you see stars? lightning bolts . . .
    ¿Ve estrellas? relámpagos . . .
    before the pain?
    antes del dolor?
    during the pain?
    durante el dolor?
    after the pain?
    después del dolor?

94. Do you have difficulty speaking . . .
    ¿Tiene dificultad al hablar . . .
    before the pain?
    antes del dolor?

during the pain?
durante el dolor?
after the pain?
después del dolor?

95. Do noises bother you . . .
    ¿Le molestan los ruidos . . .
    before the pain?
    antes del dolor?
    during the pain?
    durante el dolor?
    after the pain?
    después del dolor?

96. Do you experience numbness or weakness. . .
    ¿Tiene alguna parte entumecida o débil . . .
    before the pain?
    antes del dolor?
    during the pain?
    durante el dolor?
    after the pain?
    después del dolor?

97. Do you have pain in one eye?
    ¿Sufre de dolor de un ojo?
    ¿Le duele un ojo?

98. Does your nose get stuffed up?
    ¿Se le tapa la nariz?

99. Does the pain hit you when you are sleeping?
    ¿Le pega el dolor cuando duerme?

100. Is the pain better in the morning?
    ¿Es mejor el dolor por la mañana?

101. Is the pain worse in the afternoon or evening?
    ¿Es peor el dolor por la tarde o por la noche?

102. Do you feel depressed?
    ¿Se siente deprimido (deprimida)?

REVIEW *REPASO*

Practice the following dialogue.

DOCTOR: Do you have any bleeding problems, Mr. Gómez?

MR. GÓMEZ: No, Doctor, I don't have any bleeding problems if I cut myself.

DOCTOR: How long have you had this rash on your face?

MR. GÓMEZ: I've had it for a month.

DOCTOR: Does it irritate you much?

MR. GÓMEZ: Yes, it itches me, but I don't scratch.

DOCTOR: Did you take anything for it?

MR. GÓMEZ: Yes, I have been using a gray ointment.

DOCTOR: Discontinue using the ointment for now.

MR. GÓMEZ: What should I use?

Practique el diálogo que sigue.

DOCTOR: **¿Tiene Vd. problemas de sangrar, señor Gómez?**

SR. GÓMEZ: **No, doctor, no tengo problemas de sangrar si me corto.**

DOCTOR: **¿Desde cuándo tiene Vd. esta erupción en la cara?**

SR. GÓMEZ: **La tengo desde hace un mes.**

DOCTOR: **¿Le irrita mucho?**

SR. GÓMEZ: **Sí, me irrita, pero, no me rasco.**

DOCTOR: **¿Ha tomado Vd. algo para curarla?**

SR. GÓMEZ: **Sí, he usado una pomada gris.**

DOCTOR: **Deje Vd. de usar la pomada por ahora.**

SR. GÓMEZ: **¿Qué debo usar?**

DOCTOR: After I do some more tests, I will give you a prescription. Do you get headaches?

MR. GÓMEZ: I do; I have an awfully bad headache now.

DOCTOR: How long do the headaches generally last?

MR. GÓMEZ: All day. The pain is especially bad over my left eye.

DOCTOR: Do you ever feel nauseated while you have a headache?

MR. GÓMEZ: Yes, Doctor, and sometimes I vomit.

DOCTOR: What do you do for the headache?

MR. GÓMEZ: I usually take two aspirins every three hours and stay in bed until I feel better.

DOCTOR: Very well, Mr. Gómez.

DOCTOR: Después de hacerle algunas pruebas más, le daré una receta. ¿Tiene Vd. dolores de cabeza?

SR. GÓMEZ: Los tengo; me duele muchísimo la cabeza ahora.

DOCTOR: Generalmente, ¿cuánto tiempo le duran los dolores de cabeza?

SR. GÓMEZ: Por lo común, todo el día. El dolor es aún más fuerte encima del ojo izquierdo.

DOCTOR: Mientras que tiene dolor de cabeza, ¿tiene náusea alguna vez?

SR. GÓMEZ: Sí, doctor, y a veces vomito.

DOCTOR: ¿Qué hace para su migraña?

SR. GÓMEZ: Por lo regular tomo dos aspirinas cada tres horas y guardo cama hasta sentirme mejor.

DOCTOR: Muy bien, señor Gómez.

EYES   *LOS OJOS*

1. Do you wear glasses?
   ¿Usa Vd. anteojos? *general term*
   ¿Usa Vd. lentes? *Mex.*
   ¿Usa Vd. espejuelos? *Cuba*

2. . . . for close-up?
   ¿para ver de cerca?
   . . . for distance?
   ¿para ver de lejos?
   . . . for reading?
   ¿para leer?
   . . . all the time?
   ¿todo el tiempo?

3. Do you wear contact lenses?
   ¿Usa Vd. lentes de contacto?

4. How long have you been wearing them?
   ¿Desde cuándo los usa?

5. Do you sometimes see things double?
   ¿Ve Vd. las cosas doble algunas veces?

6. Do you have blurred vision?
   ¿Ve Vd. borroso?

7. Do you see things through a mist?
   ¿Ve Vd. nubladas las cosas como a través de una neblina?

8. Do your eyes burn?
   ¿Le arden los ojos?

9. Do your eyes water much?
   ¿Le lagrimean mucho los ojos?

10. Your eyes seem inflamed (red).
    Sus ojos parecen inflamados (rojos).

11. Do you have eyestrain?
    ¿Tiene Vd. la vista cansada?

12. Do you have eyeaches?
    ¿Sufre Vd. de dolor en los ojos?

13. Does your (left) (right) eye hurt?
    ¿Le duele a Vd. el ojo (izquierdo) (derecho)?

14. Do both your eyes hurt?
    ¿A Vd. le duelen los dos ojos?

15. Do your eyes itch?
    ¿Tiene Vd. una picazón en los ojos?

16. Do you have a discharge from your eyes?
    ¿Le supuran los ojos?

17. Were your eyes stuck together when you awoke this morning?
    ¿Tenía los ojos pegados cuando se despertó Vd. esta mañana?

18. Does your eyeball feel as if it were swollen?
    ¿Siente como si tuviera el globo del ojo hinchado?

19. How long have your eyelids been swollen?[13]
    ¿Desde cuándo tiene Vd. los párpados hinchados?

20. When did your eyes begin to look yellow?
    ¿Cuándo empezaron sus ojos a tener este color amarillo?

21. Did you ever have trouble with your vision?
    ¿Ha tenido alguna vez dificultades con la vista?

22. Did anything get in your eyes?
    ¿Le entró algo en los ojos?

23. A splinter of metal? of wood? a liquid?
    ¿Una astilla de metal? ¿de madera? ¿un líquido?

24. Did it affect your vision?
    ¿Le afectó la vista?

25. When was the last time that you had a vision test?
    ¿Cuándo fue el último examen de la vista?

REVIEW *REPASO*

Practice the following dialogue.

DR. JONES: Hello, Mr. Garcia. Please be seated.

MR. GARCÍA: Thank you, Doctor.

DR. JONES: What seems to be your trouble?

MR. GARCÍA: My eyes hurt me.

DR. JONES: When were your eyes examined last?

MR. GARCÍA: About three years ago.

DR. JONES: Did you ever have trouble with your vision?

MR. GARCÍA: Yes, I had astigmatism in the left eye, and they gave me a prescription for glasses.

DR. JONES: Do you still wear glasses now?

MR. GARCÍA: No, I don't wear them because I lost my glasses last year, and I didn't have enough money to buy new ones.

DR. JONES: Do you feel pain in your right eye?

MR. GARCÍA: No, but my left eye hurts me, and I often have bad headaches.

Dr. Jones: Oh, really? Do you ever have eyeaches, too?

MR. GARCÍA: My left eye aches me only when I read for a long time, and only at night.

DR. JONES: Do you sometimes see things double?

MR. GARCÍA: No. When I have eyeaches, I see things as though through a mist.

DR. JONES: Do your eyes burn?

MR. GARCÍA: No.

DR. JONES: Do your eyes water much?

MR. GARCÍA: Yes, very often my eyes water a lot.

DR. JONES: Your left eye seems inflamed now. Did anything get into your eye?

MR. GARCÍA: I don't think so.

DR. JONES: Does your eyeball feel as if it were swollen?

MR. GARCÍA: I don't understand. My left eye hurts me.

DR. JONES: Very well. Let me see your eyes, and I will examine them.

Practique el diálogo que sigue.

DR. JONES: Buenas tardes, señor García. Siéntese Vd., por favor.

SR. GARCÍA: Gracias, doctor.

DR. JONES: Vamos a ver, ¿qué es lo que le molesta?

SR. GARCÍA: Me duelen los ojos.

DR. JONES: ¿Cuánto tiempo hace que se examinó la vista?

SR. GARCÍA: Hace tres años, más o menos.

DR. JONES: ¿Ha tenido alguna vez dificultades con la vista?

SR. GARCÍA: Sí, tenía astigmatismo en el ojo izquierdo, y me dieron una receta para anteojos.

DR. JONES: ¿Todavía lleva los anteojos?

SR. GARCÍA: No, no los uso porque se me perdieron los anteojos el año pasado, y no tuve bastante dinero para comprar unos nuevos.

DR. JONES: ¿Siente dolor en el ojo derecho?

SR. GARCÍA: No, pero me duele el izquierdo, y muchas veces tengo horribles dolores de cabeza.

DR. JONES: ¿De veras? ¿Sufre de dolor en los ojos también?

SR. GARCÍA: Me duele el ojo izquierdo solamente cuando leo por mucho tiempo y entonces solamente por la noche.

DR. JONES: ¿Ve Vd. las cosas doble algunas veces?

SR. GARCÍA: No. Cuando me duelen los ojos, veo nubladas las cosas como a través de una neblina.

DR. JONES: ¿Le arden los ojos?

SR. GARCÍA: No.

DR. JONES: ¿Le lagrimean mucho los ojos?

SR. GARCÍA: Sí, muy a menudo me lagrimean mucho los ojos.

DR. JONES: El ojo izquierdo parece inflamado ahora. ¿Le entró algo en el ojo?

SR. GARCÍA: Creo que no.

DR. JONES: ¿Siente el ojo hinchado?

SR. GARCÍA: No comprendo. El ojo izquierdo me duele.

DR. JONES: Muy bien. Déjeme ver sus ojos, y los examinaré.

EARS   *LOS OIDOS*

1. Do you ever have middle or inner ear infections?
    ¿Tiene Vd. alguna vez infecciones del oído medio o interno?

2. Are you (tone-deaf) hard of hearing or deaf?
    ¿Es Vd. duro de oído o sordo (sorda)?

3. Do you wear a hearing aid?
    ¿Lleva Vd. un aparato auditivo?

4. Do you have any hearing problems?
    ¿Tiene Vd. problemas de oído?

    ¿Padece Vd. de defectos de la audición?

5. Have you put anything in your ear?
    ¿Se ha puesto Vd. algo en el oído?

6. Do your ears run?
    ¿Le supuran los oídos?
    ¿Le sale algo de los oídos?

7. Do you have a discharge from your left (right) ear?
    ¿Le supura el oído izquierdo (derecho)?

8. Do you usually get earaches?
    ¿Le duelen con frecuencia los oídos?

9. Are you ears clogged?
    ¿Siente Vd. los oídos taponados? (tapados) *Mex.*?

10. Do your ears ring?
    ¿Siente Vd. un tintineo en los oídos?
    ¿Le rumban a Vd. los oídos?
    ¿Tiene Vd. como companillas en los oídos?

11. Do you have ringing in your right (left) ear?
    ¿Le rumba el oído derecho (izquierdo)?

12. Do you ever have dizzy spells?
    ¿Tiene Vd. vértigo alguna vez?
    ¿Suele Vd. tener mareos? *fam*
    ¿Tiene Vd. episodios de mareos?

13. Do you ever feel dizzy on getting up quickly from bed?
    ¿Tiene Vd. mareos al levantarse de la cama rápido?

14. When was the last time you had a hearing test?
    ¿Cuándo fue el último examen especial de los oídos?

NOSE AND SINUSES   *LA NARIZ Y LOS SENOS*

1. Do you have a stuffed nose?
    ¿Tiene Vd. la nariz obstruida?

2. Does your nose feel clogged?
    ¿Tiene Vd. la nariz taponada?
       tupida?
       mormada?
       tapada? *Mex., Arg.*

3. Do you have a cold?
    ¿Tiene Vd. un resfriado?
    ¿Tiene Vd. un catarro? [*head cold*]
    ¿Está Vd. resfriado (resfriada)?[14]
    ¿Está Vd. acatarrado (acatarrada)?[14]

4. Did you catch cold?[15]
    ¿Se ha resfriado Vd.?
    ¿Se acatarró Vd.?

5. How many colds did you have last year?
    ¿Cuántos resfríos (resfriados; catarros) ha tenido Vd. el año pasado?

6. Do you have nose bleeds?
    ¿Le sangra la nariz a veces?

7. Do you have a running nose?
    ¿Le fluye a Vd. la nariz?
    ¿Moquea Vd.? *slang*
    ¿Tiene Vd. coriza?

8. Do you have problems smelling?
    ¿Tiene Vd. problemas olfatorios?

9. Do you have sinus headaches?
    ¿Tiene Vd. jaquecas del seno nasal?

10. Breathe through your nose.
    Respire por la nariz, por favor.

MOUTH AND THROAT   *LA BOCA Y LA GARGANTA*

1. Are you frequently hoarse?
    ¿Tiene Vd. ronquera a menudo?
    ¿Está Vd. ronco (ronca) con frecuencia?

2. Does your tongue feel swollen, thick, or rough?
    ¿Siente la lengua hinchada, gruesa, o áspera/bronca?

3. Does your tongue feel furry?
    ¿Siente la lengua con costra?
    ¿Se forman incrustaciones en su lengua?

4. How long has your tongue been that color?[13]
    ¿Desde cuándo tiene la lengua de ese color?

5. Does your tongue burn?
    ¿Le arde la lengua?

6. Does your tongue feel sore?
    ¿Tiene Vd. la lengua adolorida?

7. Can you taste anything?
    ¿Puede Vd. saborear algo?

8. Do you have a sour taste in your mouth?
    ¿Siente Vd. un sabor agrio de boca?
    ¿Tiene Vd. una acidez en la boca?

9. Do you have sore throats?
    ¿Suele Vd. tener la garganta adolorida?
    ¿Suele Vd. tener dolor de garganta?
    ¿Le duele la garganta con frecuencia?

10. Does your throat hurt when you swallow?
    ¿Le duele la garganta cuando Vd. traga?
    ¿Tiene Vd. dolores o dificultades al tragar?

11. Is it just scratchy?
    ¿Le pica?

12. Can you swallow and breathe without pain?
    ¿Puede tragar y respirar sin dolor?

13. I want to take a throat culture. Open your mouth.[16]
    Quiero hacerle un cultivo de la garganta. Abra la boca, por favor.

14. This won't hurt.
    Esto no le dolerá.

15. Do you also have a cold?
    ¿Tiene catarro también?

16. Do your gums bleed frequently?[17]
    ¿Le sangran las encías frecuentemente?

17. Do you have infections of the gum?[17]
    ¿Tiene Vd. infecciones en las encías?

18. Do you have a toothache?[17]
    ¿Tiene Vd. dolor de muelas?

19. Which tooth hurts?[17]
    ¿Cuál de los dientes le duele?

20. Please point.
    Señale Vd., por favor.

21. Have you had any changes in your voice?
    ¿Ha tenido Vd. algún cambio de voz?

NECK *EL CUELLO*

1. Can you swallow?
   ¿Puede Vd. tragar?

2. Do you have difficulty swallowing?
   ¿Tiene Vd. dificultad al tragar?

3. Do you have difficulty drinking liquids?
   ¿Tiene Vd. dificultad para beber (pasar) líquidos?

4. Have you noticed swelling of the glands in your neck?
   ¿Se ha fijado en alguna hinchazón en las glándulas en el cuello?

5. Have you noticed any lumps in your neck?
   ¿Se ha fijado en algunas bolitas en el cuello?

BREASTS[18] *LOS PECHOS*

1. All women are at risk for breast cancer.
   Cada mujer está en riesgo de contraer el cáncer del seno.

2. The risk increases as they grow older.
   El riesgo aumenta a medida que va teniendo más edad.

3. The best way of protecting yourself is through detection in the early stages.
   La mejor forma de protegerse usted misma es a través de la detección en una etapa temprana.

4. All women over 20 (twenty) should have a clinical breast exam once every 3 (three) years.[19]
   Cada mujer mayor de 20 (veinte) años debe tener un examen clínico de los senos hecho por su médico cada 3 (tres) años.

5. The . . . Cancer Society recommends that you examine your breasts monthly.
   La Sociedad . . . de Cáncer le recomienda que se examine los senos mensualmente.

6. It is important to be familiar with your breasts.
   Es importante que Vd. se familiarice con los senos.

7. You will be able to recognize any change if present after you learn how the normal tissue of your breasts feels.
   Vd. podrá reconocer algún cambio si se presenta después de aprender cómo siente el tejido normal de los senos.

8. Examine your breasts once a month at the same time.
   Examínese los senos en el mismo tiempo cada mes.

9. You should examine them about a week after your period when your breasts are usually not tender nor swollen.
   Debe examinarse los senos más o menos una semana después de su período menstrual cuando los senos por lo común no estén ni doloridos ni hinchados.

10. Since you no longer are menstruating, you should examine your breasts on the first day of each month.
    Porque Vd. no menstrúa (no tiene período menstrual) más, debe examinarse los senos el primer día de cada mes.

11. When was your last breast examination?
    ¿Cuándo fue su último examen de las mamas? de los senos?

12. Were the results . . .
    ¿Fueron . . . los resultados?
    normal
    normales
    abnormal
    anormales

13. Do you know how to do breast self-examination?[20]
    ¿Sabe Vd. autoexaminarse los senos?[20]

14. Do you examine your breasts every month?
    ¿Hace Vd. un autoexamen mensual de los senos?

15. Do you look at your breasts in a mirror?
    ¿Mira Vd. los senos en un espejo?

16. Do a visual inspection of your breasts for changes in form or shape or dimples in the skin.

Haga Vd. una inspección visual de los senos en busca de cambios en la forma o el tamaño o los hoyuelos en la piel.

17. Have you noticed any lumps in your breasts?
¿Se ha fijado Vd. algún tumor en los pechos?
alguna protuberancia
algún abultamiento
¿Ha notado alguna bolita en la mama? *fam*
algún tumorcito

18. Have you noticed a change . . .
¿Se ha fijado Vd. en algún cambio . . .
in the size of your breasts?
en el tamaño de los senos?
in the shape of your breasts?
en la forma de los senos?
in the consistency of your breasts?
en la consistencia de los senos?

19. Do you have any pain or swelling . . .
¿Tiene Vd. dolor o hinchazón . . .
of your breasts?
de los senos?
under your arms?
debajo de los brazos?

20. Touch the spot.
Tóquese el lugar.

21. Have you noticed a change . . .
¿Se ha fijado Vd. en algún cambio . . .
in the size of your nipples?
en el tamaño de los pezones?
in the shape of your nipples?
en la forma de los pezones?
in the consistency of your nipples?
en la consistencia de los pezones?

22. Do your nipples hurt you?
¿Le duelen los pezones?

23. Do you have a discharge from your nipples?
¿Le supuran los pezones?

24. What color is the discharge from your nipples?
¿De qué color es el material (la supuración) que le sale de los pezones?

25. Your breasts are swollen. Do they hurt when you have your period?
Vd. tiene los pechos hinchados. ¿Le duelen durante la regla?

26. Do your breasts begin to swell before your periods?
¿Empiezan a hincharse los pechos antes de la regla?

27. How many children do you have?
¿Cuántos hijos tiene Vd.?

28. Did you breast-feed them?[21]
¿Les dio de mamar?

29. Did you nurse your child?[21]
¿Amamantó a su criatura?

30. Have you nursed your child?[21]
¿Ha dado de mamar a su criatura?

31. Are you breast-feeding now?[21]
¿Está Vd. dando de mamar ahora?
¿Amamanta Vd. ahora?

32. How long have you been nursing?
¿Desde cuándo da Vd. el pecho?

33. How long did you nurse?
¿Por cuánto tiempo dio Vd. el pecho?

34. How old are you now?
¿Cuántos años tiene Vd. ahora?

35. You should have a base-line mammogram between the ages of 35 and 39.
Vd. debe hacerse un mamograma que sirva de base de comparación para el futuro entre las edades de 35 (treinta y cinco) y 39 (treinta y nueve) años.

36. A mammogram is a special breast x-ray.
Un mamograma es una radiografía especial de los senos.

37. A mammogram can detect a cancer as small as a pin head.
Un mamograma puede detectar un cáncer tan pequeño como la cabeza de un alfiler.

38. Have you ever had a mammogram?[22]
¿Le han hecho jamás un mamograma (una mamografía)?
¿Ha tenido alguna vez un mamograma?

39. When was your last mammogram?
¿Cuándo fue su último mamograma?

40. Is there a history of breast cancer in your immediate family—mother, sister, grandmother, aunt?
¿Hay historia de cáncer del seno en familiares cercanos—madre, hermana, abuela, tía?

41. Have you ever had a breast biopsy?
¿Jamás le han hecho una biopsia de los senos?

42. Have you ever had a mastectomy?
¿Le han hecho alguna vez una mastectomía?
¿Jamás le operaron de mastectomía?

43. Have you ever had a lumpectomy?
¿Ha tenido una extirpación de un bulto?

44. Have you ever had radiation therapy to treat breast cancer?
¿Le han puesto radioterapia como tratamiento para el cáncer de los senos?

45. Have you ever had chemotherapy to treat breast cancer?
¿Le han puesto quimioterapia para tratar el cáncer de los senos?

46. Do you remember the chemotherapy drugs you were given?
¿Recuerda Vd. qué medicamentos de quimioterapia le administraron?

47. Do you remember how long you were given these medications?
¿Se acuerda Vd. por cuánto tiempo le dieron esas medicinas?

RESPIRATORY *RESPIRATORIO*

1. Can you breathe well?
   ¿Puede Vd. respirar bien?

2. Do you have any difficulty in breathing?
   ¿Tiene Vd. alguna dificultad para respirar?

3. How long can you hold your breath?
   ¿Durante cuánto tiempo puede Vd. retener la respiración?

4. Try it.
   Pruébelo.

5. Are you short of breath?
   ¿Le falta la respiración?
   . . . while exercising?
   ¿. . . al hacer ejercicios?
   . . . when you are resting?
   ¿. . . al descansar?
   . . . when you are upset?
   ¿. . . cuando está trastornado (trastornada)?

6. Do you have any difficulty in breathing . . .
   ¿Respira Vd. con dificultad . . .
   at night?
   por la noche?
   sitting down?
   sentado (sentada)?
   lying down?
   acostado (acostada)?
   standing up?
   de pie?
   exercising?
   al hacer ejercicios?
   at rest?
   al descansar?

7. Do you perspire a lot, especially at night?
   ¿Transpira Vd. mucho, sobre todo por la noche?

8. Do you or have you had frequent colds . . .
   ¿Tiene o ha tenido catarros frecuentes . . .
   in the fall?
   en el otoño?
   in the winter?
   en el invierno?
   in the spring?
   en la primavera?
   in the summer?
   en el verano?

9. Do you cough a lot?
   ¿Tiene Vd. mucha tos?
   ¿Tose Vd. mucho?

10. How long have you been coughing?
    ¿Desde cuándo tiene Vd. tos?
    ¿Desde cuándo tose Vd.?

11. Does it hurt when you cough?
    ¿Le duele cuando tose (al toser)?

12. Are you coughing from an allergy?
    ¿Tose Vd. por alguna alergia?

13. Do you cough up phlegm?
    Al toser, ¿arroja Vd. flemas?

14. What color is the phlegm?[13]
    ¿De qué color es la flema?
    clear
    incolora
    gray or white
    gris o blanca
    yellow or green
    amarilla o verde
    red
    roja
    maroon
    roja oscura
    brown or black
    marrón o negra

15. Is it a dry cough?
    ¿Es una tos seca?

16. Is it a productive cough?
    ¿Es una tos con flema (esputo)?

17. Is the phlegm foul-smelling?
    ¿Es la flema apestosa?

18. Is it abundant?
    ¿Es abundante?

19. Is it thick or foamy?
    ¿Es espesa o espumosa?

20. Do you cough up blood?
    Al toser, ¿arroja Vd. sangre?

21. Do you spit blood?
    ¿Escupe Vd. sangre?

22. Streaks of blood or clots?
    ¿Tose Vd. rayas de sangre o cuajarones?
    ¿Tose Vd. manchas de sangre o coágulos?

23. Do you spit a lot?
    ¿Escupe mucho?

24. Do you have pain when you cough?
    ¿Le duele al toser?

25. Do you breathe easier after you cough?
    ¿Respira Vd. mejor después de toser?

26. Is there any position . . .
    ¿Hay alguna posición que lo . . .
    that makes it better?
    alivie?
    that makes it worse?
    haga sentir peor?

27. Do you wheeze?
    ¿Le silba a Vd. el pecho?
    ¿Le sale un silbido al respirar?
    ¿Tiene la respiración jadeante?

28. Do you smoke?[23]
    ¿Fuma Vd.?

29. How many packs per day?[7]
    ¿Cuántos paquetes al día?
    ¿Cuántas cajetillas por día?

30. Do you smoke more than _____ cigarettes a week?[7]
    ¿Fuma Vd. más de _____ cigarillos por semana?

31. For how many years?[7]
    ¿Por cuántos años?

32. Have you had asthma, emphysema, T.B.?
    ¿Ha padecido Vd. de asma, enfisema, tuberculosis (tisis)?

33. Have you ever had bronchitis or pneumonia?
    ¿Ha tenido Vd. alguna vez bronquitis o pulmonía?

34. Do you get chills?
    ¿Le dan escalofríos?

35. Do you always feel cold?
    ¿Siempre siente Vd. frío?

36. Do you feel warm and feverish at night?
    ¿Se siente Vd. caliente y febril por la noche?

37. When was your last chest x-ray?
    ¿Cuándo tuvo su última radiografía del pecho (de los pulmones)?
    ¿Cuándo le hicieron su última radiografía de los pulmones?

38. What were the results?
    ¿Cuáles fueron los resultados?

REVIEW   *REPASO*

Practice the following dialogue.

DR. SMITH: When did your illness begin, Mrs. Navas?

MRS. NAVAS: It began Wednesday evening.

DR. SMITH: Did you have any fever?

MRS. NAVAS: Yes, I had 102.

DR. SMITH: How long did the fever last?

MRS. NAVAS: For almost two days.

DR. SMITH: Did you vomit?

MRS. NAVAS: Yes, I vomited a lot, and I also coughed quite a bit.

DR. SMITH: How long have you been coughing?

MRS. NAVAS: For about a day.

DR. SMITH: Does it hurt when you cough?

MRS. NAVAS: Yes, my chest hurts, and so does my throat.

DR. SMITH: Do you cough up phlegm?

MRS. NAVAS: Sometimes.

DR. SMITH: What color is the phlegm?

MRS. NAVAS: I am not sure. I think it's yellow.

DR. SMITH: Does anything else hurt you?

MRS. NAVAS: Right now my throat is sore.

DR. SMITH: Are you hoarse frequently?

MRS. NAVAS: Usually not.

DR. SMITH: Does your throat hurt when you swallow?

MRS. NAVAS: Yes, and it is difficult for me to swallow.

DR. SMITH: I am going to give you a prescription for two medicines. One is for lozenges. Take one every four hours. The other is for a cough medicine. Take two teaspoonsful after every meal and at bedtime. Call me tomorrow.

Practique el diálogo que sigue.

DR. SMITH: **¿Cuando empezó su enfermedad, señora?**

SRA. NAVAS: **Empezó el miércoles por la noche.**

DR. SMITH: **¿Tuvo Vd. fiebre?**

SRA. NAVAS: **Sí, ciento dos grados Fahrenheit.**

DR. SMITH: **¿Por cuánto tiempo tuvo fiebre?**

SRA. NAVAS: **Por casi dos días.**

DR. SMITH: **¿Vomitó Vd.?**

SRA. NAVAS: **Sí, vomité mucho y también tosí bastante.**

DR. SMITH: **¿Desde cuándo tose Vd.?**

SRA. NAVAS: **Hace como un día.**

DR. SMITH: **¿Le duele al toser?**

SRA. NAVAS: **Sí, me duele el pecho, y la garganta también.**

DR. SMITH: **Al toser, ¿arroja Vd. flemas?**

SRA. NAVAS: **A veces.**

DR. SMITH: **¿De qué color son las flemas?**

SRA. NAVAS: **No estoy segura. Creo que son amarillas.**

DR. SMITH: **¿Le duele algo más?**

SRA. NAVAS: **En este momento tengo la garganta dolorida.**

DR. SMITH: **¿Está Vd. ronca con frecuencia?**

SRA. NAVAS: **Generalmente no.**

DR. SMITH: **¿Le duele la garganta al tragar?**

SRA. NAVAS: **Sí, y no puedo tragar muy bien.**

DR. SMITH: **Voy a darle unas recetas para dos medicinas. Una es para pastillas. Tome una cada cuatro horas. La otra es para un jarabe para la tos. Tome dos cucharaditas después de cada comida y al acostarse. Llámeme mañana.**

CARDIOVASCULAR   *CARDIOVASCULAR*

1. Do you feel (very) weak?
   ¿Se siente (muy) débil?

2. Do you have pains in your chest?
   ¿Tiene Vd. dolores en el pecho?

3. What part of your chest hurts you?
   ¿Qué parte del pecho le duele?

4. Where in your chest does it hurt you?
   ¿Dónde en el pecho le duele?

5. In what part of the chest?
   ¿En qué parte del pecho?

6. In the middle?
   ¿En el medio?

7. More towards the left side?
   ¿Más hacia el lado izquierdo?

8. More towards the right side?
   ¿Más hacia el lado derecho?

9. Under the breastbone?
   ¿Debajo del esternón?

10. Does the pain (sometimes) extend . . .
    ¿Se extiende el dolor (algunas veces) . . .
    to the arms?
    hacia los brazos?
    to the shoulders?
    hacia los hombros?
    to the neck?
    hacia el cuello?

11. Does the pain extend to the back[24] or neck or jaw?
    ¿Se extiende el dolor hacia la espalda o el cuello o la quijada?[4]

12. Where do you feel the pain?
    ¿Dónde siente Vd. el dolor?

13. Point to where it hurts.
    Señale Vd. por favor, donde le duele.

14. Does the pain stay here in the chest or does it radiate to another part?
    ¿Se queda el dolor aquí en el pecho o corre a otra parte?

15. Does the pain stay in one place?
    ¿Se queda el dolor en un solo lugar?

16. Does the pain radiate?
    ¿Se corre el dolor?

17. Do you have pain in another part?
    ¿Tiene dolor en otra parte?
    Your shoulder?
    ¿El hombro?
    Your arm?
    ¿El brazo?
    Your neck?
    ¿El cuello?
    Your jaw?
    ¿La quijada?
    Your back?[24]
    ¿La espalda?

18. From where to where?
    ¿Hacia dónde?

19. Is it the first time that your chest hurts?
    ¿Es la primera vez que le duele el pecho?

20. When did it begin the first time?
    ¿Cuándo empezó la primera vez?
    Last year?
    ¿El año pasado?
    Last month?
    ¿El mes pasado?
    Last week?
    ¿La semana pasada?
    Two days ago?
    ¿Anteayer?
    Yesterday?
    ¿Ayer?
    Today?
    ¿Hoy?
    Three hours ago?
    ¿Hace tres horas?
    Forty minutes ago?
    ¿Hace cuarenta minutos?

21. How long have you had it?
    ¿Cuánto tiempo hace que lo tiene?

22. How often do you have pain?
    ¿Cada cuánto tiempo tiene dolor?
    Every ten minutes?
    ¿Cada diez minutos?
    Every five minutes?
    ¿Cada cinco minutos?

23. How did the pain begin the first time?
    ¿Cómo empezó el dolor la primera vez?

24. How does the pain begin?
    ¿Cómo empieza el dolor?

25. Gradually?
    ¿Poco a poco?

26. Suddenly?
    ¿De repente?

27. How long does (did) it last each time?
    ¿Cuánto le dura (duró) cuando le viene (vino)?

28. More than half an hour?
    ¿Más de media hora?

29. How often do you have the pain?
    ¿Con qué frecuencia tiene Vd. el dolor?

30. What is (was) the pain like?
    ¿Cómo es (era) el dolor?

31. Is (Was) it strong?
    ¿Es (Fue) fuerte?

32. Is (Was) it mild?
    ¿Es (Fue) leve?

33. Is (Was) it sharp?
    ¿Es (Fue) agudo?

34. Is (Was) it aching?
    ¿Es (Fue) dolorido / adolorido?

35. Was it dull and crushing like a person standing on your chest?
¿Fue sordo y oprimido como si alguien estuviese colocado sobre su pecho?

36. Is (Was) it burning?
¿Es (Fue) como ardor?

37. Is (Was) it pressure / tightness?
¿Es (Fue) como opresión?

38. Is (Was) it sharp, shooting pain?
¿Es (Fue) como punzada?

39. Is (Was) it crampy?
¿Es (Fue) como calambre?

40. Did you perspire when the pain came?
¿Transpiró cuando le vino el dolor?

41. Did you black out?
¿Se desmayó Vd.?

42. Are (Were) you nauseated with the pain?
¿Tiene (Tenía) náuseas con el dolor?

43. Do (Did) you have hiccups with the pain?
¿Tiene (Tuvo) hipos con el dolor?

44. Do (Did) you burp with the pain?
¿Eructa (Eructó) con el dolor?

45. Do (Did) you vomit with the pain?
¿Vomita (Vomitó) con el dolor?

46. Have you had it before?
¿Lo ha tenido antes?

47. Do you have pain when . . .
¿Tiene dolor cuando . . .
   you walk?
   camina?
   you run?
   corre?
   you climb stairs? / go up stairs?
   sube escaleras?
   you work?
   trabaja?
   you are resting?
   descansa?
   you get angry?
   se enoja? / se enfada?
   it is cold outside?
   hace frío afuera?

48. Can you walk?
¿Puede caminar?

49. How many blocks can you walk?
¿Cuántas cuadras puede caminar?[25]

50. Can you climb stairs?
¿Puede subir escaleras?

51. How many flights of stairs can you climb?
¿Cuántas escaleras puede subir?

52. How many blocks can you walk without having . . .
¿Cuántas cuadras[25] **puede Vd. andar sin tener . . .**
   pain in your chest?
   dolor del corazón?
   pain in your legs?
   dolores de las piernas?
   a shortness of breath?
   una sensación de ahogo?

53. How many flights of stairs can you climb without being short of breath?
¿Cuántos tramos puede Vd. subir sin que le falte el aliento?
¿Cuántas escaleras puede Vd. subir sin tener falta de aliento?

54. Does it disappear when you stop?
¿Se desaparece cuando para?

55. Do you have difficulty breathing through your nose when you walk?
¿Tiene Vd. dificultad en respirar por la nariz al caminar?

56. Have you noticed any shortness of breath lately?
¿Ha notado si le ha faltado el aliento últimamente?

57. Do you get short of breath . . .
¿Le falta el aliento cuando . . .
   when you climb stairs?
   sube Vd. por las escaleras?
   when you walk?
   cuando camina?

58. What type of regular exercise do you do?
¿Qué tipo de ejercicio hace Vd. regularmente?

59. Did you ever have shortness of breath at night?
¿Ha tenido falta de aliento por la noche alguna vez?

60. Do you awaken in the night because of shortness of breath?
¿Se despierta Vd. por la noche por falta de respiración?

61. How many pillows do you use to sleep on?
¿Cuántas almohadas usa Vd. para dormir?

62. Can you lay flat on the bed without pillows and not be short of breath?
¿Puede Vd. acostarse sobre la cama sin almohadas y no tener falta de aliento?

63. Is it better or worse . . .
¿Es mejor o peor . . .
   with food?
   con comida?
   with liquids?
   con líquidos?
   after eating?
   después de comer?
   when you breathe deeply?
   cuando respira profundo?
   when you move one arm?
   cuando mueve un brazo?
   when you rest?
   al descansar?
   with medicine?
   con la medicina?

64. Do you take medicine for this pain?[26]
    ¿Toma Vd. medicina para el dolor?

65. What is the name of the medicine?
    ¿Sabe Vd. el nombre de esta medicina?
    nitroglycerin?
    ¿nitroglicerina?
    pills that you put under your tongue?
    ¿píldoras que se ponen debajo de la lengua?
    digitalis?
    ¿digital(is)?
    water pills / diuretics?
    ¿píldoras para sacar el agua? / ¿diuréticos?

66. Do you use a (cardiac) patch?
    ¿Usa un parche (con medicina para el corazón)?

67. How many pills/tablets do you use to take away the pain?
    ¿Cuántas pastillas/tabletas usa para quitársele el dolor?

68. How many pills take away the pain?
    ¿Cuántas píldoras se le quitan el dolor?

69. How long does it take to take away the pain?
    ¿Cuánto tiempo tarda en quitarle el dolor?

70. Does the pain last less than five seconds?[27]
    ¿Le dura el dolor menos de cinco segundos?

71. Does the pain last more than thirty minutes (a half hour)?
    ¿Le dura el dolor más de treinta minutos (media hora)?

72. Does your heart beat rapidly or irregularly?
    ¿Le late el corazón rápidamente o con irregularidad?

73. Can you remember ever having had irregular heart beats, or very rapid heart beats?
    ¿Puede Vd. recordar haber tenido alguna vez latidos irregulares o palpitaciones muy rápidas del corazón?

74. When?
    ¿Cuándo?

75. Do you get palpitations? With pain?
    ¿Tiene palpitaciones? ¿Con dolor?

76. Is this the first time that the pain lasted more than a half hour?
    ¿Es ésta la primera vez que dura el dolor más de media hora?

77. Does the pain last more than a half hour when you are . . .
    ¿Dura más de media hora cuando está . . .
    lying down?
    acostado (acostada)?
    standing?
    de pie?

78. Do you have diabetes?[28]
    ¿Tiene diabetes?

79. When did it begin?
    ¿Cuándo empezó?

80. Are you taking birth control pills?[29]
    ¿Toma la píldora?
    ¿Toma pastillas anticonceptivas?

81. Do you smoke?
    ¿Fuma?

82. How much do you smoke?
    ¿Cuánto ha fumado?

83. How many years have you been smoking?
    ¿Por cuántos años ha fumado?
    ¿Cuántos años hace que fuma?

84. Are you running a fever?
    ¿Tiene fiebre?

85. Have you ever been told that you had heart trouble?
    ¿Sabe Vd. si ha tenido jamás enfermedad del corazón?

86. Do you have a heart condition?
    ¿Tiene Vd. problemas del corazón?

87. Do you have palpitations?
    ¿Tiene problemas con palpitaciones?

88. Do you faint?
    ¿Se desmaya?

89. Do you have valve problems?
    ¿Tiene problemas con la válvula?

90. Do you have problems with infections?
    ¿Tiene problemas con infecciones?

91. Have you ever had a heart attack?
    ¿Ha tenido alguna vez un ataque cardíaco?

92. How many times?
    ¿Cuántas veces?

93. When was it (were they)?
    ¿Cuándo fue (fueron)?

94. Is any part of your body swollen?
    ¿Tiene Vd. hinchada alguna parte del cuerpo?

95. How long has it been swollen like this?
    ¿Desde cuándo está hinchado así?
    ¿Cuánto tiempo hace que está hinchado así?

96. How many days?
    ¿Cuántos días?

97. How many weeks?
    ¿Cuántas semanas?

98. Are both of your legs swollen?
    ¿Tiene las dos piernas hinchadas?

99. Show me.
    Enséñemelas.

100. Are your ankles swollen in the morning when you awaken?
    ¿Tiene Vd. los tobillos hinchados por la mañana al despertarse?

101. Do you get short of breath when you . . .
    ¿Le falta el aire cuando . . .
    walk?
    camina?
    lie down?
    se acuesta?

102. Have you ever seen a bluish color in your lips?
¿Jamás ha visto Vd. que los labios se le ponen morados?[30]
    in your feet and hands?
    los pies y las manos se le ponen morados?[30]

103. Is there a coldness in your hands?
¿Tiene frío en las manos?

104. Is there a coldness in your feet?
¿Tiene frío en los pies?

105. Do you have a cough?
¿Tiene tos?

106. Do you cough up sputum?
¿Arroja flema?
¿Bota flema?

107. Is it . . .
¿Es . . .

    thick
    espesa?
    yellow?
    amarilla?
    green?
    verde?
    bloody?
    con sangre?

108. Do you have a heart murmur or hypertension?
¿Tiene Vd. un murmullo en el corazón o padece Vd. de la hipertensión?

109. When did you last have an electrocardiogram?
¿Cuándo fue la última vez que le hicieron un electrocardiograma?

110. What were the results?
¿Cuáles fueron los resultados?

GASTROINTESTINAL *GASTROINTESTINAL*[31]

1. Do you eat between meals?
¿Come Vd. algo entre comidas?

2. Do you drink a lot of liquids?
¿Toma Vd. muchos líquidos?

3. Do you drink milk?
¿Bebe Vd. leche?

4. How much? How many glasses?
¿Cuánta? ¿Cuántos vasos?

5. What type of milk do you drink?
¿Qué tipo de leche bebe Vd?
    whole milk?
    ¡leche sin desnatar?
    skim milk?
    ¡leche desnatada?
    ¡leche descremada?
    low-fat milk?
    ¡leche desgrasada?

6. Do you drink alcoholic beverages?[32]
¿Toma Vd. algunas bebidas alcohólicas?

7. How many drinks do you have?
¿Cuántas bebidas toma Vd. por día?

8. What type of alcoholic beverage do you drink?
¿Qué tipo (clase) de bebida alcohólica toma Vd.?

9. How many beers do you drink a night?
¿Cuántas cervezas toma Vd. cada noche?

10. How much coffee or tea do you drink?
¿Cuántas tazas de café o de té bebe Vd.?

11. What type of coffee do you drink, regular or decaffeinated?
¿Qué clase de café toma Vd.? ¿regular o descafeinado?

12. How much water do you drink daily?
¿Cuántos vasos de agua bebe Vd. diariamente?

13. How much pop do you drink?
¿Cuántas bebidas gaseosas toma Vd. diariamente, como una Coca-Cola?

14. What foods disagree with you?
¿Qué alimentos le caen mal?

15. Do you get gas pains?
¿Suele Vd. tener gas?

16. Do you belch (burp) a lot?
¿Eructa Vd. mucho?
¿Repite Vd. mucho? *Chicano*

17. Do you suffer from indigestion? Frequently?
¿Padece Vd. de indigestión? ¿Con frecuencia?

18. Do you get heartburn?
¿Suele tener ardor de estómago?
¿Tiene Vd. molestias en la parte superior del abdomen?

19. Do you feel some acid or food coming into the back of your throat when you lie flat?
¿Siente Vd. algún ácido o comida en el fondo de la garganta cuando Vd. está acostado(acostada)?

20. Do you have an upset stomach after eating fried or fatty foods?
¿Se siente descompuesto (descompuesta) del estómago después de comidas fritas o con grasa?

21. What exactly happens?
¿Qué le pasa exactamente?

22. Do you feel pain?
¿Siente Vd. algún dolor?

23. Show me where it hurts the most.
Muéstreme dónde le duele más.

24. How long does the pain last?
¿Cuánto tiempo le dura el dolor?

25. Describe the pain. Is it . . .
Describa el dolor. ¿Es . . .
    sharp?
    agudo?
    dull?
    sordo?

radiating?
un dolor que corre?
burning?
con ardor?
cramping?
con calambres?
deep pain?
dolor profundo?

26. What causes it?
¿Qué lo causa?

27. What aggravates it / makes it worse?
¿Qué lo agrava / hace peor?

28. What relieves it?
¿Qué lo alivia?

29. Where did the pain begin? Show me.
¿Dónde empezó el dolor? Enséñeme.

30. Where does it hurt you now?
¿Dónde le duele ahora?

31. Does another part hurt you?
¿Le duele otra parte?
Your shoulder?
¿El hombro?
Your back?[24]
¿La espalda?
Your testicles?
¿Los testículos?

32. Does the pain change position?
¿Cambia el dolor de sitio?

33. Where?
¿Adónde?

REVIEW *REPASO*

Practice the following dialogue.

Dr. Burns: What is your problem, Miss Mendoza?

Miss Mendoza: My stomach often bothers me.

Dr. Burns: How much do you weigh?

Miss Mendoza: 125 pounds.

Dr. Burns: What is your occupation?

Miss Mendoza: I am a beautician.

Dr. Burns: Do you like working in a beauty shop?

Miss Mendoza: Yes, but the hours are very long.

Dr. Burns: Generally what hours do you work?

Miss Mendoza: I work on Sundays from 10 until 3 in the afternoon, and on Tuesdays, Wednesdays and Thursdays, I work from 9 until 6. On Fridays and Saturdays I work from 9 until 10 in the evening.

Dr. Burns: How many meals do you normally eat?

Miss Mendoza: Well, I always eat a good breakfast. Orange juice, two eggs, ham, some toast and coffee.

Dr. Burns: Do you eat lunch?

Miss Mendoza: Usually I just drink black coffee all day long.

Dr. Burns: What about supper?

Miss Mendoza: I am generally too tired to cook, so I have a hamburger and french fries, and a coke, or else fried chicken and french fries.

Dr. Burns: Do you have an upset stomach after eating such a supper?

Practique el diálogo que sigue

Dr. Burns: **¿Qué le sucede a Vd., señorita?**

Srta. Mendoza: **Me molesta mucho el estómago con frecuencia.**

Dr. Burns: **¿Cuánto pesa Vd.?**

Srta. Mendoza: **Ciento veinticinco libras.**

Dr. Burns: **¿En qué trabaja Vd.?**

Srta. Mendoza: **Soy peluquera.**

Dr. Burns: **¿Le gusta trabajar en un salón de belleza?**

Srta. Mendoza: **Sí, pero las horas son larguísimas.**

Dr. Burns: **Por lo común, ¿cuáles son las horas que trabaja?**

Srta. Mendoza: **Los domingos trabajo desde las diez hasta las tres de la tarde, y los martes, miércoles y jueves, trabajo desde las nueve hasta las seis. Los viernes y los sábados trabajo desde las nueve de la mañana hasta las diez de la noche.**

Dr. Burns: **¿Cuántas veces come Vd. al día?**

Srta. Mendoza: **Pues, siempre me desayuno bien. Jugo de naranja, dos huevos, jamón, unas tostadas y café.**

Dr. Burns: **¿Almuerza Vd.?**

Srta. Mendoza: **Generalmente solamente bebo café puro todo el día.**

Dr. Burns: **¿Y para la cena?**

Srta. Mendoza: **Con frecuencia estoy tan cansada que compro una hamburguesa, papas fritas y una cola, o pollo frito con papas fritas.**

Dr. Burns: **¿Se siente descompuesta del estómago después de cenar así?**

MISS MENDOZA: Frequently my stomach hurts me after the chicken.

DR. BURNS: What exactly happens.

MISS MENDOZA: I have sharp pains here.

DR. BURNS: Do you drink milk?

MISS MENDOZA: I drink coffee because I don't like milk.

DR. BURNS: What type of coffee do you drink, regular or decaffeinated?

MISS MENDOZA: I drink regular.

DR. BURNS: How many cups do you drink daily?

MISS MENDOZA: I drink between fifteen and twenty.

DR. BURNS: How much water do you drink daily?

MISS MENDOZA: I almost never drink water.

DR. BURNS: Do you drink much pop?

MISS MENDOZA: Sometimes while I am working, I drink two or three cans of pop.

DR. BURNS: Do you burp a lot?

MISS MENDOZA: Only after drinking the pop.

DR. BURNS: Do you get heartburn often?

MISS MENDOZA: Yes, I usually have heartburn after drinking too much coffee, or late in the evening after supper.

DR BURNS: You must eat more regularly—three meals a day, and you must drink more water and less coffee. Here is a list of foods which you should eat daily.

SRTA. MENDOZA: Después del pollo muchas veces me duele el estómago.

DR. BURNS: ¿Qué le pasa exactamente?

SRTA. MENDOZA: Sufro de dolores agudos aquí.

DR. BURNS: ¿Bebe Vd. leche?

SRTA. MENDOZA: Tomo café porque no me gusta la leche.

DR. BURNS: ¿Qué clase de café toma Vd., regular o descafeinado?

SRTA. MENDOZA: Tomo regular.

DR. BURNS: ¿Cuántas tazas de café bebe Vd. al día?

SRTA. MENDOZA: Tomo entre quince y veinte.

DR. BURNS: ¿Cuántos vasos de agua bebe Vd. diariamente?

SRTA. MENDOZA: Casi nunca bebo agua.

DR. BURNS: ¿Toma Vd. muchas bebidas gaseosas?

SRTA. MENDOZA: A veces mientras trabajo, bebo dos o tres botes de soda.

DR. BURNS: ¿Eructa Vd. mucho?

SRTA. MENDOZA: Solamente después de beber soda.

DR. BURNS: ¿Suele tener ardor de estómago a menudo?

SRTA. MENDOZA: Sí, por lo regular suelo tener ardor de estómago después de beber demasiado café o muy tarde por la noche después de la cena.

DR. BURNS: Vd. debe comer con más regularidad—tres comidas al día y debe beber más agua y menos café. Aquí tiene una lista de las comidas que debe tomar diariamente.

---

34. Do you feel bloated?
    ¿Se siente aventado (aventada)?
    ¿Se siente hinchado (hinchada)?

35. Do you get sour regurgitation?
    ¿Le suben ácidos a la boca?

36. Do you have frequent stomach aches (belly-aches)?
    ¿Suele tener dolor de estómago (de vientre) a menudo?
    ¿Tiene Vd. dolor de estómago (de vientre) con frecuencia?

37. Do you have abdominal (stomach) pain?
    ¿Tiene Vd. dolor de estómago?
    ¿Le duele el estómago / el abdomen / la barriga / la panza?

38. Where is the pain?
    ¿Dónde le duele?

39. Point to where it hurts.
    Señale Vd. donde le duele.

    . . . with one finger.
    . . . con un dedo.

40. When did the pain begin?
    ¿Cuándo empezó el dolor?

41. When did the pain begin for the first time?
    ¿Cuándo empezó el dolor por primera vez?
    Last year?
    ¿El año pasado?
    Last month?
    ¿El mes pasado?
    Last week?
    ¿La semana pasada?
    Two days ago?
    ¿Hace dos días?
    Yesterday?
    ¿Ayer?
    Today?
    ¿Hoy?
    Five hours ago?
    ¿Hace cinco horas?

42. Where was the pain when it started?
    ¿Dónde le empezó el dolor?

43. What is the pain like?
    ¿Cómo es el dolor?

44. Is it strong or mild?
    ¿Es fuerte o leve?

45. Does it come and go?
    ¿Va y viene/vuelve?

46. How long does the pain last?
    ¿Cuánto tiempo hace que tiene el dolor?

47. How often do you have it?
    ¿Con qué frecuencia lo tiene?
    ¿Cada cuánto tiempo tiene dolor?
      Every ten minutes?
        ¿Cada diez minutos?

48. Do you have problems swallowing or chewing?
    ¿Tiene Vd. problemas al tragar o masticar?

49. Does eating or drinking make the pain better?
    ¿Se alivia el dolor cuando come o bebe?

50. Does eating make the pain worse?
    ¿Se empeora el dolor cuando come?

51. Is the pain better or worse with . . .
    ¿Es mejor o peor el dolor con . . .
      spicy hot food?
      comida picante?
      greasy/fatty food?
      comida que tiene grasa?
      milk?
      leche?

52. Is the pain better or worse when . . .
    ¿Es mejor o peor el dolor cuando . . .
      you are standing?
      está de pie?
      you are bent over?
      está doblado (doblada)?
      you are lying down?
      está acostado (acostada)?
      you breathe deeply?
      respira profundo?
      you move?
      se mueve?
      you cough?
      tose?

53. Do you feel nauseated?
    ¿Tiene Vd. ganas de vomitar?

54. Are you nauseated?
    ¿Tiene náusea(s)?

55. Are you going to vomit?
    ¿Va a vomitar?

56. Did you vomit? A lot? A little?
    ¿Vomitó? ¿Mucho? ¿Poco?

57. How many times did you vomit . . .
    ¿Cuántas veces vomitó . . .
      today?
      hoy?
      yesterday?
      ayer?
      last night?
      anoche?

58. How often did you vomit?
    ¿Con qué frecuencia vomitó?
    ¿Cada cuánto tiempo vomitó?

59. Every five minutes?
    ¿Cada cinco minutos?

60. Did vomiting relieve your pains?
    ¿Le aliviaron el dolor los vómitos?

61. What did you vomit?
    ¿Qué vomitó?
      Almost nothing?
      ¿Casi nada?
      Food?
      ¿Comida?
      Foul-smelling liquid?
      ¿Un líquido de mal olor?

62. What color is it?[13]
    ¿De qué color es?
      Green?
      ¿Verde?
      Brown?
      ¿Café?
      Black?
      ¿Negro?
      Orange?
      ¿Anaranjado?
      Red?
      ¿Rojo?
      Yellow?
      ¿Amarillo?

63. Do you have blood in your vomit?
    ¿Hay sangre en los vómitos?

64. When you vomit, is it . . .
    Cuando Vd. vomita, ¿es . . .
      before eating?
      antes de comer?
      (immediately) after eating?
      (inmediatamente) después de comer?
      several hours after eating?
      varias horas después de comer?
      while eating?
      mientras come?
      not related to when you eat?
      sin relación a cuando come?
      accompanied by nausea?
      acompañado de náusea?

65. Are you vomiting blood?
    ¿Vomita Vd. sangre?
    ¿Está vomitando sangre?

66. Are you vomiting something similar to what you have just eaten?
    ¿Vomita Vd. algo parecido a lo que acaba de comer?

67. Is it acidic in taste?
    ¿Es de sabor ácido?

68. Is it bitter?
    ¿Es de sabor amargo?

69. Do you keep vomiting?
    ¿Sigue Vd. vomitando?

70. Do you need a pan?
    ¿Necesita el bacín?

71. Can you hold down water without vomiting?
    ¿Puede retener agua sin vomitarla?

72. Did you begin to vomit . . . the pain began?
    ¿Empezó a vomitar . . . empezó el dolor?
    before
    antes de que
    at the same time that
    al mismo tiempo que
    after
    después de que

73. How much time before the pain began?
    ¿Cuánto tiempo antes de que empezó el dolor?

74. How much time afterwards?
    ¿Cuánto tiempo después?

75. Do you have an appetite?
    ¿Tiene apetito?

76. Are you hungry?
    ¿Tiene hambre?

77. When did you lose your appetite?
    ¿Cuándo perdió su apetito?

78. When is the last time that you ate?
    ¿Cuándo es la última vez que comió?

79. When is the last time that you ate well?
    ¿Cuándo es la última vez que comió bien?

80. When is the last time that you moved your bowels?
    ¿Cuándo es la última vez que evacuó?

81. How are your stools?
    ¿Cómo son sus evacuaciones (excrementos)?

82. Do you move your bowels regularly?
    ¿Evacúa Vd. con regularidad?
    ¿Va Vd. al inodoro con regularidad?
    ¿Obra Vd. con regularidad? *Mex.*

83. Did you move your bowels yet?
    ¿Ya evacuó Vd.?
    ¿Obró ya? *Mex.*
    ¿Hizo caca ya? *juvenile, slang*

84. When was your last bowel movement?
    ¿Cuándo fue su última evacuación (intestinal)?

85. Is there anything unusual about your bowel movements?
    ¿Hay algo raro en su excremento?

86. Are you moving your bowels normally?
    ¿Evacúa Vd. normalmente?

87. How often do you have a bowel movement?
    ¿Cada cuánto evacúa?

88. When is the last time that you passed gas?
    ¿Cuándo es la última vez que pasó gases?

89. Do you have pain when you move your bowels?
    ¿Le duele el vientre al evacuar?

90. Is the pain continuous or intermittent?
    ¿Es continuo, o va y viene el dolor? (continuo o intermitente)

91. Do you have pain after you defecate? How long does it last?
    ¿Tiene Vd. dolor después de evacuar?
    ¿Cuánto tiempo le dura?

92. Do you have rectal bleeding?
    ¿Le sale sangre por el ano?
    ¿Echa sangre del recto?

93. Do you have blood in your stools?
    ¿Tiene sangre en las deposiciones intestinales?

94. Have you noticed the color of your stools?
    ¿Se ha fijado Vd. en el color de sus evacuaciones?

95. Is your stool black or light gray?
    ¿Son sus evacuaciones negras o grises claras?

96. Is your stool black like tar?
    ¿Son sus evacuaciones negras como alquitrán?

97. Is your stool clay-colored?
    ¿Son sus heces de color de arcilla?
    ¿Son sus evacuaciones blancuzcas?

98. Is your stool normal color?
    ¿Es su excremento de un color normal?

99. Is your stool foul-smelling?
    ¿Tienen mal olor sus evacuaciones?

100. Have you noticed foamy stools?
    ¿Se ha fijado en heces espumosas?

101. Have you ever seen worms in your bowel movements?
    ¿Ha visto jamás gusanos en el excremento?

102. Do you have diarrhea?
    ¿Tiene Vd. diarrea?
    ¿Tiene el chorrillo? *slang*
    ¿Tiene la cursera? *slang*
    ¿Están sus intestinos corrientes? *Mex, Chicano*

103. Have you had diarrhea recently?
    ¿Ha tenido diarrea recientemente?

104. Since when have you had it?
    ¿Desde cuándo la ha tenido?

105. How often do (did) you have diarrhea?
    ¿Con qué frecuencia tiene (tenía) diarrea?

106. Do you have intestinal cramps with it?
    ¿Se acompaña de retortijones?

107. Do you have straining with it?
    ¿Se acompaña de pujo?

108. What is the diarrhea like?
    ¿Cómo es la diarrea?

109. Is it watery?
    ¿Es puro líquido?

110. Is it diarrhea with mucus?
     ¿Es diarrea con moco?

111. Is there mucus with it?
     ¿Hay moco en la diarrea?

112. Is the diarrhea very foul-smelling?
     ¿Es muy apestosa la diarrea?

113. Does it float on top of the water?
     ¿Flota en el agua?

114. When you finish, do you still feel as if you have to go?
     Al terminar, ¿se queda Vd. con ganas de defecar?

115. Have you ever had typhoid fever?
     ¿Ha tenido alguna vez la fiebre tifoidea?

116. Have you noticed any anal itching?
     ¿Se ha fijado en alguna picazón del ano?

117. Is this worse before or after a bowel movement?
     ¿Es peor antes o después de obrar?

118. Is the itching worse when you go to bed?
     ¿Se empeora la picazón al acostarse?

119. Does it awaken you?
     ¿Le despierta?

120. Does the anus swell? Is there a lump at the anus?
     ¿Se le hincha el ano? ¿Hay un bulto al ano?

121. Is it painful?
     ¿Le duele mucho?

122. Does the swelling have a discharge?
     ¿Tiene la hinchazón una supuración (pus)?

123. Does the rectum come out when you move your bowels?
     ¿Se le sale el recto al obrar?

124. Do you have to replace it manually or does it return by itself (spontaneously)?
     ¿Tiene Vd. que ponerlo en su sitio manualmente o se vuelve a su lugar por sí mismo (espontáneamente)?

125. Is there a history of rectal tumors or hemorrhages in your family?
     ¿Ha habido casos de tumores del recto o hemorragias en su familia?

126. Have you ever had hemorrhages?
     ¿Ha tenido Vd. hemorragias?

127. Do you have hemorrhoids?
     ¿Padece Vd. de hemorroides?
     ¿Sufre Vd. de almorranas?

128. Do you have bleeding hemorrhoids?
     ¿Tiene Vd. hemorroides sangrantes?

129. Did you ever have any kind of rectal or intestinal problem before?
     ¿Tuvo Vd. jamás alguna enfermedad del ano o del intestino antes?

130. Have you had inguinal swollen glands?
     ¿Ha tenido Vd. las glándulas hinchadas en la ingle?

131. Do you know if you have ulcers?
     ¿Sabe si tiene úlceras?

132. Since when have you had ulcers?
     ¿Desde cuándo tiene úlceras?

133. Did you used to have ulcers?
     ¿Tenía úlceras?

134. When?
     ¿Cuándo?

135. Are you constipated?
     ¿Está Vd. estreñido (estreñida)?

136. Do you take remedies?
     ¿Toma remedios?[26]

137. Do you take enemas?[33]
     ¿Usa Vd. enemas (lavativas)?

138. Do you often take laxatives?[33]
     ¿Suele Vd. tomar laxantes?
     ¿Suele Vd. tomar medicina para evacuar el vientre?

139. How often?
     ¿Con qué frecuencia?
     Every day?
     ¿Cada día?
     ¿Todos los días?
     About once a week?
     ¿Más o menos una vez por semana?
     Periodically?
     ¿De vez en cuando?

140. What laxatives do you take?
     ¿Qué purgantes toma Vd.?
     Mineral oil?
     ¿Aceite mineral?
     Ex-Lax?
     ¿Ex-Lax?
     Milk of magnesia?
     ¿Leche de magnesia?

141. Do you use suppositories?
     ¿Usa Vd. supositorios?

142. Do you use medicated suppositories for your hemorrhoids?
     ¿Usa Vd. supositorios medicinales para sus almorranas?

143. Does it relieve the pain?
     ¿Alivia el dolor?

144. Have you ever had a (an inguinal) hernia?
     ¿Ha tenido alguna vez una hernia (una quebradura) inguinal (en la ingle)?

145. Have you ever had a barium x-ray where you swallowed barium or where you had a barium enema?[34]
     ¿Le han hecho alguna vez una radiografía de bario donde Vd. tragó el bario o donde le hicieron una lavativa (enema) de bario?

146. Have you ever had a gastrointestinal x-ray?[35]
     ¿Le han hecho alguna vez una radiografía gastrointestinal?

147. Have you ever had a gallbladder x-ray?
     ¿Le han hecho alguna vez radiografía de la vesícula biliar?

148. What were the results?
     ¿Cuáles fueron los resultados?

149. Have you ever been told you have gallstones?[31]
     ¿Le han dicho a Vd. alguna vez que tiene cálculos en la vesícula biliar?

150. Did you have a gallbladder operation?
     ¿Tuvo operación de la vesícula?

151. Did you have an operation on your stomach or intestines?
     ¿Tuvo operación del estómago o del intestino?

152. Why? Did you have . . .
     ¿Por qué? ¿Sufrió de . . .

     stones?
     piedras?
     an obstruction?
     una obstrucción?
     cancer?
     cáncer?

153. Have you ever had a barium enema?
     ¿Jamás le han hecho un lavado de bario?
     ¿Ha tenido alguna vez una enema de bario?

154. Have you ever had a barium X-ray?
     ¿Le han hecho jamás una radiografía con bario?

155. What have you eaten in the last twenty-four (24) hours?
     ¿Qué ha comido en las últimas veinticuatro (24) horas?

GENITOURINARY *GENITOURINARIO*

1. Can you urinate?
   ¿Puede Vd. orinar?

2. When you urinate, do you notice a delay in beginning?
   Al orinar, ¿ha notado Vd. una demora antes de comenzar a orinar?

3. Are you unable to control your urine?
   ¿Tiene Vd. pérdidas involuntarias de orina?

4. How long has it been since you have urinated?
   ¿Desde cuándo no orina Vd.?

5. Do you feel like urinating constantly?
   ¿Tiene Vd. ganas de orinar seguido?

6. Have you ever passed urine involuntarily when you laugh?
   ¿Se le sale la orina involuntariamente cuando se ríe /al reírse?
     sneeze?
     estornuda / al estornudar?
     cough?
     tose / al toser?
     lift something?
     levanta algo / al levantar algo?

7. How frequently do you urinate?
   ¿Con qué frecuencia orina Vd.

8. How much do you urinate (at one time)?
   ¿Cuánto orina Vd. (a la vez)?

9. When you urinate, do you pass a lot or a little urine?
   Al orinar, ¿pasa mucha o poca orina?

10. How many times a day do you urinate?
    ¿Cuántas veces al día orina Vd.?

11. Do you awaken in the night to urinate?
    ¿Se despierta Vd. por la noche para orinar?
    ¿Se levanta Vd. de la cama para orinar por la noche?

12. How often?
    ¿Cuántas veces?

13. Did you urinate?
    ¿Orinó Vd.?
    ¿Hizo pipí? *juvenile, slang*

14. Do you have or have you ever had pain from your kidneys or bladder?
    ¿Tiene Vd. o ha tenido jamás dolor de los riñones o de la vejiga?

15. Where is (was) the pain?
    ¿Dónde le duele (dolía)?

16. How long have (did) you had (have) the pain?
    ¿Cuánto tiempo hace (hacía) que Vd. tiene (tenía) el dolor?

17. How long does (did) it last?
    ¿Cuánto tiempo le dura (duraba)?

18. How often do (did) you have it?
    ¿Con qué frecuencia lo tiene (tenía)?

19. What is the pain like?
    ¿Cómo es el dolor?

20. Is it painful when you begin to urinate?
    ¿Tiene dolor al empezar a orinar?

21. Is it painful the entire time you urinate?
    ¿Tiene dolor por todo el tiempo que orina?

22. Is it painful when you finish urinating?
    ¿Le duele al terminar de orinar?

23. Does it hurt when you urinate?
    ¿Le duele cuando orina Vd.?

24. Does the pain stay in one place, or does it go toward the groin?
    ¿Se queda el dolor en un lugar, o se le corre hacia la ingle?

25. Is there a burning sensation when you urinate?
    ¿Siente un ardor (quemazón) al orinar?

26. Do you have a feeling of urgency to urinate?
    ¿Siente Vd. urgencia para orinar?

27. Is there any difficulty starting to urinate?
    ¿Hay alguna dificultad para empezar a orinar?

28. Do you have to wait a long time for the urine to come out?
    ¿Tiene que esperar mucho para que le salga la orina?

29. Do you have to strain to urinate?
    ¿Tiene que hacer fuerza para orinar?
    ¿Tiene que hacer fuerza para que salga la orina?

30. Is there an interrupted flow of urine?
    ¿Hay un chorro interrumpido de orina?

31. Do you notice dribbling after urination?
    ¿Se ha fijado en un goteo al terminar de orinar?

32. Is there a decrease in the force of the flow of urine?
    ¿Hay una disminución en la fuerza del chorro de orina?

33. Is the urine flow strong and continuous?
    ¿Es fuerte y continuo el chorro de orina?

34. Are there small stones in your urine?
    ¿Orina Vd. con arenilla?

35. Have you ever had kidney stones?[36]
    ¿Ha tenido alguna vez cálculos en los riñones?

36. Have you passed any stones?
    ¿Ha pasado algunas piedras?

37. Do you usually get backaches?
    ¿Suele Vd. tener dolor de espalda?

38. Do you ever have low back pain?
    ¿Suele Vd. tener dolor de cintura?[37]

39. Have you ever had a kidney (urinary) infection?
    ¿Ha tenido Vd. una infección en los riñones (una infección urinaria) alguna vez?

40. Was it treated?
    ¿Fue tratada?

41. What color is your urine?[13]
    ¿De qué color es la orina?
    pink?
    ¿rosada?
    like Coca-Cola?
    ¿color de Coca-Cola?

42. Do you have blood in your urine?
    ¿Tiene Vd. sangre en la orina?

43. Is your urine cloudy?
    ¿Es nublosa la orina?
    ¿Es turbia la orina?

44. Does your urine look bloody?
    ¿Le parece que tiene sangre en la orina?

45. Do you have pus in your urine?
    ¿Orina Vd. con pus?
    ¿Tiene Vd. pus en la orina?

46. Do your ankles swell when you don't urinate?
    ¿Se le hinchan los tobillos cuando no orina Vd.?

47. Do you ever lose urine for no reason?
    ¿Jamás pierde Vd. orina sin ninguna razón?

48. Do you ever lose urine before getting to the toilet when you do have to urinate?
    ¿Hay veces cuando pierde orina antes de llegar al baño / retrete cuando sí tiene que orinar?

49. Have you ever had a kidney infection?
    ¿Jamás ha tenido una infección de los riñones?

50. Have you ever had prostatitis? (*for men*)
    ¿Ha tenido alguna vez problemas de la próstata? (*para los varones*)

51. Do you have a lump in your testes? (*for men*)[38]
    ¿Tiene alguna bolita en los testículos? (*para los varones*)

52. Have you ever had cystitis?
    ¿Ha tenido jamás cistitis?

53. Your kidneys aren't functioning.
    Sus riñones no funcionan.

54. Have you ever had an operation on your kidneys?
    ¿Ha tenido alguna vez una operación de los riñones?

55. Have you ever had an operation on your bladder?
    ¿Ha tenido jamás operaciones de la vejiga?

56. Have you had an operation on your ureters or urethra?
    ¿Ha tenido operaciones de los uréteres o en la uretra?

57. Have you ever suffered an injury to your spinal cord or brain?
    ¿Jamás ha sufrido algún daño a la columna vertebral o al cerebro?

58. Do you have diabetes, multiple sclerosis, or Parkinson's disease?
    ¿Sufre Vd. de diabetes, esclerosis múltiple, o enfermedad de Parkinson?

REVIEW *REPASO*

Practice the following dialogue.

Practique el diálogo que sigue.

DR. GREEN: What is your problem, Miss Ruiz?

DR. GREEN: **¿Cuál es su problema, señorita?**

MISS RUIZ: I am having problems with my urine.

SRTA. RUIZ: **Tengo problemas al orinar.**

DR. GREEN: Can you urinate?

DR. GREEN: **¿Puede Vd. orinar?**

MISS RUIZ: Oh, yes, Doctor, but I am unable to control my urine.

SRTA. RUIZ: **Ah, sí, doctor, pero tengo pérdidas involuntarias de orina.**

DR. GREEN: How long has it been since you have urinated?

DR. GREEN: ¿Desde cuándo no orina Vd.?

MISS RUIZ: About five minutes.

SRTA. RUIZ: Casi cinco minutos.

DR. GREEN: How frequently do you urinate?

DR. GREEN: ¿Con qué frecuencia orina Vd.?

MISS RUIZ: I feel like I have to urinate every few minutes.

SRTA. RUIZ: Me parece que tengo que orinar cada pocos minutos.

DR. GREEN: When you urinate, do you pass a lot or a little urine?

DR. GREEN: Al orinar, ¿pasa mucha o poca orina?

MISS RUIZ: I only pass a few drops, but I feel like I have to go.

SRTA. RUIZ: No paso más que unas gotas, pero me parece que tengo que orinar.

DR. GREEN: Does it hurt when you urinate?

DR. GREEN: ¿Le duele cuando orina Vd.?

MISS RUIZ: I don't think so.

SRTA. RUIZ: Creo que no.

DR. GREEN: Is there a burning sensation when you urinate?

DR. GREEN: ¿Siente un ardor al orinar?

MISS RUIZ: No.

SRTA. RUIZ: No.

DR. GREEN: I am going to give you a prescription for some pills. Take one pill after each meal and at bedtime. Drink two glasses of water with each pill.

DR. GREEN: Le daré una prescripción para unas píldoras. Tome una después de cada comida y antes de acostarse. Trague esta medicina con dos vasos de agua cada vez.

MISS RUIZ: Yes, Doctor.

SRTA. RUIZ: Sí, doctor.

DR. GREEN: These pills may turn your urine different colors. Do not be afraid.

DR. GREEN: Es posible que estas píldoras cambien su orina a varios colores. No se preocupe Vd.

GENITOURINARY (MEN)

GENITOURINARIO (MASCULINO)

1. Do you get pains in the testicles?
   ¿Suele Vd. tener dolores en los testículos?
      en los huevos? *slang*
      en los compañones? *slang*

2. Do you pull back the foreskin on your penis when you wash in the genital region?
   ¿Se le pela Vd. al lavarse las partes?

3. Have you ever been impotent or sterile?
   ¿Ha padecido alguna vez de impotencia o esterilidad?

4. Do you have a discharge from your penis?
   ¿Le supura el pene?

5. Have you ever had prostatitis (inflamed prostate)?
   ¿Ha padecido alguna vez de prostatitis (la próstata inflamada)?
   ¿Ha tenido alguna vez problemas de la próstata?

6. Have you had any sores on your penis?
   ¿Ha tenido Vd. llagas (úlceras) en el pene?

GENITOURINARY (WOMEN): MENSTRUATION[18]

GENITOURINARIO (FEMENINO): MENSTRUACION

1. When was your last menstrual period?
   ¿Cuándo fue su última menstruación? *general*
   ¿Cuándo fue su último período? *fam*
   ¿Cuándo fue su última administración? *Mex.*
   ¿Cuándo fue su última regla? *Mex., PR*

2. How long did it last?
   ¿Cuánto tiempo le duró?

3. How often do you get your periods?
   ¿Cada cuánto le baja a Vd. la menstruación?
   ¿Cada cuánto menstrúa Vd.?

4. How many days does it last?
    ¿Cuántos días le dura?

5. Do you have it now?
    ¿La tiene ahora?

6. Do you have a light (heavy) flow?
    ¿Sale poca (mucha) sangre?

7. How old were you when you first began to menstruate?
    ¿A qué edad tuvo su primera menstruación (regla)?

8. Have your periods always been regular up to now?
    ¿Han sido regulares sus reglas hasta ahora?

9. Have you ever had menstrual problems?
    ¿Ha tenido alguna vez desórdenes menstruales?

10. Do you have pain with it?
    ¿Ha tenido dolor con ella?

11. Do you usually have pain with your periods?
    ¿Suele Vd. tener dolor durante su regla?

12. Was it worse this time?
    ¿Fue más fuerte esta vez?

13. Was there more bleeding than usual?
    ¿Sangró Vd. más de lo común?

14. How is your mood during your menstrual flow?
    ¿En qué humor se siente durante la menstruación?

15. Describe your menstrual flow.
    Describa Vd. su flujo menstrual.

16. Do you spot between periods (or after menopause)?
    ¿Tiene Vd. manchas de sangre entre periodos menstruales? (o después de la menopausia?)

17. Do you ever see lots of dark red blood then?
    ¿Ve Vd. hemorragia con sangre obscura o sangre roja entonces?

18. Are you bleeding heavily?
    ¿Está sangrando mucho?

19. How many sanitary pads or tampons did you use during your last menstrual cycle?
    ¿Cuántas toallas higiénicas ha usado Vd. durante su última menstruación?

20. Do you gain weight during your period?
    ¿Aumenta Vd. de peso durante su período?

21. Do you have severe menstrual cramps?
    ¿Sufre Vd. de retortijones menstruales?

22. Are your breasts tender during your period?
    Con su período, ¿le duelen los senos?

REVIEW

REPASO

PRACTICE *PRACTICA*

Read the following aloud both for fluency and comprehension. Then answer the questions based on the passage.

From the age of puberty until a woman enters menopause, she menstruates monthly. Once a month, an egg is formed by the woman's ovaries and if the woman does not become pregnant, the lining of the uterus is cast off and replaced each month. This reproductive process, because it is repeated regularly every month, is called a menstrual cycle. The menstrual cycle is measured from the first day of menstruation to the first day of the next menstruation. Usually these cycles are 28 days long. Some women have longer menstrual cycles, others shorter ones. The menstrual cycle is controlled by hormones. These hormones cause one of the ovaries to produce an egg each month. The hormones also cause changes in the lining of the uterus. If an egg is fertilized by sperm from a man, the egg attaches itself to the lining of the uterus.

If the egg is not fertilized the lining of the uterus is shed, accompanied by a flow of blood. The flow of blood passes from the uterus out through the vagina. This flow lasts from three to five days. Hormone secretions begin with the next menstrual cycle.

1. How long are menstrual cycles on the average?
2. What does the ovary produce?
3. How long does the flow of blood last?

Lea lo que sigue en voz alta para fluidez y comprehensión. Entonces conteste Vd. a las preguntas que siguen.

Desde la edad de pubertad hasta el cambio de vida, una mujer menstrúa una vez al mes. Una vez por mes un óvulo se forma y a menos que la mujer esté embarazada, el forro o recubrimiento interior del útero es expulsado y reemplazado cada mes. Este proceso reproductivo, a causa de la repetición regular cada mes, se llama un ciclo menstrual. El ciclo menstrual empieza el primer día de la menstruación y dura hasta el primer día de la próxima menstruación. Generalmente estos ciclos duran veintiocho días. Para algunas mujeres estos ciclos duran más, para otras duran menos tiempo. El ciclo menstrual es controlado por hormonas.

Estas hormonas hacen que uno de los ovarios produzca un óvulo cada mes. Estas hormonas también producen cambios en el forro del útero. Si un óvulo es fertilizado por los espermatozoides de un hombre, el óvulo fertilizado se adhiere al forro del útero.

Si el óvulo no es fertilizado, el recubrimiento interior del útero es expulsado, acompañado de un flujo de sangre. El flujo de sangre pasa desde el útero hasta la vagina. El sangrado menstrual dura de tres a cinco días. La secreción de hormonas cormienza de nuevo al empezar la menstruación.

1. ¿Por cuántos días duran los ciclos menstruales por lo regular?
2. ¿Qué produce un ovario?
3. ¿Cuántos días dura el flujo sanguíneo?

SEXUAL FUNCTION

FUNCION SEXUAL

1. Are you active sexually?
   ¿Tiene Vd. relaciones sexuales?

2. Are you okay with your sex life?
   ¿Está satisfecho (satisfecha) con sus relaciones sexuales?

3. Do you use contraceptives? What?
   ¿Usa Vd. anticonceptivos? ¿Cuáles?[39]

4. Is there a change in your desire to make love to . . .
   ¿Hay un cambio en su deseo de tener relaciones sexuales con . . .
   a man
   un hombre?
   a woman?
   una mujer?

5. Have you noticed a change in your desire to masturbate?
   ¿Ha notado un cambio en su deseo de masturbarse?

6. Are you having problems with orgasm?
   ¿Tiene Vd. problemas con el orgasmo?

7. Are you reaching climax / having an orgasm?
   ¿Tiene Vd. orgasmo?

8. Is it difficult to achieve an orgasm?
   ¿Le cuesta tener orgasmo?

9. Is it painful?
   ¿Es doloroso?

10. Do you have pain during sexual intercourse . . .
    ¿Tiene Vd. dolor durante sus relaciones sexuales . . .
    before intercourse?
    antes del acto sexual?
    during intercourse?
    durante el acto sexual?
    after intercourse?
    después del acto sexual?

FOR MEN   PARA LOS VARONES

1. Are you having a problem with your erections?
   ¿Tiene problemas con la erección?

2. Is it difficult to achieve?
   ¿Le cuesta tener?

3. Is it difficult to maintain?
   ¿Le cuesta mantener?

4. Is it painful?
   ¿Es dolorosa?

5. Are you having problems with ejaculation?
   ¿Tiene Vd. problemas con la eyaculación?

6. Do you ejaculate prematurely?
   ¿Tiene eyaculación prematura?

7. Is it difficult to achieve?
   ¿Le cuesta?

8. Is it painful?
   ¿Es dolorosa?

9. Is it bloody?
   ¿Es con sangre?

10. Do you ejaculate?
    ¿Eyacula?

FOR WOMEN   PARA LAS HEMBRAS

1. Are you having a problem with the amount of genital secretions that you have?
   ¿Tiene Vd. problema con la cantidad de secreciones genitales que tiene?

2. Is it not enough?
   ¿No es bastante?
   ¿Es poca?

3. Is it excessive?
   Es excesiva?

VAGINAL DISCHARGE

SECRECION VAGINAL

1. Do you have vaginal secretions?
   ¿Tiene Vd. secreciones vaginales?

2. Are they watery?
   ¿Son aguachentas?

3. Are they thick and yellow?
   ¿Son espesas y amarillas?

4. Are they thick and white?
   ¿Son espesas y blancas?

5. Are they frothy and greenish?
   ¿Son espumosas y verdosas?

6. Is your vagina itchy?
   ¿Tiene Vd. comezón en la vagina?

7. Have you had it before?
   ¿La ha tenido antes?

8. How long has the discharge been there?
   ¿Cuánto tiempo hace que le desecha?
   ¿Cuánto tiempo hace que le sale esta descarga?

9. Do you have a yellow-greenish or a whitish frothy, foul-smelling discharge that itches?
   ¿Tiene Vd. un desecho verde-amarillo o blancuzco, espumoso, apestoso con comezón?

10. Do you have a white discharge similar to "curds" that smells like mold or bread in the oven?
    ¿Tiene Vd. un desecho blanco, parecido a un cuajo con olor a moho o pan en el horno?

11. Do you have a milky, thick discharge, with a rancid odor?
    ¿Tiene Vd. un desecho color de leche, espeso, con olor rancio?

12. Do you have a coffee-colored discharge that is watery?
    ¿Tiene Vd. un desecho color café, como agua?

13. Do you have a lead-colored discharge, streaked with blood?
    ¿Tiene Vd. un desecho color plomo, rayado con sangre?

14. Have you ever had venereal disease (VD)?
    ¿Ha tenido jamás una enfermedad venérea (VD / EV)?

15. Is your husband circumcised?
    ¿Está circunciso su esposo?
    ¿Está circuncidado su esposo?

16. Is your sexual partner circumcised?
    ¿Está circuncisa la persona con quien Vd. tiene relaciones sexuales?
    ¿Está circuncidada la persona con quien Vd. tiene relaciones sexuales?

17. Do you suffer from prolapse of the uterus?
    ¿Padece Vd. de la matriz caída?

18. When was your last pap smear?
    ¿Cuándo le hicieron un frotis vaginal para el test de Papanicolau?

19. Were the results normal (abnormal)?
    ¿Fueron normales (anormales) los resultados?

PREGNANCY

EMBARAZO[40]

1. Have you ever been pregnant?[41]
   ¿Ha estado embarazada alguna vez?
   ¿Ha estado encinta jamás?

2. How many times have you been pregnant?
   ¿Cuántos embarazos ha tenido Vd.?

3. Were all your pregnancies normal?
   ¿Fueron normales todos sus embarazos?

4. Was the birth natural or induced?
   ¿Fue el parto natural o inducido?

5. Was the delivery normal, or did they use instruments?
   ¿Fue un parto normal, o usaron fórceps?

6. Was the delivery by Caesarean section?
   ¿Fue el parto por operación cesárea?

7. How many children do you have?[42]
   ¿Cuántos hijos tiene Vd.?

8. How old is your oldest child? Your youngest?
   ¿Cuántos años tiene el (la) mayor? ¿El (La) menor (más joven)?

9. Have you ever had an abortion, induced or spontaneous, or a miscarriage?
   ¿Ha tenido alguna vez un aborto, inducido o espontáneo, o un mal parto?

10. How many?
    ¿Cuántos?

11. How many weeks pregnant were you?
    ¿Cuántas semanas de embarazo tenía Vd. cuando tuvo el aborto (inducido / espontáneo)?

12. Have you ever had a baby who died at birth? How many?
    ¿Ha tenido jamás algún niño que haya muerto poco después de nacer? ¿Cuántos?

13. Have you ever had a stillborn child?
¿Jamás ha tenido Vd. un niño que haya nacido muerto?

14. Have you ever had a child who was born with the cord wrapped around the neck?
¿Jamás ha tenido un niño que haya nacido con el cordón umbilical alrededor del cuello?

15. Have you ever had a placenta previa?
¿Jamás ha tenido Vd. placenta previa?

16. Have you ever had postpartum hemorrhage?
¿Ha tenido Vd. alguna vez desangramiento (hemorragia) después del parto?

17. How long was your labor with your first child?
¿Cuánto tiempo duró el parto de su primer hijo?
    with your other children?
    ¿de sus otros hijos?

18. What is the date of your last period?
¿Cuál fue la fecha de su última regla?

19. Are you pregnant now?
¿Está Vd. embarazada en este momento?

20. How do you know you are pregnant?
¿Cómo sabe Vd. que está en estado?
    Did you give yourself a home pregnancy test?
    ¿Se dio a sí misma una prueba del embarazo en su propia casa?
    Did you see a doctor?
    ¿Le visitó a un médico (una médica)?

21. How many months?
¿Cuántos meses?

22. Was this a planned pregnancy?
¿Se planeó este embarazo?

23. When is your baby due?
¿Cuándo va a nacer el niño?

24. Is this your first pregnancy?
¿Es su primer embarazo?

25. Have you had German measles during this pregnancy?
¿Ha tenido Vd. el sarampión de tres días (rubéola) durante este embarazo?

26. Do you have any hereditary diseases?
¿Sufre Vd. de alguna enfermedad hereditaria?

27. Do you have diabetes?
¿Sufre Vd. de diabetes?

28. Do you have high blood pressure?
¿Sufre Vd. de alta presión arterial?

29. Have you been using any medications?[26]
¿Ha tomado alguna medicina?

30. What type?
¿De qué clase?

31. What is the name?
¿Cómo se llama(n)?

32. Have you been taking drugs (narcotics) during this pregnancy?[43]
¿Ha estado tomando drogas durante este embarazo?

33. Have you been drinking during this pregnancy daily?
¿Ha tomado alcohol diariamente durante este embarazo?

34. Have you had varicose veins or hemorrhoids during the pregnancy?
¿Ha tenido Vd. várices o hemorroides durante este embarazo?

35. Do you have nausea or vomiting?
¿Tiene Vd. náusea o vómitos?

36. Tiredness or low back pain?
¿Cansancio o dolor de cintura?[37]

37. Do you want to breastfeed this child?[21]
¿Quiere Vd. amamantar a este niño?

38. Do you have any new aversion to certain foods?
¿Siente Vd. repugnancia hacia alguna comida?
    Cravings?
    ¿Antojos?

39. Do your breasts feel heavy and tight?
¿Siente los senos pesados y apretados?

40. If you see any bleeding, call me at once.
Si Vd. tiene un derrame o flujo sangriento, llámeme en seguida.

41. Call me immediately if you have any severe pain.
Llámeme en seguida si Vd. siente dolores fuertes.
    severe and persistent headaches.
    dolores de cabeza severos y persistentes.
    stomachaches that do not go away when you move your bowels.
    dolores abdominales continuos que no se alivien al evacuar.

MENOPAUSE

LA MENOPAUSIA

1. Have you noticed any change in your periods?
¿Se ha fijado en algún cambio en su período?

2. Do you have hot flashes?
¿Siente Vd. sensaciones de calor en la cara?

3. Do you have a decrease in your vaginal secretions?
   ¿Tiene Vd. una disminución de las secreciones vaginales?
4. Is there a dryness of your skin?
   ¿Tiene sequedad de la piel?
5. Are you feeling "sick" with grief, depression, nervousness?
   ¿Siente Vd. males como angustias, tristeza, nerviosidad?
6. You are going through menopause / change of life.

Vd. pasa por la menopausia / el cambio de vida.
7. These symptoms are normal for a woman between the age of 40 and 50.
   Estos síntomas son normales para una mujer entre los 40 y 50 años de edad.
8. The symptoms will pass.
   Los síntomas pasarán.
9. After menopause, the majority of women again feel well.
   Después de la menopausia, la mayoría de las mujeres vuelven a sentirse bien.

GENITOURINARY (VENEREAL)

GENITOURINARIO (VENEREA)

1. Have you ever had any veneral disease (syphilis[44], gonorrhea)?
   ¿Ha padecido Vd. alguna vez de una enfermedad venérea (sífilis, gonorrea)?
2. Have you ever had a test for . . .
   ¿Jamás le han hecho una prueba para . . .
   AIDS?
   SIDA?
   syphilis?
   sífilis?
   gonorrhea?
   gonorrea?
   herpes?
   herpes?
3. When was the (last) test?
   ¿Cuándo fue la (última) prueba?
4. What were the results?
   ¿Cuáles fueron los resultados?
   positive?
   ¿positivos?
   negative?
   ¿negativos?
5. Did you receive treatment?
   ¿Recibió tratamiento?
6. With what did they treat you?
   ¿Con qué le trataron?
7. When? Where?
   ¿Cuándo? ¿Dónde?
8. Do you have a discharge from your penis (vagina)?
   ¿Tiene Vd. supuración en el pene (la vagina)?
9. Do you have any sores on your penis (in or around your vagina)?
   ¿Tiene Vd. llagas (úlceras) en el pene (en o alrededor de la vagina)?
10. Is there genital itching?
    ¿Tiene picazón de los genitales?
11. Do you have a burning sensation of your genitals?
    ¿Siente Vd. ardor en los genitales?

12. Is there swelling or tenderness of the inguinal area?
    ¿Hay hinchazón o dolor en la ingle?
13. Does it hurt to urinate?
    ¿Le duele al orinar?
14. Do any joints hurt you—wrist, ankle, knee?
    ¿Le duelen las coyunturas—las de la muñeca, del tobillo, de la rodilla?
15. Is your genital area red?
    ¿Tiene Vd. enrojecimiento de los genitales?
16. Do you have any rash on your body?
    ¿Tiene Vd. salpullido en el cuerpo?
17. How long has this been going on?
    ¿Cuánto tiempo hace que pasa esto?
18. Have you slept with a man (woman) recently?
    ¿Ha tenido relaciones sexuales con un hombre (una mujer) recientemente?
19. Do you know if that person with whom you have had sexual relations also has these symptoms?
    ¿Sabe Vd. si esa persona con quien Vd. ha tenido relaciones sexuales también tiene estos síntomas?
20. When was the last time that you had sexual relations?
    ¿Cuándo fue la última vez que tuvo relaciones sexuales?
21. Don't have sexual relations until you are completely cured.
    No tenga relaciones sexuales hasta que esté completamente curado (curada).
22. Don't drink any alcoholic beverages until you are completely cured.
    No tome ninguna bebida alcohólica hasta que esté completamente curado (curada).
23. Avoid physical exercise.
    Evite Vd. hacer ejercicios físicos.
24. You must go to the VD clinic.
    Vd. tiene que ir a la clínica de enfermedades venéreas.

AIDS

SIDA[45]

1. Do you know what AIDS is?
   ¿Sabe lo que significa «AIDS»?

2. It is the English acronym for "Acquired Immuno-Deficiency Syndrome," the name given to a fatal disease which destroys the body's immune system and central nervous system, and ultimately destroys the body's ability to fight infections and illnesses.
   Es la sigla inglesa para el «Síndrome de Inmunodeficiencia Adquirida» o SIDA, el nombre dado a una enfermedad que destruye el sistema inmune (inmunológico) del cuerpo y el sistema nervioso central, y últimamente destruye la habilidad del cuerpo para combatir infecciones y enfermedades.

3. Presently there is no cure for AIDS nor a vaccine to avoid the HIV infection.
   Actualmente no hay cura para el SIDA ni una vacuna para evitar la infección por VIH.

4. Do you know what causes AIDS?
   ¿Sabe cuál es la causa del SIDA?

5. The cause is a virus, HIV, which stands for Human Immunodeficiency Virus.
   La causa es un virus, cuya sigla en inglés es «HIV» y en español es «VIH»,[46] que significa Virus de Inmunodeficiencia Humana.

6. HIV attacks and weakens the body's ability to fight off infection.
   El VIH[46] ataca y debilita la capacidad del cuerpo de defenderse contra infección.

7. Not everybody with this virus has AIDS.
   No todo el mundo que sufre de este virus tiene el SIDA.

8. A person can have HIV for years before developing AIDS; some never develop it.
   Una persona puede estar infectada con el VIH[46] por años antes de incubar el SIDA; algunas personas nunca lo contraen.

9. Do you know how the AIDS causing virus is transmitted from one person to another?
   ¿Sabe cómo se transmite el virus que causa el SIDA entre una y otra persona?

10. AIDS is not a disease acquired by casual contact among friends.
    El SIDA no es una enfermedad adquirida por el contacto casual entre personas.

11. We know that the virus can be transmitted by sexual contact, by using intravenous drugs and sharing a contaminated hypodermic needle, thus bringing the virus directly to the bloodstream, and although less likely, through blood or blood products, or from an infected mother to her new-born child.
    Sabemos que el virus puede ser transmitido por contacto sexual, contacto íntimo, por el uso de drogas intravenosas y compartiendo una aguja hipodérmica contaminada, así llevando el virus directamente a la sangre, o aunque menos probable, queda la posibilidad de transmitirlo por la sangre o productos de sangre, o de una madre infectada a su bebé recién nacido.

12. There are a small number of cases which do not fit in any of these categories.
    Hay un pequeño número de casos que no encaja dentro de estas categorías.

13. At this time there is no known cure for AIDS although research is continuing to try to find one and there are many helpful treatments.
    Hasta la fecha no se conoce cura para el SIDA aunque la investigación continúa en la esperanza de encontrarla y hay muchos tratamientos efectivos.

14. Patients with AIDS often have secondary illnesses and infections, called "opportunistic," like PCP, a type of lung infection, or Kaposi's sarcoma, a tumor that affects various parts of the body.
    Muchas veces pacientes con SIDA sufren de enfermedades e infecciones secundarias, llamadas «oportunistas», como PCP, un tipo de infección del pulmón, o la sarcoma de Kaposi, un tumor que afecta diferentes partes del cuerpo.

15. The patient who does not yet have AIDS but does have the virus is referred to as an "ARC."
    El paciente que todavía no sufre del SIDA pero sí tiene el virus se refiere como un «ARC»—una persona con el complejo relacionado al SIDA.

16. The patient who has AIDS is called a "PWA" which stands for a person with AIDS.
    El paciente que sufre del SIDA se llama un «PWA» que significa una persona con el SIDA.

17. There is a blood test, which is extremely accurate, which can detect whether you have been infected with HIV.
    Hay un análisis de sangre, que es muy preciso, que puede detectar si usted está infectado (infectada) por el VIH.

18. Please answer the following questions honestly.
Favor de contestar a las preguntas siguientes honestamente.

19. Have you had sex with more than one person?
¿Ha tenido sexo con más de una persona?

20. Have you had many different sexual partners?
¿Ha tenido relaciones sexuales con muchas parejas diferentes?

21. Is there more than one person with whom you are having a sexual relationship now?
¿Hay más de una persona con quien tiene relaciones sexuales ahora?

22. Do you know the person(s) with whom you have (had) sex?
¿Conoce a la(s) persona(s) con quien(es) tiene (tuvo) sexo?

23. Have you had sex with someone who uses (intravenous) drugs?
¿Ha tenido relaciones sexuales con alguien que usa drogas intravenosas?

24. Have you ever had sex with someone who has been infected with HIV or who has contracted AIDS?
¿Ha tenido relaciones sexuales jamás con alguien que se haya infectado con el VIH o haya contraído el SIDA?

25. Where does this person live?
¿Dónde vive esta persona?

26. Have you ever had a sexual relationship with anyone who could have had a sexual relationship with a person of that same sex?
¿Ha tenido relaciones sexuales alguna vez con una persona que pudiese haber tenido relaciones sexuales con una persona de ese mismo sexo? ¿una persona bisexual?

27. Have you ever been sexually abused or raped?
¿Le (La) han abusado sexualmente o violado?

28. Have you ever had sexual contact with a person of your sex?
¿Jamás ha tenido contacto sexual con una persona de su sexo?

29. Have you ever had sex with a prostitute?
¿Ha tenido relaciones sexuales alguna vez con una prostituta?

30. Have you ever paid anyone to have sex with you?
¿Jamás le ha pagado a alguien para tener sexo con Vd.?

31. Have you ever had sex with other men? other women?
¿Ha tenido relaciones sexuales alguna vez con otros hombres? con otras mujeres?

32. Do you use a condom when you have sexual relations?
¿Usa un condón cuando tiene relaciones sexuales?

33. Do you always use a condom?
¿Siempre usa usted un condón?

34. You must use a condom when you have sexual relations.
Vd. tiene que usar un condón cuando tiene relaciones sexuales.

35. Do you know how to use a condom?[47]
¿Sabe cómo usar un condón / profiláctico?[47]

36. You must be extremely careful not to infect your mate with HIV.
Vd. tiene que tener muchísimo cuidado para no infectar a su compañera (compañero) con el VIH.

37. When was the last time that you had sex?
¿Cuándo fue la última vez que tuvo relaciones sexuales?

38. Was the contact genital or oral?
¿Fue el contacto por los genitales o por la boca?

39. Did you have anal sex?
¿Tuvo sexo por el ano?

40. Did you have oral sex?
¿Tuvo sexo oral? ¿por la boca?

41. Have you ever had a blood transfusion?
¿Jamás le han hecho una transfusión de sangre?

42. When was it? Was it before 1985?
¿Cuándo fue? ¿Ocurrió antes de mil novecientos ochenta y cinco (1985)?

43. Have you received any blood products since 1985?
¿Ha recibido algún producto de sangre desde mil novecientos ochenta y cinco?

44. Do you use intravenous drugs?
¿Usa Vd. drogas intravenosas?

45. Have you ever shared needles with someone who uses street drugs?
¿Ha compartido jamás agujas con alguien que usa drogas corrientes de la calle?

46. Have you ever been accidentally exposed to HIV?
¿Ha sido expuesto (expuesta) por casualidad al VIH?

47. Are you getting sick more frequently?
¿Se enferma con más frecuencia?

48. Are you constantly tired?
¿Sufre de fatiga constante?

49. Do you have insomnia?
¿Sufre de insomnio?

50. Have you had recurring fevers, including night sweats?
¿Ha tenido fiebre recurrente, incluyendo «sudores nocturnos»?

51. Do you have diarrhea and a loss of appetite?
¿Padece de diarrea y pérdida de apetito?

52. Have you had a rapid loss of weight without any apparent reason?
¿Ha sufrido una rápida pérdida de peso sin razón aparente?

53. Have you noticed white spots around your mouth?
¿Se ha fijado en manchas blancas en la boca?

54. Have you noticed any changes in your skin?
¿Se ha fijado en algunos cambios en la piel?

55. Do you have pink or purplish blotches on your skin?
¿Tiene manchas rosadas o purpurinas (marrones) en la piel?

56. Have you had tuberculosis recently?
¿Ha padecido de la tuberculosis recientemente?

57. Remember that only people with whom one is intimate or shares needles are at risk for getting AIDS.
Recuerde Vd. que solamente las personas con quienes tiene relaciones íntimas (sexuales) o comparte agujas corren el riesgo de contraer el SIDA.

EXTREMITIES *LAS EXTREMIDADES*

1. Are your joints stiff in the morning?
¿Siente Vd. rígidas sus articulaciones por la mañana?
¿Están rígidas las coyunturas por la mañana?
fam

2. Have you had aches in your joints during the last year?
¿Ha tenido Vd. dolores en las articulaciones durante el año pasado?

3. Which joints are painful?
¿Cuáles son las articulaciones que le duelen?

4. Are your knees and wrists swollen or only your ankles and knees?
¿Tiene Vd. las rodillas y las muñecas hinchadas o solamente los tobillos y las rodillas hinchados?

5. Do you feel pain when you stand?
¿Siente Vd. dolor cuando se pone de pie?

6. Do you feel pain when you bend?
¿Siente Vd. dolor cuando se dobla (se agacha)?

7. Do the pains shoot down toward the legs?
¿Le baja el dolor a las piernas?

8. Is the pain sharp or dull?
¿Es agudo o sordo el dolor?

9. What part of your leg hurts?
¿Qué parte de la pierna le duele?

10. Is it deep pain?
¿Es dolor profundo?

11. Show me where it hurts you.
Enséñeme dónde le duele.

12. Is this the first time that your leg has been hurting you?
¿Es ésta la primera vez que le duele la pierna?

13. When did it begin?
¿Cuándo empezó?

14. When did it begin the first time?
¿Cuándo empezó la primera vez?

15. When did it begin this time?
¿Cuándo empezó esta vez?

16. How did (does) the pain begin?
¿Cómo empezó (empieza) el dolor?

17. How did it begin the first time?
¿Cómo empezó la primera vez?

18. Suddenly or gradually?
¿De repente o poco a poco?

19. What is the pain like?
¿Cómo es el dolor?[48]

20. Is your leg (arm) weak?
    ¿Siente débil la pierna (el brazo)?

21. Is it getting worse?
    ¿Se empeora?

22. Do you have any numb spots?
    ¿Tiene alguna parte entumecida?

23. Show me where.
    Enséñeme dónde.

24. Here?
    ¿Aquí?

25. Is it getting worse with time?
    ¿Se empeora con el tiempo?

26. Do you have tingling any place?
    ¿Tiene hormigueos en algún lugar?

27. Show me where.
    Enséñeme dónde.

28. Do you have any redness on your leg?
    ¿Tiene alguna parte roja en la pierna?

29. Do you have any bluish part on your leg?
    ¿Tiene alguna parte morada en la pierna?[30]

30. Do you have any pale place on your leg?
    ¿Tiene alguna parte pálida en la pierna?

31. Is any part of your leg cold?
    ¿Hay alguna parte fría de la pierna?

32. Is any part of your leg warm?
    ¿Hay alguna parte caliente de la pierna?

33. Is it getting worse?
    ¿Se empeora?

34. Do you have one swollen leg?
    ¿Tiene una pierna hinchada?

35. Is one leg skinnier than the other?
    ¿Tiene una pierna más flaca que la otra?

36. Are both of your legs swollen?
    ¿Tiene las dos piernas hinchadas?

37. Is it getting worse?
    ¿Se empeora?

38. Do you have shortness of breath?
    ¿Tiene una falta de aire?

39. Do you get short of breath . . .
    ¿Le falta el aire . . .
    when you walk?
    al caminar?
    when you climb stairs?
    al subir las escaleras?
    when you lie down?
    al acostarse?

40. Is the pain constant?
    ¿Es constante el dolor?

41. Is it better or worse . . .
    ¿Es mejor o peor . . .
    in the morning?
    por la mañana?
    at night?
    por la noche?
    with rest?
    al descansar?
    with exercise?
    con ejercicio?
    when you walk?
    cuando camina?
    when you lie down?
    al acostarse?
    when you run?
    al correr?
    when you are standing up?
    al estar de pie?
    with one leg up?
    con una pierna arriba?
    with the leg down?
    con la pierna abajo?
    with cold?
    con el frío?
    with heat.
    con el calor?
    with the rain?
    con la lluvia?

42. Can you walk?
    ¿Puede caminar?

43. How many blocks can you walk?
    ¿Cuántas cuadras puede caminar?
    Without pain?
    ¿Sin dolor?
    Without getting tired?
    ¿Sin cansarse?

44. Can you climb stairs?
    ¿Puede subir escaleras?

45. How many stairs can you climb?
    ¿Cuántas escaleras puede subir?
    Without pain?
    ¿Sin dolor?
    Without getting tired?
    ¿Sin cansarse?

46. Do you have to stop then?
    ¿Tiene que parar entonces?

47. How long?
    ¿Por cuánto tiempo?

48. Do your legs get tired?
    ¿Se le cansan las piernas?

NEUROLOGICAL *NEUROLOGICO*

Motor Coordination *Movilidad-coordinación*

1. Do you feel (very) weak?
    ¿Se siente (muy) débil?

2. Do you ever feel dizzy (giddy)?
    ¿Tiene Vd. vértigo alguna vez?
    ¿Suele Vd. Tener mareos? *fam*

3. Do you spin around?
    ¿Da Vd. vueltas?

4. Do objects spin around you?
    ¿A Vd. le dan vueltas los objetos?

5. Do you ever lose your coordination?
    ¿Pierde Vd. jamás su coordinación?

6. Do you ever lose your balance?
    ¿Pierde Vd. jamás su equilibrio?

7. Do you feel like falling?
    ¿Se siente Vd. como si se cayese / cayera?

Sensory   *Sensibilidad*

8. Do you ever have trouble . . .
    ¿Tiene Vd. algunas veces dificultad . . .
        feeling heat on your skin?
        en distinguir el calor en la piel?
        feeling cold on your skin?
        en distinguir el frío en la piel?

9. Do you ever lose your sense of touch?
    ¿Le falta jamás la sensibilidad táctil?

10. Do you have tingling sensations?
    ¿Tiene Vd. hormigueos?

11. Do you have numbness in your hands or feet?
    ¿Tiene Vd. entumecimiento (calambres) en las manos o los pies?

12. Have you been sleeping on your arm?
    ¿Ha estado durmiendo Vd. sobre el brazo?

13. Are some of the fingers numb?
    ¿Tiene Vd. algunos de los dedos adormecidos?

14. Come see me if your fingers become numb.
    Venga a verme si se le adormecen los dedos.

Convulsions and Headaches[49]   *Convulsiones y dolores de cabeza*

15. Do you have fainting spells?
    ¿Ha tenido Vd. desmayos?
    ¿Suele Vd. tener desvanecimientos?

16. Are you subject to them?
    ¿Se desmaya Vd. con frecuencia?

17. Do you have convulsions?
    ¿Le ha ocurrido a Vd. tener convulsiones o haber estado inconsciente?
    ¿Suele Vd. tener convulsiones?

18. When was your most recent one?
    ¿Cuándo fue la última?

19. When was your first one?
    ¿Cuándo fue la primera?

20. How often do you have them?
    ¿Con qué frecuencia las tiene Vd.?

21. Have you ever lost consciousness?
    ¿Perdió Vd. el sentido alguna vez?

22. For how long?
    ¿Por cuánto tiempo?

23. How frequently does this happen?
    ¿Con qué frecuencia ocurre?

24. When you have convulsions, do you ever bite your tongue?
    Cuando tiene Vd. convulsiones, ¿jamás se muerde la lengua?

25. Are the convulsions preceded by any warning, like an odor, a strange feeling, pain, a vision, etc?
    ¿Precede las convulsiones algún aviso, como un olor, una sensación rara, un dolor, una visión, etc.?

26. Are you disoriented afterwards?
    ¿Está Vd. desorientado (desorientada) después?

27. Do you take medicine for the convulsions?
    ¿Toma Vd. medicina para las convulsiones?

28. What kind?
    ¿De qué tipo?

29. Do you have headaches?
    ¿Sufre Vd. de dolores de cabeza?

30. What type—mild, moderate, migraines?
    ¿Cómo son—leves, moderados, migrañas?

31. Describe the pain.
    Describa Vd. el dolor de la cabeza.

Special   *Especial*

32. Do you ever have trouble speaking clearly?
    ¿Tiene Vd. algunas veces dificultad en hablar claramente?

33. Do you ever have trouble when you read or write?
    ¿Tiene Vd. algunas veces problemas al leer o al escribir?

34. Do you ever have trouble understanding what someone asks?
    ¿Tiene Vd. algunas veces dificultad en entender cuando alguien le pregunta algo?

35. Have you ever had memory defects?
    ¿Ha tenido Vd. defectos de memoria?

36. Have you ever had difficulty remembering . . .
    ¿Ha tenido alguna vez dificultad para recordar . . .
        past events?
        acontecimientos pasados?

recent events?
acontecimientos recientes?

37. Have you ever had a loss of . . .
¿Ha tenido jamás una pérdida del control para . . .

bladder control?
orinar?

bowel control?
defecar?

38. Are you unable to urinate?
¿Se le tapa la orina?

39. How did the pain begin?
¿Cómo empezó el dolor?

Cranial Nerves   *Nervios craneales*

40. Do you see double?
¿Ve Vd. doble?
¿Ve Vd. las cosas doble?
¿Ve Vd. bizco? *C.A.*

41. Do you have blurred vision?
¿Ve Vd. borrosamente?
¿Ve Vd. borroso?

42. Do you ever see spots before your eyes?
¿Ve Vd. jamás manchas (moscos) volantes delante de los ojos?

43. Do you ever have pain behind your eyes?
¿Tiene Vd. jamás dolor que parece estar detrás de los ojos?

44. Has it gotten better?
¿Se ha mejorado?

45. Has it gotten worse?
¿Se ha empeorado?

46. Have you ever had a problem distinguishing colors?
¿Ha tenido algunas veces problemas en distinguir los colores?

47. Have you ever had trouble smelling?
¿Ha tenido jamás problemas con el sentido olfatorio?

48. Have you ever had a sensation of . . .
¿Ha tenido alguna vez una sensación de . . .
strange odors?
olores extraños?
unpleasant odors?
olores desagradables?

49. Have you ever had a change in taste sensations?
¿Ha tenido jamás un cambio en el sentido del gusto?

50. Have you ever had difficulty chewing?
¿Ha tenido jamás dificultad para masticar?

51. Have you ever had trouble swallowing?
¿Ha tenido alguna vez dificultad para tragar?

52. Since when?
¿Desde cuándo?

53. Have you ever had a loss of feeling in your face?
¿Ha tenido jamás pérdida de la sensibilidad en la cara?

54. Did it develop . . .
¿Se inició . . .
slowly?
lentamente?
suddenly?
de repente?

55. Have you ever had difficulty in hearing?
¿Ha tenido jamás dificultad para oír?

56. Since when?
¿Desde cuándo?

57. How did it begin—slowly or suddenly?
¿Cómo empezó—lentamente o de repente?

58. Have you ever had a ringing in your ears?
¿Ha tenido jamás un zumbido en los oídos?

MUSCULOSKELETAL   *MUSCULAR-ESQUELÉTICO*

1. Do you have any swelling?
¿Se le hincha a Vd. alguna parte del cuerpo?

2. Do you have a herniated disc?
¿Tiene Vd. una hernia del disco intervertebral?

3. Do you have varicose veins?
¿Tiene Vd. las venas inflamadas (várices o venas varicosas)?

4. Have you had any pain in your back?[24]
¿Ha tenido Vd. (algún) dolor de espalda?

5. What part of your back hurts?
¿Qué parte de la espalda le duele?

6. Does your lower back hurt?
Le duele la cintura?[37]
le duelen los riñones?[50]

7. Where? Show me where it hurts. Show me with one finger where it hurts.
¿Dónde? Enséñeme donde le duele. Enséñeme con un sólo dedo donde le duele.

8. How often do you have pain?
¿Con qué frecuencia tiene dolor?

9. Does the pain stay here in the back or does it radiate to another spot?
¿Se queda el dolor aquí en la espalda o corre a otra parte?

10. Does your leg hurt you?
    ¿Le duele la pierna?

11. Does your foot hurt?
    ¿Le duele el pie?

12. Does your big toe hurt?
    ¿Le duele el dedo grande?

13. Does your stomach hurt?
    ¿Le duele el estómago?

14. Do you have any numb spots?
    ¿Tiene alguna parte entumecida?

15. Show me where.
    Enséñeme dónde.

16. Here?
    ¿Aquí?

17. Is it getting worse with time?
    ¿Se empeora con el tiempo?

18. Do you have tingling any place?
    ¿Tiene hormigueos en algún lugar?

19. Show me where.
    ¿Enséñeme dónde.

20. Are you unable to urinate?
    ¿Se le tapa la orina?

21. Do you have a loss of bowel control?
    ¿Se ensucia de excremento?

22. Do you soil yourself with urine?
    ¿Se ensucia de orina?

23. How did the pain begin?
    ¿Cómo empezó el dolor?

24. Gradually?
    ¿Poco a poco?

25. Suddenly?
    ¿De repente?

26. What is the pain like?
    ¿Cómo es el dolor?

27. Is it mild or strong?
    ¿Es leve o fuerte?

28. Is the pain constant or does it come and go?
    ¿Es constante el dolor o va y viene?

29. Do you have lower back pain when . . .
    ¿Se queda el dolor de cintura[37] cuando . . .
    you are lying down?
    se acuesta?
    you are resting?
    descansa?

30. Is it better, worse, or the same when you . . .
    ¿Se mejora, se empeora, o es igual cuando . . .
    sneeze?
    estornuda?
    cough
    tose?
    move your bowels?
    evacua?
    walk?
    camina?

move?
se mueve?
twist?
se tuerce?
bend?
se dobla?
lie down?
se acuesta?
rest?
descansa?

31. Is there a position in which it improves?
    ¿Hay una posición en que se mejora?

32. Show me.
    Enséñeme.

33. Do you know what caused the pain?
    ¿Sabe qué causó el dolor?
    Did you have an accident?
    ¿Tuvo un accidente?
    Did you fall?
    ¿Se cayó?
    Did you hurt yourself?
    ¿Se hizo daño?

34. Do you lift heavy items in your work?
    ¿Levanta muchas cosas pesadas en su trabajo?

35. Did you lift something heavy one time in particular?
    ¿Levantó algo muy pesado una vez en particular?

36. When?
    ¿Cuándo?

37. Did you hurt yourself ever?
    ¿Se hizo daño jamás?

38. How?
    ¿Cómo?

39. Did you fall?
    ¿Se cayó?

40. How?
    ¿Cómo?

41. How do you relieve the pain?
    ¿Cómo se alivia el dolor?

42. Do you take medicine?
    ¿Toma medicinas?

43. What medicines do you take? Aspirin? Something else?[26]
    ¿Qué medicinas toma? ¿Aspirina? ¿Algo más?

44. Do you use heat?
    ¿Usa calor?

45. Rest?
    ¿Descanso?

46. Do you reduce the pain with exercises?
    ¿Se alivia el dolor con ejercicios?

47. Have you been bothered recently by muscle spasms?
    ¿Ha tenido Vd. recientemente molestias o dolor en los músculos?

48. Have you had muscle weakness?
    ¿Ha tenido Vd. debilidad muscular?

49. Have you had pain in your . . .
    ¿Ha tenido dolor en . . .
    muscles?
    los músculos?
    bones?
    los huesos?
    joints?
    las coyunturas
    fingers?
    los dedos?
    knees?
    las rodillas?
    hips?
    las caderas?
    ankles?
    los tobillos?
    wrists?
    las muñecas?

50. Where do you have pain in your joints?
    ¿Dónde le duelen las articulaciones?

51. Do you take medicine? What?
    ¿Toma medicina? ¿Qué?

Aspirin?
¿Aspirina?
Herbs?
¿Hierbas?[51]
Cortisone?
¿Cortisona?
Prednisone?
¿prednisona?

52. Which hand do you use more?
    ¿Qué mano usa Vd. más?
    the left?
    ¿la izquierda?
    the right?
    ¿la derecha?
    both equally?
    las dos iqualmente?

53. Have you had any trouble getting up out of a chair?
    ¿Ha tenido problemas alguna vez para levantarse de una silla?

54. Have you had any problems with your legs climbing the stairs?
    ¿Ha tenido algunos problemas con las piernas para subir las escaleras?

ENDOCRINE   *ENDOCRINO*

1. Has there been a significant change in your weight recently? A gain? A loss?
   ¿Ha habido un gran cambio en su peso recientemente? ¿Ha engordado? ¿Ha adelgazado?

2. Are you eating more than usual but not gaining weight?
   ¿Come Vd. más de lo común pero no engorda?

3. Has there been any change in your facial features?
   ¿Ha habido algún cambio en las facciones de la cara?

4. Has there been any change in your skin?
   ¿Ha habido algún cambio en la piel?

5. Is it darker?
   ¿Es más oscura?

6. Is it a finer texture?
   ¿Es más áspera?

7. Has there been any change in your hair—either in texture, color, or quantity?
   ¿Ha habido algún cambio en el cabello—o en cuanto a la textura, el color o la cantidad?

8. Have you noticed a change in the placement of your hair?
   ¿Ha notado un cambio en la localización del pelo?

9. Have you noticed a change in your voice?
   ¿Se ha fijado en algún cambio en su voz?

10. Is it lower?
    ¿Es más baja?

11. Is it higher?
    ¿Es más alta?

12. Have you noticed any change in your desire to have sexual relations?
    ¿Se ha fijado en algún cambio en sus deseos de tener relaciones sexuales?

13. Have you noticed that you are more intolerant to heat than usual?
    ¿Ha notado Vd. que no aguanta el calor tanto como siempre?

14. Have you noticed that you can't tolerate the cold?
    ¿Ha notado que no aguanta el frío?

15. Are you more nervous than before?
    ¿Se pone Vd. más nervioso (nerviosa) que antes?

16. Have you noticed that you are more tired than usual?
    ¿Ha notado que se cansa más de lo común?

17. Have you noticed that you perspire more than usual?
    ¿Ha notado que transpira más de lo común?

18. Are you thirstier than usual?
    ¿Tiene Vd. más sed de lo normal?

19. Have you noticed a problem concentrating?
    ¿Ha notado Vd. un problema en concentrarse?

20. Have you noticed a problem sleeping?
    ¿Ha notado un problema en dormir?

21. Do you urinate more than usual?
    ¿Orina Vd. más de lo normal?

22. When you were young, did you ever receive radiation to . . .
    Cuando era joven, ¿jamás recibió radiación . . .

    your neck?
    al cuello?
    your head?
    a la cabeza?

23. Have you ever noticed a lump in your neck?
    Se ha fijado alguna vez en una masa en el cuello?

Notes *Notas*

1. Bear in mind that the metric system is used in all Spanish-speaking countries. Consequently, some Spanish-speaking patients may have difficulty with or not fully understand discussions of weights and measures that do not utilize metrics. See Chapter 4, pages 92–95.
2. See note 1, page 9, Chapter 1 for a complete discussion on Spanish names.
3. In some places the literal translations, *está caliente* and *está frío* are vulgar and have sexual connotations.
4. See Chapter 3, "Anatomic and Physiological Vocabulary," for other body parts.
5. See also page 188 below.
6. See Chapter 7, page 150, note 10.
7. See Chapter 4, page 187 for the numbers.
8. See above, pages 155–156, questions 17–25.
9. If the patient is 30 or younger, skip questions 51–62.
10. Patients from South America might substitute *la nieve*, which means "snow" for ice cream.
11. There is a high correlation with diet, obesity, and diabetes in the Hispanic population. Many Hispanics chose a diet that is frequently high in saturated fats although as people become more aware of health risks and proper nutrition, this type of diet preference is changing. Studies have shown that almost 30% of Hispanic males and 39% of females of Mexican-American descent are overweight as are 25% of males and 37% of females of Puerto Rican heritage, and 29% of males and 34% of females of Cuban descent. These same studies show that Mexican Americans tend to have higher levels of cholesterol and triglycerides. See G. Marks, *et al.*, "Health Risk Behaviors of Hispanics in the United States: Findings from HHANES, 1982–84" *American Journal of Public Health*, 1990; 80 (Supplement): 20–26.
12. See Chapter 16, pages 350–351 for nouns of family relationship.
13. For a listing of colors, see Chapter 16, p. 353.
14. *Constipado (constipada)* also can be used. It means either "to have a cold" or "to be constipated."
15. When a person sneezes, many Spanish-speaking people often say *¡Jesús!* The phrase originated in the Middle Ages as a supplication for divine help in time of trouble. See Chapter 6, page 134, notes 6 and 10.
16. For additional information, see Chapter 12, page 254, "Throat Culture," 'Cultivo de la garganta."
17. Refer to Chapter 13 for Dental Conversations.
18. It is important for health care practitioners to be sensitive to the embarrassment and discomfort of Hispanic women when asked to discuss matters of sex or reproduction, or the organs associated with them, especially with a male doctor. This is not unique to Hispanic women, however.
19. Survey results gathered by the American Cancer Society indicate that Hispanics who were queried (age 40 and over), responded that 13.4% had never heard of a clinical breast exam, 14.7% had heard of it but never had one, and of those who had had the procedure, 45% had had the C.B.E. within 1 year of the survey, and 11.7% had had the procedure within 1–3 years of the survey.
20. See below, Chapter 12, pages 264–265.
21. There appears to be a rather low percentage of Hispanic mothers living in the United States who breast-feed their babies for any length of time. This may be in part to the way the obstetrician discusses the subject with the woman during her prenatal visits; it may also reflect a cultural attitude held by many, but not all, Hispanics that a fat baby is healthy. Because many breast-fed infants tend to be skinnier than bottle-fed babies, many are reluctant to breast-feed. Research indicates that 31%–60% of Mexican-American women are likely to breast-feed, compared to 12% of Cuban American mothers and 10% to 11% of Puerto Rican mothers. (S. Guendelman, *et. al*, "Generational Differences in Perinatal Health among the Mexican American Population: Findings from HHANES 1982–84," *American Journal of Public Health*, 1990; 80 (Supplement): 61–65.
22. Statistics compiled by the American Cancer Society indicated that of the Hispanic population age 40 and over who were surveyed, 31.6% had never heard of mammography, 42.2% had heard of it but had never had a mammogram. Of the respondees who had had the procedure, the percentages were extremely low: 3.1% had had a mammogram 1–3 years earlier, and 12.9% had had a mammogram within the year. See also L. Suárez, "Pap Smear and Mammogram Screening in Mexican-American Women: The Effects of Acculturation," *American Journal Public Health.* 1994; 84:742–746, *Cancer Statistics Review 1973–1986 [Including a Report on the Status of Cancer Control, May 1989]* Washington, DC: NCI; 1989. 1151-1153 and S.A. Fox, "The Effect of Physician-Patient Communication on Mammography Utilization by Different Ethnic Groups, *Med Care*, 1991; 29:1065–1082.
23. For additional questions on smoking and drinking, see Chapter 9, page 197.
24. See Chapter 7, page 150, note 11.
25. *Cuadra* is a word understood by all as "city block." *Manzana* is a synonym. *Bloque* is a colloquial word, extremely popular among Puerto Ricans. Its usage has been widely accepted by U.S. Hispanics living in urban areas.
26. See Chapter 1, page 20 for discussion about this Hispanic custom of borrowing and lending medications.
27. It is a good idea for the health care practitioner to tap out a five second interval so that the patient will realize how long five seconds of pain is.
28. See Chapter 7, page 150, notes 12 and 18, and also Chapter 15, pages 316–324.
29. See Chapter 12, pages 270–271.
30. Although *morado* literally means "purple," it is used here to describe the color produced by a lack of oxygen, known as "cyanotic."
31. Because of their diet and their lifestyle, gastrointestinal problems are very common among Hispanics. Of particular concern for Hispanics is the high incidence rate of gallstones. See Chapter 15, pages 324–326.

32. Alcoholism and cirrhosis are serious health problems which continue to plague the U.S. Hispanic population. Most affected within the population are the Mexican American and Puerto Rican segments. See K. Markides, *et al.*, "Acculturation and Alcohol Consumption in the Mexican American Population of the Southwestern United States: Findings from HHANES 1982–84," *American Journal of Public Health*, 1990; 80 (Supplement): 42–46.

33. Many Hispanics as well as members of many other ethnic groups that originated in Europe believe that periodic "cleanings," or *purgas* are necessary in order to keep the body healthy. In addition to the "scientific" aids, castor oil, tea of senna leaves, and camomile tea are used as *remedios caseros* for this purpose. See Chapter 1, pages 17–25 and below, note 40 for further discussion.

34. See Chapter 12, pages 262–263.

35. See Chapter 12, page 262.

36. See Chapter 15, pages 326–328, "Kidney Stones."

37. See Chapter 7, page 150, note 13.

38. See Chapter 12, pages 265–266, for instructions on Testicular Self-Examination.

39. See Chapter 12, pages 267–272, for a discussion on Contraceptive Methods for Family Planning.

40. Hispanos regard pregnancy and childbirth as a woman's normal obligation. When pregnant, a woman may be **enferma con niño** (*ill with child*); when she delivers, **se sana** (*she is healed*) (M. Kay, "Health and Illness," p. 155). Hispanic women generally do not have early prenatal medical help unless they experience complications such as elevated blood pressure, kidney disease, or prolonged dizziness and nausea. This is because they look to the female members of their family for advice.

Much of a pregnant woman's behavior is culturally prescribed to assure an easy birth. Pregnancy is thought to be a dangerous time for the fetus, and so the pregnant woman avoids distress whenever possible. Hispanic women may be careful to avoid "hot" foods or medication during this period in order to prevent their baby from being born with an "irritation" (a rash or red skin). These women may "refresh" themselves with "cool" medicines such as milk of magnesia or commercial antacids, especially during the first and second trimesters. (See A. Harwood, "Hot Cold Theory of Disease," *Journal of American Medical Association*, Vol. 216, No.7, p. 1157.) Iron tablets, calcium pills, and other essential medicines are often shunned by pregnant women as a consequence of the avoidance of "hot" substances during pregnancy. These women should be encouraged to "neutralize" these needed medicines with fruit juice or herb tea, which are considered "cold." (See N. Galli, "The Influence of Cultural Heritage on the Health Status of Puerto Ricans," *Journal of School Health*, Vol. XLV, No. I, p. 13.) Traditional beliefs suggest that the mother-to-be not gain too much weight, lest the baby be too big, or "stick" to the sides of the womb, and need to be delivered with instruments. It is felt that if the mother sleeps too much, the baby will also "stick" to the uterus. Finally, sexual activity is encouraged until labor is imminent "to keep the birth canal lubricated" (M. Kay, "Health and Illness in a Mexican American *Barrio*", in E.H. Spicers (edi): *Ethic Medicine in the Southwest*, Arizona: University of Arizona Press, 1977, p. 154). Massages and castor oil purges become a regular part of the pregnancy, increasing in frequency toward the last stages. Hispanic women in general tend to be "embarrassed" by the final months of pregnancy and prefer the privacy of their homes, frequently attempting to conceal their condition.

In rural areas and small towns of Latin America, *parteras*, or midwives, are used with great regularity because of a lack of doctors. Nonetheless, in general even in large cities Hispanic women often prefer home deliveries to hospital ones. This is in part attributed to the presence of the midwife who stays by the side of the new mother from the beginning of labor until after delivery and administers tea, gives oil massages for relaxation, and shows warm concern. Recent licensing requirements in the southwestern United States have resulted in a decline of this type of practitioner who had had an important role in the health of Spanish-speaking women. (See M. Kay, "Health and Illness," p. 152.)

A Mexican tradition involves rubbing the new mother's back with warm olive oil and powdered sulphur in order to assure healthy breasts and a good milk supply. It is believed that the colostrum is not good for the baby, and babies are given olive oil or castor oil, to promote evacuation. Nursing is encouraged, and many feel that bottle feeding causes children to suffer from stomach trouble later in life. Most babies, however, are soon given formula during the day and only nursed at night, often past a year of age. (If the pediatrician puts the baby on a formula that contains "hot" evaporated milk as a base, many mothers will put their baby on "cold" whole milk or, after feeding the baby formula, "refresh" the child's stomach with various cool foods, like weak tea, barley water, or magnesium carbonate. This often is a source of diarrhea in infants because some of these substances act as diuretics.) (See A. Harwood, "Hot-Cold Theory," p. 1155–1156; M. Kay, "Health and Illness," p. 156.)

41. Studies indicate that, with the exception of Cuban Americans, approximately only sixty percent of Hispanic women living in the U.S. begin prenatal care during the first trimester of their pregnancy. Additionally, in comparison with the general population, Hispanics are three times as likely to receive no prenatal care. Within the Hispanic sub-groups, Puerto Rican females receive whatever prenatal care they obtain later and less often. Nevertheless, it must be noted that Hispanic females in general, and the Mexican American sub-group in particular, have lower rates of premature deliveries and low birth weights than the general population.

42. As has already been established in Chapter 1, page 8, Hispanic women have a much higher fertility rate than the general population; moreover, they give birth to children at younger ages, and have more children.

43. The word *drogas* refers to narcotics and other illegal substances; it does not refer to prescription medications.

44. There is a segment of the Hispanics population that believes that syphilis comes from mere physical contact.

45. AIDS is a devastating problem for the Hispanic population which constitutes 10.7% of the total U.S. population as of 1996, yet accounted for 14% of all reported AIDS cases. This disease has affected Hispanic women (about one fifth of all cases are within the Hispanic population) and children. Twenty-two percent of all pediatric AIDS cases are Hispanic children. Although no one knows exactly why Hispanics are so affected by this, it has been posited that where they tend to live and their use of intravenous drugs are significant factors. Nearly half of the reported Hispanic cases are heterosexuals. See Chapter 1 for additional information.

46. Use the Spanish pronunciation of the letters.

47. See Chapter 12, pages 268–269 for instructions on how to use a condom.

48. See above, pages 155–156 questions 17–25.

49. See above, pages 155 f.

50. See Chapter 7, page 150, note 12.

51. The singular form, *hierba*, may refer to a weed. It is also a slang way of saying "marijuana."

CHAPTER 9

Conversations for Health Professionals: Personal, Social, and Family History

Conversaciones para personal médico y paramédico: Historiales personal, social, y familiar

PERSONAL HISTORY

HISTORIAL PERSONAL

IDENTIFICATION   IDENTIFICACION

1. What is your name?[1]
   ¿Cómo se llama Vd.?

2. Where do you live?[2]
   ¿Dónde vive Vd.?

3. What is your telephone number?[3]
   ¿Cuál es el número de teléfono de su casa, por favor?

4. Is there somebody who lives near you with a telephone if you do not have one?
   ¿Hay alguien que viva cerca de usted con teléfono si usted no tiene uno?

5. What is that number?
   ¿Cuál es ese número?

6. How old are you?
   ¿Cuántos años tiene Vd.?
   ¿Qué edad tiene Vd.? fam

7. What is your birthdate?[4]
   ¿Cuál es la fecha de su nacimiento?

8. Where were you born?
   ¿Dónde nació Vd.?

9. When did you come to this country?
   ¿Cuándo vino Vd. a este país?

10. Are you single or married?
    ¿Es Vd. soltero (soltera) o casado (casada)?

11. Are you single but living with your girlfriend (boyfriend)?
    ¿Es Vd. soltero (soltera) pero vive con su novia (novio)?
    ¿Está Vd. amancebado (amancebada)? P.R.

12. Are you divorced?
    ¿Es Vd. divorciado (divorciada)?

13. Are you a widow?
    ¿Es Vd. viuda?

14. Are you a widower?
    ¿Es Vd. viudo?

15. Are you separated?
    ¿Está Vd. separado (separada)?

16. Have you been married before?
    ¿Ha estado casado (casada) antes?

17. How long have you been married to your spouse?
    ¿Desde cuándo está Vd. casado (casada) con su esposa (esposo)?

18. Are you happy with your spouse?
    ¿Es Vd. feliz con su esposa (esposo)?

19. Is your spouse in good health?
    ¿Goza de buena salud su esposo (esposa)?

20. Do you have any children?
    ¿Tiene Vd. (algunos) hijos?

21. How many?
    ¿Cuántos?

22. How old is she / he (are they)?
    ¿Cuántos años tiene(n)?
    ¿Qué edad tiene(n)?

23. Are your children in good health?
    ¿Gozan de buena salud sus hijos?

24. Do you consider yourself to be . . .
    ¿Se considera . . .
    heterosexual?
    heterosexual?
    homosexual?
    homosexual?
    bisexual?
    bisexual?

25. How many different (sexual) partners do you have in a month?
    ¿Cuántos (¿Cuántas) amantes tiene Vd. por mes?

26. Do you have anal intercourse?
    ¿Practica coito anal?

JOB DATA   INFORMACION DEL EMPLEO

1. What do you do? (How do you earn a living?)
   ¿Cómo se gana Vd. la vida?
   ¿Qué clase de trabajo tiene Vd.?

2. What is your occupation?[5]
   ¿En qué trabaja Vd?

3. Where do you work?
   ¿Dónde trabaja Vd.?

4. How long have you worked there?
   ¿Desde cuándo trabaja Vd. allí?

5. What was your first job?
   ¿Cuál fue su primer empleo?

6. What other jobs have you had?
   ¿Qué otros empleos ha tenido Vd.?

7. How long did you work at each?
   ¿Cuánto tiempo trabajó Vd. en cada uno de estos empleos?

8. Why did you change jobs?
   ¿Por qué cambió Vd. de empleo?

9. Are you happy in your work?
   ¿Está Vd. satisfecho (satisfecha) en el trabajo?

10. Do you work with . . .
    En su empleo, ¿usa Vd. . . . (¿está Vd. en contacto con . . .)

paints?
pinturas?
insecticides?
insecticidas?
lead?
plomo?
plastics?
plásticos?
other synthetic materials?
otros materiales sintéticos?
drugs?
drogas?
dusts?
polvos?
chemicals?
productos químicos?

11. How long are you in contact with them?
    ¿Por cuánto tiempo tiene Vd. tal contacto?

12. Do you take any precautionary measures?
    ¿Toma Vd. precauciones?

13. What?
    ¿Cuáles son?

14. What is your religion?[6]
    ¿Cuál es su religión?

15. What is your nationality?[7]
    ¿Cuál es su nacionalidad?

16. How much education do you have?
    ¿Cuántos años de escuela completó Vd.?
    grade school?
    ¿educación primaria?
    high school?
    ¿educación secundaria?
    occupational education?
    ¿educación especializada?
    college?
    ¿educación universitaria?
    graduate school?
    ¿educación pos-graduada?
    professional school?
    ¿facultad profesional?

ALLERGY *ALERGIA*

1. Do you have allergies?
   ¿Tiene Vd. alergias?

2. What causes your allergies?
   ¿Qué le causa las alergias?

3. Are you allergic to any medication? To any food? To dust or pollen?
   ¿Es Vd. alérgico (alérgica) a alguna medicina? ¿a alguna comida? ¿a polvo o a polen?

4. Do you have hay fever?
   ¿Tiene Vd. fiebre de heno?

WEIGHT CHANGE *CAMBIO DE PESO*

1. How much do you normally weigh?
   Por lo regular, ¿cuánto pesa Vd.?

2. Have you gained or lost much weight recently, suddenly?
   ¿Ha engordado o adelgazado últimamente, de repente?

3. Have you had a problem with your weight most of your life?
   ¿Ha tenido problema de peso casi toda su vida?

DIET *DIETA*

1. Do you have a good appetite?
   ¿Tiene Vd. buen apetito?

2. During the last year have you noticed an increase in your desire for sweets?
   ¿Ha observado Vd. durante el año pasado un aumento de apetito por dulces?

3. Do you have any problems chewing?
   ¿Tiene Vd. problemas al masticar?

4. How many meals do you eat daily?
   ¿Cuántas veces come Vd. al día?
   ¿Cuántas comidas toma Vd. al día?

5. Do you wear dentures?
   ¿Usa dentadura postiza?

6. Do they fit correctly?
   ¿Le sientan bien?

7. Do you have to eat softened or pureed food?
   ¿Tiene que tomar comida ablandada o en puré?

8. What do you eat for breakfast? lunch? dinner?[8]
   ¿Qué toma Vd. para el desayuno? ¿para el almuerzo? ¿para la cena?

9. Do you eat between meals?
   ¿Toma Vd. algo entre comidas?

10. How much butter do you eat daily?
    ¿Cuánta mantequilla come Vd. al día?

11. How many eggs do you eat weekly?
    ¿Cuántos huevos come Vd. por semana?

12. Do you drink coffee or tea?
    ¿Toma Vd. café o té?

13. How much coffee and tea do you drink a day?
    ¿Cuántas tazas de café o de té bebe Vd. al día?

14. Do you drink regular or decaffeinated coffee?
    ¿Toma Vd. café regular o descafeinado?

15. How much water do you drink daily?
    ¿Cuántos vasos de agua bebe Vd. al día?

16. Are you on a diet at home?
    ¿Sigue dieta en casa?

17. Why are you on that diet?
    ¿Por qué sigue esa dieta?

18. Are you hungry?
    ¿Tiene Vd. hambre?

19. Are you full?
    ¿Está satisfecho (satisfecha)?

SMOKING, DRINKING   *EL FUMAR, EL BEBER*

1. Do you drink alcoholic beverages?
   ¿Toma Vd. (algunas) bebidas alcohólicas?

2. Have you been drinking a lot?[9]
   ¿Ha estado tomando mucho alcohol?

3. What type of alcoholic beverage do you generally buy?
   ¿Qué tipo de bebida alcohólica compra Vd. por lo regular?

4. How long does a bottle of alcohol last you?
   ¿Cuánto tiempo le dura una botella de alcohol?

5. How often during the week do you drink alcoholic beverages?
   ¿Cuántas veces durante la semana toma Vd. bebidas alcohólicas?

6. Do you sleep well?
   ¿Duerme Vd. bien?

7. What time do you go to bed?
   ¿A qué hora se acuesta por la noche, por lo regular?

8. What time do you get up in the morning?
   ¿A qué hora se despierta por la mañana?

9. It is important to rest more.
   ¿Es importante descansar más.

10. Do you walk a lot at home?
    ¿Camina Vd. mucho en casa?

11. Do you walk a lot outside of the house?
    ¿Camina Vd. mucho afuera de la casa?

12. How many blocks do you walk on the average during the day?
    ¿Cuántas manzanas camina Vd. promedio durante el día?[10]

13. Do you do your own shopping?
    ¿Hace las compras Vd. mismo (misma)?

14. Do you smoke?
    ¿Fuma Vd.?

15. How many cigarettes do you smoke each day?
    ¿Cuántos cigarrillos fuma Vd. al día?

16. If you smoke (or have smoked), how many years have you been smoking?
    Si Vd. fuma (o ha fumado antes), ¿por cuántos años viene haciéndolo?

17. I advise you to stop smoking or at least to reduce it to a minimum.
    Le aconsejo que deje de fumar o que lo reduzca a un mínimo.

DRUGS[11]   *USO DE DROGAS*[12]

1. Do you use drugs regularly?
   ¿Es Vd. adicto (adicta) al uso de drogas?
   ¿Acostumbra Vd. tomar alguna droga?
   ¿Toma Vd. alguna droga?

2. Are you a drug addict?
   ¿Es Vd. drogadicto (drogadicta)?
   ¿Es Vd. un adicto (una adicta)?

3. Have you taken illegal drugs?
   ¿Ha tomado Vd. drogas ilegales?

4. How much money do you spend daily on your drug habit?
   ¿Cuánto dinero gasta Vd. por día en sus drogas?

5. Do. you smoke marijuana?
   ¿Fuma Vd. la mariguana?[13]

6. Do you take morphine?
   ¿Ingiere Vd. morfina?
   ¿Se administra Vd. morfina?
   ¿Es Vd. adicto (adicta) a morfina?

7. Do you use heroin, cocaine, LSD?
   ¿Toma Vd. heroína, cocaína, drogas alucinantes (LSD)?[14]

8. Do you use amphetamines?
   ¿Usa Vd. anfetaminas?

9. Are you using barbiturates without medical supervision?
   ¿Toma Vd. barbitúricos sin supervisión médica?

10. When was your last fix?
    ¿Cuándo fue su último filerazo?

11. Where do you shoot the drugs?
    ¿Dónde se pone Vd. las drogas?

12. Have you ever overdosed on drugs?
    ¿Se ha sobredrogado jamás?
    ¿Ha tomado alguna vez una dosis excesiva de drogas?

13. Have you ever been through a detoxification program?
¿Ha sufrido jamás un programa de desintoxicación?

14. Have you ever taken methadone?
¿Jamás ha tomado metadona?

15. Have you taken methadone during detoxification treatment?
¿Ha tomado metadona durante el tratamiento para desintoxicarse?

16. Have you ever had hepatitis?
¿Ha sufrido jamás de hepatitis?

MEDICATION *MEDICACION*

1. Do you use . . . ?
¿Ha tomado Vd. . . .?
  antihistamines?
  antihistamínicos?
  aspirin?
  aspirinas?
  sleeping pills?
  píldoras para dormir (sedantes)?
  birth control pills?
  píldoras anticonceptivas?
  diet pills?
  píldoras para régimen (dieta)?
  laxatives?
  laxantes?
  diuretics?
  píldoras diuréticas?
  medication for diabetes?
  medicamento para diabetes?
  digitalin or nitroglycerin?
  digitalina o nitroglicerina?

  antacids?
  antiácidos?
  antibiotics?
  antibióticos?
  tranquilizers?
  tranquilizantes?
  vitamins?
  vitaminas?
  thyroid pills?
  medicamento para tiroides?
  cortisone?
  cortisona?

2. How many pills do you take?
¿Cuántas píldoras toma Vd.?

3. Do not take more than ___ a day at most.
No tome más de ___ cada día en total.

4. How would you describe the feelings that you experience during coitus?
¿Cómo describiría Vd. las sensaciones que tiene durante el coito (relaciones sexuales)?

EXERCISE *EJERCICIO*

¿Cómo se dice en español?

1. I normally weight 168 pounds.
2. Paul drinks two bottles of beer daily.
3. We never drink milk.
4. The man drinks decaf coffee, but I drink tea.
5. They have been smoking for many years.
6. Now I get up at 6:15 in the morning.
7. Carlos gets up at midnight because he works during the night.
8. Do you smoke cigarettes now?
9. Why do you use amphetamines?
10. The widow has seven sons and a daughter.

SOCIAL HISTORY

HISTORIAL SOCIAL

GENERAL BACKGROUND *ANTECEDENTES GENERALES*

1. Do you live alone?
¿Vive solo (sola)?

2. Do you live with . . .[15]
¿Vive Vd. con . . .
  your parents?
  sus padres?
  your mother?
  su madre?
  your father?
  su padre?
  your spouse?
  su esposo? su esposa?

  your son? your daughter?
  su hijo? su hija?
  your grandparents?
  sus abuelos?
  your grandmother?
  su abuela?
  your aunt and uncle?
  sus tíos?
  a cousin?
  un primo? una prima?
  a friend?
  un amigo? una amiga?

3. Where do you live?
   ¿Dónde vive Vd.?

4. How long have you lived there?
   ¿Desde cuándo vive Vd. allí?

5. Is this an apartment or a house?
   ¿Es un departamento (apartamento) o una casa particular?

6. On what floor do you live?
   ¿En qué piso vive Vd.?[16]

7. How many rooms do you have?
   ¿Cuántos cuartos tiene Vd.?

8. How many people live in your apartment?
   ¿Cuántas personas viven en su apartamento?[17]

9. How many are adults? Children?
   ¿Cuántos son adultos? ¿Niños?

10. How many people sleep in one room?
    ¿Cuántas personas duermen en un cuarto?

11. How many beds are there in one room?
    ¿Cuántas camas hay en un cuarto?

12. Is there a bathroom in your apartment?
    ¿Hay cuarto de baño en su apartamento?

13. Do you share the bathroom?
    ¿Comparte Vd. el baño con otros?

14. Is there hot and cold water inside your house?
    ¿Hay agua caliente y fría en su casa?

15. Are there any insects or rodents in your apartment?
    ¿Hay insectos o ratas en su apartamento?

ECONOMIC AND INSURANCE DATA
INFORMACION FINANCIERA Y DE SEGUROS

1. Who lives at home with you?
   ¿Quién vive en casa con Vd.?

2. Are you on relief?
   ¿Recibe Vd. auxilio social?
   ¿Está Vd. en relief? *fam*

3. Do you receive workmen's compensation?
   ¿Recibe Vd. compensación de obreros?

4. Do you support yourself?
   ¿Se mantiene Vd. a sí mismo (misma)?

5. What do you earn per week, approximately?
   ¿Cuánto gana Vd. por semana, más o menos?

6. Are you the sole financial support of your family?
   ¿Es Vd. el único (la única) que sostiene a su familia?

7. What is the name of the person who supports you?
   ¿Cómo se llama la persona que le (la) mantiene?

8. Is this person a relative? a friend?
   ¿Es un pariente esta persona? ¿un amigo (una amiga)?

9. How many people in the family work for money?[18]
   ¿Cuántas personas en la familia perciben dinero?

10. Do the people in the family who work contribute financially to the household?
    ¿Contribuyen a los gastos del hogar las personas que trabajan en su familia?

11. How many children attend school?
    ¿Cuántos niños asisten a la escuela?

12. Do you have money from other sources?
    ¿Recibe Vd. ayuda financiera de otras entradas?

13. Are there any city or religious agencies helping you or your family?
    ¿Hay algunas agencias municipales o religiosas que le ayuden a Vd. o a su familia?

14. Do you have any savings? bonds? bank accounts?
    ¿Tiene Vd. ahorros? ¿bonos? ¿cuentas de banco?

15. Do you rent or own your own house?
    ¿Alquila Vd. o tiene casa propia?

16. How much rent do you pay?
    ¿Cuánto paga Vd. de alquiler?

17. How much is the mortgage?
    ¿Cuánto es la hipoteca?

18. Does anyone in your family own property?
    ¿Tiene propiedad alguien de su familia?

19. Do you have any unusual expenses?
    ¿Tiene Vd. gastos extraordinarios?

20. Do you have . . .
    ¿Tiene Vd. seguros . . .[19]
    health insurance?
    médicos / de salud?
    hospitalization insurance?
    para el hospital?
    accident insurance?
    para accidentes?
    life insurance?
    de vida?
    disability insurance?
    por incapacidad?

Blue Cross?
de Blue Cross?
Blue Shield?
de Blue Shield?

21. Does your insurance cover psychiatric treatment and hospitalization?
¿Cubre su seguro tratamiento psiquiátrico y hospitalización?

22. Do you have Medicare / Medicaid Card?
¿Tiene Vd. tarjeta de Medicare / Medicaid?

23. Are you receiving Social Security?
¿Recibe Vd. Seguro Social?

24. Are you receiving Public Aid?
¿Recibe Vd. ayuda pública /bienestar público?

25. You don't have any insurance?[19]
Vd. no tiene ningún seguro, ¿verdad?

26. We need to set up a payment plan for you.[20]
Necesitamos establecerle un plan de pagos.

27. Can you afford $____/ month?
Vd. puede pagar $____ [dólares] por mes, ¿verdad?

28. On what date can we expect your monthly payments?
¿En qué fecha del mes podemos esperar su pago?

29. Do you have a Visa / Mastercard to pay your bill with?
¿Tiene Vd. una tarjeta de crédito—o Visa o Mastercard—que pueda usar para pagar su cuenta?

EXTRACURRICULAR   *EXTRACURRICULAR*

1. Do you have many friends?
¿Tiene Vd. muchos amigos?

2. Do you have a large extended family?
¿Tiene Vd. una familia grande?

3. Do you enjoy the company of your friends/family?
¿Le gusta a Vd. la compañía de sus amigos/su familia?

4. Are you a member of a parish?
¿Pertenece a una parroquia?

5. Are you a member of any community club?
¿Pertenece Vd. a algún club o sociedad en la comunidad?

6. Do you belong to any sports organization?
¿Pertenece Vd. a algún grupo de deportes?

7. Who will take care of you when you leave the hospital?
¿Quién va a cuidarle (cuidarla) cuando salga del hospital?

FAMILY HISTORY

HISTORIAL FAMILIAR

1. Are your parents alive?
¿Todavía están vivos sus padres?
¿Todavía viven sus padres?

2. How old are they?
¿Cuántos años tienen?

3. What did your mother die from?
¿De qué murió su madre?

4. How is / was your mother's health?
¿Cómo es / fue la salud de su madre?

5. What did your father die from?
¿De qué murió su padre?

6. How is / was your father's health?
¿Cómo es / fue la salud de su padre?

7. How old was s/he when s/he died?
¿Cuántos años tenía al morir?

8. Is there anyone in the family with the same problems?
¿Hay alguien en la familia con los mismos problemas?

9. How old were your grandparents when they died, or are they still alive?
¿Cuántos años tenían sus abuelos cuando murieron, o viven todavía?
¿A qué edad murieron sus abuelos, o están vivos todavía?

10. What did your grandmother die from?
¿De qué murió su abuela?

11. What did your grandfather die from?
¿De qué murió su abuelo?

12. What was your mother's maiden name?
¿Cuál era el nombre de soltera de su madre?

13. Where were you born?
¿Dónde nació Vd.?

14. Where were your parents born?
¿Dónde nacieron sus padres?

15. Do you have any brothers? Sisters?
¿Tiene Vd. algunos hermanos? ¿hermanas?

16. How many?
¿Cuántos? (¿Cuántas?)

17. Have any of your siblings died?
    ¿Ha muerto alguno de sus hermanos (hermanas)?

18. How old was he (she)?
    ¿Cuántos años tenía?

19. Of what did he (she) die?
    ¿De qué murió?

20. Is there any family history of blood disease?
    ¿Hay algún caso de enfermedades de la sangre en su familia?

21. Is there anyone in the family with . . .
    ¿Hay alguien en la familia con . . .
    hemophilia?
    la hemofilia?
    AIDS?
    el SIDA?[21]
    sickle cell anemia?
    anemia de glóbulos falciformes?

22. Is there a history of lung trouble or diabetes?
    ¿Hay algún caso de problemas pulmonares o de diabetes?

23. Does anyone in your family suffer from asthma or hay fever?
    ¿Padece alguien de su familia de asma o de fiebre del heno?

extreme obesity[22]
obesidad extremada
cancer or leukemia
cáncer o leucemia
heart attack
ataque al corazón
angina (pectoris)
angina del pecho
chronic anemia
anemia crónica (sangre pobre *slang*)
stroke
parálisis
thyroid problems
enfermedad de la tiroides
stomach or duodenal ulcers
úlceras de estómago o duodenales
peptic ulcer
úlcera péptica
gall stones
cálculos en la vesícula
kidney stones
cálculos en los riñones (cálculos renales)

24. Whom can we call in case of emergency?
    ¿A quién podemos llamar en caso de emergencia?

Notes   *Notas*

1. See Chapter 1, pp. 9–10 for discussion about the nomenclature.
2. See Chapter 4, p. 91.
3. Spanish speakers answer the telephone in a variety of ways, depending on their nationality. In Spain a telephone call is answered with «*Diga*» or «*Dígame.*» The person calling will say «*Oiga*» ("Listen" and may add «*¿Con quién hablo?*» ("Who is this?/With whom am I speaking?"). The answer to this question is «*Habla el doctor Fulano*» (Dr. So-and-so speaking"). In the Western Hemisphere answering the telephone seems informal or casual. In Puerto Rico and Chile people say «*Aló.*» In Argentina the response is «*Hola,*» while in Cuba people answer «*Digo*» or «*¿Qué hay?*» Mexicans will say «*Bueno.*» In Colombia the correct response is «*¿A ver?*» which means "Let's see." It is elliptical for «*Vamos a ver.*» One can speculate that it came into being shortly after telephones were installed in Colombia when people were still probably intrigued by this invention and expressed their curiosity by saying "Let's see (who's on the other end of the line)."
4. In Spanish-speaking countries, it is customary to celebrate both one's birthday and one's saint's day, the **dia de su santo,** the day of the saint after whom one is named.
5. See Chapter 16 for a listing of **Occupations,** pages 353–355.
6. See Chapter 16 for a listing of **Religions,** pages 353–354.
7. See Chapter 16 for a listing of **Nationalities,** page 354.
8. See Chapter 11, pages 247 and Chapter 16, pages 356f.
9. Hispanics view being able "to hold one's liquor" as a highly masculine virtue. Hispanic society places strict restraints and sanctions on excessive alcohol consumption and inebriation. This apparently accounts for the low rate of alcoholism among the unacculturated Hispanics, especially the Mexican-Americans, and the higher rates among those who are actively seeking to reject the ethnic ways of the past and adopt "American" ways. (See A. Kiev, *Curanderismo: Mexican-American Folk Psychiatry,* New York: The Free Press, 1968, p. 100.)
10. *Cuadra* is a word understood by all as "city block." *Manzana* is a synonym. *Bloque* is a colloquial word, extremely popular among Puerto Ricans. Its usage has been widely accepted by U.S. Hispanics living in urban areas.
11. See Chapter 16 for Selected **Drug Abuse Vocabulary,** pages 343–345.
12. The Spanish word *drogas* refers to narcotics and other illegal substances; it does translate as "prescription medications."
13. I have followed the spelling given in the *Diccionario de la lengua española,* RAE, 21st edition, 1990. Spanish does recognize variations using **j** and **h.**
14. Self-reporting survey results from the HHANES indicate that 21.5% of Puerto Ricans reported having used cocaine. The percentages were significantly lower for Mexican Americans and Cuban Americans at 11.1% and 9.2% respectively.
15. See Chapter 1, pages 8, 10, 12 for discussion on Hispanic families.
16. In Spain el **piso bajo** or **planta baja** is the ground floor, el **piso principal** is the first floor, and **el primer piso** usually corresponds to the second or third floor in the United States. In Spanish America, however, floors are usually counted the way they are in the United States.

17. Vocabulary varies widely for the word "apartment." In Spain the word *piso* refers to a large apartment or condominium. There an *apartamento* is similar in space, but smaller. In various countries in Hispanic America, however, the word *condominio* refers to *propiedad horizontal*. Other terminology used for a condo would include *apartamento* and *departamento*.

18. See Chapter 1, page 6f, for a demographic profile of Hispanics.

19. Recent research appears to indicate that whether or not Hispanics use health care services depends greatly upon their socioeconomic status and the type of employment that they have. Uninsured Hispanics are less likely to have a regular source of health care, and it is quite unlikely that they will have seen a physician in the past year or have had a routine physical exam. See Chapter 1, page 25 and Chapter 5, pages 104, 108 for additional information and conversations.

20. For additional conversation regarding insurance and payment plans, see Chapter 5, page 105.

21. See Chapter 8, page 184–186 for the section about AIDS and HIV.

22. See Chapter 7, page 150, note 17 and Chapter 8, page 192, note 10.

Conversations for Health Professionals: Physical Examination

Conversaciones para personal médico y paramédico: Reconocimiento físico

PREPARATION FOR PHYSICAL EXAMINATION

PREPARACION PARA EL RECONOCIMIENTO FISICO

1. Take off your clothes, please.
   Desvístase Vd., por favor.
   Favor de desvestirse.

2. Take off your clothes except for your underwear, please.
   Desvístase Vd. por favor, menos la ropa interior.

3. Please take off your clothes down to your waist.
   Desvístase Vd. hasta la cintura, por favor.
   Quítese Vd. la ropa hasta la cintura, por favor.

4. Please take off your clothes from the waist down.
   Desvístase Vd. de la cintura para abajo, por favor.

5. Please take off your girdle and bra.
   Quítese Vd. la faja y el sostén / ajustador / portabustos *slang,* **por favor.**

6. Lower your trousers, please.
   Bájese Vd. los pantalones, por favor.

7. Please hang your clothes over there.
   Cuelgue Vd. la ropa ahí, por favor.

8. Put on the gown, please.
   Póngase Vd. la bata, por favor.

9. Sit on the table, please.
   Siéntese Vd. sobre la mesa, por favor.

10. Please lie down on the examining table.
    Acuéstese Vd. sobre la mesa de reconocimiento, por favor.

11. Lie on your back.
    Acuéstese Vd. boca arriba, por favor.

12. Turn over.
    Dése vuelta, por favor.

13. Lie on your stomach.
    Acuéstese Vd. boca abajo, por favor.

14. Turn on your right (left) side.
    Dé media vuelta al lado derecho (izquierdo), por favor.

15. Lie on your right (left) side.
    Acuéstese sobre el lado derecho (izquierdo), por favor.

16. Lie still.
    Quédese quieto (quieta), por favor.

17. Sit up now.
    Incorpórese ahora, por favor.

18. Sit up straight, please.
    Póngase derecho (derecha), por favor.

19. Lean forward.
    Inclínese hacia adelante, por favor.

20. Lean backwards.
    Inclínese hacia atrás, por favor.

21. Stand up.
    Levántese, por favor.

22. Bend down.
    Dóblese hacia adelante, por favor.

23. Bend over backwards.
    Dóblese hacia atrás, por favor.

24. Don't talk.
    No hable, por favor.

25. Please turn face up.
    Póngase Vd. boca arriba, por favor.

26. Please turn face down.
    Póngase Vd. boca abajo, por favor.

27. The doctor will examine you now.
    El doctor / La doctora le (la) examinará ahora.

28. I am going to examine you now.
    Voy a examinarle (examinarla) ahora.

PHYSICAL EXAMINATION

RECONOCIMIENTO FISICO

HEAD *LA CABEZA*

1. I am going to examine your head.
   Voy a examinarle la cabeza.

2. Bend your head to the right, please.
   Doble Vd. la cabeza a la derecha, por favor.

3. Bend your head to the left, please.
   Doble Vd. la cabeza a la izquierda, por favor.

4. Bend your head forward.
   Doble Vd. la cabeza hacia adelante.

5. Bend your head backwards.
   Doble Vd. la cabeza hacia atrás.

6. Turn your head.
   Gire Vd. la cabeza.

7. Turn your head . . .
   Mueva la cabeza . . .
   Vuelva Vd. la cabeza . . .
      to the right.
      a la derecha.
      hacia la derecha.
      to the left.
      a la izquierda
      hacia la izquierda.

8. Don't move your head.
   No mueva la cabeza, por favor.

EYES   *LOS OJOS*

1. Let me see your eyes, please.
   Déjeme verle los ojos, por favor.
   Déjeme mirarle los ojos.

2. I am going to examine your eyes (them).
   Voy a examinarle los ojos.
   Voy a examinárselos.

3. Look up.
   Mire Vd. hacia arriba.
   Mire Vd. para arriba.

4. Look down.
   Mire Vd. hacia abajo.
   Mire Vd. para abajo.

5. Look to the right.
   Mire Vd. para la derecha.

6. Look to the left.
   Mire Vd. para la izquierda.

7. Look here.
   Mire aquí, por favor.

8. Look into the light.
   Mire la luz, por favor.

9. Don't blink.
   No parpadee, por favor.

10. Don't move your eyes.
    No mueva los ojos.

11. Look at my finger.
    Mire Vd. mi dedo.

12. Look at this.
    Mire Vd. esto.

13. Look at the (red) light.
    Mire Vd. la luz (roja).

14. Keep looking at my nose.
    Siga mirándome la nariz.

15. Keep looking here (there).
    Siga mirando aquí (allí).

16. Follow my finger with your eyes without moving your head.
    Siga Vd. mi dedo con los ojos sin mover la cabeza.

17. Open your eyes more (wider).
    Abra Vd. más los ojos.

18. Can you see this?
    ¿Puede Vd. ver esto?

19. Do you see this?
    ¿Ve Vd. esto?

20. How many fingers do you see?
    ¿Cuántos dedos ve Vd.?

21. Squeeze my fingers.
    Apriéteme los dedos.

22. Where do you see my finger?
    ¿Dónde ve Vd. mi dedo?

23. Cover your eye like this.
    Tápese Vd. el ojo así.

24. Don't blink.
    No parpadee Vd., por favor.

25. Open your eyes.
    Abra Vd. los ojos.

26. Close your eyes.
    Cierre los ojos.

27. There is something in your eye.
    Hay algo en su ojo.
    Tiene algo en el ojo.

28. I am going to try to get it out.
    Voy a tratar de quitárselo.

29. Look up.
    Mire arriba.

30. Look down.
    Mire abajo.

31. Look to the side.
    Mire el lado.

32. I am going to touch your eye with this instrument.
    Voy a tocarle el ojo con este instrumento.

33. Don't be afraid; open your eyes.
    No tenga miedo; abra los ojos.

34. I am going to put some drops (medicine) in your eye.
    Voy a ponerle gotas (medicina) en el ojo.

35. It will burn for a moment.
    Va a arderle por un momento.

36. I am going to patch your eye.
    Voy a ponerle un parche sobre el ojo.

37. Leave it on for twenty-four (24) hours.
    Déjeselo Vd. por veinticuatro (24) horas.

38. I want to see your eye again tomorrow.
    Quiero examinarle el ojo de nuevo mañana.

AT THE OPHTHALMOLOGIST'S OFFICE

	Doctor:	I am going to check your visual acuity today, Max. How old are you now?
	Patient:	Almost eight.
	Doctor:	Mrs. Ortiz, is Max wearing an occluder?
	Mrs. Ortiz:	Yes.
5	Doctor:	How long does he wear it, and for how long has he been wearing it?
	Mrs. Ortiz:	He wears the patch all day until he goes to bed. He has been wearing the patch for about six months now.

	Doctor:	Okay, Max. Let's take your glasses off now. Look at my finger . . . Good. Mrs. Ortiz, has he had surgery?
10	Mrs. Ortiz:	No. Our other doctor said that it wouldn't be necessary.
	Doctor:	Let's put this patch over your eye. Take a look at the end of the room. Can you read this line?
	Patient:	Yes. "E," "G," "N."
	Doctor:	Now this one.
15	Patient:	"F," "Z," "B."
	Doctor:	Now this.
	Patient:	"O," "T," "L," "C."
	Doctor:	Let's take it off this eye and put it on the other. What can you read now?
	Patient:	"F," "C," "B."
20	Doctor:	Now this.
	Patient:	"E," "V," "Q," "T."
	Doctor:	Very good. Now, let's put the patch back on and the glasses, too. What does that say?
	Patient:	"A," "P," "B," "O."
25	Doctor:	Dr. Maya will check you now.
	Dr. Maya:	Dr. Martín tells me that you are seeing better than you ever have before. Are these the same glasses that Max had last time?
	Mrs. Ortiz:	Yes.
	Dr. Maya:	Well, the vision has remained at least the same, if not better than last time. Max has gained
30		back the line of vision that he lost last time. Max, are you wearing your glasses all the time?
	Patient:	I don't wear them when I take a bath.
	Dr. Maya:	Let's try these glasses with a red and green lens. We'll see how well you see. How many dots?
35	Patient:	Four.
	Dr. Maya:	Look at the end of the room. Now, how many dots and what color are they?
	Patient:	Three green dots and a lighter green one.
	Dr. Maya:	Okay. Look right here now. Keep your eye on that parrot. Do you see him now?
40	Patient:	Yes.
	Dr. Maya:	Do any of these animals stand out?
	Patient:	No.
	Dr. Maya:	Does the fly?
	Patient:	No.
45	Dr. Maya:	Take your glasses off for a minute. Now does the fly stick up?
	Patient:	Yes.
	Dr. Maya:	Put on these dark glasses. Do you see any animals here?
	Patient:	No.
	Dr. Maya:	Do you see any buttons in the box?
50	Patient:	No.
	Dr. Maya:	Do you still see four dots?
	Patient:	Yes.
	Dr. Maya:	What do you see down there?
	Patient:	Four dots.
55	Dr. Maya:	Now put these glasses on. Look at the red dot. Look at the bottom dot. Keep looking. Did it move?
	Patient:	Yes. It changed colors.
	Dr. Maya:	What color is it?
	Patient:	Red.
60	Dr. Maya:	Look at the red dot. Watch it. Okay. Hold your hand over your right eye. Look at the chart. Can you read the numbers?
	Patient:	"6," "3," "9," "5."
	Dr. Maya:	There are five numbers. Which one did you miss?
	Patient:	"2."
65	Dr. Maya:	Okay. Can you read any numbers on this line?
	Patient:	Yes. "3," "5," "2," "8," "3," "4."
	Dr. Maya:	All right. These glasses that Max has are fine. They don't need to be changed. Everything else is doing okay. Next week you will be eight. We have to continue to patch. I want to see you again in six months.
70	Mrs. Ortiz:	What is Max' vision?
	Dr. Maya:	20-40, which he was in May.
	Mrs. Ortiz:	Does Max have to wear the patch?

Dr. Maya:		Yes, he should wear it for several hours every day. When he went for two months without it, he lost vision. We now know that he will lose the vision again if he doesn't keep this on. Okay? We are not going to refract your eyes this time. See you.
Patient & Mrs. Ortiz:		Good bye, and thank you.

Situation

**You are the orthoptist. Explain to the parents why they must have the young child's vision checked before age five.

**You are the parent of a five year old child whose eyes are not straight (*tiene ojos con visión distorsionada*). Tell the doctor that there is a family history of strabismus (*estrabismo*). Ask about treatment.

EN EL CONSULTORIO DEL OFTALMOLOGO

	Doctor:	Voy a examinar tu agudeza visual hoy, Max. ¿Cuántos años tienes ya?
	Paciente:	Casi ocho años.
	Doctor:	Señora Ortiz, ¿lleva Max un parche?
	Sra. Ortiz:	Sí.
5	Doctor:	¿Por cuánto tiempo lo lleva, y desde cuándo lo lleva?
	Sra. Ortiz:	Lleva el parche todo el día hasta que se acueste. Hace seis meses que lleva el parche.
	Doctor:	Bueno, Max. Quitemos los anteojos ahora. Mira tú el dedo. Bien. Sra. Ortiz, ¿le han operado?
10	Sra. Ortiz:	No. Nuestro otro oftalmólogo dijo que no sería necesario.
	Doctor:	Pongamos este parche sobre el ojo. Echa una mirada hacia el otro lado del cuarto. ¿Puedes leer esta línea?
	Paciente:	Sí. «E,» «G,» «N.»
	Doctor:	Ahora, ésta.
15	Paciente:	«F,» «Z,» «B.»
	Doctor:	Ahora ésta.
	Paciente:	«O,» «T,» «L,» «C.»
	Doctor:	Vamos a quitártelo de este ojo y ponértelo en el otro. ¿Qué puedes leer ahora?
	Paciente:	«F,» «C,» «B.»
20	Doctor:	Ahora ésta.
	Paciente:	«E,» «V,» «Q,» «T.»
	Doctor:	Muy bien. Ahora vas a ponerte el parche y los anteojos a la vez. ¿Qué dice ésa?
	Paciente:	«A,» «P,» «B,» «O.»
25	Doctor:	La doctora Maya te examinará.
	Dra. Maya:	El doctor Martín me dice que ves mejor que nunca. ¿Son éstos los mismos anteojos que llevó Max la última vez?
	Sra. Ortiz:	Sí.
	Dra. Maya:	Pues, la visión ha quedado por lo menos si no mejor, igual que la última vez. Max
30		ha ganado de nuevo la línea de visión que perdió la última vez. Max, ¿llevas los anteojos todo el tiempo?
	Paciente:	No los llevo cuando me baño.
	Dra. Maya:	Pruébate estos anteojos de un lente rojo y otro verde, y veremos qué bien ves. ¿Cuántos puntos ves?
35	Paciente:	Cuatro.
	Dra. Maya:	Echa la mirada hacia el otro lado del cuarto. Ahora, ¿cuántos puntos ves y de qué color son?
	Paciente:	Tres puntos verdes y otro verde más claro.
	Dra. Maya:	Bien. Mira aquí ahora. Ten los ojos puestos en ese loro. ¿Lo ves ahora?
40	Paciente:	Sí.
	Dra. Maya:	¿Resaltan algunos de estos animales?
	Paciente:	No.
	Dra. Maya:	¿Y la mosca?
	Paciente:	No.
45	Dra. Maya:	Quítate los anteojos un minuto. ¿Resalta ahora la mosca?
	Paciente:	Sí.
	Dra. Maya:	Pónte/Pruébate estos anteojos con los lentes negros. ¿Ves algunos animales aquí?
	Paciente:	No.

50	Dra. Maya:	¿Ves algunos botones en la caja?
	Paciente:	No.
	Dra. Maya:	¿Todavía ves cuatro puntos?
	Paciente:	Sí.
	Dra. Maya:	¿Qué ves por allí?
55	Paciente:	Cuatro puntos.
	Dra. Maya:	Ahora, pónte estos anteojos. Mira tú el punto rojo. Mira el botón al fondo. Sigue mirando. ¿Se movió?
	Paciente:	Sí. Cambió de color.
	Dra. Maya:	¿De qué color es?
60	Paciente:	Rojo.
	Dra. Maya:	Mira el punto rojo. Está atento. Bien. Cubre el ojo derecho con la mano. Mira la gráfica. ¿Puedes leer los números?
	Paciente:	«Seis,» «tres,» «nueve,» «cinco.»
	Dra. Maya:	Hay cinco números. ¿Qué se te escapó?
65	Paciente:	«Dos.»
	Dra. Maya:	Bien. ¿Puedes leer algunos números de esta línea?
	Paciente:	Sí. «Tres,» «cinco,» «dos,» «ocho,» «tres,» «cuatro.»
	Dra. Maya:	Muy bien. Estos anteojos de Max le sirven bien. No es necesario cambiarlos. Todo lo
70		demás va muy bien. La semana que viene tendrás ocho años. Tenemos que seguir usando el parche. Quiero verte de nuevo de hoy en seis meses.
	Sra. Ortiz:	¿Cuál es la visión de Max?
	Dra. Maya:	Veinte-cuarenta, lo que tenía en mayo.
	Sra. Ortiz:	¿Tiene que llevar Max el parche?
	Dra. Maya:	Sí. Debe llevarlo varias horas cada día. Cuando pasó Max dos meses sin llevarlo, se le
75		escapó la visión (un poco). Ahora sabemos que perderá la visión otra vez si no sigue llevándolo. ¿Comprenden? No vamos a hacerte una refracción de los ojos esta vez. Hasta luego.

Paciente y Sra. Ortiz: Adiós, y gracias.

Preguntas

1. ¿Cuántos años tiene Max?
2. ¿Por qué tiene que llevar Max un parche?
3. Max parece sufrir de una condición llamada «ambliopia de supresión.» Se llama ambliopia a una disminución de visión producida por el no usar uno de los ojos. ¿Cómo se llama esta condición en inglés?
4. La Dra. Maya le hizo a Max una prueba para verificar la fusión de los ojos. (Usó anteojos hechos de un lente rojo y un lente verde.) ¿Parece que Max los usa juntos?
5. Parece que a Max le falta la percepción de profundidad (estereopsia), ¿verdad?
6. ¿Cuándo tendrá Max que volver?

EARS *LOS OIDOS*

1. I am going to examine your ears.
   Voy a examinarle los oídos.

2. I am going to touch you with an instrument.
   Voy a tocarle con un instrumento.

3. Do you hear this tuning fork vibrating?
   ¿Oye Vd. vibrar este diapasón?

4. Tell me if it seems sharper to you on the left side than on the right.
   Dígame Vd. si le parece más agudo en el lado izquierdo que en el derecho.

5. Tell me when you can(not) hear this.
   Dígame Vd. por favor, cuando (no) pueda oír esto.

6. Is this the same in both ears?
   ¿Es esto igual en ambos oídos?

7. Is this louder in the right ear than in the left?
   ¿Oye Vd. mejor en el oído derecho que en el izquierdo?

8. Is this softer in one ear?
   ¿Es más suave en un oído?

9. Is there any difference?
   ¿Hay alguna diferencia?

10. Call me if there is any change.
    Avíseme Vd. si hay algún cambio.

11. You have an ear infection.
    Vd. tiene una infección del oído.

12. I am going to give you eardrops.
    Voy a darle gotas para el oído.

MOUTH AND THROAT   *LA BOCA Y LA GARGANTA*

1. I am going to examine your mouth (throat).
   Voy a examinarle la boca (garganta).

2. Can you open your mouth?
   ¿Puede Vd. abrir la boca?

3. Open your mouth, please.
   Abra Vd. la boca, por favor.

4. Say "ah."
   Diga «ah.»

5. Close it, please.
   Ciérrela Vd., por favor.

6. Stick out your tongue.
   Saque Vd. la lengua, por favor.

7. I am going to take a throat culture.[1]
   Voy a tomarle un cultivo de la garganta.

8. Today when you cough, please collect in this jar all the phlegm that comes up, so that we can examine it.
   Hoy, cuando tosa, ponga todo el esputo (la flema) en este vaso, para que lo (la) examinemos.

9. Breathe deeply through your mouth.
   Respire hondo por la boca.

10. Take acetaminophen (Tylenol) every four (4) hours for fever.
    Tome acetaminofena (Tylenol) cada cuatro (4) horas para la fiebre.

11. Call me immediately if the symptoms change.
    Llámeme inmediatamente si cambian los síntomas.

NECK   *EL CUELLO*

1. I am going to examine your neck.
   Voy a examinarle el cuello.

2. Does it hurt you when I bend your neck?
   ¿Le duele cuando le doblo a Vd. el cuello?

3. Please swallow.
   Trague Vd., por favor.

4. Again, please.
   Otra vez, por favor.

5. Your neck seems enlarged?
   El cuello parece agrandado.

6. I can feel a lump in your neck.
   Puedo sentir una masa (bolita) en el cuello.

BREASTS   *LOS PECHOS*

1. I am going to examine your breasts.
   Voy a examinarle los pechos.

2. I am going to teach you how to do breast self-examination (BSE).[2]
   Voy a enseñarle cómo hacer el autoexamen de los senos. (la autoexploración mamaria).

3. This is a model of the female breast.
   Este es un modelo del seno femenino.

4. The anatomy of the female breast has different parts: lobules, ducts, lactiferous cavities.
   La anatomía del seno femenino tiene diferentes partes: lóbulos, lobulillos, conductos, cavidades lactíferas.

5. Some parts have a distinct form and also feel different to the touch.
   Algunas partes tienen una forma distinta y también se sienten distintas al tacto.

6. You have to get used to the feel of your breasts.
   Vd. tiene que acostumbrarse al tacto de los senos.

7. Breast tissue can have somewhat of a lump or protuberance before the menstrual cycle or during pregnancy.
   El tejido del seno puede estar con algo de abultamientos o protuberancias antes de la menstruación o durante el embarazo.

8. If a lump persists, tell your physician.
   Si persiste un abultamiento, dígaselo a su médico (médica).

9. Remember, the majority of breast lumps (protuberances) turn out to be non-malignant.
   Recuerde Vd. que la mayoría de los abultamientos en los senos no resultan ser cancerosos.

RESPIRATORY-CARDIOVASCULAR   *RESPIRATORIO-CARDIOVASCULAR*

Vital Signs   *Signos vitales*

1. I am going to examine your lungs.
   Voy a examinarle los pulmones.

2. I am going to examine your heart.
   Voy a examinarle el corazón.

3. I want you to have an electrocardiogram.[3]
   Quiero que le hagan un electrocardiograma.

4. I am going to listen to your chest.
   Voy a escucharle el pecho.

5. Take a deep breath.
   Respire Vd. profundo.

6. Breathe slowly.
   Respire Vd. al paso. *fam*
   Respire Vd. lento.

7. Breathe rapidly.
   Respire Vd. rápido.

8. Raise both arms over your head.
   Levante Vd. los dos brazos sobre la cabeza.

9. Lower your arms.
   Baje Vd. los brazos.

10. Breathe through your mouth.
    Respire por la boca.

11. Breathe deeply in and out through your mouth.
    Respire Vd. fuertemente hacia dentro y hacia fuera, por la boca.

12. Don't be afraid.
    No tenga Vd. miedo.

13. Cough, please.
    Tosa Vd. por favor.

14. Again.
    Otra vez.

15. Once more.
    Una vez más.

16. Say "thirty three (33)."
    Diga «treinta y tres (33).»

17. Please don't breathe for one minute.
    Favor de no respirar por un minuto.

18. Hold your breath.
    Mantenga Vd. la respiración.

19. Hold it.
    No saque el aire.

20. Now you can breathe.
    Ya Vd. puede respirar.

21. Inhale.
    Inspire Vd.
    Inhale Vd.

22. Exhale.
    Exhale Vd.

23. Breathe normally.
    Respire Vd. normalmente.

24. Climb these stairs.
    Suba estas escaleras.

25. Everything is OK.
    Todo está bien.

26. Everything will be OK.
    Todo va a estar bien.

27. Calm down.
    Cálmese Vd.

28. Relax.
    Descanse Vd.
    No se apure Vd. *Chicano*

29. Don't worry.

No se preocupe Vd.
No se apure Vd. *Chicano*
No se apene Vd. *Chicano*

30. I am going to take your blood pressure.
    Voy a tomarle la presión (de la sangre).

31. Roll up your sleeves.
    Arremánguese, por favor.
    Súbase las mangas, por favor.

32. Relax (physically).
    Afloje Vd. el cuerpo, por favor.

33. Bend your elbow.
    Doble Vd. el codo, por favor.

34. Make a fist.
    Haga Vd. un puño, por favor.
    Cierre Vd. el puño, por favor.

35. Your blood pressure is normal.
    Su presión arterial es normal.

36. Your pressure is too low.
    Su presión está demasiado baja.

37. Your pressure is quite high.
    Su presión arterial está bastante alta.

38. Your pressure is too high.
    Su presión está demasiado alta.

39. Your pressure is higher than normal.
    Su presión está más alta que lo normal.

40. We have to try to determine why you have high blood pressure although sometimes this is not possible.
    Debemos tratar de determinar por qué tiene Vd. la presión alta aunque a veces no se puede hacer esto.

41. Here is a prescription to reduce your blood pressure.
    Aquí tiene Vd. una receta para reducir la presión arterial.

42. Fill the prescription at the nearest pharmacy.
    Llene la receta a la farmacia más cercana.

43. Take one pill every day after breakfast.
    Tome Vd. una píldora todos los días después de desayunarse.

44. Let me feel your pulse.
    Déjeme tomarle el pulso.

45. Your pulse is too rapid.
    El pulso está demasiado rápido.

46. Please step on the scale.
    Súbase Vd. en la balanza, por favor.
    Párese Vd. en la balanza, por favor.

47. Do you feel dizzy?
    ¿Se siente mareado (mareada)?

Temperature   *La Temperatura*

1. I am going to take your temperature.
   Voy a tomarle la temperatura.

2. Let me take your temperature.
   Permítame tomarle la temperatura.

3. Moisten your lips, please.
   Por favor, humedézcase Vd. los labios.
   Favor de humedecerse los labios.

4. Please keep the thermometer in your mouth, under the tongue.
Por favor, mantenga el termómetro en la boca, bajo la lengua.

Favor de mantener el termómetro en la boca, bajo la lengua.

5. Open your mouth.
Abra Vd. la boca, por favor.

6. Don't be afraid.
No tenga Vd. miedo.

7. You have a high fever.
Vd. tiene fiebre alta.

8. You have a slight fever.
Vd. tiene un poco de fiebre.

9. How long have you had fever?
¿Desde cuándo tiene Vd. fiebre?

10. Did you have fever last night? Yesterday?
¿Tuvo Vd. fiebre (calentura) anoche? ¿ayer?

11. How much?[4]
¿Cuánta?

12. Did you take any medicine before coming to the hospital?
¿Tomó Vd. alguna medicina antes de venir al hospital?

13. What type?
¿Qué clase?

14. How much?
¿Cuánta?

GASTROINTESTINAL   *GASTROINTESTINAL*

Abdominal Exam   *Reconocimiento abdominal*

1. I am going to examine your abdomen (stomach).
Voy a examinarle el estómago.

2. Sit up and don't cross your legs.
Siéntese Vd. y no cruce las piernas.

3. Relax please.
Cálmese Vd., por favor.

4. Lie down.
Acuéstese, por favor.

5. Lie on your right (left) side.
Acuéstese, por favor, sobre el lado derecho (izquierdo).

6. Extend one leg and bend the other.
Estire Vd. una pierna y doble la otra.

7. Does it hurt when I press here?
¿Le duele cuando le aprieto aquí?

8. Does it hurt when I let go?
¿Le duele cuando le suelto?

9. Suck in your stomach.
Succione Vd. el estómago.

Meta Vd. el estómago.

10. Inflate it.
Inflelo Vd.

11. Relax.
Descanse Vd.

Rectal Exam[5]   *Reconocimiento Rectal*

1. I am going to examine you rectally.
Voy a examinarle el recto.

2. Are you comfortable?
¿Está cómodo (cómoda)?

3. I am sorry if this makes you uncomfortable.
Lo siento si esto le molesta.

4. This won't hurt.
Esto no le dolerá.

5. Please kneel.
Póngase Vd. de rodillas, por favor.

6. Turn on your left side and draw your knees up to your chin.
Póngase Vd. del lado izquierdo y doble Vd. las rodillas hasta la barbilla.

7. Pull your legs toward you.
Encoja Vd. las piernas.

8. Stay on your back.
Póngase Vd. boca arriba.

9. Don't cross your legs.
No cruce las piernas.

10. Does this hurt?
¿Le duele esto?

11. Can you feel this?
¿Puede sentir esto?

12. Hold still, please.
No se mueva, por favor.

13. It will only take a minute more.
No durará más de un minuto.
Sólo tardará un minuto más.

14. That's enough.
Basta.
Suficiente.

15. Just relax.
Relaje Vd. el cuerpo.
Relájese Vd.[6]

16. I am going to do a proctoscopic examination.
Voy a hacerle un examen proctoscópico.

17. Bear down as if you were going to move your bowels.
Puje[7] Vd. como si fuera a obrar.

18. I am going to examine your rectum with an instrument that I am now putting in.
Voy a examinarle el recto con un instrumento que le voy a introducir.

19. It will probably only be slightly irritating.
    Le molestará un poco solamente.

20. Push. (Bear down.)
    Puje Vd., por favor.[7]

21. Don't move.
    No se mueva Vd.

22. I have finished.
    He terminado ya.

23. You have . . .
    Vd. tiene . . .
    ulcerations
    ulceraciones
    an inflammation
    inflamación
    fissures

grietas (partiduras)
polyps
pólipos
fistulas
fístulas
an abscess
un absceso (apostema)
a foreign body
un cuerpo extraño
a prolapsed rectum
un prolapso del recto

24. You will also need a stool culture.[8]
    También Vd. necesita un cultivo de materia fecal.

GENITOURINARY *GENITOURINARIO*

Female Genitalia *Los órganos genitales femeninos*

1. I have to examine you internally.[9]
   Tengo que examinarle por dentro.

2. I am going to do a pelvic examination.
   Voy a hacerle ahora un examen de la pelvis.

3. Have you ever had a pelvic exam before?
   ¿Ha tenido jamás un examen pélvico antes?

4. I am going to insert my fingers into your vagina in order to examine you internally.
   Voy a introducirle mis dedos en la vagina para hacerle un examen por dentro.

5. This will not hurt.
   Esto no le va a doler.
   Esto no va a dolerle.

6. Please lie on your back.
   Acuéstese de espaldas, por favor.

7. Put your feet in these stirrups.
   Ponga Vd. los pies en estos estribos.

8. Scoot closer to the edge of the table.
   Acérquese al borde de la mesa.

9. Bend your legs more.
   Doble Vd. las piernas más.

10. Spread your knees and legs apart.
    Abra Vd. las rodillas y las piernas.

11. Let your legs relax.
    Relaje las piernas.

12. Try to relax.
    Aflójese un poco.

13. Relax your muscles.
    Relaje los músculos.

14. Don't tighten up.
    No se atiese Vd.
    No se ponga tiesa.

15. I am going to insert an instrument called a speculum into your vagina to help me examine your uterus and cervix better.
    Voy a introducirle un instrumento que se llama un espéculo en la vagina para ayu-
    darme a examinarle mejor el útero y el cuello de la matriz (la cérvix).

16. The instrument may feel a bit cold. I'm sorry.
    Sentirá el instrumento un poco frío. Lo siento.

17. I am going to insert a speculum into your vagina in order to do the Pap smear.
    Voy a introducirle un espéculo (espéculum) en la vagina para hacerle el examen de Pap.

18. I am going to take a sample of cells from the cervix and the area around it, with a cotton swab (with a spatula).
    Voy a extraer unas células del cuello del útero y sus alredededores con un hisopillo (con una espátula).

19. It may be a little uncomfortable, but it won't last long.
    Se sentirá un poco incómoda, pero no durará mucho tiempo.

20. Place your arms at your side and leave them there.
    Acomode los brazos al lado del cuerpo y déjelos allí.

21. The cells are normal (abnormal).
    Las células son normales (anormales).
    Las células son sanas (contienen cáncer).

22. I want to do another Pap test.
    Quiero hacerle otro examen de Pap.

23. We are going to order an ultrasound of your uterus.
    Vamos a ordenar una prueba de ultrasonido del útero.

24. I am going to do a colposcopy (a visual examination of the cervix with a special magnifying instrument—a colposcope).
    Voy a hacerle una colposcopia (un examen visual del cuello uterino con un instrumento especial de aumento—un colposcopio).

25. You need a uterine biopsy.
    Vd. necesita una biopsia del útero.

26. I advise you to have a "cone biopsy"/conization.
    Le aconsejo que le hagan una biopsia del cono del cuello uterino / una conización.

27. Return in six months (next year) for another Pap.
    Vuelva Vd. en seis meses (el año que viene) para otro examen de Pap (otro Papanicolau).

28. Stay quiet.
    Esté Vd. tranquila.

29. Now I am going to insert my finger into your rectum.
    Ahora voy a ponerle mi dedo en su recto.

30. Relax. It will not hurt.
    Relájese Vd.[6] No va a dolerle.

31. You can slide back now and sit up.
    Vd. puede deslizarse hacia atrás e incorporarse.

32. I have finished.
    He terminado.

33. You can get dressed now.
    Vd. puede vestirse ahora.

34. You should not have sexual intercourse for a while.
    No debería Vd. tener relaciones sexuales durante algún tiempo.

35. Do not use any douche.
    No se dé Vd. duchas vaginales.

Male Genitalia   *Los Organos Genitales Masculinos*

1. I am going to examine your testicles.
   Voy a examinarle los testículos.

2. You should also examine your testicles every month.[10]
   También Vd. debe examinarse los testículos una vez por mes.

3. I am going to examine you for hernias.
   Voy a examinarle para ver si tiene hernias inguinales.

Urinary   *Urinario*

1. I am going to examine your kidneys.
   Voy a examinarle los riñones.

2. Lean forward, please.
   Inclínese hacia adelante, por favor.

3. I am going to order some tests on your urine.[11]
   Pediré unas pruebas de su orina.

MID-STREAM URINE COLLECTION

	Dr. López:	Do you have any complaints that you want to tell me of?
	Mrs. Peña:	When I urinate, I feel a slight burning. Also, I feel that I have to urinate every five minutes, even though I am unable to pass more than a few drops of urine.
	Dr. López:	When did this begin?
5	Mrs. Peña:	Two nights ago.
	Dr. López:	Well, Mrs. Peña, I want to order a special type of urinalysis in order to determine if you have a kidney or bladder infection, or not. Before we continue with your examination, I want you to take this kit and go to the bathroom. Do you know where it is?
10	Mrs. Peña:	Yes, it is down the hall, the first door on the right.
	Dr. López:	No, it is the third room on the left. After you have locked the door, wash your hands very carefully with soap and water. Open the package and remove all the small packets that contain towelettes.
	Mrs. Peña:	Shall I remove the container, too?
15	Dr. López:	No, leave the container in the kit. Your hands will be clean. Take out the towelettes, open them up, one at a time, and clean the perineal area.
	Mrs. Peña:	I am very sorry, doctor. I do not understand what you mean.
	Dr. López:	Wash the area between your legs where you urinate. Separate the lips/folds of your vagina with your forefingers. Clean the area inside with the towelettes. Wipe downward only—toward your rectum. Do **NOT** wipe upwards, from the rectum to the urinary opening. This could cause further problems. Keep the labia separated during urination. Now remove the container. Do not touch the inside of the container. Leave the cap inside the kit.
20		
25		Begin urinating into the toilet. Remember, separate the lips of your vagina with one hand. After a few seconds, stop and bring the container between your legs. Continue urinating, this time into the container. In this way you will obtain what is called "a clean voided specimen."
	Mrs. Peña:	Should I fill the little container with clean urine?
	Dr. López:	No, fill the container only half way. Then remove the cap from the package with your thumb and forefinger. Do not touch the inside of the cap. Screw the cap on the container and place the self-adhering label on the jar. Wipe yourself with toilet paper, wash your hands again, and return here with the specimen. We will then continue the exam.
30		

Questions

1. What is Mrs. Peña complaining about? What are her symptoms?
2. What can a midstream urinanalysis indicate which, generally, a regular urinanalysis does not?
3. Where is the perineum (the perineal area)?
4. Why is it necessary to use a backward movement when wiping oneself?
5. Should the flask be filled immediately upon urinating?
6. How much urine is needed for this test?

ORINA RECOGIDA A LA MITAD DE LA MICCION

	Dra. López:	¿En qué puedo servirla? ¿De qué se queja?
	Sra. Peña:	Cuando orino, siento un ardor [quemazón]. También, me parece que tengo que orinar cada cinco minutos [me parece que tengo una urgencia para orinar], aun cuando no pueda pasar más que unas gotitas de orina.
5	Dra. López:	¿Cuándo empezó esto?
	Sra. Peña:	Hace dos noches.
	Dra. López:	Bueno, señora Peña. Quiero pedir un tipo especial de urinálisis para averiguar si Vd. tiene o no una infección de los riñones o de la vejiga de la orina. Antes de continuar su examen, quiero que coja este recipiente y que vaya al cuarto de baño. ¿Conoce Vd.
10		dónde está?
	Sra. Peña:	Sí, está derecho por el pasillo, la primera puerta a la derecha.
	Dra. López:	No, es el tercer cuarto a la izquierda. Después de cerrar la puerta con llave, lávese las manos cuidadosamente con jabón y agua. Abra el paquete y saque todas las toallitas.
15	Sra. Peña:	¿Debo quitar el frasco también?
	Dra. López:	No, deje el frasco en el recipiente. Con las manos limpias, saque las toallitas, ábralas, una por una, y límpiese el área perineal.
	Sra. Peña:	Lo siento mucho, doctora. No comprendo lo que quiere decir.
	Dra. López:	Lávese el área entre las piernas donde orina. Con los dedos, separe los labios / el
20		doblez de la vagina. Limpie esta área de adentro con las toallitas. Emplee un movimiento suave hacia abajo—hacia el recto, solamente. No emplee un movimiento hacia arriba, del recto a la abertura urinaria. El hacer esto causaría más problemas. Coloque el frasco para que la orina caiga dentro. Mantenga los labios de la vagina separados cuando orina. Ahora, quite el frasco. No lo toque por dentro. Deje la tapa dentro del recipiente.
25		Empiece a orinar dentro del inodoro. Recuerde, separe Vd. los labios de la vagina con una mano. Después de unos segundos, pare y ponga el frasco entre las piernas. Siga orinando, esta vez dentro del frasco. De esta manera obtendrá lo que se llama «una muestra limpia de orina.»
	Sra. Peña:	¿Debo llenar todo el frasco de claro espécimen?
	Dra. López:	No, llene sólo la mitad. Entonces, quite la tapa del paquete con el pulgar y el índice. No toque dentro de la tapa tampoco. Enrosque la tapa sobre el frasco y fije la etiqueta. Séquese con papel higiénico, lávese las manos otra vez, y vuelva aquí con la
30		muestra. Entonces, continuaremos el reconocimiento físico.

Preguntas

1. ¿De qué se queja la señora Peña? ¿Cuáles son sus síntomas?
2. ¿Qué puede indicar la orina recogida a la mitad de la micción que, en general, un urinálisis común no indica?
3. ¿Dónde está el perineo (el área perineal)?
4. ¿Por qué es necesario usar un movimiento hacia el recto al limpiarse?
5. ¿Debe llenar el frasco inmediatamente al orinar?
6. ¿Cuánta orina se necesita para esta prueba?

4. I am going to order a cystoscopy in order to determine what is causing the infection / inflammation / bleeding in your urinary tract.[12]
    Pediré una cistoscopia para determinar lo que está causando la infección / la inflamación / el flujo de sangre en sus vías urinarias.[12]

5. I am going to order an intravenous pyelogram. You will have to follow a special diet the day before the IVP.[13]
    Voy a pedirle un pielograma intravenoso.[13] Usted tendrá que seguir una dieta especial el día antes del PIV.

MUSCULOSKELETAL AND EXTREMITIES   *MUSCULAR-ESQUELETICO Y LAS EXTREMIDADES*

1. Please stand up.
   Levántese Vd., por favor.

2. Please sit down.
   Siéntese Vd., por favor.

3. Walk a little.
   Camine Vd. un poco.

4. Come back, please.
   Vuelva Vd., por favor.
   Regrese Vd., por favor.

5. Walk backwards.
   Camine Vd. hacia atrás.

6. Walk on your toes.
   Camine Vd. sobre los dedos.

7. Walk on your heels.
   Camine Vd. sobre los talones.

8. Bend over.
   Dóblese Vd. hacia adelante.

9. Bend backwards.
   Dóblese Vd. hacia atrás.

10. Bend your trunk forward as far as you can.
    Doble Vd. el tronco hacia adelante todo lo que pueda.

11. The doctor wants to examine your arm.
    El doctor quiere examinarle el brazo.

12. Close your hand.
    Cierre Vd. la mano.

13. Open it.
    Abrala Vd., por favor.

14. Close your fist.
    Cierre Vd. el puño.

15. Open it.
    Abralo Vd., por favor.

16. Grip my hands tightly.
    Apriete Vd. mis manos con fuerza.

17. Can't you do it better than that?
    ¿No puede Vd. hacerlo más fuerte?

18. Push against my hand as hard as you can.
    Empuje[7] mi mano tan fuerte como pueda.

19. Squeeze my fingers as hard as you can.
    Apriete fuerte mis dedos tanto como pueda.

20. Don't let me move your _____ .
    No me deje mover su _____ .
    head
    cabeza
    arm
    brazo
    leg
    pierna

21. Relax and let me move your _____ .
    Relájese[6] y déjeme mover su _____ .
    Relaje el cuerpo y déjeme mover su_____ .
    arm
    brazo
    foot
    pie
    leg
    pierna

22. Raise your arms.
    Suba Vd. los brazos.
    Levante Vd. los brazos.

23. Higher.
    Más alto.

24. Raise your arms all the way up.
    Levante Vd. los brazos completamente.
    Suba Vd. los brazos completamente.

25. Lower.
    Más bajo.

26. Raise your left (right) leg.
    Levante Vd. la pierna izquierda (derecha).
    Suba Vd. la pierna izquierda (derecha).

27. Can you move that arm?
    ¿Puede Vd. mover ese brazo?

28. Can you lift that arm?
    ¿Puede Vd. levantar ese brazo?

29. Can you move that leg?
    ¿Puede Vd. mover esa pierna?

30. Can you lift that leg?
    ¿Puede Vd. levantar esa pierna?

31. When did you sprain _____ ?
    ¿Cuándo se torció _____ ?

NEUROLOGICAL EXAM   *RECONOCIMIENTO NEUROLOGICO*

Coordination   *Coordinación*

1. Close your eyes and cross your left leg over your right one.
   Cierre los ojos y cruce Vd. la pierna izquierda sobre la derecha.

2. Now cross the right leg over the left.
   Ahora cruce Vd. la pierna derecha sobre la izquierda.

3. Bend your right (left) knee.
   Doble Vd. la rodilla derecha (izquierda).

4. Hold your arms out straight.
   Extienda los brazos al frente.

5. Bend your right (left) elbow.
   Doble Vd. el codo derecho (izquierdo).

6. Move a little over to the right.
   Muévese Vd. un poco hacia la derecha.

7. Does it hurt?
   ¿Le duele?

8. Where?
   ¿Dónde?

9. Turn your ankle.
   Gire el tobillo.

10. To the right.
    A la derecha.

11. To the left.
    A la izquierda.

12. This way.
    Hacia acá.

13. Walk heel to toe—like this.
    Camine con un pie delante del otro—así.

14. Put one foot directly in front of the other—like this.
    Ponga un pie directamente enfrente del otro—así.

15. Walk in a straight line toward the door.
    Camine en una línea recta hacia la puerta.

16. Turn around and come back to me.
    Dé la vuelta y regrese hacia mí.
    Vuélvase y venga hacia mí.

17. Touch your right (left) heel to your left (right) ankle.
    Toque el tobillo izquierdo (derecho) con el talón derecho (izquierdo).

18. Run your heel up and down your leg.
    Deslice Vd. el talón sobre la pierna.

19. Do it faster.
    Hágalo más rápido.

20. Touch your right knee with your left heel.
    Toque la rodilla derecha con el talón izquierdo.

21. Run your right heel down the front of your left shin to the ankle.
    Deslice el talón derecho sobre la espinilla izquierda hasta el tobillo.

22. Do the same thing with the other leg.
    Hágalo con la otra pierna.

23. Stand up.
    Levántese, por favor.

24. Keep your eyes closed.
    Mantenga los ojos cerrados.

25. Hop on one foot.
    Salte a la pata coja *fam.*
    Brinque en un pie.

26. Hop on the other foot.
    Usando el otro pie, salte a la pata coja *fam.*
    Brinque en el otro pie.

27. Stand with your feet together.
    Párese con los pies juntos.

28. Extend your arms in front of you with your palms up.
    Extienda los brazos enfrente con las palmas arriba.

29. Keep your eyes closed and your arms extended.
    Mantenga los ojos cerrados y los brazos extendidos.

30. Stretch your fingers.
    Estire Vd. los dedos.

31. Grasp this object between your fingers.
    Apriete Vd. este objeto entre los dedos.

32. Push against my hand.
    Empuje[7] contra mi mano.

33. Push harder.
    Empuje[7] más fuerte.

34. Flex your wrist against my hand.
    Flexione la muñeca contra mi mano.

35. Touch my finger with yours and then touch your nose.
    Toque mi dedo con el de Vd. y entonces toque la nariz.

36. Keep on touching my finger and your nose using your left (right) index finger.
    Siga tocando mi dedo y su nariz usando el índice izquierdo (derecho).

37. Do it faster.
    Hágalo más rápido, por favor.

38. Sit down here and stretch your legs.
    Siéntese aquí y estire Vd. las piernas.

39. Lift your leg up and don't let me push it down.
    Levante la pierna y no me deje bajarla.

40. Try harder.
    Trate más.

41. Push your feet against my hands.
    Empuje[7] los pies contra mis manos.

42. More.
    Más.

43. Extend your leg against my hand.
    Extienda la pierna contra mi mano.

44. Bend your toes towards you keeping your legs straight.
    Dóblese los dedos del pie hacia usted, manteniendo rectas las piernas.

45. Flex your feet.
    Flexione Vd. los pies.

46. Now move your head but not your shoulders . . .
    Ahora, mueva la cabeza pero no los hombros hacia . . .
    to the left.
    la izquierda.
    to the right.
    la derecha.
    forward as much as possible.
    adelante lo más que se pueda.
    backward—like this.
    atrás—así.

Motor *Movilidad*

1. Relax.
   Relájese,[6] por favor.

2. Repeat the words that I am going to say.
   Repita las palabras que voy a decirle.

3. I am going to check your reflexes.
   Voy a revisarle sus reflejos.

4. Relax your . . .
   Relaje . . .
   arms.
   los brazos.
   wrists.
   las muñecas.
   legs.
   las piernas.

5. Squeeze my fingers in your right (left) hand as hard as you can.
   Apriete mis dedos en la mano derecha (izquierda) lo más fuerte que pueda.

6. Raise your arm toward your shoulder.
   Suba el brazo hacia el hombro.

7. I am going to touch your knee with an instrument.
   Voy a tocarle la rodilla con un instrumento.

8. Once more.
   Una vez más.

9. Very good.
   Muy bien.

10. Thank you.
    Gracias.

Sensory *Sensibilidad*

1. Close your eyes and keep them shut.
   Cierre Vd. los ojos por favor y manténgalos cerrados.

2. Try to close your eyes now.
   Trate de cerrar los ojos ahora, por favor.

3. Tell me when you feel something.
   Dígame cuando sienta algo.

4. Can you feel it when I touch you with this . . .
   ¿Puede sentirlo cuando le toco con este . . .
   piece of cotton?
   algodón?
   pin?
   alfiler?

5. I am going to use the pin to test your sensations.
   Voy a usar este alfiler para revisar las sensaciones.

6. Close your eyes and tell me if I am sticking you with the point of the pin or with the head.
   Cierre los ojos y dígame si le pincho con la punta o con la cabeza del alfiler.

7. The point of the pin is sharp.
   La punta del alfiler es aguda.

8. The head of the pin is dull.
   La cabeza del alfiler es sorda.

9. Tell me when you feel something.
   Dígame cuando sienta algo.

10. Where do you feel it?
    ¿Dónde lo siente?

11. Tell me if it feels sharp or dull each time that I touch you.
    Dígame si siente agudo o sordo cada vez que le toco.

12. Do you feel something like a prick?
    ¿Siente Vd. algo como un pinchazo?

13. Is it moving upward?
    Se mueve hacia arriba?

14. Is it moving downward?
    ¿Se mueve hacia abajo?

15. Keep your eyes closed and tell me if I am sticking you with one (1) point or with two (2) points.
    Mantenga los ojos cerrados y dígame si le pincho con una (1) punta o con dos (2) puntas.

16. Does this feel hot (cold)?
    ¿Siente esto caliente (frío)?

17. Do you feel it more on the right side than on the left?
    ¿Lo siente más en el lado derecho que en el izquierdo?

Cranial Nerves *Nervios craneales*

1. What does this smell like?
   ¿A qué huele esto?
   ¿Cómo huele esto?

2. Does it smell like . . .
   ¿Huele a . . .
   alcohol?
   alcohol?
   cinnamon?
   canela?
   cloves?
   clavos?
   mint?
   menta?
   tobacco?
   tabaco?

3. Can you hear this?
   ¿Puede oír esto?

4. Don't let me open your mouth.
   No me permita abrirle la boca.

5. Clench your teeth.
   Apriete los dientes.

6. Smile.
   Sonría, por favor.

7. Whistle.
   Silbe, por favor.

8. Open your mouth and say "ah."
   Abra la boca y diga «ah.»

9. Stick out your tongue.
   Saque la lengua, por favor.

10. Move it from side to side.
    Muévala de un lado a otro.
    Muévala de lado a lado.

11. With your eyes closed, tell me if you can feel this on your face.
    Con los ojos cerrados, dígame si puede sentir esto en la cara.

12. Shrug your shoulders.
    Encójase de hombros.
    Levante los hombros.

13. I want to examine your eyes.
    Quiero examinarle los ojos.

14. Close your eyes and don't let me open them.
    Cierre Vd. los ojos por favor y no me deje abrirlos.

15. Cover one eye and look at my nose.
    Tápese un ojo y mire mi nariz.

16. How many fingers do you see?
    ¿Cuántos dedos ve?

17. Without moving your head, look . . .
    Sin mover la cabeza, mire . . .
    to the right.
    la derecha.
    to the left.
    la izquierda.
    up.
    arriba.
    down.
    abajo.

18. Cover your right eye and read this.
    Tápese el ojo derecho y lea esto.

19. Cover your left eye and read this.
    Tápese el ojo izquierdo y lea esto.

20. You may get dressed now.
    Vd. puede vestirse ahora.

21. I want to talk with you when you are dressed.
    Quiero hablar con Vd. cuando se haya vestido.

22. The doctor will speak with you when you are finished.
    El médico (La médica) hablará con usted cuando termine.

Exercise   *Ejercicio*

Statements 1–6 in the above Neurology Section are polite commands. Several acceptable substitutes exist for the polite command. These involve using some form of *please* and the infinitive. In Spanish several forms of *please* may be used:

haga Vd. el favor de
favor de
tenga la bondad de
sírvase

Rewrite all polite commands in the musculoskeletal and neurological exam sections using the above ways to say *please*.

Bend your head to the right, please. **Doble Vd. la cabeza a la derecha, por favor.**
(**Haga Vd. el favor de**) _____

Haga Vd. el favor de doblar la cabeza a la derecha.
(**Favor de**) _____

Favor de doblar la cabeza a la derecha.
(**Tenga la bondad de**) _____

Tenga la bondad de doblar la cabeza a la derecha.
(**Sírvase**) _____

Sírvase doblar la cabeza a la derecha.

Continue in this fashion with all the commands listed.

Notes   *Notas*

1. See Chapter 12, page 254, "Throat Culture" *Cultivo de la garganta.*
2. See Chapter 12, pages 264–265 for "Breast Self-Examination" «Autoexploración Mamaria».
3. See Chapter 12, page 256 for "Electrocardiogram" «Electrocardiograma».
4. Remember, many Spanish-speaking people use centigrade temperatures. See Chapter 4, page 92F for a conversion table.

5. Hispanics may be hesitant to have their children examined too often rectally. This combined with an excessive use of enemas, they worry, may incline a child toward homosexuality. Some believe that masturbation leads to a decrease in strength, and often to insanity. They also believe that insanity may also be caused by inadequate sexual gratification and that excessive sexual gratification deteriorates the nerves. Some Hispanics believe that pent-up sexual energy may lead to epilepsy.

6. This expression means to physically relax; in rural New Mexico and Southern Colorado **relájese** is not used because it means "*get embarrassed.*"

7. *Pujar*—to push (as in labor or in evacuating the bowels or bladder).

   Empujar—to push, bring (external) pressure on (something).

8. See Chapter 12, page 254 for "Stool Culture," «Cultivo de excemento»

9. Before beginning a pelvic exam or any other type of test which requires "intimate" touching, it is extremely important to obtain the *Latina/Hispanic* patient's cooperation and understanding. This is even more important should the patient be very young, a virgin, or unmarried. Therefore, it is essential to reinforce the reasons why such an exam is necessary in order to calm her anxiety.

10. See Chapter 12, pages 265–266 "Testicular Self-Examination," «*Autoexploración testicular*»

11. See Chapter 12, page 257 "Urine and Kidney Test," «*Pruebas de la orina y los riñones*»

12. See Chapter 12, pages 257–259, for the Cystoscopy Procedure *el Procedimiento para hacer cistoscopia.*

13. See Chapter 12, pages 259–260, "Intravenous Pyelogram [IVP]," «*Pielograma intravenoso* [PIV].»

Conversations for Health Professionals:
Labor & Delivery, Surgery, Medication,
Diet, Treatments, Drug Overdose,
and Accidental Poisonings

Conversaciones para personal médico y paramédico: el parto, cirugía, medicación, dieta, tratamientos, la dosis excesiva de drogas, y envenenamientos accidentales

LABOR AND DELIVERY

EL PARTO

1. When is your expected delivery date? How many more weeks?
   ¿Cuál es la fecha anticipada (esperada) del parto? ¿Cuántas semanas le quedan?

2. Do you have / Are you having sharp pains in your hip—in the lumbar region?
   ¿Tiene Vd. dolor agudo de la cadera—de la espalda en la region lumbar?

3. Are you having uterine contractions (abdominal pains) now?
   ¿Tiene Vd. contracciones uterinas (dolores abdominales) ahora?

4. Do the pains come at regular intervals—for example, every 10 minutes?
   ¿Le vienen los dolores (de parto) a intervalos regulares—como, por ejemplo, cada diez minutos?

5. Do the pains decrease when you walk?
   ¿Se disminuyen las contracciones uterinas (los dolores abdominales) al caminar?

6. How close together are they? (How many minutes apart are they?)
   ¿Con qué frecuencia le vienen?
   ¿Cuántos minutos hay entre las contracciones (los dolores)?
   20-30 (twenty to thirty) minutes?
   ¿de 20-30 (veinte a treinta) minutos?
   10-20 (ten to twenty) minutes?
   ¿de 10-20 (diez a veinte) minutos?
   5-10 (five to ten) minutes?
   ¿de 5-10 (cinco a diez) minutos?
   2-3 (two to three) minutes?
   ¿cada dos a tres minutos?
   less than 2 (two) minutes?
   ¿menos de cada dos minutos?

7. How long do they last?
   ¿Cuánto tiempo le duran?

8. Since this is your first baby, you should come to the hospital when the contractions are five minutes apart.
   Puesto que va a tener su primer bebé, le aconsejo que venga al hospital cuando las contracciones uterinas vengan cada cinco minutos.

9. Since this is not your first baby, I advise you to come to the hospital when your contractions are ten minutes apart.
   Puesto que éste no es su primer bebé, le aconsejo que venga al hospital cuando las contracciones uterinas vengan cada diez minutos.

10. Have your waters broken?
    ¿Se ha roto la bolsa membranosa (que contiene el bebé y el líquido que le rodea)?
    ¿Se le ha quebrado la bolsa de aguas?
    ¿Se rompió la fuente?
    ¿Se reventaron las aguas?

11. Have you noticed a bloody show?
    ¿Se ha fijado en una secreción mucosa mezclada con sangre procedente de la vagina?[1]
    ¿Había ya una muestra de sangre (un tapón de moco)?

12. You are in the first stage of labor—the dilation stage.
    Vd. está en la primera etapa del parto—el período de dilatación.

13. Come to the emergency room entrance and tell the receptionist that you are in labor.
    Venga al hospital, por la entrada de emergencia e indique a la recepcionista que Vd. está de parto.

14. You will be sent to the labor area in a wheelchair.
    A Vd. le enviarán en seguida a la sala de parto en una silla de ruedas.

15. The nurse will take you to the prep room where you will undress and put on a hospital gown.
    La enfermera la llevará al cuarto de preparación donde Vd. se quitará la ropa (se desvestirá) y se pondrá una bata de hospital.

16. The nurse will ask you for a urine specimen and will ask you to lie down on the bed so that she will be able to take your blood pressure, pulse, and temperature and check your breathing.
    La enfermera le pedirá que le dé una muestra de orina, y que se acueste en una cama de modo que pueda tomarle la presión arterial, el pulso, la temperatura y respiración.

17. Do you feel like urinating?
    ¿Tiene Vd. deseos de orinar?

18. Do you feel like having a bowel movement?
    ¿Siente Vd. ganas de vaciar el intestino?

19. I am going to take a blood sample that will be sent to the laboratory for routine admission tests.[2]
    Voy a sacarle una muestra de sangre para enviarla al laboratorio para exámenes rutinarios de admisión.

20. I am going to shave you.
    Voy a rasurarla.

21. I am going to shave the lower part of your vulva, which is where you will have an episiotomy.
    Voy a afeitarle la parte inferior de la vulva donde será el sitio para hacer la episiotomía (el corte de las partes).

22. I am going to give you an enema.[3]
    Voy a ponerle una enema (un lavado intestinal).[3]

23. Try to relax.
    Trate de relajarse.[4]

24. Your doctor will do a vaginal examination to determine the progress of your labor.
    Su doctor(a) le hará un examen vaginal para determinar el progreso de su parto.

25. I need to examine you.
    Necesito examinarla.

26. Please lie down on your back.
    Acuéstese, por favor, boca arriba.

27. You are six centimeters dilated.
    Vd. tiene seis centímetros de cuello.
    La cérvix está dilatada seis centímetros.

28. We have to prepare for the delivery.[5]
    Tenemos que prepararnos para el parto.

29. Did you have anesthesia for your last delivery?
    ¿Tuvo Vd. anestesia para tener su último bebé?

30. What kind of anesthesia did you have? Do you know?
    ¿Qué tipo de anestesia tuvo Vd?
    ¿Sabe Vd.?

31. Would you like something to relieve the pain?
    ¿Quisiera algo para aliviar el dolor?

32. We can give you an injection.
    Podemos ponerle una inyección.

33. We can anesthetize you . . .
    Podemos anestesiarle . . .
    using caudal anesthesia.
    usando la anestesia caudal.
    using epidural anesthesia.
    usando la anestesia epidural.
    using spinal anesthesia.
    usando la anestesia espinal / anestesia raquídea.
    using general anesthesia.
    usando la anestesia general.

34. Are you going to have natural childbirth?
    ¿Va a tener el parto natural?

35. Try to relax and do the breathing exercises.
    Trate de calmarse y hacer los ejercicios de respiración.

36. The child's head is completely down in the birth canal.
    La cabecita del niño está completamente abajo en el canal vaginal (canal de nacimiento).

37. Your husband may stay with you during your labor.
    Su esposo puede estar aquí a su lado durante su parto.

38. Your cervix is completely dilated and the baby's head is crowning.
    La cérvix se abre (se dilata) completamente y la cabecita del niño está asomándose.

39. You are going to feel a tremendous pushing sensation.
    Va a tener una sensación tremenda de pujo.

40. Do abdominal breathing when you have contractions.
    Respire lentamente con el abdomen cuando haya contracciones.

41. Don't push.
    No puje Vd.[6]

42. At the end of the first stage of labor you may feel nauseated. Don't be frightened; it indicates transition to the second stage.
    Al fin de la primera etapa del parto, puede sentir náuseas. No se asuste; indica la transición a la segunda etapa.

43. A positive mental attitude is important—concentrate on something pleasant.
    Una mentalidad positiva es importante—concéntrese en algo agradable.

44. The best person to help you during this period is your husband (the baby's father).
    La persona más indicada para ayudarla es su esposo (el padre del niño).

45. He can rub your back.
    Puede sobarle la espalda.

46. During the first stage, concentrate on squeezing his hand; don't push.
    Durante la primera etapa, concéntrese Vd. en apretar fuerte la mano del esposo; no puje.[6]

47. Pant—breathe shallowly and rapidly. This helps to prevent tearing.
    Jadee Vd.—respire corto y rápido. Esto ayuda a evitar que se desgarre la abertura.

48. If you anticipate the contractions, you will not feel them so much.
    Si Vd. anticipa la presión, no se siente tanto.

49. At the beginning of the contraction take a deep breath, let it out, and then breathe deeply, slowly, and evenly for the remainder of the contraction.
    Al principio de la contracción haga una aspiración completa y expúlsela (exhálela) y luego respire profunda, lenta y rítmicamente por el resto de la contracción.

50. Abdominal breathing helps keep the abdominal walls relaxed and helps keep them from touching the uterus.
    La respiración abdominal ayuda a mantener las paredes abdominales relajadas y mantener el útero sin tocar (presionar) contra la cavidad abdominal (contra ellas).

51. We are going to move you to the delivery room now that you are dilated.
    Vamos a trasladarla a la sala de partos ya que el cuello de la matriz está completamente dilatado.

52. You are now in the second phase of labor—the expulsion period.
Vd. está en la segunda etapa del parto—el período de expulsión.

53. It is a short phase.
No dura mucho tiempo.

54. With the second stage of labor the muscles of the perineum are flattened or stretched out, the coccyx is pushed back.
Cuando viene la segunda etapa del parto, los músculos del perineo se extienden, el cóccix está bien atrás.

55. When the head is crowning, the doctor does an episiotomy—a simple incision in the area between the vagina and the anus.
Cuando la cabecita está asomando, el doctor (la doctora) le hace la episiotomía—una incisión sencilla en el área entre la vagina y el ano.

56. The episiotomy prevents the rupture or tearing of the perineum and gives the baby more room.
El corte de las partes (la episiotomía) evita la ruptura o un desgarramiento irregular de los tejidos y proporciona más espacio para el bebé.

57. In the delivery room there is a lamp that has a type of mirror so that you can see the child's birth.
En la sala de partos hay una lámpara que contiene una especie de espejos para que Vd. pueda ver cómo aparece el niño.

58. Don't push until you are told.
No puje[6] hasta que se lo diga.

59. Push hard.
Puje[6] con fuerza.

60. Push with the contraction.
Puje[6] con la contracción.

61. Rest between contractions.
Descanse cuando no tenga contracciones.

62. Get ready for another contraction.
Prepárese que ya viene otra contracción.

63. I am going to give you a shot of a local anesthetic which will help you a lot.
Voy a ponerle una inyección de anestesia local que le ayudará mucho.

64. Normally the baby's head comes out with the face downward.
Normalmente la cabeza sale con la cara hacia abajo.

65. I can see the baby's head.
Puedo ver la cabecita del bebé.

66. Your baby is coming in a good position.
Su bebé ya viene en buena posición.

67. The baby's body is turning in order to allow the shoulders to come out.
El cuerpecito del bebé se ladea para dejar salir los hombros.

68. It is a boy!
¡Es varón (niño)!
It is a girl!
¡Es niña!

69. Everything is turning out fine.
Todo sale bien.

70. The nurses will clean the baby up and put an ID on his (her) ankle.
Las enfermeras limpiarán al (a la) bebé y le pondrán identificación en el tobillo.

71. Your uterus is going to contract again now that you are in the third phase of labor—the expulsion of the placenta.
El útero va a contraerse de nuevo ahora que está en la tercera etapa del parto—la expulsión de la placenta (el período placentario).

72. Push.
Puje.[6]

73. You have to push a little bit more still to push out the placenta.
Vd. tiene que pujar[6] un poco más todavía para hacer salir la placenta.

74. I am going to sew you up.
Voy a reparar la incisión ahora.
Voy a coserla ahora.

75. I am going to use dissolving stitches.
Voy a emplear suturas absorbibles.
Voy a utilizar puntos que se absorben.

76. It will not be necessary to remove them.
No hará falta quitarlas.
No será necesario levantarlos.
No será preciso sacarlas.

77. Are you going to nurse the baby?
¿Piensa darle el pecho?
¿Va a amamantarle?

78. If you are going to bottle feed her (him), I am going to give you an injection to dry up your milk.
Si Vd. va a darle biberón, voy a ponerle una inyección para que los senos se sequen y no tengan leche.

79. Your breasts will swell and fill with milk.
Los senos se le hincharán y se llenarán de leche.

80. Wear a good nursing bra both for support and for convenience.
Póngase un buen sostén para amamantar tanto para comodidad como para buen sostén de los pechos.

81. During the first days after birth, you will produce colostrum.
En los primeros días después del parto, le saldrá un líquido de los pezones llamado calostro.

82. Ask the nurse for help.
Pídale ayuda a la enfermera.

83. Your breasts will become painful, and it will help you to wear a breast binder.
Los senos le dolerán, y va a ayudarle a llevar una faja para los pechos.

84. You will need a caesarean.
Necesitará una operación cesárea.

85. I recommend a C (caesarean) section.
Recomiendo una operación cesárea.

86. We are going to have to perform a caesarean.
Tendremos que efectuar una operación cesárea.

87. The baby will be born through an incision in the abdomen, instead of through the birth canal.
Su bebé nacerá a través de una incisión en su abdomen en lugar de por el conducto natal.

88. Your pelvis is too small.
Vd. tiene la pelvis demasiado pequeña.

89. It is a case of placenta previa.
Se trata de placenta previa.
Es un caso de placenta previa.

90. You will have to stay in the hospital a few extra days.
Vd. tendrá que permanecer en el hospital unos días más.

91. After the baby is born, you will be taken to the recovery room.
Después de nacer su niño, se la llevará a la sala de recuperación.

92. When you are back in your own room, tell the nurse if you want to eat, or if the food is no good.[7]
Cuando vuelva a su propio cuarto, dígale a la enfermera si quiere comer o si la comida no le gusta.

93. The dietician will try to plan foods for you to eat that you will like.[7]
La dietista tratará de planear una dieta para Vd. que le guste.

94. You need to begin to think about family planning.[8]
Vd. necesita empezar a pensar en la planificación de familia.

Practice   *Práctica*

Translate into Spanish:

1. You should see an obstetrician.
2. While you are pregnant you should eat a balanced diet.
3. When are you going to give birth?
4. The doctor has the results of your tests.
5. You should avoid strenuous activity.
6. She is having contractions every three minutes.

Tradúzcase al inglés:

1. **Nunca he tenido aborto.**
2. **Tiene que respirar profundamente.**
3. **Pienso darle el pecho a mi nene.**
4. **Vd. debe visitar a su obstétrica regularmente.**
5. **El uso de drogas no recetadas por su médico le hace daño al feto.**
6. **No hay efectos secundarios.**

POSTPARTUM DIALOGUE

Nurse: Good morning, Mrs. López. I am Anita, one of your nurses and a Spanish student. I want to teach you something about cord care for your baby. First, you will need these towelettes or some clean cotton balls and rubbing alcohol.

5   You should clean the umbilical cord well each time that you change her diaper. Clean it from the back, using your fingers in order to move the skin, like this. You do it now, please.

Mrs. Lopez: Like this?

Nurse: Yes. Very good. You may notice that the baby's umbilical cord is purple. Don't worry. During the first hours of life they apply a special medicine called "Tripe Dye" to prevent infection. The cord is going to fall off within two weeks. You should not bathe the baby in water until the cord falls off.

10   You can give the baby a sponge bath until it falls off. Do you have any questions?

Mrs. López: No. Thank you.

DIALOGO POSTPARTO

Enfermera: **Buenos días, señora López. Me llamo Anita. Soy una de sus enfermeras y una estudiante de español. Quiero enseñarle algo acerca del cuidado del cordón del ombligo de su bebé. Primero, Vd. necesita estas toallitas o unas bolas de algodón limpias y alcohol**

5   de fricción. Debe limpiarlo bien cada vez que cambie el pañal. Límpielo desde el fondo utilizando los dedos para mover la piel, así. Ahora, hágalo Vd., por favor.

Señora López: ¿De esta manera?

Enfermera: Sí. Muy bien. Puede notar que el cordón del ombligo de su bebé es de color morado. No se preocupe. Durante las primeras horas de vida, se aplica una medicina especial que se llama «Tripe Dye» (tinta triple) para prevenir infección. El cordón va a caerse dentro de dos semanas. Vd. no debe meter a la bebé en una tina de agua hasta que se caiga el cordón. Puede bañar a la bebé con una esponja hasta que se caiga el cordón.

10   ¿Tiene Vd. preguntas?

Señora López: No. Gracias.

SURGERY

CIRUGIA

PRE-OP *ANTES DE LA OPERACION*

1. You need an operation.[9]
   Vd. necesita una operación.

2. It is not a serious operation.
   No es una operación grave.

3. It is a very serious operation.
   Es una operación muy grave.

4. We have to operate on your ____[10] so that you will get well.
   Es necesario hacerle una operación de ____ para que se mejore.

5. There can be no delay. We have to operate on you/him/her immediately.
   No puede haber demora. Tenemos que operarle [operarla] inmediatamente.

6. Your surgery is scheduled for ____.
   La operación está programada para el + *day of week*.[11]

7. We are going to sew up your wound.
   Vamos a coserle la herida.

8. We are going to remove your appendix.
   Vamos a sacarle el apéndice.

9. We think that we may have to remove part of your stomach.
   Pensamos que es preciso sacarle una parte del estómago.

10. We have to amputate your leg (arm, finger).
    Tenemos que amputarle la pierna (el brazo, el dedo).

11. We cannot do this unless you give us your written permission.[12]
    No podemos operar sin su permiso escrito. Hay que firmar el permiso para operar.

12. This should be a rather simple operation.
    Esta operación va a ser bastante sencilla.

13. We expect that everything will be fine, but we cannot be absolutely sure.
    Esperamos que todo esté bien, pero no se puede estar completamente seguro.

14. Do you understand?[13]
    ¿Me comprende Vd.?

15. Are you certain that you understand me? Do you have any questions?
    ¿Está seguro (segura) de que me comprende? ¿Tiene Vd. algunas preguntas para mí?

16. Please sign your name here.[12]
    Firme Vd. su nombre aquí, por favor.

17. I am going to make arrangements with the hospital.
    Voy a hacer los arreglos en el hospital.

18. You will go to the hospital on ___[11]
    Vd. se internará en el hospital el ____.

19. Do you have any X-rays to bring?
    ¿Tiene Vd. algunas radiografías?

20. Take your hospitalization and insurance papers with you.
    Lleve Vd. sus papeles de hospitalización y seguros consigo.

21. We will notify your family of the approximate time that your operation is scheduled.
    Le avisaremos a su familia de la hora aproximada en que está programada la operación.

22. Your family may come to see you before the operation and accompany you to the surgical floor.
    Su familia puede venir a verle antes de la operación y acompañarle al piso quirúrgico.

23. Would you like me to call your family to tell them about your operation?
    ¿Quiere Vd. que yo avise a su familia (acerca) de su operación?[9]

24. We intend to operate tomorrow, but we may have to postpone it until the next day.
    Pensamos operar mañana, pero quizás sea necesario cambiarla hasta el día siguiente.

25. The surgery will be at 6 A.M., and you will be in the recovery room by 9 A.M.
    La cirugía será a las seis de la mañana, y Vd. estará en la sala de recuperación a eso de las nueve de la mañana.

26. We do not know exactly how long the surgery will take; it could be several hours.
    No sabemos exactamente cuánto tiempo durará la cirugía; podría ser un par de horas.

27. I am going to prepare you for the operation.
    Voy a prepararle (prepararla) para la operación.

28. The nurse will give you an enema.
    La enfermera le pondrá una enema.[14]

29. You will feel better after the enema.[15]
    Vd. se sentirá mejor después de la enema.

30. I have to shave you.
    Tengo que rasurarle (rasurarla).

31. I am going to shave you.
    Voy a rasurarle (rasurarla).

32. The patient is in a lot of pain.
    El (La) paciente tiene mucho dolor.

33. This injection will stop your pain.
    Esta inyección le quitará el dolor.

34. You won't feel the pain.
    Vd. no sentirá el dolor.

35. Just relax.
    No se apure.

36. You can't have these injections too often.
    No se le pueden poner estas inyecciones con demasiada frecuencia.

37. We are going to take you to the operating room on this gurney.
    Vamos a llevarlo (llevarla) al quirófano (a la sala de operaciones) con esta camilla.

38. We have to move you onto this gurney now.
    Necesitamos moverlo (moverla) a esta camilla ahora.

39. Don't try to help. We will move you.
    No trate de ayudar. Lo (La) moveremos.

40. Has someone already taken a sample of your blood?
    ¿Le sacaron una muestra de sangre ya?

41. Did you get a shot/injection before coming to the operating room?
    ¿Le pusieron una inyección antes de venir al quirófano?

42. Have you removed your . . .
    ¿Se quitó . . .
    dentures?
    la dentadura postiza?
    nail polish?
    su esmalte para las uñas?

43. Have you taken out your contact lenses?
    ¿Se le quitaron los lentes de contacto?

44. Are you wearing any jewelry? You must take them off.
    ¿Usa alhajas/joyas? Debe quitárselas.

45. Are you cold?
    ¿Tiene frío?

46. Do you need another blanket?
    ¿Necesita otra manta?
    ¿Le falta otra frazada?

47. How are you feeling?
    ¿Cómo se siente?

48. Don't be nervous.
    No se ponga nervioso (nerviosa).

49. Don't be afraid.
    No tenga miedo.

50. You will feel fine . . .
    Vd. se sentirá bien . . .
    soon.
    dentro de poco.
    during the procedure.
    durante el procedimiento.
    after the operation.
    después de la operación.

51. Don't worry if you cannot urinate after the operation; the nurse will empty your bladder.
    No se apure Vd. si no puede orinar después de la cirugía; la enfermera le vaciará la vejiga.

52. We will put a tube in your bladder so that you can urinate.
    Le pondremos un tubo en la vejiga para que pueda orinar.

53. I am going to start these fluids in your vein.[16]
    Voy a ponerle estos flúidos (este suero) en la vena.

54. You will feel a little stick.
    Vd. va a sentir un piquete.

55. It may hurt a little, but we have to do it in order to help you.
    Puede dolerle un poco (Sentirá la aguja un poco), pero tenemos que hacerlo para ayudarle (ayudarla).

56. This IV is in your arm in order to feed you.
    Tiene este suero en el brazo para alimentarle (alimentarla).

57. This IV in your arm is to give you sugar, water, and salt through your veins.
    Este suero en el brazo es para darle azúcar, agua y sal por las venas.

58. The IV must stay there for a while after the operation.
    El suero tiene que quedarse ahí por algún tiempo después de la operación.

59. Please do not remove it.
    No se lo quite, por favor.

60. After the operation the IV must stay in your arm until you begin to eat and drink.
    Después de la cirugía, el suero tiene que quedarse en el brazo hasta que empiece a comer y beber.

61. If you do not eat (drink), we will have to put the IV back into your arm.
    Si Vd. no come (bebe), tendremos que ponerle el suero en el brazo de nuevo.

62. After the operation you may have a tube in your stomach so you will not vomit.
Después de la operación, es posible que tenga un tubo en el estómago para que no vomite.

63. The surgeon has just arrived.
El cirujano (La cirujana) acaba de llegar.

ANESTHESIA   *ANESTESIA*

1. The anesthesiologist will be here soon to discuss what anesthesia (s)he is going to give you.
El anestesiólogo (La anestesióloga) estará aquí dentro de poco para discutir qué anestesia va a ponerle.

2. I am Dr. ____ from the Anesthesiology Department at ____ Hospital.
Soy el (la) Dr(a). ____ del Departamento de Anestesiología al Hospital de ____.

3. I have to ask you some questions about your health in order to be able to make decisions about the anesthesia for your surgery.
Tengo que hacerle unas preguntas acerca de su salud para poder tomar una decisión en cuanto a la anestesia para su cirugía.

4. Have you had surgery before?
¿Ha tenido una cirugía antes?
¿Ha tenido alguna operación anteriormente?

5. For what? When was it? Where was it?
¿Para qué? ¿Cuándo fue? ¿Dónde ocurrió?

6. What type of anesthesia have you had?
¿Qué clase de anestesia ha tenido Vd.?
General anesthesia?
¿Anestesia general?
Local anesthesia?
¿Anestesia local?
Epidural anesthesia?
¿Anestesia epidural?
Spinal anesthesia?
¿Anestesia espinal?

7. Have you or anyone in your family ever had problems with anesthesia?
¿Ha tenido Vd. o algún miembro de su familia problemas con anestesia?

8. Are you taking any medicine? What type? What for?
¿Toma medicina? ¿Qué tipo? ¿Para qué?

9. What are the names of the medicines?
¿Cuáles son los nombres de las medicinas?

10. What is the name of the medicine?
¿Cuál es el nombre de la medicina?

11. What are the medicines for?[17]
¿Para qué son las medicinas?

12. What is the medicine for?[17]
¿Para qué es la medicina?

13. Do you have any difficulty taking medication?
¿Tiene difficultades al tomar las medicinas?

14. Do you have any allergies?
¿Tiene Vd. alergias?

15. Are you allergic to anything?
¿Es Vd. alérgico (alérgica) a algo?
Penicillin?
¿Penicilina?
Any medicines?
¿Cualquier medicina?
Any medication?
¿Algún medicamento?
Foods?
¿Alimentos?
Insect bites?
¿Picaduras de insectos?

16. Do you smoke? What do you smoke? How many do you smoke each day?
¿Fuma Vd.? ¿Qué fuma? ¿Cuánto fuma por día?

17. Do you drink alcohol?
¿Toma Vd. alcohol?

18. How many drinks a day do you have?
¿Cuántos tragos por día toma Vd.?

19. Do you have . . .
¿Sufre . . .
AIDS?
del SIDA?
diabetes?
de diabetis?
epilepsy or seizures?
de epilepsia o ataques?
heart trouble?
del corazón?
chest pains?
de dolores del pecho?
breathing problems?
de problemas al respirar?
asthma?
de asma?
high blood pressure?
de la presión alta?
kidney problems?
del riñon?
thyroid disease?
de enfermedad de la tiroide?

20. Do you take or have you taken steroids recently?
¿Toma o ha tomado esteroides recientemente?

21. Do you have a cold?
¿Tiene Vd. resfriado?

22. How tall are you?
¿Cuánto mide Vd.?

23. How many feet?
¿Cuántos pies de altura?

24. How many inches?
    ¿Cuántas pulgadas?

25. How much do you weigh?
    ¿Cuánto pesa Vd.?

26. Do you have a(ny) . . .
    ¿Tiene Vd. . . .
    loose teeth?
    dientes flojos?
    false teeth?
    dientes postizos?
    glass eye?
    ojo postizo?
    removable bridges?
    puentes movibles?
    crowns / caps
    coronas / casquillos dentales?

27. We will try to be careful, but sometimes false teeth, bridges, or caps/crowns get damaged under anesthesia.
    Vamos a tratar de tener mucho cuidado, pero a veces los dientes postizos, los puentes, o los casquillos/las coronas dentales se dañan con la anestesia.

28. I have to listen to your chest.
    Tengo que auscultarle el pecho.

29. Breathe deeply.
    Respire profundo.

30. Inhale.
    Inspire Vd.
    Inhale Vd.

31. Exhale.
    Exhale Vd.

32. Very good.
    Muy bien.

33. Here is a list of instructions that you must follow for your surgery.[18]
    Aquí tiene Vd. una lista de instrucciones que tiene que seguir para la cirugía.

34. When was the last time you ate?
    ¿Cuándo fue la última vez que comió?

35. Do not eat or drink anything after midnight by mouth.
    No coma ni beba nada por la boca después de medianoche.

36. You must not eat or drink anything after midnight.
    Vd. no debe ni comer ni beber nada después de medianoche.

37. We are going to give you a sedative before taking you to the operating room.
    Vamos a darle un calmante antes de llevarle (llevarla) a la sala de operaciones.

38. I am going to give you a pill to make you sleep.
    Voy a darle una píldora para hacerle dormir.

39. I am going to put you to sleep while the doctors perform the operation.
    Voy a ponerle a dormir mientras que los médicos realicen la operación.

40. You will wake up when the surgery has finished.
    Vd. va a despertarse cuando la cirugía se haya terminado.

41. When you awaken after the operation, you may have a tube in your throat to help you breathe.
    Al despertarse después de la cirugía, es posible que tenga un tubo en la garganta para ayudarle (ayudarla) a respirar.

42. When you wake up, your throat may feel a little sore, but it will get better.
    Al despertarse, su garanta podrá estar un poco dolorida, pero se mejorará.

43. We are taking you to the operating room now.
    Le (La) llevamos al quirófano ahora.

44. Can you move onto this gurney?
    ¿Puede moverse para esta camilla?

45. We are going to move you onto this gurney.
    Vamos a moverle (moverla) para esta camilla.

46. Move over here, please.
    Muévase para acá por favor.

47. Move up.
    Muévase hacia arriba.

48. Move down.
    Muévase hacia abajo.

49. A little more.
    Un poco más.

50. Lie down.
    Acuéstese, por favor.

51. Uncross your legs.
    Descruce las piernas, por favor.

52. Raise your head.
    Levante la cabeza.

53. Lower your head.
    Baje la cabeza.

54. I am going to put a blood pressure cuff on your arm.
    Voy a ponerle alrededor del brazo un instrumento para medir la presión arterial (la presión sanguínea).

55. It will be taking your blood pressure during the surgery.
    Va a medirle la presión arterial durante la cirugía.

56. This is going to feel tight for just a few minutes.
    Esto va a sentirle apretado por solamente unos minutos.

57. Try to relax. Don't worry. We will take (very) good care of you.
    Trate de relajar. No se preocupe. Vamos a cuidarle (cuidarla) (muy) bien.

58. I am going to give you oxygen with this little mask.
Voy a administrarle oxígeno con esta mascarilla.

59. It won't bother you.
No le molestará.

60. I am going to give you a drug through this mask.
Voy a ponerle una droga por medio de esta máscara.

61. Breathe naturally through the mask.
Respire Vd. naturalmente por la máscara.

62. Take a deep breath.
Respire Vd. profundo.

63. Again.
Otra vez.

64. You will fall asleep soon and be asleep during the surgery.
Vd. se dormirá dentro de poco y estará dormido (dormida) durante la cirugía.

65. You are going to start to feel sleepy.
Va a empezar a tener sueño.

66. Do you feel sleepy?
¿Se siente con sueño?

67. You are going to sleep now.
Vd. va a dormir ahora.

68. Count backwards from one hundred.
Cuente del uno al cien al revés.

69. One hundred, ninety-nine, ninety-eight . . .
Ciento, noventa y nueve, noventa y ocho . . .

70. Perhaps I will use a local anesthetic.
Tal vez usaré anestesia local.

71. I am going to give you a local anesthetic—a shot so that you will feel no pain during the operation.
Voy a ponerle un anestésico local—una inyección para que no sienta ningún dolor durante la operación.

72. I am going to give you some medicine to put your ____ to sleep so the doctors can perform the surgery.
    arm
    legs
    body
Voy a poner alguna medicina que le adormecerá(n) ____ para que los médicos puedan realizar la cirugía.
    brazo
    piernas
    cuerpo

73. You will not feel any pain.
Usted no sentirá ningún dolor.

74. You will be awake in the operating room, but you will not feel any pain.
Estará despierto (despierta) en el quirófano (la sala de operaciones), pero no sentirá ningún dolor.

75. Perhaps I will give you spinal anesthesia.
Tal vez le pondré anestesia espinal.

76. You will not be able to move. Do not be afraid. It is only temporary.
Usted no podrá moverse. No tenga miedo. Es solamente algo transitorio.

77. I am going to give you a spinal anesthetic (an epidural, a caudal).
Voy a ponerle anestesia espinal (anestesia epidural, anestesia caudal).

78. I am going to inject a drug into your back so that you will not feel pain during the operation, but you will not be asleep.
Voy a inyectarle una droga en la espalda, para que no sienta ningún dolor durante la operación, pero Vd. no estará dormido (dormida).

79. Please turn on your right (left) side at the edge of your bed.
Acuéstese Vd. sobre el lado derecho (izquierdo), muy cerca del borde de la cama.

80. Bend forward.
Dóblese hacia adelante.

81. Bring your knees up to your chest and bend your head down, so that your chin rests on your chest.
Doble Vd. las rodillas junto al pecho e incline la cabeza de modo que la barbilla esté junto al pecho.

82. Push your back out toward me (the doctor).
Empuje[6] la espalda hacia mí (el doctor/la doctora).

83. That's right.
Así. Bien.

84. Hold still.
No se mueva, por favor.
Quédese inmóvil.

85. That is all.
Eso es todo.

86. You may relax now.
Vd. puede relajarse[4] ahora.

87. Can you feel your legs?
¿Puede sentir las piernas?

88. Do your legs feel normal?
¿Siente Vd. las piernas normales?

89. Have your legs gone numb?
¿Se le han dormido las piernas?

90. Can you feel this?
¿Puede sentir esto?

91. Is this sharp?
¿Es esto agudo?

92. Can you move your feet?
¿Puede mover los pies?

93. Can you wiggle your toes?
¿Puede menear (mover) los dedos de los pies?

94. We are going to put your legs up.
    Vamos a levantarle las piernas.

95. I will be at the operation.
    Asistiré a la operación.

96. I will come to see you after the operation.
    Vendré a verle (verla) después de la operación.

97. Stretch your legs.
    Extienda las piernas.

98. Is this painful?
    ¿Le duele esto?

99. Is this more painful than this? The same? More? Less?
    ¿Le duele esto más que esto? ¿Lo mismo?
    ¿Más? ¿Menos?

100. Tell me when you feel pain, not just pressure.
     Dígame cuando sienta dolor, no sólo presión.

101. I am going to place a ground plate under your hip.
     Voy a ponerle una placa antieléctrica debajo de la cadera.

102. I am sorry that it is cold and sticky.
     Siento que estará fría y pegajosa.

103. It will warm up soon and you won't realize it is there.
     Se calentará pronto y no se dará cuenta de que está allí.

PRE-ANESTHETIC CONFERENCE

	Anesthesiologist:	Good evening, Mr. Rojas. I am Dr. Martínez. I will be giving you the anesthesia for your hernia operation tomorrow.
	Patient:	Good evening, doctor.
5	Anest.:	I have a few things that I would like to discuss with you, and also some questions. Have you ever had surgery before?
	Pat.:	Yes, doctor. I had my gallbladder removed.
	Anesthesiologist:	When was your gallbladder removed, and do you know what type of anesthesia you were given?
10	Pat.:	It was five years ago. They put me to sleep. It was done at the ABC Hospital in Mexico City.
	Anesthesiologist:	Were there any complications—either from anesthesia or from surgery?
	Pat.:	Well, I had a sore throat and was hoarse for about two days.
	Anesthesiologist:	That was probably due to the endotracheal tube which was inserted into your windpipe right after you went to sleep, and withdrawn just before you were awakened.
15	Pat.:	Will that happen again?
	Anesthesiologist:	It is unlikely, but always a possibility. I am an expert when it comes to intubation—that is, putting the tube in the larynx. Were there any other complications?
	Pat.:	No.
	Anesthesiologist:	Okay. Are you allergic to any medicines, foods, or drugs?
20	Pat.:	I am allergic to penicillin.
	Anesthesiologist:	What happens when you take penicillin?
	Pat.:	I break out in a rash on my body.
	Anesthesiologist:	Have you ever had any heart problems?
25	Pat.:	Yes. I suffered a heart attack 2 years ago. I was hospitalized in CICU for 9 days, and in a regular room for another week. Also, from time to time I suffer from angina.
	Anesthesiologist:	Are you under a doctor's care now? And do you take any medicine?
	Pat.:	Yes, I see Dr. Cárdenas every month. I take Inderal four times a day.
	Anesthesiologist:	How many milligrams?
	Pat.:	20 milligrams.
30	Anesthesiologist:	Do you take other medications?
	Pat.:	I take two Lasix tablets (80 mgs) at 8:00 A.M. and at 2:00 P.M. I take an additional tablet. I also take two Isordil pills when I suffer an angina attack or when I'm in a situation which I think will cause an attack.
	Anesthesiologist:	How many milligrams do you take?
35	Pat.:	I don't remember.
	Anesthesiologist:	Don't worry. What color are the pills?
	Pat.:	They're pink.
	Anesthesiologist:	Do your ankles swell?
40	Pat.:	Yes, sometimes at the end of the day. My feet swell when it is warm, or when I sit for a long time.
	Anesthesiologist:	Does the swelling go away in the morning?
	Pat.:	Yes.

	Anesthesiologist:	You do use pillows at night, don't you?
	Pat.:	Yes. I sleep with 2 pillows under my head and shoulders.
45	Anesthesiologist:	Do you wake up during the night feeling as if you can't breathe?
	Pat.:	Yes, but when I sit up, it goes away almost immediately.
	Anesthesiologist:	How many times do you get up to go to the bathroom after you've gone to bed?
	Pat.:	Four times, usually.
	Anesthesiologist:	When you walk, do you have cramps or pains in your legs?
50	Pat.:	Occasionally. But only when I climb stairs or go uphill. The pains stop when I stop to rest.
	Anesthesiologist:	Do you get these pains when you are in bed?
	Pat.:	No.
	Anesthesiologist:	Have you had any other major medical problems? Have you ever had problems with your lungs, muscles, tumors, etc.?
55	Pat.:	No.
	Anesthesiologist:	Do you smoke?
	Pat.:	A little bit.
	Anesthesiologist:	How many cigarettes do you smoke per day?
	Pat.:	Only 1 or 2 since the heart attack.
60	Anesthesiologist:	Well, you must not do any smoking before your surgery. I would like you to walk down the hall with me. . .Fine. Now, let's walk up a flight of stairs. . . Okay. Let's go back to your room and talk more.
65		Mr. Rojas, frankly, it is my opinion that it would be a risk for you to have an operation now. There are some aspects of your health that should be first. I would like to postpone this surgery for a week until we can stabilize your heart problems.
	Pat.:	Does that mean that I can go home?
	Anesthesiologist:	No. You will remain here in the hospital. We are going to change your medicine and digitalize you. We will give you Lanoxin until your heart is working better. Then we will reschedule the surgery. Your internist will give you more information about the new medicines.
70	Pat.:	Thank you, doctor.

[A week later Dr. Martínez is back in Mr. Rojas' room.]

	Anesthesiologist:	I want to explain to you a little more about what will be happening before and after the surgery which will be tomorrow at 11:00. You may not eat or drink anything after midnight tonight. There will be a sign on your bed, and the nurses will not give you anything until after the operation. This is VERY IMPORTANT. If you disobey and eat or drink anything after midnight, tomorrow when you are under the anesthesia, what you have eaten or drunk may be regurgitated into your mouth and then breathed into your lungs. This could cause pneumonia, and even be fatal. Tomorrow morning you will not get breakfast. A nurse will awaken you about 6:30 A.M. You will go to the bathroom, brush your teeth, shower, and then get back into bed by 7:00 A.M. Someone will come to shave your abdominal area. Later someone will give you an enema. The nurse will start an IV. The glucose serum will give you liquid nourishment. Are you right-handed or left?
75		
80		
	Pat.:	Right.
	Anesthesiologist:	Then, we will try to use your left arm for the IV. I will also prescribe a shot to sedate you. This will be given either in your arm or in your buttocks. The orderlies will take you down to the waiting area outside the O.R.
85		
	Pat.:	What will happen then?
	Anesthesiologist:	They will bring you into the O.R. and move you onto the operating table. I will be in there near your head at all times. I will have a mask on. When you are on the operating table, I will attach a blood-pressure cuff to your right arm so that I can take your blood pressure. I will also put E.C.G. leads on your chest. In this way I will be able to watch your heart rhythm. I will inject the anesthetics into the IV to put you to sleep.
90		
	Pat.:	I don't understand what you mean, doctor.
	Anesthesiologist:	I will put a drug called sodium pentothal into the tube. You will go to sleep within seconds. Then I will add other drugs that you get through the (IV) tubing. This will keep you asleep during the operation. I will awaken you by reversing or withdrawing the drugs. Before you are awake, I will take out the tube in your windpipe.
95		
	Pat.:	How long will I be asleep?
	Anesthesiologist:	Between 45 minutes and 1 hour. After the operation you will be placed on a gurney and brought to the recovery room. You will be there several hours. There the nurses will check your reactions every 15 minutes, encourage you to cough and take deep breaths. It
100		

is important for you to expand your lungs. You will probably have post-operative pain. If it hurts too much, ask the nurse for something to stop the pain (a painkiller).

	Pat.:	Will you give me a pill to take?
105	Anesthesiologist:	No, you might throw up from the pill and water. You will either get the pain medicine through the tube or via a shot intramuscularly. Don't worry! It is normal. When we are sure that you are stable, you will return to your room.
	Pat.:	Is this a very dangerous operation? Will I die while I'm in the O.R.?
110	Anesthesiologist:	I don't think so. The operation itself is a simple repair. Do you want me to discuss the risks and problems that could occur?
	Pat.:	No, thank you, doctor. I'd rather not know. Oh, will I be able to eat food if I am hungry?
115	Anesthesiologist:	Your physician will probably order a liquid diet for you at first. He may keep the IV going until he is certain that you can take a sufficient amount of fluids orally. Gradually you will return to your normal diet, which in your case is low salt and low fat. Do you have any other questions?
	Pat.:	No, thank you for your explanation.
	Anesthesiologist:	Well, then, I'll see you in the morning, Mr. Rojas. Don't worry. Everything will be all right.

UNA CONFERENCIA PRE-ANESTETICA

	Anestesiólogo:	Buenas tardes, Sr. Rojas. Soy el Dr. Martínez. Mañana le administraré la anestesia para la operación de su hernia.
	Paciente:	Muy buenas, doctor.
5	Anestesiólogo:	Quisiera hablar con Vd. acerca de algunos asuntos. También quiero hacerle unas preguntas. ¿Ha tenido alguna operación anteriormente?
	Paciente:	Sí, doctor. Me operaron la vesícula biliar.
	Anestesiólogo:	¿Cuándo fue que le operaron la vesícula biliar? ¿Sabe qué tipo de anestesia le dieron?
10	Paciente:	Fue hace cinco años. Me durmieron. (Me dieron una anestesia general.) Lo hicieron en el hospital ABC en la Ciudad de México.
	Anestesiólogo:	¿Hubo complicaciones o en la anestesia o en la cirugía?
	Paciente:	Pues, me dolió la garganta y estuve ronco por dos días más o menos.
	Anestesiólogo:	Eso sería por el tubo [endotráqueo] que le fue introducido en la tráquea tan pronto como Vd. se durmió y quitado poco antes de que le despertaran.
15	Paciente:	¿Eso sucederá de nuevo?
	Anestesiólogo:	No es probable, pero siempre es una posibilidad. Me especializo en la intubación—eso es, insertar el tubo en la laringe. ¿Tuvo otras complicaciones?
	Paciente:	No.
	Anestesiólogo:	Está bien. ¿Es Vd. alérgico a algunas medicinas, alimentos o drogas?
20	Paciente:	Soy alérgico a la penicilina.
	Anestesiólogo:	¿Qué le pasa cuando Vd. la toma?
	Paciente:	Me brotan granos por todo el cuerpo.
	Anestesiólogo:	¿Alguna vez ha tenido problemas cardíacos?
25	Paciente:	Sí, sufrí un ataque cardíaco hace dos años. Estuve en la unidad de cuidados intensivos coronarios por nueve días, y en un cuarto ordinario por una semana adicional. También, de vez en cuando sufro de angina.
	Anestesiólogo:	¿Le atiende ahora un médico? ¿Y toma medicina?
	Paciente:	Sí, tengo turnos con el Dr. Cárdenas cada mes. Tomo Inderal cuatro veces al día.
	Anestesiólogo:	¿Cuántos miligramos?
30	Paciente:	Veinte miligramos.
	Anestesiólogo:	¿Toma Vd. otras medicinas?
35	Paciente:	Tomo dos tabletas de Lasix (80 mgs.) a las ocho de la mañana y a las dos de la tarde tomo otra tableta adicional. También tomo dos píldoras de Isordil cuando sufro un ataque de angina o cuando estoy en una situación la cual creo que me causará un ataque.
	Anestesiólogo:	¿Cuántos miligramos toma Vd.?
	Paciente:	No me acuerdo.
	Anestesiólogo:	No se preocupe. ¿De qué color son estas píldoras?
	Paciente:	Son rosadas.
40	Anestesiólogo:	¿Se le hinchan los tobillos?
	Paciente:	Sí, algunas veces al final del día. Se me hinchan los pies cuando hace calor o cuando me siento por mucho tiempo.

	Anestesiólogo:	¿Se va la hinchazón por la mañana?
	Paciente:	Sí.
45	Anestesiólogo:	Vd. usa almohadas por la noche, ¿no?
	Paciente:	Sí, duermo con dos almohadas debajo de la cabeza y los hombros.
	Anestesiólogo:	¿Se despierta por la noche con la sensación de no poder respirar?
	Paciente:	Sí, pero cuando me levanto, se me quita casi en seguida.
	Anestesiólogo:	¿Cuántas veces se levanta para ir al baño después de acostarse?
50	Paciente:	Cuatro veces, por lo general.
	Anestesiólogo:	Cuando Vd. anda, ¿tiene calambres o dolores en las piernas?
	Paciente:	A veces, pero sólo al subir escaleras o al ir cuesta arriba. Los dolores se van cuando me detengo a descansar.
	Anestesiólogo:	¿Ocurren estos dolores cuando Vd. esté en la cama?
55	Paciente:	No.
	Anestesiólogo:	¿Ha tenido otros problemas médicos importantes? ¿Jamás ha tenido problemas con los pulmones, músculos, tumores, etc.?
	Paciente:	No.
	Anestesiólogo:	¿Fuma Vd.?
60	Paciente:	Un poco.
	Anestesiólogo:	¿Cuántos cigarillos o puros fuma Vd. por día?
	Paciente:	No fumo más de 1 o 2 cigarillos diarios desde el ataque cardíaco.
	Anestesiólogo:	Pues, tiene que dejar de fumar antes de su operación. Quiero que Vd. ande por el pasillo conmigo . . . Bien. Ahora. Subamos un tramo de escalera . . . Bien. Regresemos a su cuarto y hablemos más.
65		
		Francamente, Sr. Rojas, es mi opinión que sería un riesgo para Vd. tener una operación ya. Hay algunos aspectos de su salud que deben ser mejorados antes. Quisiera aplazar esta operación por una semana hasta poder estabilizar sus problemas cardíacos. Pare de fumar hasta después de la cirugía, por favor.
	Paciente:	¿Eso quiere decir que me voy a casa?
70	Anestesiólogo:	No. Vd. se quedará aquí en el hospital. Vamos a cambiar su medicina y digitalizarle (hacerle una cura de digital a la dosis y por el tiempo que sea necesaria para la producción de sus efectos terapéuticos). Le daremos Lanoxin hasta que funcione mejor el corazón. Entonces, fijaremos de nuevo la hora de la cirugía. Su internista le dará más informes acerca de las medicinas nuevas.
75	Paciente:	Gracias, doctor.
		(Una semana más tarde el doctor está de nuevo en el cuarto del Sr. Rojas.)
	Anestesiólogo:	Quiero explicarle un poco más respecto a lo que pasará antes y después de la operación que será mañana a las once de la mañana. Se le prohibe comer o beber algo esta noche después de medianoche. Habrá un aviso en su cama, y las enfermeras no le darán nada hasta después de la operación. Esto es importantísimo. Si desobedece y come o bebe algo después de medianoche, mañana cuando se le anestesie, le podrá venir a la boca lo que haya tomado y esto puede ser aspirado y alojado en los pulmones. Esto puede provocar la pulmonía y aun podrá ser fatal. Mañana por la mañana no desayunará. Una enfermera le despertará a eso de las seis y media. Vd. irá al baño, se cepillará los dientes, se duchará y volverá a acostarse antes de las siete. Alguien vendrá a afeitarle el abdomen. Más tarde se le pondrá una enema. La enfermera le colocará un suero intravenoso. El suero de glucosa le dará alimento líquido. ¿Usa Vd. la mano derecha o la izquierda?
80		
85		
	Paciente:	Uso la derecha.
90	Anestesiólogo:	Por eso trataremos de usar el brazo izquierdo para el suero. También, recetaré una inyección para hacerle dormir. Se le pondrá esta inyección o en el brazo o en la nalga. Los asistentes (del hospital) le llevarán al área de espera afuera del quirófano.
	Paciente:	¿Qué sucederá después?
	Anestesiólogo:	Le llevarán dentro del quirófano y le pondrán sobre la mesa de operaciones. Estaré allí cerca de su cabeza todo el tiempo. Llevaré puesto una máscara. Cuando Vd. esté encima de la mesa de operaciones, le pondré un instrumento para medir la presión arterial alrededor del brazo derecho [para medir la presión sanguínea.]. También le pondré los terminales del electrocardiograma sobre el pecho. Así podré revisar el ritmo del corazón. Entonces le pondré una inyección de anestesia por vía intravenosa para hacerle dormir en seguida.
95		
100		

	Paciente:	No entiendo lo que Vd. quiere decir, doctor.
	Anestesiólogo:	Pondré una droga llamada pentotal de sodio en el tubo del suero. Se dormirá casi en seguida. Entonces, añadiré otras drogas que Vd. recibe por el suero. Esto le mantendrá dormido durante toda la operación. Le despertaré al invertir o quitarle las drogas. Antes de que Vd. se despierte, le sacaré el tubo de la tráquea.

105

	Paciente:	¿Por cuánto tiempo dormiré?
	Anestesiólogo:	Entre cuarenta y cinco minutos y una hora. Después de la operación, le trasladarán a una camilla de ruedas y le llevarán a la sala de recuperación. Vd. se quedará allí por varias horas. Allí las enfermeras estarán al tanto de sus reacciones cada quince minutos, le aconsejarán que tosa y respire profundamente. Es importante que Vd. dilate los pulmones. Es probable que Vd. tenga dolor después de la operación. Si le duele demasiado, pida algo que detenga el dolor (un remedio contra el dolor) a la enfermera.
	Paciente:	¿Me dará una píldora para tomar?
	Anestesiólogo:	No. Vomitaría de la píldora y el agua. Vd. recibirá la medicina para el dolor o por el tubo o por una inyección intramuscular. No se preocupe. Esto es normal. Cuando estemos seguros de que Vd. está estable, regresará a su cuarto.
	Paciente:	¿Es ésta una operación muy peligrosa? ¿Me moriré en el quirófano?
	Anestesiólogo:	No hay mucha posibilidad. La operación es una reparación sencilla. ¿Quiere que le explique los riesgos y los problemas que puedan ocurrir?
	Paciente:	Gracias, pero no, doctor. Prefiero no saber. A propósito, ¿podré tomar comida sólida si tengo hambre?
	Anestesiólogo:	Su médico probablemente le indicará una dieta de líquidos al principio. El puede continuarle el suero hasta estar seguro de que Vd. pueda tomar una cantidad suficiente de líquidos por la boca. Poco a poco volverá a su dieta normal, que es, en su caso, dieta con escaso contenido de sal y escaso contenido graso. ¿Tiene Vd. algunas otras preguntas?
	Paciente:	No, gracias por sus explicaciones.
	Anestesiólogo:	Pues, entonces le veré mañana por la mañana, Sr. Rojas. No se preocupe. Todo saldrá bien.

110 — 115 — 120 — 125

Preguntas

1. ¿Cuál es el problema del Sr. Rojas? ¿Por qué está en el hospital?
2. ¿Cuándo piensan hacerle la operación?
3. ¿Quién es el Dr. Martínez? ¿Por qué habla con el Sr. Rojas?
4. ¿Tiene el Sr. Rojas alguna alergia?
5. ¿Es grave la condición cardíaca del Sr. Rojas?
6. ¿Qué píldoras toma para su problema cardíaco? ¿Cuánto le toma generalmente?
7. ¿Qué le pasa al Sr. Rojas al subir las escaleras?
8. ¿Qué decide hacer el anestesiólogo?
9. ¿Le darán el desayuno la mañana de la operación? ¿Por qué no?
10. ¿Hasta qué hora podrá comer?
11. ¿Qué le recetará el anestesiólogo antes de bajarle a la sala de operaciones.
12. ¿En qué parte del cuerpo van a ponerle la inyección?
13. ¿Qué piensa determinar el anestesiólogo con los terminales del electrocardiograma?
14. ¿Qué le pasará al paciente al recibir pentotal de sodio?
15. ¿Cuánto tiempo durará la operación?
16. ¿Habrá efectos secundarios de la anestesia? ¿Cuáles pueden ser?
17. ¿Qué hacen las enfermeras en la sala de recuperación?

Situations

**You are an anesthesiologist. Your patient is a child. Find out about allergies, reactions, and previous illnesses and operations from the parent.

**You are going to have an operation tomorrow. Tell the anesthesiologist what you are allergic to, about your previous operations and a little medical history.

POST-OP *DESPUES DE LA OPERACION*

1. The operation turned out all right.
   La operación salió bien.

2. Wake up.
   Despiértese.

3. You are waking up.
   Vd. está despertándose.

4. You will feel better soon.
   Vd. se sentirá mejor dentro de poco.

5. The patient is out of danger.
    El (La) paciente está fuera de peligro.

6. You are out of danger.
    Vd. está fuera de peligro.

7. The patient is not expected to live.
    No se cree que el (la) paciente vaya a vivir.

8. The patient is going to live.
    El (La) paciente va a vivir.

9. You are going to live.
    Vd. va a vivir.
    Vd. vivirá.

10. The patient has been taken to the Recovery Room.
    El paciente ha sido llevado a la sala de recuperación.

11. The patient has been taken to the Intensive Care (Cardiac Care) Unit.
    La paciente ha sido llevada a la Unidad del Cuidado Intensivo (del Cuidado Cardíaco).

12. He (She/You) will leave Intensive Care tomorrow.
    Saldrá del Cuidado Intensivo mañana.

13. They are not going to operate on him (her/you) any more.
    No le van a operar más.

14. You are in the Recovery Room.
    Vd. está en la sala de recuperación.

15. When you are fully awake, you will be taken to your room.
    Cuando Vd. esté completamente despierto (despierta), le (la) llevarán a su cuarto.

16. You cannot have anything to eat (drink) yet because the anesthesia may make you vomit.
    Vd. no puede comer (beber) nada todavía porque la anestesia puede hacerle vomitar.

17. You may only have a few chips of ice.
    Vd. puede tomar solamente unos pedacitos de hielo triturado.

18. You must lie flat.
    Debe extenderse completamente.

19. Has the anesthesia worn off yet?
    ¿Se le ha pasado la anestesia ya?

20. Can you move your toes?
    ¿Puede mover los dedos del pie?

21. Do your legs still feel numb?
    ¿Todavía siente adormecidas las piernas?

22. Do you have a metallic taste in your mouth?
    ¿Tiene Vd. un sabor a lata en la boca?

23. Can you feel this?
    ¿Puede Vd. sentir esto?

24. Is it sharp or dull?
    ¿Es agudo o sordo?

25. Which is sharper? This or this?
    ¿Cuál es más agudo? ¿Esto o esto?

26. Do you feel nauseated?
    ¿Tiene Vd. náuseas?

27. Are you in (a lot of) pain?
    ¿Tiene Vd. (mucho) dolor?

28. We can give you some medicine to make it hurt less.
    Podemos ponerle más medicina para que le duela menos.

29. I must check your incision for bleeding.
    Debo revisarle su incisión para verificar si sangra.

30. I am going to check your IV.
    Voy a revisar su suero.

31. I am going to take your temperature.
    Voy a tomarle la temperatura.

32. Open your mouth.
    Abra la boca, por favor.

33. Keep your mouth closed.
    Mantenga la boca cerrada.

34. Your temperature is normal.
    Su temperatura es normal.

35. You have a slight fever.
    Vd. tiene un poco de fiebre.

36. You have a high fever.
    Vd. tiene una temperatura alta.

37. I am going to take your blood pressure.
    Voy a tomarle la presión arterial.

38. Relax.
    Cálmese.
    Relájese.[4]

39. Your blood pressure is normal.
    Su presión (sanguínea) es normal.

40. Your blood pressure is rather high.
    Su presión (arterial) está un poco alta.

41. I am going to listen to your lungs.
    Voy a escucharle los pulmones.

42. Take a deep breath.
    Respire profundo.

43. Breathe slowly.
    Respire despacio.

44. You have fluid in your lungs.
    Vd. tiene un líquido en los pulmones.

45. You have to cough strongly to keep your lungs working.
    Vd. tiene que toser fuertemente para que los pulmones puedan seguir funcionando.

46. You must breathe deeply and cough to help prevent pneumonia.
    Vd. debe respirar profundamente y toser para ayudar a prevenir la pulmonía.

47. I know that it hurts when you take a deep breath.
    Sé que le duele cuando respire profundo.

48. Use this pillow to help you breathe.
    Use esta almohada para ayudarle a respirar.

49. Press the pillow firmly against your incision when you cough (or sneeze).
    Apriete la almohada fuerte sobre la incisión (herida) al toser (o estornudar).

50. Cough deeply.
    Tosa fuertemente.

51. This machine will help you expand your lungs.
    Esta máquina le ayudará a expander los pulmones.

52. Put this tube in your mouth and blow.
    Ponga este tubo en la boca y sople.

53. Try to get all the balls to rise to the top of the machine when you blow.
    Trate de hacer subir todas las bolas a la parte de arriba de la máquina al soplar.

54. Blow again.
    Sople otra vez.

55. You must practice blowing vigorously on this machine several times each day. Each time you must blow a minimum of _____ times.[19]
    Vd. debe practicar soplando fuertemente con esta máquina varias veces cada día. Cada vez debe soplar un mínimo de _____ veces.[19]

56. You have to make the balls rise higher.
    Tiene que hacer subir las bolas un poco más.

57. Blow again but harder.
    Sople de nuevo, pero con más fuerza.

58. That's better.
    Mejor.

59. Your family is waiting outside.
    Su familia está esperando afuera.

60. The doctor has told them that the operation is over.
    El doctor le ha dicho que la cirugía se acabó.

61. You can see your family (husband, wife) when you are back in your room.
    Vd. puede ver a su familia (esposo, esposa) cuando haya vuelto a su cuarto.

62. They can only visit five minutes.
    Pueden visitarle (visitarla) no más de cinco minutos.

63. I am going to remove this tube as soon as you don't need it any longer.
    Voy a quitarle este tubo (esta sonda) en cuanto no lo (la) necesite más.

64. Your doctor is going to remove your stitches today.

Su doctor va a quitarle los puntos hoy.
Su médico va a quitarle las puntadas hoy.

65. Tomorrow the doctor will probably change your dressing.
    Mañana el doctor probablemente le cambie el vendaje.

66. You are doing very well.
    Vd. va muy bien.

67. When the stitches are taken out, you may have a scar.
    Cuando le quitemos los puntos, quizás tenga una cicatriz.

68. Don't remove your dressing.
    No se quite el vendaje.

69. We must know how much liquid you are putting out.
    Debemos saber cuánto líquido produce.

70. We have to measure how much you drink.
    Tenemos que medir cuánto bebe.

71. We have to measure how much you urinate.
    Tenemos que medir cuánto orina.

72. You must urinate into the aparatus.
    Debe orinar en el aparato.

73. Do not flush; I have to check the amount of your urine.
    No tire de la cadena; tengo que analizar la cantidad de su orina.

74. Stick to the diet that we gave you.
    Siga Vd. la dieta que le dimos.

75. Don't drive a car for a month.
    No conduzca Vd. un coche por un mes.

76. Don't do any heavy work for two months (weeks).
    No haga ningún trabajo pesado por dos meses (semanas).

77. When cancer is too far advanced, it is incurable.
    El cáncer, cuando está avanzado, es incurable.

78. Your case is difficult, but you are going to get better and recover.
    Su caso es difícil, pero Vd. va a mejorarse y sanar.

79. The patient should (not) know his/her diagnosis.
    El (La) paciente (no) debiera conocer su diagnóstico.

80. Worries can affect your/his/her life.
    Las preocupaciones pueden afectar su vida.

MEDICATION *MEDICACION*

1. Whose medicine is this?[20]
   ¿De quién es esta medicina?

2. Whose vaccine is that?
   ¿De quién es esa vacuna?

3. Give me the medicine, please.
   Favor de darme la medicina.

4. Take the medicine today.
   Tome Vd. la medicina hoy.

5. Don't take the medicine tomorrow.
   No tome Vd. la medicina mañana.

6. I am going for the medicine.
   Voy por la medicina.

7. Are you taking the medicine?
    ¿Toma Vd. la medicina?

8. You have to take your medicine, Ma'am.
    Vd. tiene que tomar su medicina, señora.

9. You must take your medicines, or you will not get better.
    Es preciso que Vd. tome sus medicinas, porque si no, no se recuperará.

10. If you don't take them, it will take a long time for you to get well.
    Si no las toma, no se recuperará por mucho tiempo.

11. Take your medicines regularly at the same hour, if possible.
    Debe tomar sus medicinas regularmente, a la misma hora, si es posible.

12. Take only what the nurse gives you.
    Tome Vd. solamente las (medicinas) que le dé la enfermera.

13. Do not take any medicine from home.
    No tome Vd. ninguna medicina traída de su casa.

14. Do not take any medicine before coming to the hospital.
    No tome Vd. ninguna medicina antes de venir al hospital.

15. When was your last tetanus shot?
    ¿Cuándo fue su última inyección (vacuna) contra el tétano?

16. I am going to give you an injection.
    Voy a ponerle una inyección.

17. Here is your prescription.
    Aquí tiene Vd. su receta.

18. This is a prescription for your medicine.
    Esta es una receta para su medicina.

19. The doctor will give you a prescription.
    El doctor (La doctora) le dará una receta.

20. You can have it filled at any drugstore.
    Puede comprarla en cualquier farmacia.[21]

21. You can renew it ___ times.[19]
    Vd. puede usarla ___ veces.

22. Take the prescription to your druggist.[22]
    Lleve Vd. esta receta a su farmacéutico/ farmacólogo.

23. Take this to the hospital pharmacy.
    Lleve Vd. ésta a la farmacia del hospital.

24. Who is taking your prescriptions to the pharmacy?
    ¿Quién lleva las recetas a la farmacia?

25. The pharmacy is open . . .
    La farmacia está abierta . . .
    Monday through Friday.
    de lunes a viernes.
    everyday.
    todos los días.
    on Saturdays and Sundays.
    los sábados y domingos.
    on holidays.
    los días feriados.
    los días festivos.
    from 9:00 A.M. until 10:00 P.M.
    de las nueve de la mañana a las diez de la noche.
    from noon to 6:00 P.M.
    de mediodía a las seis de la tarde.

26. The medicine will have a label which will tell . . .
    La medicina tendrá una etiqueta que dirá . . .
    your name.
    su nombre.
    your doctor's name.
    el nombre de su médico (médica).
    the date the prescription was dispensed.
    la fecha en que se recetó.
    the generic name of the medicine.
    el nombre genérico de la medicina.
    the name of the medicine.
    el nombre de la medicina.
    the dosage.
    la dosis.
    the quantity.
    la cantidad.
    the expiration date.
    la fecha de caducidad.

27. Come back if you don't feel better.
    Regrese Vd. si no se siente mejor.

28. Call me if you need more.
    Llámeme Vd., por favor, si necesita más.

29. Call the office if you have any questions.
    Llame Vd. al consultorio si tiene alguna pregunta.

30. Call me if you feel worse.
    Llámeme si Vd. se siente peor.

31. Stop the medicine immediately if you have any reactions.
    Deje de tomar la medicina si Vd. tiene cualquier molestia.

32. If you have a bad reaction to the medicine, go to the hospital immediately.
    Si reacciona mal a la medicina, vaya inmediatamente al hospital.

33. You may have side effects from the medication.
    Puede tener efectos secundarios de la medicina.

34. You may have a dry mouth.
    Vd. puede tener la boca seca.

35. You may be depressed or irritable.
    Vd. puede tener depresión o irritabilidad.

36. You may be nauseated.
    Vd. puede tener náuseas.

37. You may have blurred or double vision.
    Vd. puede tener visión nublada o vista doble.

38. You may have a bad taste in your mouth.
Vd. puede tener un sabor desagradable en la boca.

39. You may lose your appetite.
Vd. puede perder el apetito.
Vd. puede tener falta de apetito.

40. You may have insomnia.
Vd. puede tener insomnio.

41. You may be constipated.
Vd. puede estar estreñido (estreñida).
Vd. puede tener estreñimiento.

42. You may have diarrhea.
Vd. puede tener diarrea.

43. You may be thirsty or hungry.
Vd. puede tener sed o hambre.

44. Do you have this medicine in the house?
¿Tiene esta medicina en casa?

45. Have you ever taken it before?
¿Jamás la ha tomado antes?

46. When? How much?
¿Cuándo? ¿Cuánto? ¿Qué cantidad?

47. Did it help (you)?
¿Le (La) alivió?

48. Did you have any reactions to it?
¿Sufrió Vd. algunas reacciones?
¿Tuvo algunas molestias?

49. These pills are for pain.
Estas píldoras son para el dolor.

50. Take this every time you feel pain.
Tome Vd. esto cada vez que sienta dolor.

51. Take these pills only if you feel pain.
Tome Vd. estas píldoras solamente si siente dolor.

52. Take this only when absolutely necessary because it is habit-forming.
Tome esta medicina solamente cuando sea absolutamente necesario (cuando la necesite muchísimo) porque puede enviciarse.

53. This medicine is not habit-forming.
Esta medicina no envicia.

54. Follow the instructions carefully.
Siga las instrucciones con cuidado.

55. Take these pills two (2) times a day [BID] for ten (10) days.
Tome Vd. estas pastillas dos (2) veces al (por) día durante diez (10) días.

56. Take these pills three (3) times daily [TID] for a week.
Tome Vd. estas píldoras tres (3) veces al (por) día por una semana.

57. Take this medicine four (4) times a day [QID] until you finish it.
Tome esta medicina cuatro (4) veces al día hasta terminarla.

58. Take two (2) pills twice a day.
Tome Vd. dos (2) píldoras dos veces al día.

59. Instead of taking two (2) pills, you can take only one (1).
En vez de tomar dos (2) píldoras, puede tomar solamente una (1).

60. Three times a day.
Tres veces al día.

61. Every four hours.
Cada cuatro horas.

62. Every other day.
Cada tercer día.

63. When you get up in the morning.
Al levantarse.

64. One half (1/2) hour after meals.
Media (1/2) hora después de cada comida.
Media (1/2) hora después de comer.

65. One (1) hour before meals.
Una (1) hora antes de cada comida.
Una (1) hora antes de comer.

66. Take a tablespoonful of this.
Tome una cucharada de esto.

67. Take a teaspoonful of this.
Tome Vd. una cucharadita de esto.

68. Whenever it hurts you.
Cuando le duela.

69. Put this pill under your tongue and let it dissolve in your mouth.
Ponga esta píldora debajo de la lengua hasta que se disuelva en la boca.

70. Take this without food.
Tome esto sin comida.

71. Take this medicine before meals.
Tome Vd. esta medicina antes de las comidas.
before breakfast.
antes de desayunarse.
before lunch.
antes de almorzar.
before dinner.
antes de cenar.

72. Take one capsule at breakfast.[23]
Tome Vd. una cápsula con el desayuno.

73. Take one of these tablets before bedtime.
Tome Vd. una de estas pastillas antes de acostarse.

74. After meals.
Después de comer.
Después de cada comida.

75. Take them with a glass of water, juice, milk.
Tómelas con un vaso de agua, jugo, leche.

76. I am going to put some medicina in your ____.
Voy a ponerle medicina en ____.

77. Drink a full glass of orange juice or have a banana every day while you are taking this medicine.

Tome un vaso de jugo de naranja o una ba-nana (un plátano) cada día mientras toma esta medicina.

78. Drink more water when you are taking this medication.
    Beba más agua mientras toma esta medicina.

79. Be careful of your diet when you are taking this medication.
    Tenga cuidado con su dieta al tomar esta medicina.

80. Don't eat dairy products or take antacids with this medication.
    No tome productos lácteos o antiácidos con esta medicina.

81. Don't take with milk.
    No tome con leche.

82. Don't take this with (fruit) juices.
    No tome ésta con jugos (de frutas).

83. Take this medication on an empty stomach one (1) hour before or two to three (2-3) hours after meals.
    Tome esta medicina con el estómago vacío una (1) hora antes o dos a tres (2-3) horas después de comer.

84. Take this medication one half (1/2) hour before meals.
    Tome esta medicina media (1/2) hora antes de cada comida.

85. This medication may discolor your urine or feces.
    Esta medicina puede teñir la orina o las heces.

86. Keep the medicine . . .
    Guarde la medicina . . .
    in the refrigerator.
    en el refrigerador (nevera).
    away from heat.
    fuera del calor.
    out of direct (strong) light.
    donde no haya mucha luz (fuerte).

87. Keep in a cool, dry place.
    Consérvese en un lugar fresco y seco.

88. Do not keep in the freezer.
    No la guarde en el congelador.

89. Keep out of children's reach.
    No se deje al alcance de los niños.

90. This medicine may cause drowsiness.
    Esta medicina puede causarle sueño.
    Esta medicina puede causar somnolencia.

91. Don't drive a car after taking this.
    No conduzca Vd. después de tomar esto.

92. Don't operate machinery after taking this.
    No use maquinaria después de tomar esto.

93. Don't operate machinery while you are taking this medicine.
    No opere maquinaria mientras tome esta medicina.

No maneje ninguna máquina mientras esté tomando esta medicina.

94. Avoid other depressants.
    Evite otros depresores/deprimentes.

95. Don't drink alcohol with this.
    No tome Vd. alcohol con esto.

96. Let this lozenge dissolve in your mouth.
    Deje que esta tableta se disuelva en la boca.

97. Let these melt on (under) your tongue.
    Deje Vd. que se le derritan en (debajo de) la lengua.

98. Chew them.
    Mastíquelas Vd.

99. Don't chew them.
    No las mastique Vd.

100. Swallow this without chewing.
     Trague Vd. ésta sin masticar.

101. Finish all of the medicine prescribed.
     Termine toda la medicina recetada.

102. Take all the medicine in this prescription.
     Tome toda la medicina indicada en la receta.

103. Do not stop taking this medication suddenly.
     No deje de tomar esta medicina de repente.
     No cese de tomar esta medicina de súbito.

104. Shake well before using.
     Agite Vd. bien antes de usar.

105. I am going to give you the medicine.
     Voy a darle la medicina.

106. This medicine is not to be taken orally—by mouth.
     No se toma esta medicina por boca.

107. It is poisonous if taken by mouth.
     Es venenosa si se toma por boca.

108. The medicine will burn for a moment; then it will feel better.
     La medicina va a arderle por un momento; después, va a sentirse mejor.

109. I will give you a cream.
     Voy a darle una crema.

110. Apply this to the affected area.
     Aplíquese esto en la parte afectada.

111. Apply the ointment without rubbing.
     Aplíquese la pomada sin frotarse.

112. Put this over the rash / burn / wound.
     Póngase esto en el sarpullido / en la quemadura / en la herida.

113. Put two drops in each ear / in each eye / in each nostril.
     Póngase dos gotas en cada oído / en cada ojo / en cada ventana de la nariz.

114. Dissolve one tablet in eight (8) ounces of distilled water.
     Disuelva Vd. una tableta en ocho (8) onzas de agua destilada.

115. Mix two (2) tablespoons of the powder with two (2) cups of water.
Mezcle Vd. dos (2) cucharadas de polvo con dos (2) tazas de agua.

116. Dissolve a teaspoon of Epsom salts in a large glass of water.
Disuelva Vd. una cucharadita de sulfato de magnesio [sal de Epsom/sal de la Higuera/sal inglesa] en un vaso grande de agua.

117. Drink the medicine.
Tome Vd. la medicina.
Beba Vd. la medicina.

118. Drink it.
Tómela Vd.
Bébala Vd.

119. Gargle with this medicine for the pain.
Haga Vd. gárgaras con esta medicina para el dolor.

120. Soak your ____ [24] in the dissolved powder.
Remójese Vd. ____ en el polvo disuelto.

121. Inhale through your nose.
Inhale (Aspire/Inspire) Vd. por la nariz.

122. Use the spray in your nasal passages daily.
Use Vd. el spray (atomizador) en las ventanas de la nariz todos los días.

TREATMENTS

TRATAMIENTOS

1. I want you to apply heat to your back.
Quiero que Vd. se aplique calor a la espalda.

2. You must keep the area clean at all times.
Vd. tiene que mantener el área limpia todo el tiempo.

3. Change the bandages every day.
Cámbiese Vd. los vendajes todos los días.

4. Apply a hot, wet compress every hour.
Póngase Vd. una compresa caliente y húmeda cada hora.

5. Mix this package of medicine with one (1) quart of very warm water and soak the compress in the solution; then apply it to the affected area.
Mezcle este paquete de medicina con un (1) litro de agua caliente y remoje la compresa en la solución; entonces aplíquela a la parte afectada.

6. Apply a wet bandage every two hours.
Póngase una venda húmeda cada dos horas.

7. Apply a hot water bag over the ____.[24]
Aplique una bolsa de agua caliente sobre ____.

8. Put your ____ in warm water.[24]
Ponga ____ en agua tibia.

9. Bathe with warm (cold) water.
Báñese con agua tibia (fría).

10. Rub yourself with alcohol.
Frótese con alcohol.

11. You must wear an elastic bandage.
Debe llevar una venda elástica.

12. Put on an elastic stocking during the day.
Póngase Vd. una media elástica durante el día.

13. Paint the swelling with this.
Es preciso que Vd. pinte la hinchazón con esto.

14. Take hot sitz baths every ____ hours.
Dése Vd. un caliente baño de asiento (semicupio) cada ____[19] horas.

15. Is there anyone in your house who knows how to give an injection?
¿Hay alguien en su casa que sepa poner inyecciones?

16. Use one of these suppositories every evening.
Póngase uno de estos supositorios (una de estas calillas) cada noche.

17. Insert one of these suppositories ____ using this applicator.
Introdúzcase uno de estos supositorios (una de estas calillas) ____ por medio de este aplicador.
rectally
por el recto
vaginally
por la vagina

18. You will need a cast.
Vd. va a necesitar un yeso (un calote).

19. You are going to need a bandage.
Vd. va a necesitar un vendaje (una venda).

20. I have to give you a sling.
Tengo que ponerle un cabestrillo (una honda para el brazo).

21. Keep your arm in it.
Mantenga el brazo en él (ella).

22. You have a sprained ankle which you should keep elevated as much as possible to reduce the swelling.
Vd. tiene una dislocadura (torcedura) del tobillo, el cual debe mantener lo más elevado posible para reducir la inflamación (la hinchazón).

23. Apply ice to the torn ligament (pulled muscle) at intervals of 30 minutes for the first 24 hours after the initial injury.

Aplique Vd. hielo al ligamento roto (músculo jalado / rasgado) en intervalos de treinta minutos durante las primeras veinticuatro horas.

24. Stay in bed with your foot elevated.
Guarde Vd. cama con una almohada debajo de la pierna.

25. Leave the strapping on until you see the doctor.
Conserve Vd. el vendaje hasta que vea al (a la) doctor(a).

26. Don't get the tape (bandage) wet.
No deje mojarse la cinta (venda).

27. If the Ace bandage over the tape becomes loose, remove it and rewrap it starting at the base of the toes.
Si el vendaje de Ace se suelta, quíteselo y póngaselo de nuevo comenzando con la base de los dedos del pie.

28. Loosen the Ace bandage if numbness, tingling, swelling, or discoloration occurs.
Suelte el vendaje de Ace si hay adormecimiento, hormigueos, hinchazón, o descoloración de la piel.

29. Your finger needs to be put in a splint.
Hay que entablillar el dedo.

30. Elevate the affected hand in order to avoid/reduce the swelling.
Llevante Vd. la mano afectada para evitar / reducir la hinchazón.

31. Leave the splint on until the doctor sees it.
Conserve Vd. el entablillado hasta que lo vea el doctor (la doctora).

32. Call me if the pain, swelling, and numbness increase.
Avíseme en seguida si le duele más, o se le hincha, o se le entumece.

33. Notify me immediately if there is a change in the skin color of the fingers.
Avíseme Vd. en seguida si hay un cambio en el color de la piel de los dedos.

34. The doctor will put the broken arm in a cast.
El doctor (La doctora) le pondrá el brazo roto en un yeso.

35. Notify the doctor immediately if there is pain, numbness, or blue color of the fingers.
Avise Vd. al doctor (a la doctora) en seguida si hay dolor, adormecimiento o si los dedos se ponen morados.[25]

36. The cast will remain on for six weeks.
Vd. tiene que dejarse puesto el yeso por seis semanas.

37. If the cast hurts you, come back at once.
Si le duele el yeso, vuelva Vd. inmediatamente.

38. Don't get the cast wet.
No permita que se moje el yeso.

39. Keep the injured arm elevated and exercise the fingers to reduce the swelling.
Mantenga el brazo lastimado levantado y haga ejercicios con los dedos para reducir la hinchazón (la inflamación).

40. Don't stay on your feet much with a broken leg.[26]
No se quede Vd. de pie con la pierna rota (quebrada).

41. Walking casts need to be completely dry before they can bear weight. This takes forty-eight hours.
Las enyesaduras para caminar necesitan secarse por completo antes de poder aguantar el peso. Esto requiere cuarenta y ocho horas.

42. You will have to use crutches for a while.
Vd. tendrá que usar muletas por algún tiempo.

43. The nurse will show you how to use them even after the cast is removed.
La enfermera le enseñará cómo usarlas aún después de que se le quite el yeso.

44. You will have to come to physical therapy for diathermy twice a week.
Vd. tendrá que volver a la (clínica de) fisioterapia para la diatermia dos veces por (a la) semana.

45. You have to massage this leg daily and do an exercise like this.
Vd. tiene que darle masajes a esta pierna todos los días y también hacer un ejercicio así.

46. Observe your wound to see if bleeding or drainage develops that was not there before.
Observe su herida y llame al doctor (a la doctora) si aparece hemorragia o secreción (drenaje) que no existía antes.

47. I am putting you on a respirator.
Voy a unirle (unirla) a un respirador.

48. The respirator is to help you breathe.
El respirador es para ayudarle (ayudarla) a respirar.

49. Relax.
Cálmese Vd., por favor.
Relájese[4] Vd., por favor.

50. Breathe slowly—with the machine.
Respire Vd. despacio—con la ayuda del aparato.

51. Don't breathe so fast.
No respire Vd. tan rápido.

52. The tube that is in your throat is to help you breathe.
El tubo que tiene en la garganta es para ayudarle (ayudarla) a respirar.

53. It must stay in for a while.
Tiene que quedarse allí (por) un rato.

Exercise   *Ejercicio*

Substitution Drill. Using the cue given in parenthesis, give the correct instructions for taking medication:

Tome Vd. la medicina.
(hoy)

_____

Tome Vd. la medicina hoy.
(mañana)

_____

Tome Vd. la medicina mañana.
(No)

_____

No tome Vd. la medicina mañana.
(ninguna medicina)

_____

No tome Vd. ninguna medicina mañana.
(alcohol)

_____

No tome Vd. ningún alcohol mañana.

_____

Tome Vd. esta medicina cuatro veces al día.
(dos píldoras)

_____

Tome Vd. dos píldoras cuatro veces al día.
(tres veces)

_____

Tome Vd. dos píldoras tres veces al día.
(cada cuatro horas)

_____

Tome Vd. dos píldoras cada cuatro horas.
(cápsulas)

_____

Tome Vd. dos cápsulas cada cuatro horas.
(estas pastillas)

_____

Tome Vd. estas pastillas cada cuatro horas.
(antes de cada comida)

_____

Tome Vd. estas pastillas antes de cada comida.
(esta medicina)

_____

Tome Vd. esta medicina antes de cada comida.
(después de las comidas)

_____

Tome Vd. esta medicina después de las comidas.
(cuando le duela)

_____

Tome Vd. esta medicina cuando le duela.
(con un vaso de agua)

_____

Tome Vd. esta medicina con un vaso de agua.
(un vaso de jugo)

_____

Tome Vd. esta medicina con un vaso de jugo.
(un vaso de leche)

_____

Tome Vd. esta medicina con un vaso de leche.

_____

DRUG OVERDOSE

LA DOSIS EXCESIVA DE DROGAS

1. It is important for you to recognize the signs and symptoms of drug abuse in emergencies.
    Es importante que las señales y los síntomas del abuso de drogas sean identificados por Vd. en casos de emergencia.

2. Did he (you, she) take some pills? capsules?
    ¿Tomó pastillas (píldoras)? ¿cápsulas? ¿Pildoreó?

3. What kind of pills did you (he, she) take?[27]
    ¿Qué tipo de píldoras tomó?
    ¿Qué tipo de pastillas ingirió?

4. How many did you (he, she) take?
    ¿Cuántas tomó?

5. What color were they?[28]
    ¿De qué color (colores) eran?

6. What shape were they?
    ¿De qué forma eran?

round?
¿redondas?
oval?
¿ovales?
cylindrical?
¿cilíndricas?
triangular?
¿triangulares?
rectangular?
¿rectangulares?
square?
¿cuadradas?
pentagonal?
¿pentagonales?
hexagonal?
¿hexagonales?

7. Were they large or small?
    ¿Eran grandes o chiquitas (pequeñas)?

8. Were they flat?
   ¿Eran llanas?

9. Do you know the name of what you took?
   ¿Sabe Vd. el nombre de lo que ha tomado?

10. What time did you (he, she) take them?
    ¿A qué hora las ingirió?

11. Did you (he, she) inject something?
    ¿Se inyectó con algo?
    ¿Se picó? *fam*
    ¿Se dio un piquete? *slang*

12. Did you find anything that would indicate
    what was taken—like a teaspoon, wrapping
    paper, a medicine dropper, a hypodermic
    needle, ampules, empty gelatinous capsules,
    needle marks on the skin?
    **¿Encontró Vd. algo que le indicara / indicase
    los tipos de drogas ingeridas—como una
    cucharadita, papel de envolver, un cuentago-
    tas, una aguja hipodérmica / un jaipo, am-
    pollas, cápsulas gelatinosas vacías, o marcas
    de una aguja hipodérmica en la piel?**

13. Call the nearest Drug Abuse Center whose
    number is listed in the phone book.
    **Llame al Centro de Abusos de Drogas más
    cercano cuyo número de teléfono encontrará
    en la guía telefónica.**

14. Save the bottle (hypo) and bring it for exami-
    nation when you come.
    **Guarde el envase / la botella (la aguja) y trái-
    galo (tráigala) para examinarlo (examinarla)
    cuando venga.**

15. You (He, She has) have taken too much, and
    we are going to try to empty your stomach to
    prevent your body from absorbing the drugs.
    **Ha tomado demasiado y vamos a hacer un
    esfuerzo para vaciarle el estómago a fin de
    prevenir que su cuerpo absorba las drogas.**

16. Do you (Does he, she) have any of the follow-
    ing characteristic symptoms?
    **¿Tiene algunos de los siguientes síntomas
    característicos?**
    convulsions?
    ¿convulsiones?
    nausea and vomiting?
    ¿náusea y vómitos?
    increase in blood pressure?
    ¿aumento de la presión sanguínea?
    dilated pupils?
    ¿dilatación (agrandamiento) de las pupilas?
    contracted pupils?
    ¿pupilas reducidas?
    increased / elevated body temperature
    ¿aumento de la temperature del cuerpo?
    increased palpitations?
    **¿aumento de las palpitaciones del
    corazón?**
    reddishness in the face?
    ¿la cara rojiza (coloradota)?

increased nervousness?
¿aumento de nerviosidad?
total loss of emotional control?
pérdida completa de control emocional?
deep depression?
¿depresión profunda?
tension and anxiety?
¿tensión y ansiedad?
paranoid illusions?
¡ilusiones paranoicas?
hallucinations?
¿alucinaciones?
respiratory difficulty?
¿dificultad respiratoria?
irritation of respiratory passages?
¿irritación de las vías respiratorias?
loss of balance?
¿pérdida del equilibrio?
lethargy and reduction of activity?
**¿letargo y reducción de actividad y
conocimiento?**
sleepiness, even prolonged unconsciousness?
¿sueño, aun inconsciencia prolongada?
muscle pains as well as sharp pains in the
legs, back, stomach?
**¿dolores musculares así como dolores pun-
zantes en las piernas, espalda y abdomen?**
loss of appetite, loss of weight?
¿pérdida de apetito, pérdida de peso?
confusion?
¿confusión?
disorganization?
¿desorganización?
fear?
¿temor?
aggressiveness and harmful types of
antisocial behavior?
**¿agresividad y conducta antisocial que
puede causar peligro a otros?**
irritability?
¿irritabilidad?
insomnia?
¿insomnio (no duerme)?
catatonia?
¿catatonia?
drainage (of the nose)?
¿goteo (de la nariz)?
dry mouth?
¿boca seca?
dryness (of the mucous membranes or mucosa)?
¿resequedad (de las mucosas)?
fitful sleep?
¿sueño sobresaltado?
giggling?
¿risa tonta? (¿risa falsa?)
goose pimples?
¿carne de gallina? (¿piel erizada?)
in a stupor?
¿atolondrado? (¿atolondrada?)

nodding?
¿cabeceo?
self-control?
¿autodominio?
loss of self-control?
¿pérdida del autodominio?
thirst?
¿sed?
an abnormal walk?
¿una marcha anormal?
yawning?
¿bostezo?

17. Are his (her, your) eyes bloodshot and/or glassy?[29]
¿Tiene los ojos inyectados de sangre y/o vidriosos?

18. Are the pupils constricted?[30]
¿Están encogidas las pupilas?

19. Pinpointed?
¿Están como un punto?
¿Del tamaño de un punto?

20. Are the eyes clear?
¿Están claros (limpios) los ojos?
watery?
¿acuosos? (¿llorosos?)

21. Does he (she) lurch when walking?
¿Anda con un paso vacilante?
¿Se balancea hacia un lado u otro o hacia adelante?

22. Doe he (she) stumble?
¿Tropieza?

23. Does he (she) sway?
¿Se bambolea?
¿Se tambalea?

24. Does he (she) weave?
¿Serpentea?
¿Zigzaguea?

25. Does he (she) veer?
¿Cambia de dirección de modo repentino?
¿Se desvía?

26. Is his (her) speech slurred?
¿Habla arrastrando las palabras?
¿Habla con pronunciación indistinta?

27. Is his (her) speech incoherent?
¿Es incoherente su modo de hablar?

28. Is his (her) speech hesitant?
¿Es titubeante su modo de hablar (su lenguaje)?

ACCIDENTAL POISONINGS
ENVENENAMIENTOS ACCIDENTALES

HISTORY   *HISTORIA*

1. Did you eat or drink something that disagreed with you?
¿Comió o bebió algo que le ha sabido mal?

2. What did you (he, she) eat?
¿Qué comió?

3. Something from a can?
¿Productos enlatados?
¿Comidas de lata?

4. What did you (he, she) drink?
¿Qué bebió?

5. What did you (he, she) swallow?
¿Qué tomó?
¿Qué tragó?

6. Do you (Does he, she) know?
¿Sabe?

7. Was it lead from paint?
¿Fue plomo de pintura?

8. Was it lead from batteries?
¿Fue plomo de baterías?

9. Was it hair dye?
¿Fue tinte para el pelo?

10. When did you (he, she) swallow it?
¿Cuándo lo (la) tragó?

11. How much was swallowed?
¿Cuánto tragó?

12. The whole bottle?
¿La botella entera?

13. Do you still have the bottle that the liquid (pills) came in?
¿Todavía tiene la botella en la que vino el líquido (en la que vinieron las píldoras)?

14. Bring me the bottle that it (they) came in.
Tráigame la botella en la que vino (vinieron).

15. This is very important.
Esto es importantísimo.

16. Were you (he, she) exposed to dangerous (poisonous) chemicals at work?
¿Se expuso a químicas peligrosas (venenosas) donde trabaja?

17. Have you (he, she) breathed anything poisonous?
¿Ha respirado algo venenoso?

18. Did you (he, she) breathe the vapors of the substance?
¿Inhaló los vapores de la substancia?

19. Do you (Does he, she) know the name of the substance?
¿Sabe el nombre de la substancia?

20. Did you (he, she) swallow the substance?
¿Tragó la substancia?

21. Are there any burns around the lips or mouth?
¿Hay quemaduras alrededor de los labios o la boca?

22. Did the substance get on your (his, her) skin?
¿Tocó la substancia la piel?

23. Did the substance get in your (his, her) eyes?
¿Entró la substancia en los ojos?

24. Are your (the victim's) pupils contracted or dilated as the result of poison or an overdose?
¿Se contraen las pupilas de los ojos (de la víctima) como consecuencia del veneno o la dosis excesiva de morfina u otra droga?

25. Is there a chemical odor on the breath?
¿Hay un mal olor químico en el aliento?

26. Do you (Does he, she) feel nauseated?
¿Tiene náuseas?

27. Do you (Does he, she) have a burning sensation?
¿Tiene ardor?

28. Are you (Is he, she) dizzy?
¿Tiene mareos?

29. Are you (Is he, she) breathing okay?
¿Está respirando bien?

30. Do you (Does he, she) have any other complaints?
¿Se queja de otro problema?

DRUG OVERDOSE TREATMENT[31]   *TRATAMIENTO PARA SOBREDOSIS DE DROGAS*

1. How old are you (is he, she)?
¿Cuántos años tiene?

2. How much do you (does he, she) weigh?
¿Cuánto pesa?

3. Dilute the poison with a glass of water or milk if the victim is conscious and not having convulsions.
Diluya Vd. el veneno haciendo que la víctima ingiera un vaso de agua o leche si está consciente y no tiene convulsiones.

4. Induce vomiting in the victim by causing him (her) to retch or by giving him (her) a liquid to drink which causes nausea such as mustard water, soapy water, or milk of magnesia and water.
Hágale vomitar[32] a la víctima haciéndole cosquillas con su dedo en la garganta de la víctima (arcadas) o dándole a beber un líquido que provoque náuseas, como agua con mostaza, agua jabonosa, o agua y leche de magnesia.

5. Induce vomiting . . .
Provóquese Vd. el vómito . . .
     with your finger.
     con el dedo.
     with this syrup of ipecac.
     con este jarabe de ipecacuana.

6. Give the patient syrup of ipecac according to the instructions on the bottle along with a glass of water.
Dé al (a la) paciente jarabe de ipecacuana según las instrucciones que se hallan en la botella junto con un vaso de agua.

7. The syrup of ipecac will produce vomiting in twenty to thirty (20-30) minutes.
El jarabe de ipecacuana producirá vómitos en veinte a treinta (20-30) minutos.

8. The dosage will produce vomiting a total of three or four (3 or 4) times.
La dosis producirá vómitos un total de tres o cuatro (3 o 4) veces.

9. Each time he/she vomits, give him/her another glass of water.
Cada vez que vomite, déle otro vaso de agua.

10. Bring him/her to the hospital after administering the medicine.
Llévele al hospital después de administrar el medicamento.

11. This prevents additional absorption of the poison (toxin) because it begins the vomiting.
Esto impide más absorción del veneno (de la toxina) porque empieza los vómitos.

12. Have you (has he/she) vomited?
¿Ha vomitado?

13. What did you (he/she) vomit?
¿Qué vomitó?

14. Save the vomited material for analysis.
Conserve Vd. una muestra del vómito y tráigala para hacer análisis.

15. If you have taken an overdose of drugs that contain opium or alcohol, drink strong coffee or tea.
Si Vd. ha tomado una dosis excesiva de drogas que contienen opio o alcohol, beba café o té fuerte.

16. Do not give him (her) any fluids or induce vomiting if the victim is unconscious or having convulsions.
No le administre (dé) líquidos por vía oral ni provoque vómitos (le haga vomitar) si la víctima está inconsciente o tiene convulsiones.

17. Do not induce vomiting if you (the victim) have (has) swallowed a strong acid, alkali, or petroleum product.
No se provoque vómitos si Vd. / (No provoque vómitos si la víctima) ha ingerido un ácido fuerte, un álcali fuerte, o productos derivados del petróleo.

18. Turn the victim on his (her) side or on his (her) stomach if he (she) is vomiting and is unconscious (and has just had a convulsion).

Coloque Vd. a la víctima hacia un lado
o sobre el estómago si vomita y si está inconsciente (y si acaba de tener convulsión).

19. Turn his (her) head so that the vomit drains
from his (her) mouth and does not reenter the
airway or throat.
**Dóblele Vd. la cabeza de modo que el ve-
neno vomitado no pueda reentrar en las vías
respiratorias o los pasajes alimenticios.**

20. Call the poison-control center nearest you that
is listed in the telephone book.

Llame Vd. al centro de control de envenenamiento (intoxicantes) más cercano cuyo
número encontrará en la guía de teléfonos.

21. Stay calm.
Manténgase / Quédese tranquilo (tranquila).

22. Keep the victim quiet and covered.
**Mantenga Vd. a la víctima quieta y
abrigada.**

SNAKE BITES *MORDEDURAS POR CULEBRAS*

1. Immobilize the extremity bitten by the snake
in such a way that it is at or below heart level.
**Inmovilice Vd. la extremidad que la víbora (cu-
lebra) mordió de tal manera que esté al nivel o
debajo del nivel del corazón de la victima.**

2. Apply a constrictive bandage 2 (two) to 4
(four) inches (5 [five] to 10 [ten] cm) above
the bite if to an extremity. (The bandage
should allow a finger to be slipped underneath
if it is in place properly.)
**Aplique Vd. una venda constrictiva de 2
(dos) a 4 (cuatro) pulgadas (5 [cinco] a 10
[diez] centímetros) arriba de la mordedura
si es a una extremidad. (Al estar en su lugar,
la venda debe permitir que un dedo pueda
deslizarse debajo.)**

3. Make a straight incision (not cross-cut) along
the length of the limb, cutting only the skin.
**Haga Vd. una incisión seguida (no cruzada)
en el eje mayor del miembro, cortando
solamente la piel.**

4. Suck the poison from the affected area, either
with a suction cup or with your mouth.
**Chupe el veneno de la herida o haciendo
succión con una ventosa o usando la boca
para chuparlo y escupirlo.**

5. Do this for 30 (thirty) to 60 (sixty) minutes.
**Siga la succión de 30 (treinta) a 60 (sesenta)
minutos.**

6. Wash the bitten area with soap and water, dry-
ing it well.
**Lave Vd. la herida con agua y jabón, secán-
dola bien.**

7. Do not give any medicines that contain aspirin.
**No dé ninguna medicina que contenga
aspirina.**

8. Come immediately to the nearest (this) hospital.
**Venga Vd. inmediatamente al hospital más
cercano (a este hospital).**

9. Bring him (her) immediately to the hospital.
Tráigale (Tráigala) en seguida al hospital.

10. Call the Fire Department.
Llame Vd. al Departamento de Bomberos.

11. Get medical assistance as soon as possible.
**Procure Vd. asistencia médica tan pronto
como sea posible.**

12. Take the victim to a place in the fresh air.
Lleve Vd. a la víctima a un lugar de aire fresco.

13. Try to get an ambulance immediately.
**Procure Vd. obtener una ambulancia inme-
diatamente.**

STOMACH PUMP *BOMBA GASTRICA*

1. I have to put this tube through your nose, into
your stomach.
**Tengo que ponerle este tubo por la nariz
dentro del estómago.**

2. It will go through your nose to your stomach
so that I can clean out your stomach.
**Pasará por la nariz al estómago para que yo
pueda lavarle el estómago.**

3. I need your help for this.
Necesito su ayuda a insertar este tubo.

4. Calm down.
Tranquilícese Vd.

5. Swallow.
Trague Vd., por favor.

6. Take a sip of water.
Tome Vd. un traguito de agua.

7. Now, swallow again.
Ahora, trague Vd. otra vez.

8. Relax!
Cálmese Vd.

9. Very good. That was fine.
Muy bien. Excelente.

10. You have to (The child has to) stay in the hospital overnight.
**Vd. (El niño / La niña) tiene que quedarse
en el hospital esta noche.**

11. When you get home, if you have any questions,
don't hesitate to call and ask me.
**Después de haber salido del hospital (con-
sultorio), si se le ocurren a Vd. más preguntas, no titubee en llamarme y preguntarme.**

ADVICE *CONSEJOS*

1. Medicines cause more poisonings among children under five than any other product.
   Las medicines causan más envenenamientos entre los niños menores de cinco años, que cualquier otro producto químico.

2. Keep all medicines and other poisonous things away from children.
   Guarde Vd. (Almacene Vd.) todas las medicinas y cosas peligrosas (tóxicas) fuera del alcance de los niños.

3. Keep all medicines and other dangerous products in a cabinet that locks with a key.
   Guarde Vd. (Almacene Vd.) todas las medicinas y otros productos peligrosos en un gabinete cerrado con llave.

4. Never leave any medicine out when you go to answer the phone or the door.
   Nunca deje ninguna medicina al alcance de la mano cuando vaya a contestar al teléfono o abrir la puerta.

5. Always give a child the correct prescribed dosage.
   Siempre déle al niño (a la niña) la cantidad recetada.

6. Read the labels carefully on over-the-counter (OTC) medicines and ask either your pharmacist or your doctor if they are safe for children, should you have any doubts.
   Lea cuidadosamente las etiquetas de las medicinas que se venden sin receta (reme-
   dios caseros; medicinas patentadas; medicinas auto-prescritas) y consulte a su farmacéutico (farmacéutica) o médico (médica) para saber si deben darse o no a los niños si Vd. tiene alguna duda.

7. Ask for a child-proof bottle if your pharmacist doesn't use one automatically because the law requires that most medicines and other potentially dangerous products should be packaged in child-proof bottles.
   Pídale Vd. a su farmacéutico (farmacéutica) un envase de seguridad si él (ella) no lo usa generalmente porque la ley requiere que la mayoría de las medicinas, tanto las recetadas como las que se compran sin receta, así como muchos otros productos químicos que puedan ser peligrosos en potencia, estén envasados en forma tal que sólo un adulto pueda abrirlos.

8. When giving a child medicine, never tell him (her) that it is "candy" or that it is something that he (she) may like. When the child is alone, he (she) may try to take more by himself (herself).
   Cuando tenga que darle medicina a un niño (una niña), nunca le diga que es un «dulce» o algo que le guste. Cuando esté solo (sola), podrá tratar de tomar más por sí mismo (misma).

EXERCISE *EJERCICIO*

Rewrite all polite commands in this section using the acceptable substitutes of *please* plus the infinitive:

Please { Favor de
{ Haga Vd. el favor de
{ Tenga la bondad de
{ Sírvase

No se ponga nervioso, por favor.
(Haga Vd. el favor de)

_____

Haga Vd. el favor de no ponerse nervioso.
(Favor de)

_____

Favor de no ponerse nervioso.
(Tenga la bondad de)

_____

Tenga la bondad de no ponerse nervioso.
(Sírvase)

_____

Sírvase no ponerse nervioso.

_____

DIET

DIETA

1. What type of work do you do?[33]
   ¿Cómo se gana Vd. la vida?

2. What are your working hours?
   ¿Cuántas horas trabaja Vd. por día?

3. How many days a week do you work?
   ¿Cuántos días por semana trabaja Vd.?

4. At what time do you get up in the morning?
   ¿A qué hora se despierta por la mañana?

5. Where do you eat breakfast, at home or in a restaurant?
   ¿Dónde se desayuna Vd? ¿en casa? ¿o en un restorán?

6. What do you eat for breakfast?[34]
   ¿Qué se desayuna?

7. Do you carry lunch?
   ¿Lleva su almuerzo?

8. What do you eat for lunch? for dinner?
   ¿Qué come Vd. para el almuerzo? ¿para la cena?

9. What do you eat between meals?
   ¿Qué come Vd. entre comidas?

10. Do you eat while you watch television?
    ¿Come Vd. mientras mira la televisión?

11. What do you eat before going to bed?
    ¿Qué come antes de acostarse?

12. Have you ever been on a diet before?
    ¿Ha estado Vd. a dieta antes?

13. You will have to follow a ____ diet.[35]
    Vd. tendrá que seguir una dieta ____.

14. There are many diets available to patients.
    Hay muchas dietas para los pacientes.

15. You should select what you eat according to the Food Pyramid.
    Vd. debe escoger lo que consume según la Pirámide de Comestibles/Alimentos.

Food Pyramid   *La pirámide de Alimentos*

Food guide pyramid
A guide to daily food choices

La Guía pirámide de alimentos
Una Guía para la selección diaria de alimentos

Key/Clave
○ Fat (naturally occurring and added)/ Grasas (naturales y agregadas)
▽ Sugars (added)/Azúcares (agregados)
These symbols show fat and added sugars in foods/ Estos símbolos indican grasas y azúcares agregados en alimentos.

Fats, oils, & sweets
Use sparingly

Grasas, aceites y dulces
Úselos con moderación

Milk, yogurt & cheese group
2-3 Servings

Grupo de leche, yogurt y queso
2-3 Porciones

Meat, poultry, fish, dry beans, eggs, & nut group
2-3 Servings

Grupo de carne, aves, pescado, frijoles secos, huevos y nueces
2-3 Porciones

Vegetable group
3-5 Servings

Grupo de verduras/ vegetales
3-5 Porciones

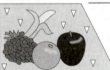

Fruit groups
2-4 Servings

Grupo de frutas
2-4 Porciones

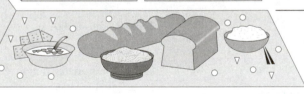

Bread, cereal, rice, & pasta group
6-11 Servings

Grupo de pan, cereal, arroz y pasta
6-11 Porciones

Source: U.S. Department of Agriculture/U.S. Department of Health and Human Services

Note: The food guide was developed for healthy people 2 years of age and older who eat a typical American diet.

Nota: La guía de alimentos fue desarrollada para personas saludables de dos años en adelante que consumen una dieta estadounidense típica.

16. Eat three (3) meals a day.
    Coma Vd. tres (3) comidas al día.

17. Do not skip meals. It is very important.
    No se salte Vd. comidas. Es muy importante.

18. Drink milk between meals and before going to bed.
    Tome Vd. leche entre las comidas y antes de acostarse.

19. Do not overeat raw vegetables of any kind.
    No coma Vd. en exceso ninguna legumbre cruda.

20. Do not use pepper or spice.
    No use Vd. ni pimienta ni especies.

21. Do not use sugar or sweets.
    No use Vd. ni azúcar ni dulces.

22. Do not use salt or baking soda.
    No use Vd. ni sal ni bicarbonato.

23. Use only sweet unsalted butter or margarine.
    No use Vd. más que mantequilla sosa o margarina sin sal.

24. Do not eat gravies or sauces.
    No coma Vd. salsas de ninguna clase.

25. Do not eat fried foods.
    No coma Vd. nada frito.

26. Some dairy products cause hives.
    Algunos productos lácteos producen urticaria.

27. Do you have any questions about your diet?[36]
    ¿Tiene Vd. preguntas acerca de su dieta?

28. Do you want to describe the meals that you are used to eating during the day?
    ¿Quiere Vd. describirme las comidas que Vd. acostumbra comer durante el día?

29. I will be able to help you plan your meals better (plan your substitutions) when you return home if I have this information.
    Podré ayudarle (ayudarla) a planificar mejor sus comidas (su lista de intercambios) cuando Vd. vuelva a casa si me da esta información.

Notes   Notas

1. Many Hispanic women may not know the word **vagina.** They may use **las partes privadas, verijas,** or some similar expression. They may not be too aware of what is occurring in **las partes privadas** because it is not considered "nice" to know.

2. See Chapter 12, pages 252–253.

3. See Chapter 12, pages 260–261 and page 272, notes 4 and 10.

4. See Chapter 10, page 219, note 6.

5. See **Anesthesia** *Anestesia* below, page 227f.

6. See Chapter 10, page 219, note 7.

7. In many parts of Latin America, but especially in Mexico, women strongly believe in the observance of the postpartum **cuarentena dieta,** which is thought to restore the mother to "normal health." Today in the United States, only those young women who are directly under their mother's or mother-in-law's supervision follow all customs of **la dieta.** This is the forty-day convalescence period following delivery during which there is a prolonged period in bed, much freedom from household responsibilities, and abstention from sexual intercourse.

   Modern women find it difficult to observe all of the prohibitions and precautions, which in some ways include the same taboos observed during menstruation, such as avoiding bathing and eating foods that are "too acid," or "cool." Many women avoid cool foods after delivery on the grounds that they "impede the blood flow and the emptying of the uterus." To help prevent this blockage, which many once believed caused nervousness or even insanity, women take "hot" substances to strengthen the womb. One such tonic is made of chocolate, garlic, cinnamon, rue, rum, and pieces of cheese. (See A. Harwood, "Hot and Cold Theory of Disease," pp. 1153–1158; N. Galli, "The Influence of Cultural Heritage," pp. 10–16). Postpartum Hispanic patients frequently complain that the foods on their hospital trays are either "too hot" or "too cold." If dieticians could substitute more familiar choices for these patients, or at least serve these food "taboos" less often, these mothers would not be forced either to violate their food prohibitions or to go hungry.

   With regard to bathing, most women who have had their babies in the hospital have become used to bathing within a few hours after delivery. There are still some who "because my mother so accustomed me" will go into the shower room, turn on the water, but avoid getting wet. Thus they satisfy both the hospital staff and their own socio-cultural pressures (M. Kay, "Health and Illness," p. 155).

8. See Chapter 12, pages 267–272 for a discussion on Contraceptive Methods for Family Planning.

9. See Chapter 1, pp. 25–28 for additional information about cultural differences.

10. See Chapter 3, Anatomic and Physiologic Vocabulary.

11. See Chapter 4, page 99.

12. See Chapter 14, Authorizations & Signatures, pages 290–296.

13. When working with Hispanic patients with limited English skills, it is very important for health care practitioners to be aware of the fact that very frequently the patient will nod in agreement when speaking to a health care practitioner. This nodding, nonetheless, does not always mean that the patient understands. There are many times when the Hispanic patient is too polite or too embarrassed to say that he/she does not.

14. See Chapter 12, page 272, note 4.

15. See Chapter 8, page 193, note 33.

16. See Chapter 12, page 257.

17. See Chapter 1, pages 17–25 for further discussion about *remedios caseros.*

18. See Chapter 12, pages 263–264.

19. See Chapter 4, page 87 for numbers.

20. See Chapter 1, page 20, for discussion about the Hispanic custom of borrowing and lending medication.

21. In most of Latin America as well as in Spain the large "super" drugstores that are so common throughout the United States, are not to be found. The *droguería* ("drugstore") is a place to go to purchase perfume, sanitary products, cosmetics, kleenex, and other items that are found in U.S. pharmacies but not medicines. Instead, people frequent their neighborhood *farmacia*, usually a small specialty shop where one can purchase items for personal care such as soap, toothpaste, shampoo, cough syrup, and vitamins, and of course, medications of all sorts, including antibiotics which in the United States are only available by prescription. In fact, in the Hispanic world, pharmacists not only recommend or prescribe medicines, but they often give shots.

   Even though there are usually several *farmacias* in each neighborhood, they work together in cooperation to provide service by taking turns staying open all night. They are called *farmacias de turno/farmacias de guardia*. The newspapers publish lists of which pharmacy's turn it is to be open all night. Additionally, either a sign is posted in the window or on the door of each neighborhood shop indicating the schedule so those in need know where to go.

22. The word for "druggist" in Spanish is *farmacéutico/farmacéutica*. Occasionally the word *farmacólogo* is used. However, the word *droguero/droguera* is NOT a cognate. It is used to refer to the person who uses or sell illicit drugs. See Chapter 16, pages 343–345.

23. In the southwestern part of the United States, breakfast is often **almuerzo** and lunch is **comida de mediodía.**

24. See Chapter 3, pages 60f for parts of the body.

25. See Chapter 8, page 192, note 29.

26. See Chapter 3, page 70 for examples of types of broken bones.

27. See Chapter 16, pages 343–345, for Selected **Drug Abuse Vocabulary.**

28. For a listing of colors, see Chapter 16 page 353.

29. Marijuana makes the eyes appear this way.

30. Opiates (heroin and opium) or downers (amytal, numbutal) constrict pupils. Stimulants or uppers (amphetamines, bennies, cocaine, dexies, whites, etc.) dilate the pupils.

31. Also see above, **Drug Overdose** *La dosis excesiva de drogas.*

32. This is directed to a third party, rather than to the patient.

33. See Chapter 16, pages 354–355 for a listing of **Occupations.**

34. See Chapter 16, pages 356–360 for section on foods.

35. See Chapter 16, page 356, **Special diets** *Dietas especiales.*

36. It might be helpful if hospitals made "Hispanic" foods more readily available to those Hispanic patients who are not on a restricted diet. Serving Spanish rice, pinto beans, tortillas, and hot chili sauce, for example, would liven the taste for these patients.

Medical Therapy, Laboratory Tests, and Patient Instructions

Terapia médica, pruebas laboratorias, e instrucciones para el paciente

LABORATORY PROCEDURES

PROCEDIMIENTOS DE LABORATORIO

CHECK-IN   *INSCRIPCION*

1. Would you please sign in.
   Quisiera que firmara el registro.

2. May I have your health insurance card?
   Favor de darme su tarjeta de seguros de salud.

3. Will you take it out and give it to me.
   Favor de sacarla y entregármela.

4. Please sign this so that we can bill your insurance.
   Firme esto aquí para que podamos pasar la factura para la compañía de seguros.

5. Do you have a (written) lab form from your doctor?
   ¿Tiene Vd. un formulario (escrito) para el laboratorio de su médico (médica)?

6. Please have a seat.
   Siéntese Vd., por favor.
   Favor de sentarse.

7. How do you spell your last name?
   ¿Cómo se escribe su apellido?
   ¿Cómo se deletrea su apellido?

8. How do you pronounce your last name?
   ¿Cómo se pronuncia su apellido?

9. Your name will be called as soon as possible.
   Llamaremos su nombre tan pronto como sea posible.

PRELIMINARIES   *LAS PRELIMINARES*

1. Mr./Mrs./Ms. _____ , please follow me.
   Señor/Señora/Señorita _____ , sígame, por favor.

2. Good morning (good afternoon), I am the technician.
   Buenos días (buenas tardes), yo soy el técnico (la técnica).

3. Do you have the doctor's written orders?
   ¿Tiene Vd. las instrucciones escritas del doctor (de la doctora)?

4. May I see the doctor's orders?
   ¿Puedo ver las instrucciones del médico (de la médica)?

5. This test must be done on an empty stomach.
   Tiene que hacerse esta prueba (este análisis) con el estómago vacío (sin haber comido nada).

6. Are you fasting?
   ¿Viene Vd. en ayunas?

7. Have you eaten since midnight?
   ¿Ha tomado algo desde la medianoche?

8. Are you chewing gum now?
   ¿Mastica Vd. chicle ahora?

9. I cannot do the test because of the gum.
   No puedo hacerle el análisis a causa del chicle.

10. Come back tomorrow fasting.
    Vuelva Vd. mañana en ayunas.

11. This test requires you to have eaten something.
    Esta prueba requiere que Vd. haya comido algo.

12. Eat something and come back in 2 (two)/3 (three) hours.
    Toma algo y vuelva en 2 (dos)/3 (tres) horas.

13. Eat a hearty breakfast—orange juice, toast, eggs or cereal, and a cup of coffee or tea, or a glass of milk. Then come back here an hour later for the test.
    Tome un bueno desayuno—jugo de naranja, pan tostado, huevos o cereal, y una taza de café o té, o un vaso de leche. Entonces regrese aquí una hora después para la prueba.

SPECIMEN COLLECTION   *COLECCION DE MUESTRAS*

Venipuncture   *Venipuntura/Sacar sangre de la vena*

1. What type of test are you here for?
   ¿Para qué clase de análisis vino Vd. aquí?
   Blood count?
   ¿Biometría hemática?
   Blood chemistry (analysis of the blood)?
   ¿Análisis de sangre?
   Prothrombin time?
   ¿Análisis de la coagulación de la sangre?
   (del tiempo de protrombina)?
   White cell count?
   ¿Un recuento de los glóbulos blancos (leucocitos)?
   Triglycerides?
   ¿Un examen de triglicéridos?
   ¿Una prueba de triglicéridos?
   Hematocrit?
   ¿Un análisis del hematócrito?

Differential blood count?
¿La fórmula que indica la proporción de cada tipo de leucocitos?
Glucose tolerance test?
¿Un examen de tolerancia para la glucosa?
Lipids?
¿Un análisis de la distribución de lípidos en la sangre?

2. You need some blood tests.[1]
Vd. necesita unos análisis de sangre.

3. I am going to take a sample of your blood.[1]
Voy a tomarle una muestra de sangre.

4. I need to take a few drops of blood from your finger.
Necesito sacarle unas gotas de sangre del dedo.

5. I need to take a few drops of the baby's blood.
Necesito sacarle unas gotas de sangre a la bebé.

6. I am going to take the blood from the baby's heel.
Voy a sacarle la sangre del talón a la bebé.

7. Please remove the baby's bootie/sock and shoe.
Favor de quitarle al (a la) bebé el borceguí (el patín)/el calcetín y el zapato.

8. Hold the baby. Don't let him/her move.
Favor de agarrar al (a la) bebé. No permita que se mueva.

9. I need to take some blood from your arm.
Necesito sacarle alguna sangre del brazo.

10. Which arm do you want me to use?
¿Cuál de los brazos quiere que use?

11. Have you ever had a blood test before?
¿Jamás le han hecho un análisis de sangre?
¿Ha tenido Vd. un análisis de sangre alguna vez?

12. Don't be nervous.
No se ponga nervioso (nerviosa).

13. Don't be afraid.
No tenga miedo.

14. I draw blood from patients many times every day.
Saco sangre de pacientes muchas veces todos los días.

15. Roll up your sleeve.
Súbase la manga.
Arremánguese.

16. Stretch out your arm.
Extienda el brazo.

17. Make a fist, please.
Cierre Vd. el puño, por favor.

18. Keep your hand closed.
Mantenga Vd. la mano cerrada.

19. I am going to tie this tourniquet around your arm.
Voy a atar este torniquete alrededor del brazo.

20. I am going to squeeze.
Voy a apretarle.

21. Try to hold still.
Trate de estar inmóvil.

22. I am going to clean your arm with a little alcohol.
Voy a limpiarle el brazo con un poco de alcohol.

23. I am going to wait until the alcohol dries.
Voy a esperar hasta secarse el alcohol.
Esperaré hasta que se seque el alcohol.

24. It will not hurt.
No le dolerá.

25. This will hurt a little.
Esto le dolerá un poquito.

26. I can't find the vein.
No puedo encontrar la vena.

27. I am sorry, but I have to stick you again.
Lo siento, pero tengo que pincharle otra vez.

28. I wasn't able to get enough blood the first time.
No pude sacarle bastante sangre la primera vez.

29. Don't move, please.
No se mueva, por favor.

30. Open your hand.
Abra Vd. la mano, por favor.

31. I am going to remove the tourniquet.
Voy a quitarle el torniquete.

32. Fold your arm.
Double Vd. el brazo, por favor.

33. Press your finger here so that the bleeding stops.
Apriete aquí con los dedos para parar el sangramiento.

34. Keep this Band-Aid on for a few minutes.
Déjese Vd. esta curita por unos minutos.

35. Do you feel dizzy?
¿Se siente mareado (mareada)?

36. Please, lean forward, and put your head down between your legs for a few minutes.
Favor de inclinarse hacia adelante y poner la cabeza entre las piernas por unos minutos.
Por favor, inclínese Vd. hacia adelante y coloque Vd. la cabeza entre las piernas por unos minutos.

37. You may call your doctor's office for the results on _____ .[2]
Vd. puede telefonear al consultorio de su médico (médica) para los resultados.

STOOL CULTURE *CULTIVO DEL EXCREMENTO*

1. You need a stool culture.
   Vd. necesita un cultivo de heces (un cultivo del excremento).

2. Bring me a (recent) specimen of your stools in this container.
   Tráigame una muestra (reciente) de su excremento (sus evacuaciones) en este frasco.

THROAT CULTURE *UN CULTIVO DE LA GARGANTA*

1. Where are the doctor's lab instructions?
   ¿Dónde están las instrucciones del médico (de la médica) para el laboratorio?

2. S/He has ordered a throat culture.
   Ha pedido un cultivo de la garganta.

3. It will not hurt.
   No le dolerá.

4. Stick your tongue out and say "ah."
   Saque Vd. la lengua y diga «ah.»

5. This is a curette.
   Esta es cureta.

6. I am going to use its cotton end to swab the back of your throat and your tonsils.
   Voy a usar su punta con algodón para frotarle la parte trasera de la garganta y las amígdalas.

7. Don't be afraid if you feel like gagging.
   No tenga miedo si siente que se atraganta.
   No tenga miedo si tiene ganas de arquear.

8. It is normal to gag.
   Es normal atragantarse/arquear.

9. It is a little uncomfortable.
   Es un poco incómodo.

10. When I finish swabbing your throat, I will put the curette back into this container and send it to the lab.
    Cuando termine de frotar la garganta, repondré la cureta en este envase y la enviaré al laboratorio.

11. The lab will examine it to see if there are any bacteria growing on it, especially streptococcus.
    El laboratorio la examinará para ver si hay bacteria que crece, especialmente estreptococo.

12. It will take between twenty-four (24) and forty-eight (48) hours to grow.
    Requiere entre veinticuatro (24) y cuarenta y ocho (48) horas para crecer.

13. The result will be positive if you have streptococcus.
    El resultado será positivo si Vd. tiene estreptococo.

14. In that case we will give you some medicine.
    En este caso le daremos medicina.

15. If the result is negative, you probably have a virus which will last about a week.
    Si el resultado es negativo, es probable que tenga virus que dure unos siete días.

16. The doctor will call you with the results of the test.
    El médico (La médica) le (la) llamará con los resultados de la prueba.

17. In the meantime, gargle with warm salt water and suck on throat lozenges.
    Entretanto, haga gárgaras con agua tibia salada y chupe pastillas para la garganta.

OTHER TESTS *OTRAS PRUEBAS*

1. We have to do some tests.
   Tenemos que hacerle algunos análisis.

2. You need . . .
   Vd. necesita . . .
   a cardiac function test.
   una prueba de función cardíaca.
   a cardiac catheterism.
   un cateterismo cardiovascular.
   angiography.
   una radiografía de los vasos sanguíneos (una angiografía).
   a mammogram.
   un mamograma (una radiografía del seno; una mamografía).[3]
   a CAP test.
   una prueba de CAP para identificar los cambios biotérmicos de los senos (un colorgrama).
   bronchoscopy.
   un examen bronquial directo con un aparato óptico (una broncoscopia).
   a pulmonary function test.
   una prueba funcionaria de los pulmones.
   a serology test.
   una prueba serológica.
   a sputum test.
   un análisis de esputos.
   sigmoidoscopy.
   una inspección del colon con un espéculo rectal (una sigmoidoscopia).
   gastroscopy.
   una gastroscopia (una endoscopia gástrica).
   an upper GI series.
   pruebas del sistema gastrointestinal superior.

a brain scan.
un gammagrama del cerebro.
a liver scan.
un gammagrama del hígado.
a liver function test.
una prueba funcionaria hepática (una prueba de la función hepática).
a proctoscopic examination.
un examen proctoscópico (una inspección del recto).
a biopsy.
una biopsia.
a culture of your vaginal secretions.
un cultivo de las secreciones vaginales.
kidney function test.
una prueba para funcionamiento renal.
a Pap smear.
los untos de Papanicolaou.
los frotis de Papanicolaou.
el test de Papanicolaou.
a pancreatic function test.
una prueba funcional pancreática.
una prueba de tolerancia para la glucosa.
a thyroid function analysis.
una prueba funcional tiroidea.
un análisis de la función del tiroides.

MAMMOGRAM *MAMOGRAMA*

1. Your doctor wants you to have a mammogram.
   Su médica (médico) quiere que tenga una radiografía del seno (una mamografía; un mamograma).

2. You need to make an appointment for a mammogram.
   Vd. tiene que hacer un turno para un mamograma.

3. Have you ever had a mammogram?
   ¿Ha tenido alguna vez un mamograma?

4. Where and when was it?
   ¿Dónde se lo hicieron y cuándo fue?

5. Here is a list of what you should not do on the day of your mammogram.
   Aquí tiene una lista de lo que Vd. no debe hacer el día de su mamograma.

6. Don't use any deodorants.
   No use desodorantes.

7. Don't use any powders.
   No use polvos.

8. Don't use any creams.
   No use cremas.

9. Deodorants, powders, or creams can interfere with the mammography equipment.
   Los desodorantes, polvos, o cremas pueden interferir con el aparato para mamografía.

10. Please remove all of your necklaces and other jewelry.

3. I want to explain them to you.
   Quiero explicárselos a usted(es).

4. You have to go to the clinic (laboratory) for the tests.
   Vd. tiene que ir a la clínica (al laboratorio) para los análisis.

5. Tomorrow they will give you a special test.
   Mañana le harán un análisis especial.

6. You cannot eat or drink anything after midnight.
   Vd. no puede comer ni tomar nada después de medianoche.

7. Don't eat or drink anything before the test.
   No coma ni beba nada antes del análisis.

8. It is important to come to the laboratory without eating.
   Es importante venir al laboratorio sin comer.

9. Don't eat anything.
   Venga en ayunas.

10. Have you eaten or drunk since midnight?
    ¿Ha comido o bebido desde la medianoche?

11. We will bring you breakfast after the test.
    Le traeremos el desayuno después del análisis.

Quítese Vd. los collares y otras joyas, por favor.

11. Please undress to your waist.
    Desvístase, por favor, hasta la cintura.
    Desnúdese de la cintura para arriba.

12. Here is a gown.
    Aquí tiene Vd. una bata de hospital.

13. Put it on with the opening in the front.
    Póngasela con la abertura hacia adelante.

14. Please stand in front of this machine.
    Favor de pararse delante de esta máquina.

15. In order to take the mammogram, I need to compress your breasts as much as possible.
    Para hacerle el mamograma, tengo que comprimirle los senos lo más que se pueda.

16. I am going to put your right (left) breast between these plates to flatten it as much as I can.
    Voy a poner el seno derecho (izquierdo) entre estas placas para aplastarlo tanto como sea posible.

17. Breast compression allows me to take the most accurate X-rays of your breasts using the least amount of radiation.
    La compresión de los senos me permite hacerle radiografías más precisas de sus senos con un mínimo uso de radiación.

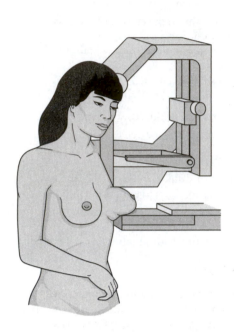

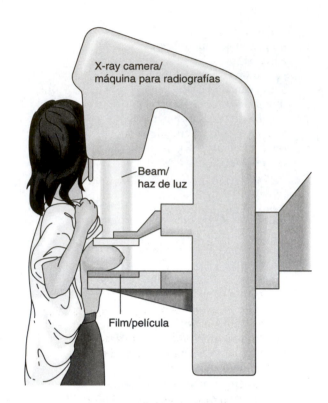

X-ray camera/
máquina para radiografías

Beam/
haz de luz

Film/película

18. Compression decreases the volume of the breast and increases its density.
   La compresión disminuye el volumen del seno y aumenta su densidad.

19. I know that this is uncomfortable and may hurt a bit, but it is only momentary.
   Sé que esto es incómodo y pueda dolerle un poco, pero es solamente momentáneo.

20. Raise your arm like this, and lean in toward the machine.
   Levante Vd. el brazo así, e inclínese hacia la máquina.

21. Hold it.
   Manténgalo.

22. After I take the last X-ray, I want you to wait before you get dressed.
   Después de que saque la última radiografía, quiero que espere antes de vestirse.

23. I must check the X-rays.
   Debo revisar las radiografías.

24. We may have to repeat some X-rays, but don't worry.
   Quizás tengamos que repetir algunas radiografías, pero no se preocupe.

ELECTROCARDIOGRAM   *ELECTROCARDIOGRAMA*

1. You need an electrocardiogram, and I am going to take it.
   Vd. necesita un electrocardiograma, y voy a hacérselo.

2. This machine will record your heartbeats.
   Este aparato (esta máquina) registrará las palpitaciones (los latidos) del corazón.

3. The test will only take 30 (thirty) minutes.
   La prueba durará solamente 30 (treinta) minutos.

4. Please lie still.
   Quédese inmóvil, por favor.

5. I am going to put some cream (jelly) on different parts of your body.
   Voy a ponerle un poco de crema (jalea) en diferentes partes del cuerpo.

6. This helps these leads (wires) to transmit the electricity that comes from the heart.
   Esto ayuda a que estos conductores (cordones) conduzcan la electricidad que viene del corazón.

7. These wires will not hurt you.
   Estos cordones no le (la) dañarán.

8. I am going to put them loosely on your skin.
   Voy a ponérselos sin apretar sobre la piel.

INJECTION   *INYECCION*

1. I am going to give you a shot.[4]
   Voy a ponerle una inyección (un chot *Chicano*).

2. Stretch out your arm.
   Extienda Vd. el brazo, por favor.

3. Roll over on your side.
Póngase Vd. de costado, por favor.
Voltéese Vd. de lado, por favor.

4. The needle will prick a little, but it is for your pain.
Vd. sentirá un poco esta aguja, pero es para aliviarle el dolor.

IV   *SUERO*

1. I am going to start an IV (intravenous feeding) on you.
Le voy a aplicar suero.

2. The IV will go into your veins through this needle.
El alimento intravenoso entrará en sus venas a través de esta aguja.

3. It is not painful once it is in place.
No duele cuando está en su sitio (una vez que está en su sitio).

4. The IV in your arm is to give you food—sugar, salt, and water.
El suero en el brazo es para darle de comer—azúcar, sal, y agua.

5. If necessary, we can also give you medicine through the IV.
Si es necesario, también podemos administrarle medicina por medio del suero.

URINE & KIDNEY TESTS   *PRUEBAS DE LA ORINA Y LOS RIÑONES*

1. The doctor wants you to have a urine culture.
El doctor (La doctora) quiere que le hagan un cultivo de orina.

2. I am going to do a urinalysis.
Voy a hacerle un urinálisis (un análisis de la orina).

3. I need a urine specimen from you.
Necesito una muestra de orina de Vd.

4. You must drink lots of liquids.
Vd. debe tomar muchos líquidos.

5. When you urinate, fill up this bottle and give it to the nurse on duty.
Cuando Vd. orine, llene este frasco y déselo a la enfermera de guardia.

6. Collect and bring your urine of the previous 24 (twenty-four) hours.
Recoja y traiga la orina de las últimas 24 (veinticuatro) horas.

7. Call when you have to go to the toilet.
Llame Vd. cuando tenga que ir al inodoro (a los servicios).

8. Go to the bathroom.
Vaya Vd. al inodoro (a los servicios/al cuarto de baño).

9. Did you urinate?
¿Orinó Vd.?

10. I want you to give me a midstream urine specimen.[5]
Quiero que me dé una muestra recogida a la mitad de la micción.

11. You need a renal function test.
Vd. necesita una prueba funcional renal (una prueba para funcionamiento renal; un análisis de la función de los riñones).

12. We have to do a cystoscopy and an intravenous pyelogram (IVP).[6]
Tenemos que hacerle una cistoscopia (un examen visual de la vejiga urinaria) y un pielograma intravenoso (PIV).

13. We are going to take a K.U.B. (kidneys, ureters, bladder), which is an x-ray of your abdomen.
Vamos a sacarle un R.U.V. (riñón, uréter, vejiga), lo que es una radiografía del abdomen.

14. You do not have to prepare for this.
Vd. no tiene que prepararse para ésta.

15. It is used in the diagnosis of urinary system diseases and disorders.
Se usa para diagnosticar enfermedades y trastornos del sistema urinario.

16. It is also used to locate foreign bodies in the digestive tract.
También se usa para encontrar cuerpos extraños en el canal digestivo.

CYSTOSCOPY   *CISTOSCOPIA*

1. I am going to perform a cystoscopy on you.
Voy a hacerle una cistoscopia.

2. I want to look into your bladder in order to find the reason for your bleeding, infection, pain, etc.
Quiero examinarle la vejiga para descubrir la razón del sangrar, de la infección, del dolor, etc.

3. You must sign a permit for me to do the cystoscopy, the name of this procedure.
Vd. tiene que firmar el permiso para que le haga la cistoscopia, que es el nombre de este procedimiento.

4. Please undress and put on this gown.
Desvístase, por favor, y póngase esta bata.

5. Get up on the table and put your feet in the stirrups. Lie back.
    Súbase a la mesa y ponga los pies en los estribos. Acuéstese.

6. Someone will wash you with an antiseptic solution.
    Alguien le lavará con una solución antiséptica.

(For Females)   *(Para hembras)*

7. The nurse will inject some medicine (topical anesthetic) into your urethra and then cover the opening with a cotton swab to keep the medicine (anesthesia) in. This will make you feel more comfortable during this procedure.
    La enfermera le jeringará algún medicamento (una anestesia local) en la uretra y entonces colocará un hisopillo en la abertura para que el medicamento (la anestesia) se quede. Esto le hará sentirse más cómoda durante este procedimiento.

8. I am going to examine your bladder with this instrument.
    Voy a examinarle la vejiga con este instrumento.

9. You will feel pressure while I am inserting it.
    Sentirá presión mientras que lo introduzca.

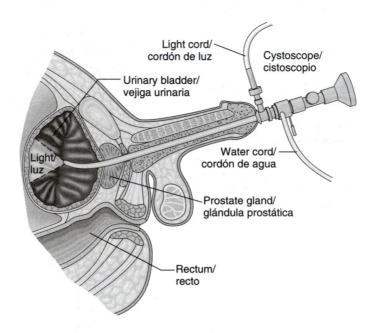

Light cord/ cordón de luz

Cystoscope/ cistoscopio

Urinary bladder/ vejiga urinaria

Light/ luz

Water cord/ cordón de agua

Prostate gland/ glándula prostática

Rectum/ recto

(For Males)   *(Para varones)*

10. The nurse will inject a topical anesthetic into your urethra and then put a clamp on your penis in order to keep the anesthetic in. This will not hurt and you will feel more comfortable during the procedure.
    El enfermero le jeringará una anestesia local en la uretra y entonces le pondrá una grapa en el pene para que se quede la anestesia. Esto no le dañará y le hará sentirse más cómodo durante el procedimiento.

11. I am going to insert this instrument through the opening in your penis.
    Voy a introducirle este instrumento por la abertura del pene.

12. You will feel some pressure in the urethra and discomfort as the instrument passes through your prostate.
    Sentirá una sensación de presión en la uretra y molestia mientras que el instrumento pase por la próstata.

13. Breathe deeply and try to relax.
    Respire profundo y trate de calmarse.

(For Both)   *(Para los dos)*

14. In order to find out the cause of your problem, I have to fill your bladder with water.
    Para averiguar la causa de su problema, tengo que llenarle la vejiga con agua.

15. The water expands your bladder and lets me see the bladder through the instrument.
    El agua amplía la vejiga y me permite observar la vejiga por medio del instrumento.

16. If there is not enough water in your bladder, it will collapse around the cystoscope (instrument).
Si no hay bastante agua en la vejiga, se caerá alrededor del cistoscopio (instrumento).

17. I can let some water out through the instrument if you feel too uncomfortable, but I cannot let much out or I will not be able to see inside.
Puedo vaciar un poco de agua por el instrumento si se siente demasiado incómodo (incómada), pero no puedo vaciar mucho o no podré ver adentro.

18. I am giving you a prescription for an antibiotic which you must take *twice* daily for *five* days to prevent infection.[7]
Le daré una receta para antibióticos que debe tomar *dos* veces por día por *cinco* días.

19. You may have some burning when you urinate and you may notice some blood in your urine today. It is normal.
Puede sufrir de ardor cuando orine y puede observar un poco de sangre en la orina hoy. Es normal.

20. If the burning, discomfort, or bleeding continue, please call me at the office.
Si el ardor, la molestia, o la sangría sigue, llámeme/avíseme al consultorio, por favor.

INTRAVENOUS PYELOGRAM [IVP] *PIELOGRAMA INTRAVENOSO [PIV]*

1. I am going to take an IVP, which is a special X-ray of your kidneys.
Voy a hacerle un pielograma intravenoso, que es una radiografía especial de los riñones.

2. It will tell us if you have cysts or kidney stones, and it also lets us look at the structures of the urinary system.
Nos avisará si usted tiene quistes o piedras (cálculos) en los riñones, y también nos permite mirar las estructuras del aparato urinario.

3. The day before the test you may eat only a limited amount of food, and it must be restricted in both fat and residue.
El día antes del examen usted puede comer solamente una cantidad limitada de comida, y debe ser restringida tanto en grasas como en resido.

4. At midday on the day before the test eat clear juice, clear broth, a piece of turkey or chicken without the skin, plain jello, some bread or toast, and a glass of milk.
Al mediodía el día antes de la prueba, tome jugo claro, caldo claro, tajadas de pavo o pollo sin pellejo, gelatina sola, unas rebanadas de pan o tostado, y un vaso de leche.

5. That evening eat only clear liquids—bouillon, clear juice, tea, and jello.
Esa tarde solo tome líquidos claros—caldo, jugo claro, té, y gelatina.

6. Do not drink milk of any kind.
No beba ningún tipo de leche.

7. The day before the test take four (4) ounces of Neoloid or three (3) Dulcolax five (5) milligram tablets from 2:00–4:00 PM.
El día antes de la prueba tome cuatro (4) onzas de Neoloid o tres (3) tabletas de cinco (5) miligramos de Dulcolax entre las dos (2) y las cuatro (4) de la tarde.

8. After an early evening meal, you may drink water only until midnight.
Después de una temprana comida de la noche, puede tomar agua solamente hasta medianoche.

9. After midnight, do not eat or drink anything by mouth if the test is scheduled before 11:00 AM.
Después de la medianoche, no coma ni beba nada por boca si la prueba se planea antes de las once.

10. If the test is scheduled after 11:00 AM, you may have half a cup of black coffee, a small amount of clear juice, a poached egg, a slice of toast or a muffin, some jelly, and sugar and salt.
Si la radiografía está planeada después de las once (11) de la mañana, puede tomar media taza de café solo, una pequeña cantidad de jugo claro, un huevo escalfado, una tajada de pan tostado o un pan inglés, alguna jalea clara, y azúcar y sal.

11. Are you allergic to iodine.[8]
¿Es Vd. alérgico (alérgica) a yodo? ¿Tiene Vd. alergia a yodo?

12. Are you allergic to seafood?[8]
¿Tiene Vd. alergia a mariscos y pescado de mar comestibles?

13. Have you received premedication with prednisone and Benadryl?
¿Le han recetado premedicación de prednisona y Benadril?[9]

14. Please lie down on this table.
Favor de acostarse en esta mesa.

15. Before beginning the test, we are going to take an X-ray of your abdomen.
Antes de empezar la prueba, vamos a hacerle unos rayos equis del abdomen.

16. I am going to inject an iodine dye in your arm.
Le inyectaré una tinta de yodo en el brazo.

17. This will take about twenty to thirty minutes. It may take forty-five minutes, however.
Esto durará unos veinte a treinta minutos. Sin embargo, puede requerir cuarenta y cinco minutos.

18. As the dye passes through your veins going into your kidneys, you will feel a hot flush.
Al pasar la tinta por las venas yendo hacia los riñones, se sentirá un sofoco de calor.

19. You may also experience a salty or metallic taste in your mouth.
Es posible que también sienta un sabor salado o metálico en la boca.

20. A sterile catheter may be inserted into the bladder through the urinary meatus.
Una sonda estéril puede insertarse en la vejiga por el orificio externo de la uretrao el meato urinario.

21. It will be a little painful, but I will be as careful and gentle as possible.
Va a dolerle un poco, pero lo haré lo más gentil y cuidadosamente que pueda.

22. Then I am going to take some X-rays of your kidneys.
Después, voy a sacarle unas radiografías (unos rayos X) de los riñones.

23. We are going to take X-rays at specific times: after 1, 5, 10, 15, 20, and 30 minutes.
Vamos a hacerle rayos equis a intervalos específicos: después de 1, 5, 10, 15, 20, y 30 minutos.

24. Can you urinate?
¿Puede Vd. orinar?

25. Don't worry. I am going to put this tube into your bladder to drain your urine.
No se preocupe. Voy a ponerle este tubo en la vejiga para drenar la orina.

26. We are going to take another film now that there is no urine in your bladder.
Vamos a hacerle otra película (otro rayo e-quis) ya que no hay orina en la vejiga.

27. This procedure is called an intravenous pyelogram.
Este procedimiento se llama un pielograma intravenoso.

28. Because you are allergic to iodine (shellfish), we are going to do a Retrograde Pyelogram using a non-iodine dye.

Porque tiene alergia a yodo (mariscos y pescado de mar comestibles), vamos a hacerle un pielograma intravenoso retrógrado usando una tinta hecha sin yodo.

29. With the Retrograde Pyelogram a certain instrument (a cystoscope) is used to guide special catheters into the ureters and then into the renal pelvis.
Con el pielograma intravenoso retrógrado se usa un cierto instrumento (un cistoscopio) para guiar catéteres especiales por los uréteres y entonces por el bacinete (la pelvis) renal.

30. You must drink at least three eight-ounce glasses of liquid to flush your kidneys.
Vd. debe beber por lo menos tres vasos de ocho onzas de líquido para limpiar los riñones.

X-Ray: Intravenous Pyelogram (IVP)
Radiografía: Pielograma intravenoso (PIV)

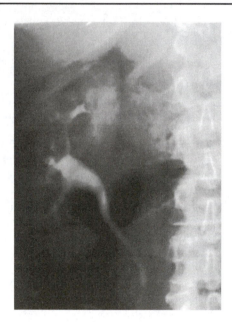

ENEMA PROCEDURE *PROCEDIMIENTO PARA UN ENEMA*

1. Give yourself an enema before coming.
Póngase una enema antes de venir.[4,10]

2. (Don't) Take a laxative the night before.
(No) Tome Vd. un laxante la noche anterior.

3. You have to give yourself at least three tap water enemas before coming to the hospital the morning of your test.
Vd. tiene que administrarse (darse) por lo menos tres enemas hechas con agua corriente antes de venir al hospital la mañana de su prueba.

4. Go to your pharmacy or drugstore and buy an enema bag kit.
Vaya a su farmacia o droguería y compre un botiquín de enemas.

5. Do not buy a Fleets enema.
No compre una lavativa de Fleets.

6. Fill the enema bag with lukewarm water.
Llene el saco de enemas con agua tibia.

7. Run a little of the water through the tubing to expel air.
Pase un poco del agua por la tubería para expeler el aire.

8. In order to give yourself an enema you should lie on your left side with your right knee bent and your arms at rest. (A)

Para ponerse una enema (una lavativa) Vd. debe acostarse al lado izquierdo con la rodilla derecha doblada y los brazos en reposo. (A)

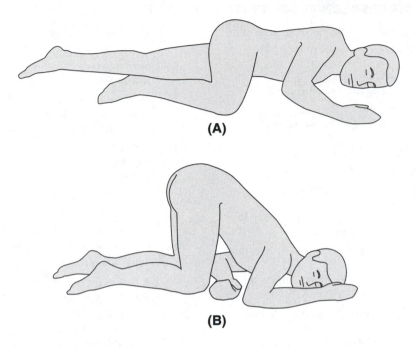

(A)

(B)

9. If that position is not comfortable, kneel. Then lower your head until the left side of your face is resting on the same surface as your knees. Position your arms comfortably. (B)
   Si esa posición no es cómoda, póngase de rodillas. Entonces baje la cabeza hasta que el lado izquierdo de la cara se apoye en la misma superficie que las rodillas. Coloque los brazos a su gusto. (B)

10. Hang the enema bag on something (i.e., a door knob) using the hanger provided or a clothes hanger.
    Cuelgue el botiquín de enemas en algo (por ejemplo, un tirador) usando el colgadero incluido o una percha.

11. Lubricate about two inches of the tubing starting at the tip.
    Lubrique dos pulgadas más o menos de la tubería comenzando a la punta.

12. Gently insert the lubricated tip into your rectum.
    Suavemente introduzca la punta lubricada en el recto.

13. The fluid should flow slowly.
    El flúido debe correr lentamente.

14. You can adjust the flow rate with the tubing clamp.
    Puede modificar la velocidad de flujo con la grapa de la tubería.

15. Breathe slowly and deeply to relax the abdominal muscles.
    Respire despacio y profundo para aflojar los músculos abdominales.

16. Try to hold as much water as you can, the whole bag if possible.
    Trate de retener tanta agua como pueda, el saco entero si es posible.

17. Expel the liquid into the toilet.
    Expele el líquido en el inodoro.

18. If you cannot hold all the water, give yourself as many enemas as necessary to equal three bags of water.
    Si no puede retener toda el agua, póngase tantos enemas como necesario hasta igualar la cantidad de tres sacos de agua.

20. Give yourself at least 3 enemas until the water expelled is clear.
    Póngase por lo menos tres enemas hasta que el agua expelada esté clara.

MORE RADIOGRAPHY   *RADIOGRAFIA ADICIONAL*

1. You need an x-ray.
   Vd. necesita (tomarse) una radiografía.

2. Someone will come to take you to x-ray.
   Alguien le (la) llevará al cuarto de rayos X.

3. The x-rays will be taken tomorrow.
   La radiografía se hará mañana.

4. Lie down on the x-ray table.
   Acuéstese Vd. sobre la mesa radiográfica.

5. It may be a little cold.
   Es posible que esté un poco fría.

6. Let me put you in the right position.
   Déjeme ponerle (colocarle) en la postura correcta.

UPPER GI *LA PARTE SUPERIOR DEL SISTEMA DIGESTIVO*

1. You need a barium swallow to try to determine if you have ulcers or a tumor in your digestive tract.
   Vd. necesita un trago de bario para tratar de determinar si tiene úlceras o un tumor en el sistema/aparato digestivo.

2. In order to take the x-ray you must swallow this mixture.
   Para sacarle la radiografía, Vd. tiene que tomar (tragar) esta mezcla.

3. Hold the cup up, and every time that I say "Drink," take a sip.
   Mantenga el vaso en alto, y cada vez que le diga «Beba,» tome Vd. un trago.

4. The liquid, which is called barium sulfate, may not taste good.
   Quizás el líquido, que se llama sulfato de bario, no tenga un buen sabor.

5. Don't drink all the mixture now. Drink only half.
   No tome Vd. toda la mezcla ahora. Beba solamente la mitad.

6. Stand here and place your chest against this plate.
   Párese Vd. aquí y apoye el pecho contra esta placa.

7. Let me put you in the right position.
   Permítame colocarle en la postura correcta.

8. Move a little over to the right (left).
   Muévase Vd. un poco hacia la derecha (izquierda).

9. Rest your chin here.
   Apoye Vd. la barbilla (el mentón) aquí.

10. Put your hands on your hips with the palms facing out, like so.
    Póngase Vd. las manos en las caderas con las palmas hacia afuera, así.

11. Take a deep breath and hold it.
    Respire Vd. profundamente y sostenga la respiración.

12. Don't move, please
    No se mueva Vd., por favor.

13. Now you may breathe.
    Ahora Vd. puede respirar.

14. Turn your body slowly to the left; to the right.
    Gire Vd. el cuerpo lentamente hacia la izquierda; hacia la derecha.

15. Breathe in.
    Aspire Vd.[11]

16. Breathe out.
    Exhale Vd.

17. Stand perfectly still.
    Párese Vd. perfectamente quieto (quieta).

18. We have to take another film.
    Tenemos que sacarle otra placa.

19. I have to press your stomach.
    Tengo que apretarle el estómago.

20. It probably will not hurt, but you may have cramps and be constipated.
    Probablemente no va a dolerle, pero puede tener calambres y estar estreñido (estreñida).

21. Thank you for your cooperation.
    Gracias por su cooperación (colaboración).

22. Your doctor will tell you the results.
    Su doctor (doctora) le dirá los resultados.

23. Sit down on the wheelchair and wait for the orderly.
    Siéntese Vd. en la silla de ruedas y espere al ayudante.

24. The orderly will take you back to your room.
    El ayudante le (la) llevará a su cuarto.

25. Come back Thursday at 9:00 AM.[2]
    Vuelva Vd. el jueves a las nueve de la mañana, por favor.

26. You have an appointment for Monday.
    Vd. tiene una cita para el lunes.

LOWER GI *LA PARTE INFERIOR DEL SISTEMA DIGESTIVO*

Barium Enema *Enema de bario*

1. Please get undressed and put on a hospital gown.
   Favor de desvestirse y ponerse una bata de hospital.

2. Put the gown on with the ties in the front.
   Póngase la bata con las cuerdas enfrente.

3. Put the gown on with the ties in the back.
   Póngase la bata con las cuerdas detrás.

4. You need a barium enema.
   Vd. necesita un enema de bario.

5. Have you ever had a barium enema?
   ¿Jamás ha tenido una lavativa de bario?

6. I will give you an enema that contains a barium sulfate solution.
   Le pondré un enema que lleva una solución de sulfato de bario.[4]

7. Turn on your left (right) side.
Acuéstese Vd. sobre el lado izquierdo (derecho).

8. Turn over.
Voltéese Vd. del otro lado, por favor.
Dése vuelta.

SPINAL TAP *LA PUNCION LUMBAR*

1. I have to do a spinal tap/lumbar puncture.
Tengo que hacerle una punción lumbar (punción raquídea).

2. I am going to draw some fluids from your spine.
Voy a sacarle flúido de la columna vertebral.

3. In order to do that, I will inject some medicine directly into your back in order to numb it.
Para hacer eso, le inyectaré medicina/le pondré una inyección de medicina directamente en la espalda para entumecerla.

4. It will sting for a little while.
Le picará durante algún tiempo.

5. Please lie on your side near the edge of the bed.
Acuéstese de un lado, por favor, cerca del borde de la cama.

6. Bring your knees up to your chest, and bend your head down so that your chin rests on your chest, if possible.
Doble Vd. las rodillas junto al pecho y baje la cabeza de manera que la barbilla descanse sobre el pecho, si es posible.

7. That's it. Lie perfectly still.
Así. Quédese perfectamente quieto (quieta).

8. Don't move at all.
No se mueva nada.

9. I am going to apply a brown liquid all over your back.
Voy a aplicarle un líquido marrón en todas partes de la espalda.

10. Now I am going to make a mark on your lower back where I am going to insert the needle.
Ahora voy a marcar el lugar en la cintura donde pienso introducir la aguja.

11. Now I am going to inject your skin with Lidocaine, a local anesthetic, so that you will not feel the pain of the needle.
Ahora voy a inyectar un poco de Lidocaína, un anestético local, para que no sienta el dolor de la aguja.

12. Do you feel the needle?
¿Siente la aguja?

13. Please don't move.
Favor de no moverse.
No se mueva, por favor.

14. Now I am going to insert the needle into the space between your vertebrae.
Ahora voy a introducir la aguja en el espacio entre las vértebras.
Ahora introduciré la aguja en el espacio entre las vértebras.

15. I am going to withdraw the needle.
Voy a quitarle la aguja.
Leguitaré la aguja.

16. I am all finished.
Ya terminé.

17. You are going to feel a bit of pressure on your back; it's my finger.
Va a sentir un poco de presión en la espalda; es mi dedo.

18. I am going to clean off your back.
Voy a limpiarle/Le limpiaré la espalda.

19. I have just put a bandage on your back.
Acabo de ponerle una venda en la espalda.

20. You may relax and move.
Vd. puede relajarse[12] ahora y moverse.

21. I suggest that you stay in bed today as much as possible.
Sugiero que se quede acostado (acostada) en cama hoy tanto como sea posible.

22. You will have a horrible headache if you try to get up.
Va a sufrir una jaqueca increíble si trata de levantarse.

23. Call the office if you feel pain or tingling in either one of your legs.
Llame al consultorio si siente algún dolor u hormigueo en cualquiera de las piernas.

24. If you develop a headache, take something for pain like aspirin or acetaminophen and lie down.
Si empieza a sufrir de un dolor de cabeza, tome algo para el dolor como aspirina o acetaminofén y acuéstese.

9. The x-rays will help us determine if you have ulcers in your lower digestive tract.
Las radiografías van a ayudarnos a determinar si tiene úlceras en la parte inferior del sistema digestivo.

INSTRUCTIONS FOR OUTPATIENT SURGERY *INSTRUCCIONES PARA PACIENTES EXTERNOS*

1. Please arrive thirty minutes (two hours) prior to your surgery.
Favor de llegar treinta minutos (dos horas antes de su cirugía.

2. You CANNOT come alone. A responsible adult must accompany you to drive you home afterward.

Vd. NO PUEDE venir solo (sola). Un adulto responsable tiene que acompañarle (acompañarla) para conducirle (conducirla) a casa después.

3. Except for medications, DO NOT EAT OR DRINK ANYTHING AFTER MIDNIGHT before surgery.
Con excepción de medicamentos, NO COMA NI BEBA NADA DESPUES DE MEDIANOCHE antes de la cirugía.

4. If you are taking medicines for high blood pressure, heart problems, or breathing problems, take your morning medicines with a sip of water on the day of the surgery.
Si toma medicinas para la alta presión, problemas cardíacos, o problemas de respirar,

tome las medicinas matutinas con un traguito de agua el día de la cirugía.

5. Bring all your medications with you.
Lleve todos los medicamentos consigo.

6. Do no smoke marijuana or use cocaine for 48 hours before surgery.
No fume mariguana ni use cocaína por 48 horas antes de la cirugía.

7. Leave all money and jewelry at home.
Deje todo su dinero y todas las joyas en casa.

8. Do not drive a car or make important legal decisions for the remainder of the day after your surgery.
No conduzca un coche ni haga decisiones legales importantes durante el resto del día de su cirugía.

BREAST SELF-EXAMINATION *AUTOEXPLORACION MAMARIA*

1. Undress from the waist up and stand in front of a mirror, first with your arms at your side and then with your arms raised.
Desnúdese de cintura para arriba y ante un espejo párese primero con los brazos caídos y luego levantados.

2. Look at both breasts carefully for irregularity of the breast surface, its shape, or the nipples.
Fíjese Vd. cuidadosamente en cualquier deformación de la superficie mamaria, de su contorno, o del pezón.

3. In front of the mirror, check both breasts for a nipple discharge, a puckering, or a dimpling.
Delante del espejo, revísese para ver si encuentra un derrame o una supuración espontánea de los pezones, un arrugamiento, u hoyuelo en la piel.

4. Lean forward to check for any abnormalities in shape.
Agáchese hacia adelante para ver si encuentra alguna anormalidad en la forma.

5. Clasp your hands behind your head, tightening the chest muscles. Repeat a careful visual inspection.
Eche Vd. las manos alrededor de la cabeza, estirando los músculos del pecho. Repita una inspección visual cuidadosa.

6. Press your hands firmly down on your hips, again tightening your chest muscles. Repeat a careful visual inspection of your breasts.
Apóyese las manos firmemente en las caderas, estirando de nuevo los músculos del pecho. Repita una inspección visual cuidadosa.

7. Remember that it is normal for one breast to look a little different from the other.
Recuerde que es normal si un seno parece un poco diferente del otro.

8. Examine your breasts while you bathe or shower when your skin is humid and lumps can be felt more easily.
Examínese los senos mientras se baña o se ducha cuando la piel está húmeda y los abultamientos pueden ser más fáciles de sentir.

9. While standing (in the shower), raise your left arm in the air.
De pie (en la ducha), levante Vd. el brazo izquierdo.

10. Use three or four fingers on your right hand to explore the left breast for any unusual lump under the skin.
Use tres o cuatro dedos de la mano derecha para explorar cuidadosamente el seno izquierdo y averiguar si siente algún abultamiento o dureza no común debajo de la piel.

11. Press with the flat part of your fingertips in a circular motion beginning at the top outside edge to look for lumps.
Apriete Vd. la yema de los dedos usando una moción circular empezando al borde exterior superior para buscar algún abultamiento.

12. Repeat the process, moving in a clockwise fashion.
Repita el proceso, usando un movimiento de reloj.

13. Make each circle smaller as you move toward the nipple.
Haga más pequeño cada círculo al moverse hacia el pezón.

14. You should make at least four concentric circles or more to cover each breast.
Vd. debe hacer por lo menos cuatro círculos concéntricos o más para examinar cada seno.

15. Then repeat the procedure on the right side with the left hand.

Entonces, repita el procedimiento con el lado derecho y la mano izquierda.

16. Lie on your back with your left hand behind your head putting a pillow under your left shoulder.
    Acuéstese Vd. de espaldas con la mano izquierda detrás de la cabeza poniéndose una almohada bajo el hombro izquierdo.

17. This position helps flatten the breast tissue.
    Esta posición ayuda a allanarse o aplanar el tejido del seno.

18. Using the flat tips of the middle three fingers of your right hand, press gently down to feel the breast tissue with in small circular clockwise motions.
    Usando la yema de los tres dedos del centro de la mano derecha, haga presión con la suficiente firmeza para sentir los diferentes tejidos del seno haciendo un movimiento circular.

19. Work inward toward the nipple. Check the area surrounding the breast, beginning with the underarm.
    Tiente el seno presionando hacia el pezón. Revise las áreas que rodean los pechos, empezando por las axilas.

20. Some women and their physicians prefer to use an up and down method, others prefer the wedge. Most use a circular (clockwise or oval) method, however, to check their breasts.
    Algunas mujeres y sus médicos prefieren usar un procedimiento de lista vertical, otros prefieren el de cuña. Sin embargo, la mayoría usan el circular (de reloj u ovalado), para examinarse los senos.

21. Finally, squeeze the nipple of the left breast gently between the thumb and index finger of the right hand.
    Oprima el pezón del seno izquierdo suavemente entre el pulgar y el índice de la mano derecha.

22. Report any discharge, clear or bloody, to your doctor.
    Hágale un informe sobre cualquier supuración, clara o sangrienta, a su médico (médica).

23. Repeat the procedure on the other side.
    Repita el procedimiento con el lado opuesto.

Breast Self-Examination *Autoexploración mamaria*

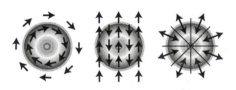

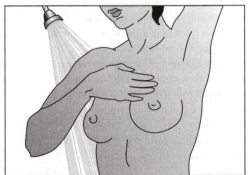

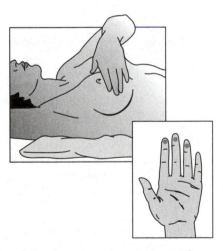

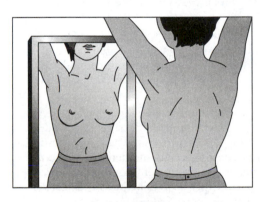

(Courtesy of the American Cancer Society).

TESTICULAR SELF-EXAMINATION *AUTOEXPLORACION TESTICULAR*

1. Every man should examine his testicles monthly to be able to find any abnormality in its earliest stages.
   Todos los hombres deben examinarse los testículos una vez por mes para poder descubrir cualquier anomalía en su etapa precoz.

2. It is ideal to do this immediately after a bath or warm shower when the skin of your body is relaxed.
    Es ideal hacer esto inmediatamente después de un baño o una ducha templada cuando la piel del cuerpo estará relajada.

3. Stand naked or undress from the waist down and stand in front of a mirror.
    Párese desnudo o desnúdese de la cintura para abajo y párese delante un espejo.

4. Look for any swelling on the skin of the scrotum.
    Busque cualquier hinchazón en la piel del escroto.

5. With one hand lift your penis and look at your scrotum remembering that the left side may be slightly lower than the right.
    Con una mano levante el pene y mire el escroto recordando que el lado izquierdo del escroto puede estar un poquito más abajo que el derecho.

6. With the penis raised, observe the scrotum and testicles carefully to see if there are any distended, red veins or any change in their shape or size.
    Con el pene levantado, observe los testículos con cuidado para ver si hay venas distendidas y rojas o algún cambio en su forma o tamaño.

7. Feel your testicles for any lumps, nodules, swelling, or change in their consistency.
    Palpe los testículos para bultos, nódulos, hinchazón, o cualquier cambio en su consistencia.

8. When examining your right testicle, place your right thumb on the front part and the index and middle fingers on the back of the testicle.
    Al examinar el testículo derecho, ponga el pulgar en la parte del frente y el índice y el dedo mayor (dedo del corazón) detrás del testículo.

9. Squeeze and roll the testicle gently trying to touch your thumb to the other two fingers. Your fingers should meet.
    Apriete y empuje el testículo suavemente tratando de hacer juntar el pulgar con los otros dos dedos. Los dedos deben encontrarse.

10. Feel all parts of the testicle.
    Palpe todas las partes del testículo.

11. Repeat the procedure on the left testicle using your left hand.
    Repita el procedimiento con el testículo izquierdo usando la mano izquierda.

12. You should be able to move the testicles.
    Vd. debe poder mover los testículos.

13. Your testicles should feel slightly tender, smooth, and gummy.
    Los testículos deben sentirse levemente sensibles, tersos, y gomosos.

14. Find the epididymis on the right testicle, which is like a string on the top and back of the testicle.
    Encuentre el epidídimo del testículo derecho, que es como un tipo de cordón ubicado en la parte posterior del testículo.

15. The spermatic cord begins at the epididymis and goes into (the inguinal duct in) the body. It contains veins, arteries, nerves, lymphatics, and sperm which it stores and transports through a(n excretory) duct.
    El cordón espermático se extiende desde el epidídimo hacia el conducto inguinal del cuerpo. Contiene venas, arterias, nervios, linfáticos, y esperma que acumula y transporta por un conducto (excretorio).

16. Examine the spermatic cord with the thumb, index, and middle finger of your right hand for lumps or masses by squeezing it gently.
    Examine el cordón espermático usando el pulgar, el índice y el dedo mayor de la mano derecha para bultos o masas al oprimirlo suavemente.

17. Do the same thing with the spermatic cord of your left testicle, using your left hand.
    Haga la misma cosa con el cordón espermático del testículo izquierdo, usando la mano izquierda.

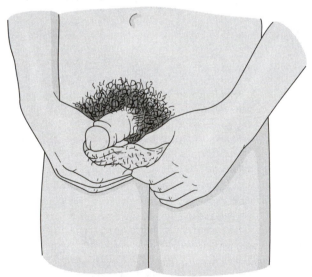

Testicular self-examination/
Autoexploración testicular

18. Call your doctor if you find any lump, nodule, or swelling or any change.
    Llame a su médico (médica) si encuentra cualquier bulto, nódulo, o hinchazón o algún cambio.

CONTRACEPTIVE METHODS FOR FAMILY PLANNING[13]

LOS METODOS ANTICONCEPTIVOS PARA LA PLANIFICACION FAMILIAR

1. Are you interested in talking about birth control?
    ¿Le interesa hablar de los métodos anticonceptivos (de la prevención del embarazo)?

2. Do you know about birth control?
    ¿Sabe Vd. (algo) de los métodos para no tener hijos (del control de la natalidad)?

3. Are you interested in using some form of birth control?
    ¿Le interesa usar alguna forma de anticoncepción (contracepción)?

4. Have you ever used it?
    ¿La ha usado Vd. alguna vez?

5. Do you use contraception now?
    ¿Usa Vd. anticonceptivos ahora?
    ¿Usa Vd. contracepción ahora?

6. Would you like to use them?[14]
    ¿Quisiera Vd. usarlos?

7. Are you satisfied with your present method?
    ¿Está Vd. satisfecha (satisfecho) con su método actual?

8. Would you like to have (more) children?
    ¿Quiere Vd. tener (más) hijos?

9. Do you want to discuss this with your husband (boyfriend)?
    ¿Quiere Vd. discutir esto con su esposo (novio)?

10. Do you want to talk about this with your husband (boyfriend) present?
    ¿Quiere Vd. hablar de esto en la presencia de su esposo (novio)?

11. I advise you to discuss your sexual goals with your spouse (boyfriend) as well as your thoughts about spacing pregnancies, and the number of children you want.
    Le aconsejo que hable de sus metas sexuales con su esposo (novio) así como las del espaciamiento de sus embarazos y del número de hijos que quisiera.

12. You and your husband will have time to talk and choose the method that is best for you.
    Su esposo y Vd. tendrán tiempo para hablar y escoger el método que sea más satisfactorio para ustedes dos.

13. It is important to know how the reproductive system works.
    Es importante saber cómo funciona el sistema reproductivo.

14. The man has two external parts: the penis and the scrotum (balls), which is a sac that hangs under the penis and contains two testicles that produce sperm.
    El hombre tiene dos partes externas: el pene y el escroto (las bolas), que es un saco que
    cuelga por debajo del pene y contiene dos testículos que producen la esperma (las semillas).

15. When a man gets excited or "hot," his penis fills with blood and becomes hard (it produces an erection).
    Cuando un hombre se excita, o «se calienta,» el pene se llena de sangre y se pone duro (se produce una erección).

16. During sexual excitement the sperm combines with a milky liquid called semen, which is expelled by the erect penis by means of muscular contractions.
    Durante la excitación sexual la esperma se combina con un líquido lechoso, llamado semen, que es expulsado por el pene erecto mediante contracciones musculares.

17. This process of expelling semen is called ejaculation ("coming"), and the feeling of pleasure is called an orgasm.
    Este proceso de expulsar el semen se llama la eyaculación (el «venirse»), y la sensación de placer se llama un orgasmo.

18. Ejaculation can also occur during a "wet-dream," one which excites sexually, or by means of masturbation.[15]
    La eyaculación también puede producirse durante el sueño que produce una emisión seminal nocturna, uno que le excite en forma sexual, o por medio de la masturbación.

19. During sexual intercourse the penis penetrates the vagina and gives off semen.
    Durante el acto sexual el pene penetra en la vagina de la mujer y suelta el semen en ella.

20. The woman has two ovaries, each of which alternately produces an egg cell about once every 28 days.
    La mujer tiene dos ovarios, uno de los cuales produce un óvulo (o célula femenina) más o menos cada veintiocho días.

21. The egg cell moves through the fallopian tube to the uterus (womb).
    El óvulo se mueve por la trompa de falopio hasta el útero (también llamado la matriz).

22. During intercourse sperm are introduced into the vagina and travel upward into the uterus and then into the tubes.
    Durante el acto sexual la esperma se introduce en la vagina y viaja hacia arriba por el útero y de ahí a las trompas.

23. If a sperm unites with an egg cell that has been released, fertilization occurs and a baby begins to develop.

Si una esperma se encuentra con un óvulo que ha sido desprendido, ocurre la fertilización y un bebé empieza a desarrollarse.

24. If the egg is not united with a sperm, the egg and the lining of the uterus (which would have fed the fertilized egg) are eliminated in the process of menstruation (the "period"), which lasts from 3 (three) to 7 (seven) days.[16]
   Si el óvulo no se une a una esperma, el óvulo y el forro del útero (que hubiera alimentado al óvulo fertilizado) se eliminan en la menstruación (o el período de la mujer), que dura de 3 (tres) a 7 (siete) días.

25. The basic idea of birth control is to prevent the sperm from meeting the egg in the woman's body.
   La idea básica de control de la natalidad es evitar que la esperma del hombre alcance el óvulo en el cuerpo de la mujer.

FOAM AND CONDOM *ESPUMA Y CONDON*

1. You can use contraceptive foam and your husband can use a condom. These can be bought in any place where sanitary items are sold.
   Vd. puede usar la espuma anticonceptiva y su esposo puede usar un condón. Estos pueden comprarse en cualquier lugar donde se venden toallas sanitarias.

2. It is best to use foam or contraceptive cream or jelly with a condom.
   Es mejor usar la espuma o una crema o jalea anticonceptivas con un condón (un preservativo).

3. Alone they are not very safe.
   Solo (Sola) no es muy seguro (segura).

4. The cream (or foam) comes in a container that resembles a tampon.
   La crema (La espuma) viene en un frasco que se parece a un tampón.

5. Fill the applicator and insert it in the vagina no more than a half-hour before intercourse since the heat of the woman's body changes it to liquid.
   Llene el aplicador e insértelo en la vagina no más de media hora antes de tener relaciones sexuales puesto que el calor del cuerpo la vuelve líquido.

6. Use it *each* time that you have intercourse.
   Usela *cada* vez que tenga coito.

7. Do not douche for 8 hours after.
   No se dé lavaje (ducha vaginal) durante ocho horas después del coito.

8. The condom is a thin sheath of rubber (or similar material) that fits over the erect penis.
   El condón (preservatio/«la goma») es una cubierta delgada hecha de hule (goma) (o de

26. There are many methods, and they are not all equally effective.
   Hay muchos métodos, y no son todos igualmente efectivos.

27. If you are having sexual relations, use protection; otherwise you can become pregnant.
   Si tiene relaciones sexuales, use protección; de otro modo, puede quedar embarazada.

28. When you resume sexual relations after having your baby, use protection so that you do not become pregnant again immediately.[17]
   Cuando vuelva a tener relaciones sexuales después de dar luz, use protección de modo que no esté embarazada de nuevo inmediatamente.

29. You can buy some of these in a drug store and others from your doctor.
   Vd. puede comprar algunas de estas (protecciones) en una farmacia y otras por medio de su médico (médica).

un material semejante), el cual se coloca sobre el pene erecto.

9. Use a condom whenever you enter the vagina, not just before ejaculation.
   Use el preservativo cada vez que entre en la vagina, no antes de eyacular.

10. If the condom has a reservoir tip, so much the better. If not, make a tip by squeezing it.
   Si el condón tiene punta de receptáculo, tanto mejor. Si no, haga lugar para el líquido, apretándolo.

11. To put it on, place it on the head of the penis and unroll it, making sure that the tip is in the center and about 1/2 inch from the end of penis.
   Para ponérselo, colóquelo en la cabeza del pene y desenróllelo, asegurándose de que la punta esté correctamente en el centro y más o menos a media pulgada del final del pene.

12. Withdraw the penis and condom together from the vagina as soon as possible after orgasm to avoid semen escape.
   Extraiga de la vagina el pene junto con el profiláctico lo antes posible después del orgasmo, para evitar escape del semen.

13. After you come, again grab hold of the condom by its tip, and remove it carefully while your penis is somewhat erect.
   Después de eyacular, agarre el condón de nuevo por la punta, y remuévalo mientas el pene está algo erecto.

14. Use a new condom each time there is intercourse.
   Use un nuevo profiláctico cada vez que repita el acto sexual.

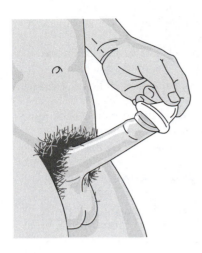
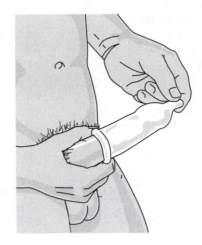
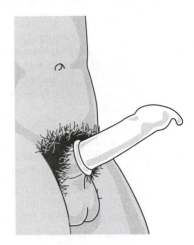

IUD   *EL DIU*

1. The IUD is best for the woman who has several children.
   El dispositivo intrauterino (DIU) es mejor para la mujer con varios hijos.

2. There are several types: those made of plastic, in forms of a loop or coil; those containing progesterone; and those made of plastic and copper.
   Hay varios tipos: los hechos de plástico en formas de lazo o rollo; los que contienen progesterona; y los hechos de plástico y cobre.

3. You must replace the plastic and plastic and copper IUDs every three years, and the IUDs with progesterone every year.
   Vd. debe cambiar el DIU hecho de plástico o de plástico y cobre cada tres años, y el DIU hecho de progesterona cada año.

4. After the IUD is fitted, it can be left in place indefinitely.
   Después de que se coloque el DIU, puede dejarse en el útero indefinidamente.

5. The IUD is inserted during your period.
   Se inserta el DIU durante el período menstrual.

6. When the IUD is well fitted, a string tied to the IUD will hang down from the cervix inside of the vagina.
   Cuando el DIU está bien colocado, un hilo atado al DIU se proyectará (colgará) de la cérvix bien adentro de la vagina.

7. You have to check to see that the IUD is in place by inserting either your index or middle finger into your vagina and touching the string, always at the same point.[18] Check once a week.
   Vd. tiene que comprobar que el DIU esté en su sitio apropiado al introducir o el dedo índice o el del corazón bien adentro en la vagina y sentir el hilo (tocar el hilo), siempre a la misma distancia. Examínese una vez por semana.

8. Do not pull the string, which could dislocate it.
   No tire Vd. del hilo, lo que podría desalojarlo.

9. If you cannot feel the string, or if you can touch the IUD itself, call the doctor, and meanwhile use other contraceptive methods.
   Si Vd. no puede sentir el hilo, o puede tocar el DIU mismo, llame al médico (a la médica), y entretanto, use otro método anticonceptivo.

10. Women with vaginal problems or tendencies toward them should not use the IUD since it increases these tendencies.
    Las mujeres con enfermedades vaginales o propensiones para ellas no deben usar el DIU puesto que aumenta estas tendencias.

DIAPHRAGM   *EL DIAFRAGMA*

1. The diaphragm is a relatively effective means of birth control.
   El diafragma es relativamente eficaz para el control de la natalidad.

2. The diaphragm is a little round rubber cup, which is used with cream or jelly.
   El diafragma es una redonda gorrita (taza) de goma que se usa con una gelatina o crema de control de la natalidad.

3. I have to measure you for the correct size.
   Tengo que medirla para recetarle el tamaño adecuado.

4. I have to show you how to properly insert the diaphragm because you have to do it yourself each time before having sexual relations.
Tengo que mostrarle cómo insertar el diafragma porque Vd. tiene que hacerlo por sí misma cada vez antes de tener relaciones sexuales.

5. Put a spoonful of cream or jelly in the middle of the diaphragm.
Unte Vd. una cucharadita de crema o jalea en el centro del diafragma.

6. Squeeze the sides until it folds; with the other hand separate the labia.
Apriete los lados hasta que se doble; con la otra mano separe los labios.

7. Insert it toward the back and then push upwards behind the pubic bone.[19]
Introdúzcalo hacia debajo y detrás y entonces, empújelo hacia arriba detrás del hueso púbico.

8. Try inserting it now.
Trate de introducirlo ahora.

9. You can put it in place two hours before sexual intercourse.
Vd. puede ponerlo en su sitio dos horas antes de tener relaciones sexuales.

10. Leave it in place at least eight hours after intercourse.
Déjelo en su lugar por lo menos ocho horas después de las relaciones.

11. Check with your finger to see that it is in place.[19]
Introduzca un dedo para saber que está en su lugar.

12. To remove it, grab the rim and pull gently.
Para quitarlo, agarre el contorno y dé un tirón suave.

13. After using it, wash it with soap and water, and dry carefully, powdering it with cornstarch.
Después de usarlo, lávelo con agua y jabón, y séquelo cuidadosamente, empolvorándolo con maicena.

THE PILL *LA PÍLDORA*[20]

1. The birth control pill is the best nonpermanent method of birth control.
La píldora (pastilla) (anticonceptiva) es el método no permanente más efectivo de prevenir el embarazo.

2. It is important to follow all instructions when you take the pill.
Es importante seguir todas las instrucciones al usar la píldora.

3. Take the pill at the same time each day. Your partner can remind you.
Tome Vd. la píldora a la misma hora cada día. Su compañero puede recordárselo.

4. If you forget to take one pill, the next day take two.
Si se le olvida tomar una píldora, el día siguiente tome dos.

5. If you forget two pills, use foam; if you forget three pills in a row, stop using them that month.
Si se le olvidan dos píldoras, use espuma; si se le olvidan tres píldoras, deje de usarlas ese mes.

6. The pill comes in two types that are prescribed frequently: packages of 21 and of 28.
La píldora viene de dos clases que se recetan con frecuencia: paquetes de veintiuna y de veintiocho.

7. The first day of your period is the first day that you bleed.
El primer día de su regla (período) es el primer día que sangra.

8. Take the first pill on the fifth day of your period.
Tome la primera píldora el quinto día de su regla.

9. Take the pills daily for 21 days.
Tome Vd. las píldoras cada día por veintiún días.

10. You will begin to menstruate on the second or third day after you finish taking all the pills.
Comenzará a menstruar (perder sangre) el segundo o tercer día después de terminar tomando todas las píldoras.

11. Stop taking the pills for an entire week before beginning to take them again.
Deje de tomar las píldoras por una semana entera antes de comenzar a tomarlas de nuevo.

12. If your period skips a month and you have been taking the pills correctly, begin the next package on the correct day as indicated.
Si se salta una menstruación un mes y si Vd. ha estado tomando las píldoras correctamente, empiece a tomar el próximo paquete el día correcto como está señalado.

13. Begin the new series of pills on the same day of the week that you began the last series.
Empiece la nueva serie de píldoras el mismo día de la semana en que comenzó la serie anterior.

14. If you have a poor memory, your doctor may prescribe a series of 28 pills for you.

Si Vd. tiene mala memoria, su médico (médica) puede recetarle una serie de veintiocho píldoras.

15. For 21 days take the white pills. For the next 7 days take the pink ones.
    Por veintiún días tome las píldoras blancas. Por los próximos siete días tome las rosadas.

16. Your period will begin on the second or third day after you begin the pink pills.
    Su regla comenzará el segundo o tercer día después de comenzar las píldoras rosadas.

17. On the eighth day begin a new pack.
    Al octavo día empiece un nuevo paquete.

18. You must take a pill daily when you use the package of 28.

Vd. tiene que tomar una píldora cada día cuando usa el paquete de veintiocho.

19. If your period does not start while you are taking the pink pills, begin a new pack anyway—the day after having taken the last pink pill.
    Si su menstruación no le viene mientras está tomando las píldoras rosadas, de todas maneras empiece un nuevo paquete de píldoras al día siguiente de haber tomado la última píldora rosada.

20. You may experience some complications, however.
    Vd. puede experimentar algunas complicaciones, sin embargo.

RHYTHM METHOD   *EL METODO DEL RITMO*

1. This is not effective for all women who are not very regular.
   No resulta efectivo para todas las mujeres que no tengan su regla puntualmente.

2. During your fertile time as well as a few days before and after, you should abstain from sexual relations because you can get pregnant.
   Durante su período fértil así como unos días antes y después, Vd. debe abstenerse de las relaciones sexuales porque puede embarazarse.

3. It is necessary to determine the "unsafe" days of the month and avoid sexual relations on them.

Hay que averiguar cuáles son los días del mes que no son «seguros» y evitarse las relaciones sexuales entonces.

4. Speak to your doctor if you intend to use this method since "safe days" vary in every woman.
   Hable Vd. con su médico (médica) si piensa utilizar este método puesto que los «días seguros» varían en cada mujer.

5. I will try to help you to determine when you are fertile.
   Trataré de ayudarla a determinar cuándo es su período fértil.

COITUS INTERRUPTUS   *EL RETIRARSE*

1. The man must withdraw his penis from the vagina before ejaculating.
   El hombre debe de retirar el pene de la vagina antes de la eyaculación.

2. This is not effective.
   Esto no es efectivo.

DOUCHING[21]   EL LAVAJE

1. The use of a vaginal douche immediately after intercourse does not prevent pregnancy.
   El uso de un lavaje para tratar de eliminar la esperma de la vagina inmediatamente

después de relaciones sexuales no evita el embarazo.

STERILIZATION   *LA ESTERILIZACION*

1. Sterilization is a *permanent* means of birth control.
   La esterilización es un medio *permanente* de control de la natalidad.

2. In a man the process is called a vasectomy:[22] the tubes through which the sperm travel (the vas deferens) are cut surgically.
   En el hombre el procedimiento se llama una vasectomía: los conductos por donde se transportan las espermas (los conductos deferentes) se cortan quirúrgicamente.

3. There is no change in the man's sexual desires, apperance, or ability to have intercourse.
   No hay ningún cambio en el instincto sexual, en la apariencia, ni en la capacidad de tener relaciones sexuales.

4. You have to use a temporary method of birth control immediately after a vasectomy to avoid pregnancy.
   Hay que utilizar un método temporal de anticoncepción inmediatamente después de una vasectomía para evitar el embarazo.

5. For a woman the procedure is called a tubal ligation:[23] the tubes through which the egg travels from the ovary to the uterus (the Fallopian tubes) are cut, separated, and tied.

Para la mujer el procedimiento se llama la ligadura de los tubos: los conductos por los que se transportan los óvulos (las trompas de Falopio) se cortan, se separan y se atan.

Notes *Notas*

1. There is a widespread Mexican belief that a person must have a large quantity of blood in order to preserve his health, that he will become ill even if he loses a small quantity. "Loss of blood for any reason, even in the small quantity necessary for laboratory tests, is thought to have a weakening effect, particularly in males, whose sexual vigor is thereby believed impaired. (L. Saunders, *Cultural Differences and Medical Care*, p. 147).

2. See Chapter 4, p. 91.

3. See below, pages 255-256.

4. Spanish uses *poner* when "give" means to administer. *Poner* is used to express the idea of putting something into a person, on a specific part of him, or under him. *Dar* is used with something for the person to take or when "give" means "to deliver to."

5. See Chapter 10, pages 213-214.

6. See immediately below.

7. See Chapter 11, pages 236-240.

8. If the patient is allergic to iodine, a retrograde pyelogram will need to be performed. See below, phrase numbers 28f.

9. If the patient has received this premedication, an IVP may be done.

10. The word "enema" may be either masculine or feminine in Spanish. Enemas can be "cleansing," as described here (*enema de limpieza*); "medicinal," (*enema medicamentoso/medicamentosa*); or "nutritive," (*enema alimenticio/alimenticia*).

11. *Respirar*—to breathe (normal process of respiration). *Aspirar*—to breathe in, inhale, breathe deeply.

12. See Chapter 10, page 219, note 6.

13. Attitudes about sex and sexuality are difficult to discuss. There are many prudish ideas prevalent, as well as considerable embarrassment. In addition, Hispanos use many euphemisms and local *modismos* (idiomatic expressions). Therefore, it might be helpful to have a native speaker present for this type of discussion. It is important that the health-care worker and the patient be of the same sex, because of the modesty and embarrassment of most Hispanic women.

 There are numerous and complex factors which influence Hispanics' attitudes about contraception. Their level of education, socioeconomic status, the strength of their religious beliefs all play a part. A significant influence, however, derives from culturally held beliefs. Motherhood and childrearing are held in extremely high regard. Also, many Hispanic males adhere strictly to the notion of *machismo*, which is associated with their masculinity, and proving their virility. An example of *machismo* can be seen in the male who is steadfast in his desire NOT to have children but who refuses to either practice birth control himself or allow his partner to use contraception. This becomes even more complicated when Roman Catholic teachings against birth control and abortion are added to the "problem."

14. Some men object to their wives using contraceptives because they think that it robs them of their "male authority." These men believe that birth control, like any other sexual matter, lies within the man's authority to determine time, form, and frequency of sexual relations. (See N. Galli, "The Influence of Cultural Heritage," pp. 10-16.)

15. Many Latin cultures believe that masturbation can lead to a decrease in strength, cause depression, and possibly even some form of insanity.

16. There are still many myths about menstruation in the Hispanic culture. Some women believe that washing their hair during menstruation may lead to death, for example.

17. According to the Hispanic culture, women who have just given birth should abstain from having sexual relations for a 40-day period, the *cuarentena*. This is not, however, always completely adhered to. (See Chapter 11, page 249, note 7).

18 Because of the tendency toward excessive modesty and reluctance to touch oneself, many Hispanic women are hesitant to touch themselves internally as is necessary on a weekly basis when using an IUD.

19. Many Hispanic women have trouble using the diaphragm because they are inhibited about touching the genital area. It is difficult for them to check the IUD on a weekly basis, but impossible for them to insert one or two fingers into the vagina to feel that the cervix is covered properly by a diaphragm both before and after intercourse.

20. A study done by the National Center for Health Statistics, popularly referred to as the HHANES Report, Hispanic Health and Nutrition Examination Survey, which was first published in 1990, indicates that Mexican American females are almost twice as likely to be using oral contraceptives as Cuban American or Puerto Rican females.

21. Many Hispanic women follow the practice of vaginal douching, common in folk medicine everywhere. A douche is indicated after each menstrual cycle and following postpartum bleeding. A homemade solution of herbs (*chicura, tlachichinole, damiana,* or rue) may be used. If bleeding is heavy, a douche is made from a solution of boiled nut shells or leaves. (See M. Kay, "Health and Illness," p. 153).

22. There are two primary cultural reasons why Hispanics seldom will choose this type of birth control: 1) the concept of *machismo*, and 2) the belief that women are supposed to be responsible for birth control. See above note 13.

23. Data from the HHANES study (See above, note 17) indicates that the largest percentage of tubal ligations among Hispanic females living in the United States occurs among Puerto Rican women. As alluded to earlier, (see above notes 13 & 14), Hispanic culture tends to place the responsibility for birth control practices on the female. The HHANES data demonstrates that 58% of all contraception in Puerto Rico is the result of tubal ligations.

Dental Conversation

Conversación dental

DENTAL OFFICE

▌ *EL CONSULTORIO DENTAL*

INITIAL DENTAL EXAMINATION[1] *PRIMER RECONOCIMIENTO DENTAL*

1. Good morning/Good afternoon/Good evening.
   Buenos días/Buenas tardes/Buenas noches.

2. My name is Dr. _____ .
   Me llamo el Dr./la Dra. _____ .

3. Please be seated in the chair and relax.
   Por favor, siéntese usted en la silla de dentista y relájese.[2]

4. Put your head back.
   Eche usted la cabeza hacia atrás.

5. You have a nice set of teeth.
   Usted tiene buena dentadura.

6. What is the matter with you?
   ¿Cuál es el problema?
   ¿Qué le sucede?
   ¿De qué se queja usted?

7. Were you in an accident?
   ¿Tuvo usted (un) accidente?

8. Do you have a toothache?
   ¿Le duelen los dientes?
   ¿Le duele un diente?

9. Do you know which tooth hurts you?
   ¿Sabe usted qué diente(s)/muela(s) le duele(n)?

10. How long have you had the pain?
    ¿Desde cuándo le duele?
    ¿Cuánto tiempo hace que le duele?
    ¿Desde cuándo tiene el dolor?

11. Are you in pain now?
    ¿Siente usted dolor ahora?

12. Is it a little or a lot?
    ¿Le duele mucho o poco?

13. Where do you feel the pain?
    ¿Dónde siente usted el dolor?

14. Show me with your finger, with your tongue.
    Muéstreme con el dedo, con la lengua.

15. Touch it with your tongue.
    Tóquelo con la lengua.

16. Does it hurt you when you eat or drink cold things?
    ¿Le duele cuando come o bebe cosas frías?

17. Does it hurt you when you eat or drink something hot?
    ¿Le duele cuando come o bebe algo caliente?

18. Does it hurt when you eat sweets?
    ¿Le duele cuando come dulces?

19. Does it hurt when you chew?
    ¿Le duele cuando mastica usted?

20. Does it hurt when you bite?
    ¿Le duele cuando muerde usted?

21. Does something sour hurt your teeth?
    ¿Le molesta algo agrio?

22. Do you feel better when you drink cold water? Hot water?
    ¿Se siente usted mejor cuando bebe agua fría? ¿agua caliente?

23. Are you worried? Don't be afraid.
    ¿Está usted preocupado (preocupada)? No tenga miedo.

24. I am going to take care of it.
    Voy a encargarme de ello.

25. When was the last time that you saw a dentist?
    ¿Cuándo fue la última vez que un/una dentista le examinó?

26. I have to examine your mouth and teeth.
    Tengo que examinarle la boca y los dientes.

27. Open your mouth, please. A little wider.
    Abra usted la boca, por favor. Un poco más.

28. Close your mouth a bit.
    Cierre usted la boca un poco.

29. Don't move.
    No se mueva usted.

30. Open your mouth wide, please.
    Abra usted bien la boca, por favor.

31. Wider.
    Más, por favor.

32. Raise your head a bit.
    Levante usted un poco la cabeza, por favor.

33. Lower it.
    Bájela usted, por favor.

34. You're doing fine.
    Está bien.
    Lo está haciendo la mar de bien.
    Está haciéndolo muy bien.

35. Try not to talk.
    Trate de no hablar.

36. It won't hurt.
    No va a dolerle.

37. This may hurt you a little.
    Esto puede dolerle un poco.

38. This is not going to hurt you at all.
    Esto no le va a doler nada.

39. Do you want a shot so that you will not feel pain?
    ¿Quiere usted que le ponga una inyección para no sentir el dolor?

40. I am going to put some medicine on the area before I give you an injection.
    Voy a ponerle una medicina en el área antes de ponerle una inyección.

41. I am going to give you a shot to put your tooth (gum) to sleep.
    Voy a ponerle una inyección para anestesiar el diente (la encía).

42. You will feel a pressure sensation.
    Usted sentirá una sensación de presión sobre el área.

43. Will you help me?
    ¿Quisiera ayudarme?

44. I will be finished soon.
    Terminaré en seguida.

45. You may rinse your mouth now.
    Ahora usted puede enjuagarse la boca.

46. I have to take some X-rays of your mouth.
    Tengo que sacarle radiografías de los dientes.

DENTAL X-RAYS   *LAS RADIOGRAFIAS DENTALES*

1. The X-rays will not hurt you.
   Las radiografías no le dañarán ni dolerán.

2. I am going to take a picture of the inside of your teeth.
   Voy a sacarle fotos del interior de los dientes con radiografías.

3. Are you pregnant?
   ¿Está usted en estado?
   ¿Está usted encinta?
   ¿Está usted embarazada?

4. Is there a possibility that you are pregnant?
   ¿Hay alguna posibilidad de que usted esté encinta?

5. I am going to put this heavy lead apron over you for protection.
   Voy a ponerle este pesado delantal de plomo encima de usted para su protección.

6. Bite down on this.
   Muerda esto.

7. Keep your mouth closed.
   Mantenga usted la boca cerrada.

8. Hold this with your index finger.
   Retenga esto con el índice.

9. Don't breathe.
   No respire usted.

10. Don't move your head. Keep it straight.
    No mueva usted la cabeza. Manténgala derecha.

11. Don't move.
    No se mueva usted.

12. Try not to gag.
    Trate de no arquear/sentir náuseas.

13. You can breathe.
    Usted puede respirar.

14. You can move now.
    Ahora usted puede moverse.

15. I have to develop the X-rays.
    Tengo que revelar las radiografías.

16. I will notify you after I look at them if I see a problem.
    Le notificaré después de examinarlas si encuentro algún problema.

RESULTS OF THE DENTAL EXAMINATION   *LOS RESULTADOS DEL RECONOCIMIENTO DENTAL*

1. You have healthy teeth.
   Usted tiene buena salud bucal.
   Usted tiene dientes buenos.

2. You have a problem here.
   Usted tiene un problema aquí.

3. You have dirty teeth.
   Usted tiene los dientes sucios.

4. You need a cleaning.
   Usted necesita una limpieza.

Cavities   *Caries*[3]

5. I don't see any cavities.
   No veo ninguna caries.

6. You have some cavities/caries.
   Usted tiene muchas cavidades/caries.

7. You have a cavity in one tooth.
   Usted tiene una cavidad en un diente.

8. You have a cavity in a molar.
   Usted tiene una caries en una muela.

9. You have three cavities.
   Usted tiene tres caries.

10. It is a very small cavity.
    Es una cavidad (picadura) muy pequeña.

11. Cavities or dental caries are the main reason that children lose their teeth.
    Las cavidades o las caries dentales son la causa principal de la pérdida de los dientes en los niños.

12. When you eat foods that contains carbohydrates (sugars and starches), the bacteria in the plaque produce acids which attack the tooth enamel.
    Cuando usted ingiere alimentos que contienen carbohidratos (los azúcares y los almidones), las bacterias en la placa producen ácidos que atacan el esmalte de los dientes.

13. The sticky plaque keeps the acids against the surface of the teeth for at least twenty minutes if you do not brush after eating.
    La placa pegajosa retiene los ácidos contra la superficie de los dientes por un mínimo de veinte minutos si no se cepilla después de comer.

14. After many such repeated acid attacks, the tooth enamel can weaken and in time will form a cavity.
Después de muchos ataques constantes del ácido, el esmalte se debilita, y con el tiempo se forma una caries.

15. In time the surface cavity goes towards the center of the tooth (the dentine), and if not treated, the decay reaches the pulp and forms an abscess at the root tip.
Con el tiempo la caries avanza de la superficie hacia el interior del diente (la dentina), y si no se trata, la caries llega a la pulpa, formándose un absceso al final de la raíz.

16. When this happens, it causes a toothache.
Cuando esto ocurre, causa dolor en el diente.

17. If this happens, you either have to have a root canal treatment (endodontia), or the tooth will have to be extracted.
Si esto sucede, o tendrá que tener una terapia de canal (tratamiento endodóntico), o el diente deberá extraerse.

18. You have a very deep cavity.
Usted tiene una caries muy profunda.

19. You have an abscess.
Usted tiene un absceso.

20. You have a nerve exposure.
Usted tiene un nervio expuesto.

21. I can (not) start today.
(No) Puedo empezar hoy.

22. Do you want me to try and save your tooth, or do you want me to extract it?
¿Quiere usted que trate de salvarle el diente, o quiere que se lo saque?

23. It is cheaper if I pull your tooth.
Es más barato si le saco el diente.

24. This will take _____ appointments.
Esto va a requerir _____ turnos/citas.

2 two	dos
3 three	tres
4 four	cuatro
5 five	cinco

25. You need to make an appointment.
Usted necesita arreglar un turno/una cita.

26. Can you come for your first appointment on _____ the _____ of _____ at _____ o'clock?[4]
¿Puede usted venir para su primer turno/primera cita el _____ , el _____ de _____ a la(s) _____ ?

Monday	lunes
Tuesday	martes
Wednesday	miércoles
Thursday	jueves
Friday	viernes
Saturday	sábado

27. I will have to fill your tooth.
Tendré que taparle el diente.

Tengo que empastarle (emplomarle *Arg.*) el diente.

28. I am going to fill the tooth/teeth / molars next week.
Voy a empastar el diente/los dientes/las muelas la semana que viene.

29. I hope that I can fill it.
Espero poder empastarlo/empastarla.

30. The cavity is very deep.
La caries está muy honda.

31. Do you want a silver filling or a gold inlay?
¿Quiere usted que use un relleno de plata o una orificación?

32. What would you like to have it filled with? A silver amalgam, gold, or porcelain?
¿Con qué quiere usted que se lo tape (empaste, calce emplome *Arg.* Ec, Col, Pan, Nic)? ¿Con platino, con oro, o con porcelana?

33. A gold inlay is the best filling because it will last the longest.
Una incrustación (de oro) es el mejor empaste (relleno, tapadura, emplomadura *Arg.*) porque le durará mucho tiempo.

34. This is not going to hurt you at all.
Esto no le dolerá nada.

35. I will give you a shot to put your tooth to sleep before I fill it.
Voy a adormecer el diente con una inyección antes de taparlo (empastarlo).

36. I am going to give you a shot to put your gum to sleep.
Voy a ponerle una inyección para anestesiar la encía.

37. You will feel only a slight prick.
No sentirá más que un leve pinchazo.

38. Don't be nervous.
No se ponga nervioso (nerviosa).

39. There is too much decay to just fill it.
Hay demasiada caries para taparlo solamente.

40. I am going to put some medicine in the tooth so that it will not hurt you.
Voy a ponerle una medicina en el diente para que no le duela.

41. Drink some water and rinse your mouth now.
Ahora beba un poco de agua y enjuáguese la boca.

42. Spit here.
Escupa aquí, por favor.

43. The cavity is too deep. You need a root canal.
La cavidad está demasiado profunda. Usted necesita un tratamiento para canalizar y sacarle el nervio del diente.

44. You will have to see a specialist.
Usted tendrá que visitar a un/una especialista.

45. It is better if you choose not to extract it and have a root canal because you can keep your tooth.
Es mejor si usted escoge no extraerlo y canalizar el diente porque usted puede salvarlo.

46. It is more expensive because you will need a crown to protect the devitalized tooth.
Es más caro porque usted necesitará una corona para proteger el diente sin nervio/el diente necrótico.

47. I am going to put a porcelain crown on your tooth because it is a front tooth.
Voy a ponerle una corona de porcelana porque el diente está en la parte anterior de la boca.

48. I am going to put a gold crown on your tooth because it is a molar and nobody will see it.
Voy a ponerle una corona de oro porque es una muela y nadie la verá.

49. I have to take impressions for the gold inlay.
Tengo que hacerle impresiones antes de orificarle el diente.

50. I must change the packing.
Tengo que cambiarle este empaque.

51. Keep your mouth wide open.
Mantenga usted la boca bien abierta, por favor.

52. Please close your mouth a little.
Cierre usted la boca un poco, por favor.

53. I am going to put some fast-hardening dental plaster in your mouth to make an exact model of the area.
Voy a ponerle en la boca yeso dentífrico que endurece rápido para hacerle un molde exacto del área.

54. Try not to gag.
Trate de no arquear/sentir náuseas.

55. You will hear a pop.
Usted oirá como un taponazo.

56. Don't be frightened.
No tenga miedo.

57. I am finished for today.
He terminado por hoy.

58. Don't eat hard foods for an hour.
No coma usted nada duro por una hora.

59. When I finish with this tooth, I am (the hygienist is) going to clean your teeth.
Cuando termine con este diente, voy (la higienista va) a hacerle una limpieza.

CLEANING YOUR TEETH AND GUMS   *COMO LIMPIARSE LOS DIENTES Y LAS ENCIAS*

1. You need to keep your teeth clean.
Usted necesita mantener los dientes limpios.

2. You should visit your dentist every six months.
Usted debe visitar a su dentista cada seis meses.

3. You must visit your dentist twice a year.
Usted tiene que visitar a su dentista dos veces por año.

4. Regular visits to your dentist let the dentist find dental problems early.
Las visitas regulares a su dentista permiten la dentección a tiempo de problemas dentales temprano.

5. Your dentist can regularly clean and examine your teeth this way.
De este modo su dentista puede limpiar y examinar sus dientes con regularidad.

6. You have too many sugary foods in your diet.
Usted tiene demasiados alimentos azucarados en su dieta.

7. You have to eat a well-balanced diet in order to have healthy teeth.
Usted tiene que comer alimentos balanceados para mantener los dientes saludables.

8. In order to have healthy teeth you must brush and floss your teeth thoroughly every day.
Para tener dientes saludables, usted debe cepillarse los dientes y usar la seda dental con mucho esmero todos los días.

9. Plaque is removed by carefully brushing and flossing.
La placa se quita al cepillarse y usar la seda dental cuidadosamente.

10. Most adults should brush their teeth at least once a day, using a toothbrush with soft, end-rounded bristles.
La mayoriá de los adultos deben limpiarse los dientes por lo menos una vez al día, u- sando un cepillo de dientes de cerdas suaves y redondeadas.

11. Children and adults who have a tendency to get cavities should brush more often, preferably after each meal.
Los niños y los adultos con una tendencia a las caries deben limpiárselos con más frecuencia, preferiblemente después de cada comida.

12. You should brush your teeth three times a day.
Usted debe cepillarse los dientes tres veces al día.

13. Brush your teeth in the morning and at bedtime, and if possible after meals.
Cepíllese usted los dientes al levantarse por la mañana y antes de acostarse por la noche, y si es posible, después de cada comida.

14. I am going to give you a toothbrush to use at home.
Voy a regalarle un cepillo de dientes para usar en casa.

15. I recommend that you buy a toothbrush small enough to fit in your mouth and which lets you clean all of your teeth.
Le recomiendo un cepillo de dientes de tamaño y forma que le quepa en la boca y que le permita limpiar todas las partes de todos los dientes y las muelas.

16. A toothbrush with soft bristles is less likely to injure the gum tissues.
Un cepillo con cerdas suaves no tiende a herir el tejido de las encías.

17. Worn-out toothbrushes should be thrown away because they may injure your gums and because they cannot properly clean your teeth.
Usted debe deshacerse de un cepillo gastado porque puede herirle las encías y porque no puede limpiarle los dientes de una manera adecuada.

18. Replace your toothbrush every three or four months.
Usted debe reemplazar su cepillo de dientes cada tres o cuatro meses.

19. Do you have an electric toothbrush?
¿Tiene usted un cepillo de dientes eléctrico?

20. Massage your gums often.
Dé masajes a las encías con frecuencia.
Masajéese las encías a menudo.
Sobe Vd. las encías a menudo.

21. I am going to scale off the calculus and clean your teeth.
Voy a quitar el cálculo de sus dientes y limpiarlos.

22. I am going to use a high speed/ultrasonic scaler on your teeth to clean them.
Voy a usar una limpiadora automática de gran velocidad/ultrasónica para hacerle la limpieza de sus dientes.

23. Before I clean your teeth, I'm going to use a disclosing solution so that you can see the plaque.
Antes de hacerle la limpieza de sus dientes, voy a usar una solución para hacer visible la tela de bacteria o placa.

24. I am going to give you a disclosing product (tablets or solutions) for you to use at home to see clearly where the plaque on your teeth is when you brush.
Voy a darle un producto revelador (tabletas o soluciones) que usará en casa cuando se cepille los dientes para que pueda ver donde hay placa.

25. In the beginning you will use the stain to disclose plaque each time that you brush, but later on, you will check for plaque only occasionally.
Al principio cuando usted esté aprendiendo la forma de quitarse la placa, es buena idea mancharse los dientes cada vez que se cepille los dientes, pero, más tarde, después de que tenga más experiencia en cepillarse bien los dientes, usted podrá verificarlo de forma ocasional.

26. The nurse is going to show you how you ought to brush your teeth to clean them well.
La enfermera (higienista) va a enseñarle (enseñarla) cómo usted debe cepillarse los dientes para limpiarlos bien.

27. Brush your teeth like this.
Cepíllese usted los dientes de este modo.

28. Place the head of the toothbrush along side of your teeth, making certain that the tooth bristles are at a 45° degree (forty-five) angle against your gumline.
Coloque el cepillo de dientes a lo largo de los dientes, asegurándose de que las cerdas están en un ángulo de 45° (cuarenta y cinco grados) contra la línea de las encías.

29. Move the brush back and forth several times with short movements, using a gentle scrubbing motion.
Mueva el cepillo hacia adelante y hacia atrás, con movimientos cortos varias veces, restregando suavemente.

30. Brush the outer surfaces of each tooth; brush both top and bottom teeth, keeping the bristles angled against the gums.
Cepille usted las superficies exteriores de cada diente; cepille tanto los dientes superiores como los inferiores, manteniendo las cerdas inclinadas contra la línea de las encías.

31. Brush down on your upper teeth.
Cepille los dientes superiores de arriba hacia abajo.

32. Brush up on your lower teeth.
Cepille los dientes inferiores de abajo hacia arriba.

33. Use the same method on the inside surfaces of your teeth and continue to use short back and forth movements.
Utilice usted el mismo método con las superficies internas de todos los dientes y siga usando los movimientos cortos hacia adelante y hacia atrás.

34. Brush the chewing surfaces of the back teeth.
Cepíllese bien las superficies de masticar de las muelas.

35. Clean the inner surface of the front teeth by tilting your brush vertically, making several up and down strokes with the tip of your toothbrush.
Limpie la superficie interior de los dientes delanteros, inclinando el cepillo verticalmente, haciendo varios movimientos hacia arriba y hacia abajo con la punta del cepillo.

36. Finish by brushing your tongue, which will freshen your breath and also remove bacteria.
Concluya cepillándose la lengua para refrescarse el aliento y quitar la bacteria.

37. You should brush your teeth as often as possible.
Usted debe cepillarse los dientes lo más frecuente posible.

38. You should brush your teeth after each meal.
Usted debe cepillarse los dientes después de cada comida.

39. You should brush your teeth before you go to bed.
Usted debe cepillarse los dientes antes de acostarse.

40. It is also important to floss your teeth every day.
También es importante usar la seda dental todos los días.

41. You should use dental floss to clean between your teeth especially where there are pockets.
Usted debe usar el hilo dental/la seda dental para limpiarse entre los dientes, sobre todo donde hay surcos gingivales (espacios anormales entre la encía y la raíz del diente).

42. Flossing removes food particles and plaque from between your teeth and near the gum line.
El uso de la seda dental quita los granos (las partículas) de comida y la placa de entre los dientes y debajo de la línea de las encías, donde no llega el cepillo de dientes.

43. You may have to practice flossing because it can be difficult at first.
Quizás usted tenga que practicar el uso correcto de la seda dental porque al principio puede ser un poco difícil.

44. Cut a strip of dental floss about 18 (eighteen) inches 45 (forty five centimeters) and wind most of it around the middle finger of your right (left) hand.
Corte una tira de seda dental de más o menos 18 (dieciocho) pulgadas (45 [cuarenta y cinco] centímetros) y enróllese la mayoría alrededor del dedo del corazón de la mano derecha (izquierda).

45. Wind the other end of the rest around the middle finger of your left (right) hand.
Enróllese la otra punta del restante de la seda dental alrededor del dedo del corazón de la mano izquierda (derecha).

46. The left (right) middle finger will take up the used, dirty floss.
El dedo del corazón izquierdo (derecho) recogerá la seda dental a medida que se use y se ensucie.

47. Using about an inch (2–3 [two to three] centimeters) of floss between your thumb and in-

dex fingers, guide the taut floss between your teeth.
Usando aproximadamente una pulgada (2–3 [dos a tres] centímetros) de la seda dental bien apretada entre el pulgare y el índice, guíe la seda dental entre los dientes.

48. Use a gentle sawing motion to insert the floss between your teeth.
Utilice un movimiento suave de vaivén para insertarla entre los dientes.

49. Never push the floss against/into your gums.
Nunca empuje[5] la seda dental contra las encías.

50. When the floss reaches the gum line, curve it into a half circle against one tooth and gently slide it into the space between the gum and the tooth until there is resistance.
Cuando la seda dental alcance las encías, colóquela en forma semi-circular contra un diente y deslícela suavemente entre la encía y el diente hasta sentir resistencia.

51. Hold the floss tightly against the tooth and scrape it up and down against the side of the tooth and away from the gum.
Mantenga la seda dental fuertemente contra el diente y raspe suavemente el costado del diente con la seda con un movimiento de arriba hacia abajo.

52. Repeat this process on the rest of your teeth.
Repita este proceso con cada uno de los dientes y las muelas.

53. Clean your bridge after every meal, if possible.
Limpie el puente después de cada comida si es posible.

54. I will show you how to clean it.
Le enseñaré cómo limpiarlo.

55. Store your dentures in a glass of water when you are not wearing them.
Guarde usted su dentadura postiza en un vaso de agua cuando no la use.

56. Buy cleaning tablets at the grocery store or at the pharmacy.
Compre las tabletas quitamanchas/tabletas de limpiar en la tienda de comestibles o en la farmacia.

57. You should take them out at night.
Usted debe quitárselos por la noche.

58. Don't take them out at night.
No se los quite por la noche.

59. Don't remove your bridge until you see me.
No se quite Vd. el puente hasta que vuelva a verme.

PERIODONTAL PROBLEMS[6] *PROBLEMAS PERIODONTALES*

1. Do you have bleeding gums?
¿Tiene usted encías que sangran?

2. Do your gums bleed a lot?
¿A usted le sangran mucho las encías?

3. My gums are bleeding a lot.
    Las encías me sangran mucho.

4. Do your gums bleed when you brush your teeth?
    ¿Tiene usted encías que sangran cuando se cepilla los dientes?
    ¿Le sangran las encías cuando se cepilla los dientes?

5. Do you have painful gums?
    ¿Le duelen las encías?

6. How long have they been bleeding?
    ¿Desde cuándo sangran?
    ¿Cuánto tiempo hace que sangran?
      Just today?
      ¿Solamente hoy?
      A couple of days?
      ¿Hace un par de días?
      A week?
      ¿Una semana?
      A month?
      ¿Un mes?

7. Do your gums get red or do they swell?
    ¿Se enrojecen las encías o se hinchan?

8. Are your gums beginning to separate from your teeth?
    ¿Están empezando a separarse las encías de los dientes?

9. Do you always have bad breath?
    ¿Tiene usted mal aliento constantemente?

10. Do you often have bad breath?
    ¿Tiene usted mal aliento con frecuencia?

11. Your gum is infected.
    Vd. tiene la encía infectada.

12. Do you have any loose teeth?
    ¿Tiene usted algunos dientes flojos?

13. Have you noticed a change in your bite?
    ¿Se ha fijado en un cambio en la mordida?

14. Has there been a change in your bridge?
    ¿Ha habido un cambio en el ajuste de puentes?

15. You have a lot of tartar.
    Usted tiene mucho sarro/tártaro.

16. You have plaque around your teeth.
    Usted tiene placa alrededor de los dientes.

17. You have too much calculus on your teeth.
    Usted tiene demasiado cálculo en los dientes.

18. Plaque and tartar can cause bad breath and pyorrhea.
    La placa y el sarro pueden causar mal aliento y piorrea.

19. You have pyorrhea. You must see a periodontist.
    Usted padece de piorrea. Debe de consultar a un(a) especialista de las encías.

20. You need gum surgery.
    Usted necesita tener cirugía en las encías.

Periodontal Disease   *Enfermedad periodontal*

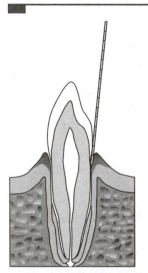 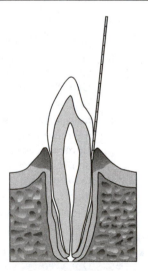 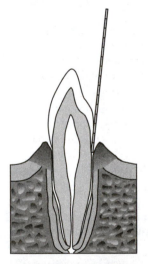 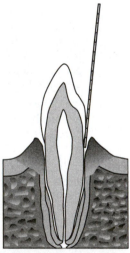

Gingivitis/Gingivitis   Early periodontitis/ Periodontitis temprana   Moderate periodontitis/ Periodontitis moderada   Advanced periodontitis/ Periodontitis avanzada

21. If you do not have it, your teeth will soon loosen and fall out.
    Si usted no la tiene, tendrá un desprendimiento de los dientes que dentro de poco se caerán.

22. Plaque is colorless and sticky, and is continuously formed on your teeth.
    La placa es incolora y pegajosa, y se forma continuamente sobre los dientes.

23. Plaque is an invisible thin layer of harmful bacteria which eventually can cause cavities.
La placa es una tela delgada e invisible de bacterias (microbios) peligrosas que, con el tiempo, puede causar cavidades/caries.

24. The bacteria in plaque are the main cause of the two most common dental problems: cavities and periodontal or gum disease (pyorrhea).
Las bacterias de la placa son la causa principal de las dos enfermedades dentales más comunes: las caries dentales y la enfermedad periodontal o la enfermedad de las encías (la piorrea).

25. Periodontal disease is a gum disease. It is also called Pyorrhea.
La enfermedad periodontal es una enfermedad de las encías. También se llama la piorrea.

26. Periodontal disease is the primary reason that adults loose their teeth.
La enfermedad periodontal es la causa mayor de la pérdida de dientes en los adultos.

27. Plaque also produces irritants which inflame the gums, redden them, or makes them bleed easily.
La placa también produce unos irritantes que inflaman las encías, las enrojecen, o hacen que sangren fácilmente.

28. If plaque is not removed every day, it will accumulate and turn into a hard deposit called calculus or tartar.
Si no se quita la placa cada día, se acumulará y se convertirá en un depósito duro que se llama cálculo o tártaro (sarro).

29. More plaque forms on top of the calculus, which irritates the gums even more.

Cuanta más placa se acumula encima de los cálculos, más se irritan las encías.

30. Inevitably the irritated gums pull away from the teeth, destroying more bone and periodontal ligaments and in the process creating pockets between the teeth and the gums.
Con el tiempo las encías irritadas pueden separarse de los dientes, destruyéndose más huesos y el ligamento periodontal y formando bolsas entre los dientes y las encías.

31. These pockets become filled with bacteria and pus.
Estas bolsas se llenan de bacterias y pus.

32. If the gums are not treated, the bone which supports the teeth will be destroyed.
Si no se tratan las encías, el hueso que soporta los dientes se destruirá.

33. The healthy teeth may loosen and fall out, or it may be necessary to remove them.
Los dientes saludables pueden aflojársele y pueden caerse o puede ser necesario sacárselos.

34. You cannot remove tartar or calculus by brushing your teeth.
Usted no puede quitar el tártaro (sarro) o el cálculo al cepillarse los dientes.

35. Only your dentist or your dental hygienist can remove it.
Sólo su dentista o su higienista dental puede quitarlo.

36. However, remember to brush and floss every day, eat a balanced diet, and visit your dentist regularly.
Sin embargo, recuerde cepillarse los dientes y usar la seda dental todos los días, alimentarse con una dieta balanceada, y visitar regularmente a su dentista.

ENDODONTAL PROBLEMS   *PROBLEMAS ENDODONTALES*

1. Your teeth are supposed to last a lifetime.
Sus dientes están destinados a durar toda su vida.

2. You have some very deep cavities.
Usted tiene unas cavidades muy profundas.

3. If you have a root canal treatment (endodontia), you can save your tooth.
Si (se) le hacen un tratamiento del conducto de la raíz/conducto radicular (un tratamiento endodóntico), puede salvar sus dientes.

4. Root canal treatment is usually done by a specialist.
Generalmente sólo un (una) especialista hace el tratamiento del conducto de la raíz/conducto radicular.

5. This dentist opens the root canal of your tooth and is able to treat the problems of the soft center known as the pulp.
Este dentista abre el conducto de la raíz y puede tratar los problemas del centro blando del diente conocido como la pulpa dentaria.

6. The pulp is a soft reddish mass which fills the center of each of your teeth and which contains the nerves, arteries, and connective tissue.
La pulpa dentaria es una masa blanda y rojiza que rellena la cavidad central del diente y contiene los nervios, las arterias y el tejido conjuntivo.

7. The pulp goes from the crown of the tooth to the tip of the root in the jawbone.
La pulpa dentaria se extiende desde la corona del diente hasta el ápice de la raíz dentaria en el hueso de las mandíbulas.

8. When the pulp is diseased or injured, it cannot be fixed and it dies.
Cuando la pulpa está morbosa o lesionada, no puede repararse y se muere.

9. The most common cause of this is a cracked tooth or a tooth with a very deep cavity.
La causa más común de la muerte de la pulpa es un diente agrietado o con una caries profunda.

10. Either of these problems allows germs (bacteria) to enter the pulp chamber.
Ambos problemas pueden dejar entrar los microbios (las bacterias) en la pulpa.

11. The germs can cause an infection inside of the tooth.
Los microbios pueden causar una infección dentro del diente.

12. If it is not treated, pus can accumulate at the tip of the root on the bone, forming a "pocket of pus" which is called an abscess.
Si no se trata, el pus se acumula en el ápice de la raíz en la mandíbula, formando una «bolsa llena de pus,» que se llama un absceso.

13. An abscess is usually painful and can harm the bone around the tooth.
Un absceso, por lo general, le duele mucho y puede dañar el hueso alrededor del diente.

14. If the pulp is not removed from the tooth, severe pain and swelling can result.
Si no se quita la pulpa infectada, pueden aparecer dolores e hinchazón.

15. Without treatment, your tooth will have to be extracted.
Sin tratamiento, deberá extraerse el diente.

16. The endodontist, which is the name of the specialist who treats problems of the pulp, completely removes the infected pulp.
El/La endodontista, que es el nombre del [de la] especialista que se especializa en los problemas de la pulpa, elimina totalmente la pulpa morbosa.

17. Then s/he cleans the pulp chamber and the root canal out and seals them with composites. This is called a pulpectomy.
Entonces limpia la cavidad de la pulpa y los conductos de la raíz y los sella con resinas compuestas, llamadas materiales compuestos o *composites*. Esto se llama pulpectomía.

18. A rubber-dam, which is a sheet of rubber, is used to isolate the tooth to be worked keeping it away from the fluids of the mouth. In order to widen the area of visibility, it is often convenient to use clips on neighboring teeth. They make it easier to isolate the area.
Un dique de goma, que es un dispositivo de caucho, es utilizado por el (la) dentista para aislar un diente enfermo de los líquidos de la boca. Cuando se desea ampliar el campo o la visibilidad, es conveniente colocar grapas en dos dientes vecinos. Facilitan el aislamiento.

19. After the area is isolated with the dam and clip and the area disinfected, access to the pulp chamber is necessary.
Después de que el área se aisla con dique y grapa y se desinfecta el campo, se abre la cámara pulpar.

20. The canals are located and the radicular pulp removed. [A]
Se localiza(n) el (los) conducto(s) y se extirpa la pulpa radicular. [A]

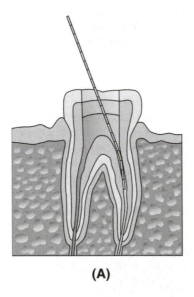

(A)

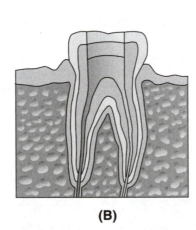

(B)

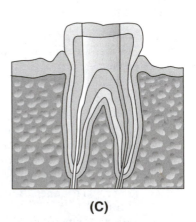

(C)

21. The canals are widened and filed, irrigated, and temporarily sealed on the first visit. [B]
Los conductos se ensanchan y liman, se lavan (con irrigación y aspiración), y se sellan temporalmente durante la primera visita. [B]

22. This process is repeated at a second session and a third if necessary.
Este proceso se repite a la segunda sesión y a la tercera si es necesario.

23. If the tooth does not have symptoms of spontaneous pain, or swelling, the canals are filled. [C]
Si el diente está asintomático, es decir, no tiene síntomas de dolor espontáneo o edema

inflamatorio, etc., se procederá a la obturación de conductos. [C]

24. If there are symptoms, the steps are repeated
again.
**Si hay síntomas, se harán los pasos indicados
de nuevo menos la obturación de conductos.**

ORAL SURGERY[6] *CIRUGIA ORAL*

1. I am going to extract your _____ tooth.
Voy a sacarle (el diente)
upper right front tooth
incisivo central superior derecho
lower left front tooth
el incisivo central inferior izquierdo
upper left lateral tooth
el incisivo lateral superior izquierdo
lower right lateral tooth
el incisivo lateral inferior derecho
upper canine/eyetooth
el canino (colmillo) superior
lower canine/eyetooth
el canino (colmillo) inferior
upper first bicuspid/premolar
el primer premolar (bicúspide) superior
upper second bicuspid
el segundo premolar (bicúspide) superior
lower first bicuspid
el primer premolar (bicúspide) inferior
lower second bicuspid
el segundo premolar (bicúspide) inferior
lower first molar
**el primer molar (la primera/muela)
inferior**
upper second molar
el segundo molar superior
upper wisdom tooth
**la muela del juicio superior
(el tercer molar superior)**
lower wisdom tooth
la muela del juicio inferior

2. I have to remove your wisdom teeth (upper
bicuspids).
**Tengo que sacarle las muelas del juicio (los
bicúspides superiores).**

3. Do you want to go to sleep?
**¿Quiere que le administro una anestesia
general?**

4. If so, you cannot eat or drink for nine hours
before the surgery.
**En este caso, no puede comer ni beber du-
rante nueve horas antes de la cirugía.**

5. Do you want local anesthesia?
¿Prefiere anestesia local?

6. Are you allergic to any medications?
**¿Es usted alérgico (alérgica) a algunos
medicamentos?**

7. Don't touch the wound with your fingers,
tongue, or toothpicks.

25. Later, the tooth is restored, usually with a
crown.
**Más tarde, se restaura el diente, por lo
común con una corona.**

**No se toque la herida con los dedos, la
lengua, o mondadientes.**

8. Bite on this gauze for an hour *without* moving it.
**Muerda Vd. a dentelladas esta gasa *sin*
moverla.**

9. If the bleeding is excessive, call me immediately.
Si (se) desangra, llámeme en seguida.

10. Only have liquids today.
Hoy no tome más que líquidos.

11. Don't use straws.
No use Vd. pajas.

12. Tomorrow begin eating a soft diet.
A partir de mañana, siga una dieta blanda.

13. Don't rinse your mouth at all for the first 24
(twenty four) hours.
**No se enjuague en absoluto la boca durante
las primeras 24 (veinticuatro) horas.**

14. Rinse your mouth with warm salt water every 4
(four) hours.
**Enjuáguese la boca con agua tibia con sal
cada 4 (cuatro) horas.**

15. You will have some pain in the form of soreness around the operated area.
**Vd. tendrá algún dolor en la forma de una
parte dolorida por toda la superficie afectada.
Vd. estará un poco dolorido (dolorida) por
toda la superficie afectada.**

16. Take two aspirins if it hurts you a lot.
Tome Vd. dos aspirinas si le duele mucho.

17. Do not change the dose or frequency of your
medication.
**No cambie ni la dosis ni la frecuencia de su
medicina.**

18. Expect some swelling for about three days.
This is normal.
**Cuente con alguna tumefacción (hinchazón)
que durará unos tres días. Es normal.**

19. Apply an ice pack as soon as possible after the
surgery.
**Póngase una bolsa de hielo tan pronto como
pueda después de la cirugía oral.**

20. Don't smoke for a few days.
No fume por unos días.

21. I want you to rest here in the office for an hour
before you leave.
**Quiero que Vd. descanse aquí en el consul-
torio (la oficina) por una hora antes de irse.**

22. Return for your next appointment in a week.
     Vuelva Vd. para su próxima cita de hoy en ocho días.

23. I will remove the stitches then.
     Voy a quitarle los puntos (las puntadas) entonces.

POST-OP AT THE ORAL SURGEON'S OFFICE

Oral Surgeon:	Mr. Mendoza, I have just removed five of your daughter's baby teeth. One of the teeth was abscessed.
Dad:	What does that mean?
Oral Surgeon:	It means that the tooth had a cavity so deep that the tooth was dying. It is possible that another tooth in her mouth may be abscessed. Therefore, I would like to see her again next week, either Tuesday or Thursday morning.
Dad:	Where is Adela now?
Oral Surgeon:	She is resting in my recovery room.
Dad:	How long will she be there? Can I see her?
Oral Surgeon:	I would like her to rest for at least a half hour. You may go in as soon as I explain the prescriptions. How old is Adela?
Dad:	She's eight years old.
Oral Surgeon:	How much does she weigh?
Dad:	She weighs 75 lbs. (seventy five pounds) (34 kgs. [thirty-four kilos]).
Oral Surgeon:	Is she allergic to any drugs?
Dad:	No.
Oral Surgeon:	I am giving you a prescription for V-cillin K. It is a liquid form of penicillin. She is to take two teaspoons immediately and then one teaspoon every four hours today. Beginning tomorrow, she may take one teaspoon after breakfast, lunch, and dinner, and another at bedtime.
Dad:	For how long does she take the medicine?
Oral Surgeon:	Until she finishes the bottle. This medicine must be kept in the refrigerator. I am writing another prescription for pain medicine. Give her one to two teaspoons as needed. Do not give her more than twelve teaspoons in twenty four hours. Do you understand?
Dad:	Yes. What about foods?
Oral Surgeon:	Here is a sheet with instructions about what she may or may not eat. Follow it closely. If her face hurts a lot, give her cold compresses immediately when you get home. By suppertime use an icebag for relief. It will stop the swelling.

EN EL CONSULTORIO DEL CIRUJANO ORAL DESPUES DE UNA EXTRACCION

Cirujano oral:	Sr. Mendoza, acabo de sacarle cinco dientes de leche a su hija. Uno de los dientes tuvo un absceso.
Padre:	¿Qué quiere decir «absceso»?
Cirujano oral:	Significa que el diente tenía una picadura tan profunda que el diente estaba muerto. Es posible que otro diente en la boca de su hija tenga absceso. Por eso, quisiera verla otra vez la semana que viene, o el martes o el jueves por la mañana.
Padre:	¿Dónde está Adela ahora?
Cirujano oral:	Descansa en mi sala de recuperación.
Padre:	¿Por cuánto tiempo se quedará allí? ¿Puedo verla?
Cirujano oral:	Quisiera que ella descansara por lo menos media hora. Vd. puede entrar tan pronto como le explique yo las recetas. ¿Cuántos años tiene Adela?
Padre:	Tiene ocho años.
Cirujano oral:	¿Cuánto pesa ella?
Padre:	Pesa setenta y cinco libras (treinta y cuatro kilos).
Cirujano oral:	¿Es alérgica a algunas medicinas?
Padre:	No.
Cirujano oral:	Le doy una receta para V-cillin K. Es una forma líquida de penicilina. Ella tiene que tomar dos cucharaditas inmediatamente y después una cucharadita cada cuatro horas hoy. Empezando mañana, ella puede tomar la cucharadita después del desayuno, del almuerzo, y de la cena, y otra al acostarse.
Padre:	¿Por cuánto tiempo debe tomar la medicina?
Cirujano oral:	Hasta terminar la botella. Esta medicina debe conservarse en el refrigerador. Le escribo otra receta para medicina contra el dolor. Déle una o dos cucharaditas cuando sea necesario. No le dé a ella más de doce cucharaditas durante un día entero (veinticuatro horas). ¿Me comprende Vd.?

Pad.:   Sí. En cuanto a los alimentos, ¿qué puede comer ella?

Cirujano oral: Aquí tiene un papel que contiene instrucciones acerca de lo que puede comer o no. Siga Vd. las instrucciones cuidadosamente. Si le duele mucho la cara, aplíquele una compresa fría tan pronto como lleguen Vds. a casa. A la hora de comer póngale una bolsa

30   de hielo para que sienta alivio. Se le quitará la hinchazón.

Preguntas

1. ¿Qué problema tuvo Adela Mendoza?
2. ¿Qué preguntas le hace el cirujano oral al padre?
3. ¿Cómo se llama la medicina que receta? ¿Cuántas veces al día tiene que tomarla?
4. ¿Qué debe hacer la chica al volver a casa?

PEDIATRIC DENTISTRY   *ODONTOLOGIA PARA NIÑOS*[7]

1. Let's have a look at you, Little One.
   A verte, m'hijo/m'hija.

2. What's your name?
   ¿Cómo te llamas?

3. How old are you?
   ¿Cuántos años tienes?

4. What's wrong (with you)?
   ¿Qué (te) pasa?

5. Who brought you today?
   ¿Quién te trajo hoy?

6. Climb up on the chair.
   Súbete a la silla.

7. Lie back.
   Acuéstate.

8. Just relax.
   Relájate.

9. Are you doing o.k.?
   ¿Estás bien?

10. The chair is going to move.
    La silla va a moverse.

11. I know that you are a good helper and a good listener.
    Sé que eres un buen ayudante/una buena ayudante y escuchas bien.

12. This is my other helper, whose name is _____ .
    Esta es mi otra ayudante, que se llama _____.

13. Open your mouth.
    Abre la boca.

14. A little more.
    Un poco más.

15. Close it a little.
    Ciérrala un poquito.

16. That's it!
    Eso es.

17. Why are you doing that?
    ¿Por qué haces eso?

18. Hop down and get something to play with (from the windowsill).
    Baja y toma algo para jugar del marco de la ventana.

19. This is my tooth counter. [explorer]
    Esta es mi herramienta para contar dientes. [un explorador]

20. It counts your teeth and tells me if there are any problems.
    Cuenta los dientes y me dice si hay algunos problemas.

21. Let's brush your teeth for you.
    Vamos a cepillarte los dientes.

22. I have a big toothbrush that I am going to show you.
    Tengo un cepillo de dientes grande que voy a mostrarte.

23. This is my scraper. [scaler]
    Este es mi cepillo de dientes especial. [un escarificador]

24. It is a special instrument that removes tartar and plaque from your teeth.
    Es un instrumento especial que quita sarro y cálculos de los dientes.

25. Do you remember my toothbrush?
    ¿Recuerda mi cepillo de dientes?

26. I am going to tickle your teeth with my toothbrush and tooth paste.
    Sentirás cosquillas en la boca cuando uso mi cepillo de dientes y la pasta dentífrica.

27. She will wash the toothpaste out for you.
    Ella te lavará la pasta dentífrica.

28. I am going to show you how you should brush your teeth.
    Voy a mostrarte cómo debes cepillarte los dientes.

29. You should brush them in the morning when you wake up, after meals, and in the evening just before you go to bed.
    Debes cepillártelos por la mañana al despertarte, después de comer, y por la noche antes de acostarte.

30. Now, let's take some special pictures of your teeth.
    Ahora, vamos a sacarte unas fotografías especiales de los dientes.

31. Do you have to go to the bathroom?
¿Tienes que ir al baño?

32. Here is a special shield for you to wear while we take the pictures.
Aquí tienes un escudo especial que usarás mientras te sacamos las fotos.

33. This is my picture card.
Esta es mi tarjeta que hace fotos.

34. These are our pillows. [mouth props]
Estas son nuestras almohadas. [un puntal especial para la boca]

35. Rest your teeth on them.
Pon los dientes en ellas.

36. Lie down.
Acuéstate.

37. Hold still.
Manténte quieto (quieta).
No te muevas.

38. Slide up in the chair.
Súbete en la silla.

39. We will check your X-rays.
Examinaremos las radiografías de tu boca.

40. I am going to give you a fluoride treatment which will help prevent cavities.
Te pondré un tratamiento de fluoruro que ayudará a prevenir las cavidades.

41. Don't eat or drink for a half hour after you leave here.
No comas ni bebas nada por media hora después de salir de aquí.

42. Do not rinse your mouth for a half hour, either.
No te enjuagues por media hora tampoco.

43. We examined the teeth, cleaned them, and gave him (her) a fluoride treatment. S/he should not eat or drink anything for one-half hour.
Examinamos los dientes, los limpiamos, y le dimos un tratamiento de fluoruro a él (a ella). No debe comer ni beber nada por media hora.

44. We took this X-ray of all the teeth.
Sacamos esta fotografía/radiografía de todos los dientes.

45. You can see all the new teeth lined up under the baby teeth.
Puede ver todos los dientes nuevos alineados por debajo de los dientes de leche.

46. S/He will keep these teeth until s/he is eleven or twelve.
Tendrá estos dientes hasta que tenga once o doce años.

47. S/He needs the teeth to chew.
Necesita los dientes para masticar.

48. S/He has _____ deep cavities.
Tiene _____ cavidades profundas.

49. Baby teeth have to be filled if they have cavities.
Es necesario empastar los dientes de leche si hay cavidades.

50. You don't want him/her to have any more toothaches.
Usted no quiere que le duelan más los dientes.
Usted no quiere que tenga más dolores de la boca.

51. S/He needs the baby teeth to hold a place for the permanent teeth.
Necesita los dientes de leche para conservar un lugar para los dientes permanentes.

52. If the baby teeth are lost too early, the space will close and the permanent teeth will be blocked.
Si los dientes de leche se pierden demasiado temprano, el espacio se cerrará y no podrán eruptar/salir los dientes permanentes.

53. If the tooth is extracted, a space maintainer will be needed to hold the space open until the new tooth erupts when s/he is eleven or twelve.
Si se le saca el diente, será necesario un aparato para mantener el espacio hasta que venga el nuevo diente permanente cuando tenga once o doce años.

54. There is too much noise here.
Hay demasiado ruido aquí.

55. Climb down and get something to play with.
Bájate de la silla y coge algo para jugar.

56. Come back to the chair.
Vuelve a la silla.

57. Open your mouth again.
Abre de nuevo la boca.

58. Don't bite my finger.
No me muerdas el dedo.

59. I am going to shake up your cheek.
Voy a sacudirte la mejilla.

60. I am going to make your tooth sleepy, but you will stay awake.
Voy a adormecerte los dientes, pero tú estarás despierto (despierta).

61. This is our buzzer.
Este es nuestro zumbador.

62. Anything else? Any other questions?
¿Algo más? ¿Tienes otras preguntas?

63. We will squirt water on your tooth and take the water out with the vacuum.
Echaremos agua sobre el diente y sacaremos el agua con la aspiradora.

64. She's being so nice to you, and you're acting so yucky!
Se está comportando tan bien contigo y tú te comportas tan mal.

65. I am going to put this ring around your tooth.
Voy a ponerte este anillo alrededor del diente.

66. That noise is the silver mixing.
 Ese ruido viene de la máquina que mezcla el empaste de plata.

67. Show Mom/Dad your teeth.
 Muéstrale los dientes a Mami/a Papi.

68. We never filled all the teeth.
 Nunca pusimos un empaste en todos los dientes.

69. Your lip and cheek are asleep. Don't play with them. You wouldn't want somebody to play with you if you were asleep.
 El labio y la mejilla están dormidos. No juegues con ellos. No te gustaría que alguien jugase contigo si tú estuvieras dormido (dormida).

70. Your mouth will feel funny for a couple of hours.
 La boca te sentirá entumida por un par de horas.

71. Don't eat or drink for an hour because you might bite your cheek or tongue.
 No comas ni bebas nada por una hora porque puedes morderte la mejilla o la lengua.

72. We never finished the treatment.
 Nunca terminamos el tratamiento.

73. Your child has a problem with her/his bite.
 Su hijo/hija tiene un problema con su oclusión o mordida.

74. We never corrected the bite.
 Nunca corregimos la mordida.
 Nunca corregimos la manera en que *fulano* muerde.

75. This side is normal.
 Este lado es normal.

76. This side is not normal.
 Este lado es anormal.

77. S/He still has a crossbite.
 Todavía tiene mordida cruzada.

78. The top teeth are inside the bottom teeth. (Class 3 occlusion)
 Los dientes superiores están dentro de los dientes inferiores. (Oclusión de la tercera clase)

79. S/He has an overbite. Notice that the upper front teeth overlap the lower front teeth when her/his jaws are closed. (Class 2 occlusion)
 Tiene una sobremordida. Fíjese usted que los incisivos superiores se superponen a los inferiores cuando muerde. (Oclusión de la segunda clase)

80. S/He has an open bite. Notice that a space exists between the upper incisors and the eye teeth and lower ones when the mouth is closed. (Apertognathia)
 Tiene una mordida abierta. Fíjese usted que los incisivos y los caninos superiores no se ponen en contacto con los inferiores creando un espacio al morder. (Apertonatia)

81. Your child needs braces.
 Su hijo/hija necesita frenos.

82. Your child needs orthodontia to correct the malocclusion of her/his teeth.
 A su hijo/hija le falta ortodoncia para corregir la maloclusión de los dientes.

83. After the treatment s/he will have a closed bite. The lower incisors will lie behind the upper incisors.
 Después del tratamiento tendrá una mordida cerrada. Los incisivos inferiores quedarán situados lingualmente en relación con los superiores.

84. Braces are necessary to keep his/her teeth straight.
 Le faltan los frenos para mantenerle derechos los dientes.

85. You need to see an orthodontist, a specialist who corrects abnormally positioned or aligned teeth, for the braces.
 Necesita consultar a un/una ortodontista, un/una dentista que se especializa en la corrección de las irregularidades y maloclusión de los dientes, para los frenos.

Notes *Notas*

1. For questions relating to a patient's health history, payment plans, and insurance, refer to Chapter 5.
2. See Chapter 10, page 219, note 6.
3. Untreated dental caries in Hispanic children and adults and the rather significant number of missing teeth in Cuban American and Puerto Rican adults compared with Mexican Americans and other Americans are the two most important oral health problems facing Hispanics today. (A.I. Ismail and S.M. Szpunar, "The Prevalence of Total Tooth Loss, Dental Caries, and Periodontal Disease among Mexican Americans, Cuban Americans, and Puerto Ricans: Findings from HHANES 1982–1984," *AJPH*, Dec. 1990, Vol. 80, pp. 66–70) See Chapter 1 pages 14–17.
4. For additional information on dates, refer to Chapter 4, page 100.
5. See Chapter 10, page 219, note 7.
6. The prevalence of gingivitis in Hispanics is higher than that found in White non-Hispanics. Puerto Rican children and adults have the highest prevalence of gingivitis among the Hispanic groups. (National Institute of Dental Research: Oral Health of United States Adults. The National Survey of Oral Health in U.S. Employed Adults and Seniors; 1985–86. National findings. NIH Pub. No. 87-2868.
7. Please note that this pediatric section of the book uses the **tú** or second person singular form of *you* when addressing the child. Spanish-speakers always use the "familiar" forms when speaking to a child. This form and its special conjugations are generally reserved for close friends, relatives, children, and pets, and sometimes, for social inferiors. The parent in this section is addressed as **usted,** the "polite" or third person singular form of *you.*

Authorizations and Signatures

Autorizaciones y firmas

This chapter contains sample hospital and dental authorization and signature forms. At crucial times patients are shown these forms. Students should practice reading them for fluency and comprehension. Key words and idioms are italicized or underscored in the texts. The following vocabulary should be helpful.

KEY WORDS AND IDIOMS FOR CONSENT FORMS
PALABRAS Y MODISMOS PRINCIPALES PARA LAS AUTORIZACIONES

abortion **aborto** *m*
  induced — **inducción del aborto** *f*
  therapeutic — **aborto terapéutico**
above (written) **arriba escrita** *adv*
above named **ya citado** *adj*
administer, to **administrar**
administration **administración** *f*
advantage **ventaja** *f*
adverse result **resultado adverso** *m*
advisable **aconsejable** *adj*
agent **representante** *m/f*
agree to, to **acceder**
agreement **convenio** *m*
AIDS **SIDA** *m*
anesthetic **anestético** *m, adj;* **anestésico**
  m, adj
apply for **solicitar admisión a**
  admission, to
appropriate **apropiado** *adj*
assistant **ayudante** *m/f*
assume, to **asumir**
assurance **aseguramiento** *m*
attending doctor **médico, (médica)**
  asistente *m/f*
authorization **permiso** *m;* **autorización**
authorize, to **autorizar**
be capable, to **ser capaz**
be desirable, to **ser conveniente**
be gowned, to **vestirse (i) de bata de**
  hospital
be guaranteed, to **ser garantizado**
be successful, to **tener éxito**
become pregnant, to **quedar**
  encinta/embarazada
blood **sangre** *f*
  blood components **componentes de**
    sangre *m;* **componentes**
    sanguíneos *m*
  blood donors **donantes de sangre**
    m/f
  blood stock **depósito de sangre** *m*
  blood transfusion **transfusión de**
    sangre *f*
  blood, whole **sangre pura**
body **cuerpo** *m;* **cadáver** *m*
certify, to **certificar**
childhood **niñez** *f*
commentary **comentario** *m*
complication **complicación** *f*
component **parte constitutiva** *f*

consent **consentimiento** *m*
consent, to **consentir (ie)**
consider, to **considerar**
cross-matching **prueba cruzada** *f*
daily **por día**
deceased **difunto** *m*
detect, to **detectar**
disposal **desecho** *m*
dispose **desechar**
educational **educativo** *adj*
effects, ill **malos efectos** *m*
8:00 P.M. **las ocho de la noche** *f*
eighteen years old **dieciocho años** *m*
element **elemento** *m*
emergency **emergencia** *f;* **urgencia** *f*
examination **examen** *m*
exception **excepción** *f*
execute (a deed, etc) **otorgar**
exempt, to (release) **eximir**
exemption (from) **exención** *f* **(de)**
fee **honorario** *m*
feeding hours **horas de alimentación** *f*
fitness (good health) **buena salud** *f*
form **formulario** *m*
free will **libre albedrío** *m*
give up (a claim), to **ceder**
guarantee, to **hacer garantías**
gynecological floor **piso**
  ginecológico *m*
have children, to **tener hijos**
hepatitis **hepatitis** *f*
  infectious ___ **hepatitis infecciosa**
  viral ___ **hepatitis viral**
hereby/by this letter, **por la presente;**
  por este medio
history **historial** *m*
incompatible **incompatible** *adj*
incompetent **incompetente** *adj*
infringement **contravención** *f*
insurance **seguro** *m*
judgment **parecer** *m*
lack **falta** *f*
law suit **pleito** *m*
make it clear, to **hacer constar**
make it known, to **hacer saber**
maternity floor **piso de maternidad**
medical purposes **fines médicos**
mentally **mentalmente** *adv*
necessary **necesario** *adj*
newborn **recién nacido** *m/f*

no one **nadie**
occasionally **de vez en cuando**
operating room **quirófano** *m*
patient **paciente** *m/f*
  in-house ___ **paciente**
    interno/interna
  out ___ **paciente**
    ambulatorio/ambulatoria
performance **ejecución** *f*
permanent **permanente** *adj*
permit **permiso** *m*
photography **fotografía** *f*
physically **físicamente**
plasma **plasma** *f*
power of attorney, durable **carta de**
  poder *f*
procedure **procedimiento** *m*
produce, to **producir**
reaction **reacción** *f*
registered nurse **enfermera titulada** *f*
release **descargo** *m;* **extención** *f*
  information ___ **divulgación de**
    información *f*
request **petición** *f;* **pedido** *m*
require, to **requerir (ie)**
restricted **restringido** *adj*
right **derecho** *m*
risk **riesgo** *m*
scientific **científico** *adj*
sterility **esterilidad** *f*
sterilization **esterilización** *f*
sterilized person **persona estéril** *f*
surgical **quirúrgico** *adj*
test **prueba** *f*
there may be **haya**
tissue **tejido** *m*
transfusion **transfusión** *f*
treatment **tratamiento** *m*
2:00 P.M. **las dos de la tarde** *f*
undersigned **abajo firmado** *adj*
understand, to **comprender**
undertaker **funerario** *m*
unexpected; unforeseen **inesperado** *adj*
virus **virus** *m*
visiting hours **horas de visita** *f*
visitor **visitante** *m/f*
warrant, to **hacer certificación**
wash one's hands, to **lavarse las manos**
witness **testigo** *m*

AUTHORIZATION FOR *SURGICAL* AND OTHER *PROCEDURES*

Date _____

Time _____

I *hereby authorize* the following operation _____

_____
(state nature and extent of operations or procedures)

to be performed upon _____
(myself, or name of patient)

under the direction of Dr. _____
(surgeon)

and whomever may be designated as his *assistants.*

I *consent* to the performance of all operations and procedures in addition to or different from those now contemplated, whether or not arising from presently *unforeseen* conditions, which the *above-named* doctor or his assistants may consider necessary or *advisable* on the basis of findings during the course of the operation.

I consent to all necessary, usual, or convenient procedures in connection with the operation including *blood transfusions,* and I consent to the administration of such *anesthetics* as may be considered necessary or advisable by the physician responsible for this service. I make the following exceptions: None: ____ or Other: ____.

I consent to the *photography* of the operation procedures to be performed including appropriate portions of my body for *medical, scientific,* or *educational purposes* provided identification is not revealed by the pictures or by descriptive texts accompanying them.

I consent to the admittance of proper professional observers to the operating room.

I consent to the *examination* of and *disposal* by hospital authorities of any *tissue* or part which may be removed during the operation.

I hereby *certify* that I have read and fully understand the above authorization for surgical *treatment* and possible blood transfusion, the reasons why these procedures are considered necessary, and the *advantages* and possible *complications,* which have been explained to me by Dr. ____. I also certify that no guarantee or *assurance* has been made as to the results that may be obtained.

Witness:_____   _____
                                                              (Signature of patient)

Name:_____   _____
                                                       (Signature of person authorized to
                                                                consent for patient)

Address:_____   _____
                                                              (Relationship to patient)

                                                       _____
                                                                      (Address)

PERMISO PARA PROCEDIMIENTOS *QUIRURGICOS* Y OTROS PROCEDIMIENTOS

Fecha _____

Hora _____

Por este medio autorizo la siguiente operación _____

_____

(Declare la naturaleza y extensión de operaciones o procedimientos)

que será ejecutada sobre _____

(mí mismo, o nombre de paciente)

bajo la dirección del doctor _____

(cirujano)

y quienes sean designados como sus *ayudantes*.

Consiento a la ejecución de todos los procedimientos y operaciones además de o diferente de los pensados, que pueda ocurrir o no, de condiciones ya *inesperadas*, que el médico ya citado, o sus ayudantes consideren *necesarios* o *aconsejables* a base de descubrimientos durante la operación.

Consiento a todos los procedimientos necesarios, comunes o convenientes con respecto a la operación incluso *transfusiones de sangre*, y consiento en *la administración* de tales *anestéticos* que el médico responsable para este servicio considere necesarios o *aconsejables*. Hago las siguientes *excepciones:* Ninguna ____ u Otra ____.

Autorizo *la fotografía* de los procedimientos quirúrgicos que serán ejecutados incluso porciones *apropiadas* de mi cuerpo para f*ines médicos, científicos* o *educativos* con tal que la identificación no sea revelada por las fotos o por *comentarios* descriptivos que las acompañen.

Autorizo la admisión de apropiados observadores profesionales al *quirófano*.

Autorizo a las autoridades de este hospital *la examinación y desecho* de cualquier *tejido*, o sus partes, que hayan sido removidos durante la operación.

Por este medio certifico que he leído y que comprendo completamente la *arriba escrita* autorización para *tratamiento quirúrgico* y para posible transfusión de sangre, las razones por las cualés estos procedimientos son considerados necesarios, *las ventajas* y *las complicaciones* posibles, que me han sido explicadas por el doctor ____. También certifico que ninguna garantía ni *aseguramiento* ha sido hecho en cuanto a los resultados que sean obtenidos.

Testigo: _____   _____

(Firma del paciente)

Nombre _____   _____

(Firma de la persona autorizada a
consentir en nombre del paciente)

Dirección _____   _____

(Parentesco al paciente)

_____

(Dirección)

CONSENT TO ANESTHETIC MANAGEMENT

Date: _____   Time: _____

1. I, _____ , hereby request that Dr. _____ or another anesthesiologist designated by the Hospital's Department of Anesthesia, administer anesthesia and provide other *required* medical care or therapeutic procedures to the above-named patient. I also understand that the *anesthetic* care shall be administered by or under the supervision of my anesthesiologist or his designate. I authorize the anesthesiologist to obtain the assistance of other physicians (including residents and interns), nurse anesthetists, or other assistants as considered *advisable*.

2. It is possible that *it may be desirable* to *administer* anesthesia by methods other than those that are planned at this time. I authorize the administration of anesthesia by such methods, with the exception of

    _____
    State the exception or "None."

3. An anesthesiologist or his designate has explained to me the nature of the anesthetic care *to be administered* and the *risks* involved in this. I have also been informed of the possible alternative methods of anesthesia, and the risks involved in these alternative methods including refusal of anesthesia. I have had an opportunity to discuss this with the anesthesiologist, or his designate, and have received answers to all the questions that I have asked.

I have read and fully understand the *Consent* to Anesthetic Management. All the blank spaces above were filled in before I signed this form.

_____   _____
Date & Time   Signature of Patient

_____   _____
Date & Time   Signature of Person *Authorized* to
                                                        Consent for *Incompetent* Patient

                                                    _____
                                                        Relationship to Patient

                                                    Patient did not sign this Consent because

                                                    _____

                                                    _____

CONSENTIMIENTO PARA LA *ADMINISTRACION* DE ANESTESIA

Fecha: _____   Hora: _____

1. Yo, _____ , *por la presente* solicito que el doctor _____ u otro anestesiólogo designado por el Departamento de Anestesia del Hospital _____, administre la anestesia y proporcione otra atención médica o procedimiento terapéutico que se *requiera* al paciente nombrado más arriba. Comprendo que la atención *anestética* será administrada por o bajo la supervisión de mi anestesiólogo o su agente. Autorizo al anestesiólogo a obtener la ayuda de otros médicos (residentes e internos inclusive), enfermeras anestesistas, u otros asistentes según lo que él considere *aconsejable*.

2. Es posible que *sea conveniente administrar* anestesia mediante otros métodos que no sean los métodos que están planeados en esta ocasión. Por la presente autorizo la administración de anestesia mediante tales métodos, con la excepción de

    _____
    indique la excepción o escriba «Ninguna.»

3. Un anestesiólogo o su agente me ha explicado el tipo de la atención *anestésica* a ser *administrado* y *los riesgos* que trae consigo. También se me informó acerca de posibles métodos alternativos de anestesia. He tenido la oportunidad de discutir esto con el anestesiólogo, o su agente, y recibido respuestas a todas las preguntas que he hecho.

He leído y comprendo completamente el *Consentimiento* para la Administración de Anestesia. Todos los espacios que aparecen en blanco han sido llenados antes de firmar yo esta forma.

_____   _____
Fecha y hora   Firma del paciente

_____   _____
Fecha y hora   o Firma de la persona *autorizada* para dar el
                                                                 Consensentimiento por un paciente *incompetente*.

                                                                 _____
                                                                 Parentesco con el Paciente

                                                                 El paciente no firmó este Consentimiento porque

                                                                 _____

                                                                 _____

STATEMENT OF PHYSICIAN

I believe that at the time the above *consent* was signed, the person who signed was capable of understanding the nature of the patient's physical condition and of the proposed treatment; the *risks* involved in the proposed *treatment* and in any reasonable alternatives to the proposed treatment; and the risks involved in the refusal of the proposed treatment.

I *certify* that I explained to the person signing this consent the items described in Paragraph 3 of the Consent to Anesthetic Management, that I answered the signer's questions about them, and that I witnessed the signature of the patient, or other person authorized to consent for the incompetent patient named above.

_____   _____

Signature of Physician   Date   Time

DECLARACION DEL MEDICO

Por la presente opino que en el momento de ser firmado el consentimiento, la persona que firmó fue capaz de comprender la naturaleza de la condición física del paciente y del *tratamiento propuesto*; los riesgos relacionados con el tratamiento propuesto y cualquier clase de alternativas razonables para el tratamiento propuesto; y los riesgos relacionados con el rechazo del tratamiento propuesto.

Certifico que expliqué al firmante de este consentimiento todo lo que está descrito en el tercer párrafo de este Consentimiento para la Administración de Anestesia, que he contestado a las preguntas del firmante relacionadas con las mismas, y que he presenciado la firma del paciente, u otra persona autorizada para dar el consentimiento por el paciente incompetente nombrado más arriba.

_____   _____

Firma del médico   Fecha   Hora

AGREEMENT AND *AUTHORIZATION* FOR EMERGENCY ROOM, *IN-PATIENT*, OR *OUTPATIENT* SERVICES

1. <u>CONSENT FOR DIAGNOSIS AND TREATMENT</u>
   I am voluntarily entering _____ Hospital for diagnostic and medical or surgical *treatment*, and I *consent* and *authorize* my physician, his assistants or designates, to carry out diagnostic procedures, as well as medical, surgical, radiographic (X-ray), nuclear, electrical, and laboratory *tests*, which, in his opinion, he may deem *necessary*. I recognize that the practice of medicine and surgery is not an exact science and I acknowledge that no guarantees have been given to me as to the result of the treatment or examination in the hospital. I *hereby authorize* _____ Hospital to retain, preserve and use for scientific or pedagogical purposes, or *to dispose* of any specimen or *tissue* which he may extract from my body during the hospitalization according to his *judgment*.

2. <u>RETENTION OF INFORMATION</u>
   I understand that _____ Hospital will record medical information as well as other types of information whether it be in electronic form or some other format. Said information is necessary during the course of my treatment and can be published by the Hospital for the purposes authorized in this *form*. I understand that part of my *medical history* may be disclosed to the appropriate nonclinical personnel for the purpose of undertaking *scientific* or statistical research, for administrative purposes, or for financial auditing. Without my explicit *consent*, I will not be identified either by name or by some other means which would personally identify me in any report of the stated research, auditing, or evaluations.

3. <u>RELEASE OF INFORMATION</u>
   I *hereby authorize* _____ Hospital *to release* all *medical records* or other information with regard to this treatment to my employers's *insurance* companies, to the health plans, to Medicare/Medicaid, to their underwriting companies or intermediaries for the purpose of reimbursing The Hospital and the physicians connected with the hospital for treatment and services which were rendered to me. I *consent* to the *release of information* pertaining to treatment, for a period which will not exceed more than one year from the date on which I am discharged from the hospital and/or from any outpatient program of the hospital. This authorization will not violate or infringe upon any internal policy of the hospital concerning the release of information, which will take precedence. It is not within the scope of this authorization to permit the release of medical history concerning my treatment for services which may require a restricted release in accordance with state or federal law, as its objective.

4. <u>ASSIGNMENT OF BENEFITS AND GUARANTEE OF PAYMENT</u>
   In consideration of the clinical and medical services which _____ Hospital has rendered to me, I *hereby assign* unto _____ Hospital, and to the physicians connected with the hospital, all *rights* and claims for reimbursement under any Medicare, Medicaid policy, or any group accident or health insurance policy, through which one has benefits for payment of services rendered. I commit myself to paying _____ Hospital and the physicians connected with the hospital, the balance of all the expenses which the aforementioned protection (with the exclusion of the expenses which cannot be collected due to Medicare regulations). This will include the costs of collection and/or reasonable attorneys' fees.

I have read the preceding clauses, 1-4, and by signing freely and voluntarily, I indicate that I am completely in agreement with what is set forth and agreed upon in the clauses, which can include treatment as a patient, subsequent to the *emergency* care or as an outpatient.

_____   _____
                     Patient   Date

_____   _____
Parent or Guardian (if the patient is eighteen)   Date

_____   _____
      (Relationship, if other than patient)   Date

_____   _____
      Insured (if other than the patient)   Date

_____   _____
                    Witness   Date

CONVENIO Y AUTORIZACION PARA SERVICIOS DE SALA DE URGENCIAS, *PACIENTE INTERNO, O PACIENTE AMBULATORIO*

1. CONSENTIMIENTO PARA DIAGNOSTICO Y TRATAMIENTO

   Ingreso voluntariamente en el Hospital _____ para fines de diagnóstico y *tratamiento* médico o quirúrgico, y *consiento* y *autorizo* a que mi médico, sus ayudantes o delegados efectúen los procedimientos de diagnóstico, así como *las pruebas* médicas, quirúrgicas, radiográficas, nucleares, eléctricas, y de laboratorio que, a su parecer, consideren necesarias. Reconozco que la práctica de la medicina y la cirugía no es una ciencia exacta y admito que no se me han dado garantías del resultado del tratamiento o examen en el hospital. *Por la presente* autorizo al Hospital _____ a retener, preservar y usar para fines científicos o pedagógicos, o a *desechar* según su *parecer* de cualquier espécimen o *tejido* que se extraiga de mi cuerpo durante la hospitalización.

2. RETENCION DE INFORMACION

   Comprendo que el Hospital _____ podrá registrar la información tanto médica como de otra índole ya sea de forma electrónica o de otra forma. Dicha información es necesaria durante el curso de mi tratamiento y podrá ser divulgada por el hospital para los fines autorizados en este *formulario*. Comprendo que parte de mi *historial* podrá ser divulgada al personal apropiado no clínico, para fines de realizar investigaciones científicas o estadísticas, para fines administrativos o de revisión financiera de cuentas. Sin mi *consentimiento* explicito, no seré identificado ni por mi nombre ni por otro modo que me identifique personalmente en ningún informe de dichas investigaciones, revisiones de cuentas o evaluaciones.

3. DIVULGACION DE INFORMACION

   Por la presente autorizo al _____ Hospital a que *divulgue* a mis compañías de *seguros* del patrón, a los planes de salud, a Medicare/Medicaid, a sus compañías aseguradoras o intermediarios, todo *historial* médico u otra información referente a este tratamiento para fines de obtener reembolso a mi nombre por el tratamiento y los servicios que me presten el _____ Hospital y los médicos relacionados con el hospital. Doy este *consentimiento* para la *divulgación de la informacion* referente al tratamiento, por un período que no se extenderá a más de un año a partir de la fecha en que se me dé de alta del hospital y/o de cualquier programa para pacientes ambulatorios del hospital. Esta autorización no estará en contravención de ninguna política interna del hospital acerca de la divulgación de información, la cual tendrá prioridad. Esta autorización no tiene como fin permitir la divulgación del historial referente a mi tratamiento, en cuanto a servicios que exijan la divulgación restringida en conformidad con la ley estatal o federal.

4. CESION DE BENEFICIOS Y GARANTIA DE PAGO

   En consideración por los servicios clínicos y médicos que me preste el _____ Hospital, por la presente *cedo* al Hospital _____, y a los médicos relacionados con el hospital, todos *los derechos* y reclamaciones de reembolso bajo cualquier póliza de Medicare, Medicaid, o póliza de seguro de grupo por accidente o salud, mediante la cual se disponga de beneficios para el pago de los servicios prestados. Me comprometo a pagarles al Hospital _____ y a los médicos relacionados con el hospital, el saldo pagadero de todos los gastos que no pague la antedicha protección (a exclusión de los gastos que no se pueden cobrar debido al reglamento de Medicare). Esto podrá incluir los gastos de cobro y/o los honorarios razonables de abogados.

He leído cada una de las precedentes cláusulas 1-4 y, al suscribir mi firma libre y voluntariamente, señalo que estoy totalmente de acuerdo con lo expuesto y convenido en ellas, lo que podrá comprender el tratamiento como paciente interno, posterior a la atención de *urgencia* o como paciente ambulatorio.

_____   _____
            Paciente   Fecha

_____   _____
Padre o guardián (si el paciente tiene   Fecha
menos de dieciocho años de edad)

_____   _____
Otro (parentesco con el paciente)   Fecha

_____   _____
El asegurado (si es distinto del paciente)   Fecha

_____   _____
            Testigo   Fecha

LIVING WILL DECLARATION

This declaration is hereby made this _____ day of _____ , _____
                                                                    (month)   (year)

I, _____ , being of sound mind, willfully and voluntarily *make known* my desires that my moment of death shall not be artificially postponed.

If at any time I should have an incurable and irreversible injury, disease, or illness judged to be a terminal condition by my *attending physician* who has personally examined me, and has determined that my death is imminent except for death delaying procedures, I direct that such procedures which would only prolong the dying process be withheld or withdrawn, and that I be permitted to die naturally with only the administration of medication, sustenance, or the performance of any medical procedure deemed *necessary* by my attending physician to provide me with comfort care.

In the absence of my ability to give directions regarding the use of such death delaying procedures, it is my intention that this declaration shall be honored by my family and physician as the final expression of my legal *right* to refuse medical or surgical treatment and accept the consequences from such refusal.

Signed _____

City, County and State of Residence _____

_____

The declarant is personally known to me and I believe him or her to be of sound mind. I did not sign the declarant's signature above for or at the direction of the declarant. At the date of this instrument I am not entitled to any portion of the estate of the declarant according to the laws of intestate succession or to the best of my knowledge and belief, under any will of declarant or other instrument taking effect at declarant's death, or directly financially responsible for declarant's medical care.

Witness: _____

Witness: _____

DECLARACION

Por medio de la presente declaro que hoy, el _____ día del _____ (mes) de _____(año), yo _____ , estando en mi sano juicio y por mi propia voluntad, *hago saber* que es mi deseo que el momento de mi muerte no sea prolongado por medios artificiales.

Si en cualquier momento yo padeciese de alguna herida, enfermedad, o condición consideradas incurables e irreversibles o mortal por mi *médico* quien me haya examinado personalmente y haya determinado que mi muerte sea inminente o muy próxima salvo que procedimientos médicos sean administrados en mi persona, sería mi voluntad que dichos procedimientos o tratamientos que servirían solamente para prolongar mi vida, no sean administrados o dejen de ser administrados y que se me permita morir de causas naturales administrando solamente procedimientos y/o medicamentos que mi médico considere *necesarios* para mi comodidad.

En caso dado que mis facultades mentales me impidan seguir dirigiendo mi tratamiento médico especialmente en caso de mi muerte, es mi deseo e intención que la presente declaración sea respetada por mi médico y mi familia como la última expresión de mi *derecho* ante la ley de rechazar tratamiento médico y/o quirúrgico y de aceptar las consecuencias de dicha denegación.

Firma _____

Ciudad, condado, y estado en donde radica _____

_____

Hago constar que conozco personalmente al (a la) declarante y que lo (la) creo que se encuentra en su sano juicio. También hago constar que la firma que aparece en este documento es la del (de la) declarante; que yo no he falsificado su firma y que no he firmado con su nombre a petición de él mismo (ella misma). Hago constar además que, a la fecha, no soy beneficiario ni tengo derecho a ninguna parte de las propiedades del (de la) declarante según las leyes de sucesión intestada vigentes o a mi leal saber y entender, en ningún testamento ni en ningún otro instrumento que entre en vigencia a la muerte del (de la) declarante, así como tampoco soy económicamente responsable por la atención médica del (de la) declarante.

Testigo: _____

Testigo: _____

DURABLE POWER OF ATTORNEY FOR HEALTHCARE

Power of Attorney made this _____ day of _____ 19_____

1. I, the *undersigned*, hereby appoint:

_____
(write name and address of agent)

as agent to act for me and in my name to make any and all decisions for me concerning my personal care, medical treatment, hospitalization and health care and to require, withhold or withdraw any type of medical treatment or procedure, even though my death may ensue. My agent shall have the same access to my medical records that I have, including the right to disclose the contents to others. My agent shall also have full power to make a disposition of any part or all of my body for medical purposes, authorize an autopsy and direct the disposition of my remains. (Neither the attending physician nor any other health care provider may act as your agent.)

2. The powers granted above shall be subject to the following rules or limitations (if none, leave blank):

_____

_____

(The subject of life-sustaining treatment is of particular importance. For your convenience in dealing with that subject, some general statements concerning the withholding or removal of life-sustaining treatment are set forth below. If you agree with one of these statements, you may initial that statement; but do not initial more than one.)

_____ I do not want my life to be prolonged nor do I want life-sustaining treatment to be provided or continued if my agent believes the burdens of the treatment outweigh the expected benefits. I want my agent to consider the relief of suffering the expense involved and the quality as well as the possible extension of my life in making decisions concerning life-sustaining treatment.

_____ I want my life to be prolonged and I want life-sustaining treatment to be provided or continued unless I am in a coma which my attending physician believes to be irreversible, in accordance with reasonable medical standards at the time of reference. If and when I have suffered irreversible coma, I want life-sustaining treatment to be withheld or discontinued.

_____ I want my life to be prolonged to the greatest extent possible without regard to my condition, the chances I have for recovery or the cost of the procedures.

3. This power of attorney shall become effective on _____.

4. This power of attorney shall terminate on _____.

Continued

5. If any agent named by me shall die, become legally disabled, resign, refuse to act or be unavailable, I name the following (each to act alone and successively, in the order named) as successors to such agent:

_____

_____

6. If a guardian of my person is to be appointed, I nominate the following to serve as such guardian (if same as agent, leave blank):

_____

7. I am fully informed as to all the contents of this form and *understand* the full import of this grant of power to my agent.

Signed_____
(Principal)

The principal has had an opportunity to read the above form and has signed the form or acknowledged his or her signature or mark on the form in my presence.

_____   Residing at_____
      (Witness)

(You may, but are not required to, request your agent and successor agents to provide specimen signatures below. If you include specimen signatures in this Power of Attorney, you must complete the certification opposite the signatures of the agents.)

Specimen signatures of agent (and successors)   I certify that the signature of my agent (and successors) are correct.

_____   _____
      (Agent)   (Principal)

_____   _____
   (Successor Agent)   (Principal)

_____   _____
   (Successor Agent)   (Principal)

                                         _____
                                           (Witness)

CARTA DE PODER PARA CUIDADO MEDICO

Carta de poder hecha el día _____ de _____ de __

1. Yo, cuyo nombre aparece aquí, por medio de *la presente,* nombro a:

_____
(escriba nombre y dirección del representante)

como mi representante para actuar en mi nombre con el fin de hacer o tomar cualquier desición con-
cerniente a mi cuidado personal, tratamiento médico, hospitalización y atención médica y para solicitar, impedir o retirar cualquier tipo de tratamiento médico o procedimiento, aún cuando el resultado
sea mi muerte. Mi representante tendrá el mismo acceso que tengo yo a mi *historial* clínico, incluyendo
el derecho de revelar el contenido a otros. Mi representante también tendrá el poder total de disponer
de cualquier parte de mi cuerpo o el cuerpo entero para propósitos médicos o *autorizar* una autopsia
y será libre de disponer de mis restos como mejor sea conveniente. (Ni el médico ni cualquier otra
persona que le preste servicios médicos puede actuar como su representante.)

2. Los poderes aquí otorgados, serán sometidos a las siguientes reglas o limitaciones: (Si no hay
   ninguna, por favor, déjelo en blanco.)

_____

_____

(El tratamiento de prolongar la vida es de suma importancia. Para que usted lo comprenda mejor, hemos enumerado algunos puntos concernientes a impedir o suspender el tratamiento para prolongar
la vida. Si usted está de acuerdo con algunos de estos puntos, escriba sus iniciales junto al mismo. Recuerde hacerlo en sólo uno de los tres puntos.)

_____ No quiero que mi vida sea prolongada ni quiero que se me provea o continúe el tratamiento
que sostiene mi vida si mi representante considera que los efectos psicológicos, morales y fi-
nancieros son más importantes que los beneficios que puedo recibir con el tratamiento.

_____ Quiero que mi representante considere el sufrimiento y el costo que implica, y la calidad de
vida que llevaré al aceptar o no aceptar el tratamiento para prolongar mi vida. Quiero que mi
vida sea prolongada y quiero que se me provea o continúe el tratamiento necesario a menos
que me encuentre en estado de coma y que mi médico considere que sea irrevocable, de
acuerdo con las normas médicas en el momento de referencia. Siempre y cuando haya sufrido
una coma irrevocable, quiero que dicho tratamiento sea retirado o descontinuado.

_____ Quiero que mi vida sea prolongada lo más posible sin que importen mi condición, las posi-
bilidades que tenga de recuperación o los costos de los procedimientos.

3. Esta carta de poder tendrá efecto a partir de _____.

4. Esta carta de poder se da por terminada en _____.

Continued

5. Si cualquier representante que nombro muere, llega a estar incapacitado, renuncia, niega a representarme o no está disponible, nombro a las siguientes personas (cada una actuará por sí mismo y en el orden nombrado como sucesor) como sus sucesores:

_____

_____

6. Si mi condición requisiese nombrar un guardián de mi persona, nombro a la siguiente como tal (si el guardián es el mismo que el representante, deje en blanco):

_____

7. Se me ha informado totalmente en cuanto al contenido de este documento y *comprendo* perfectamente el poder otorgado a mi representante.

Firma_____

(Otorgante)

El otorgante ha tenido la oportunidad de leer lo mencionado en este documento y ha firmado o reconocido su firma o marca como propia en mi presencia.

_____   Domicilio_____

(Testigo)

(No es requisito, pero se puede pedir que su representante y sucesores le provean con muestras de sus firmas en los siguientes espacios. Si incluye las firmas en esta carta de poder, es necesario llenar la certificación junto a las firmas de los representantes.)

Firmas de representante (y sucesores)

Yo certifico que las firmas de mi representante (y sucesores) son auténticas.

_____

(Representante)

_____

(Otorgante)

_____

(Sucesor)

_____

(Otorgante)

_____

(Sucesor)

_____

(Otorgante)

_____

(Testigo)

CONSENT FOR *AUTHORIZATION* TO *DIVULGE INFORMATION*

PATIENT:_____ ROOM:_____ AGE:____
ADDRESS:_____ TELEPHONE:_____

The Hospital's dedication to excellent medical attention for its patients, research, and teaching has given it a national reputation as a celebrated center for (pediatric) medical services. As such, the Hospital frequently receives requests for information about patients from agencies of the press, other medical providers, and from medical researchers. Additionally, the Hospital believes that *it is fitting* to share this information through its own publications, in order to educate the public in matters of health. Frequently such instruction is the key which permits the public to understand certain *childhood* illnesses. The availability of such information from the Hospital can also alleviate onerous *requests* from the press to the patient and his family. In order to help in these and other worthy purposes under consideration, the Hospital requests the following consents, releases, and indemnifications. Thank you very much for your help.

1. *By means of the present document* I authorize the Hospital, its employees, or affiliated physicians to divulge information to the press and medical researchers which refer to the patient or his condition or treatment, or any treatment that may be given to me or to other members of the patient's family, and I authorize them to use such information in their own publications. Such information may include (but is not limited to) age, name, sex, date of admission, name of the physician assigned as well as a description of the patient's condition, the diagnosis, the medication, the medical procedures and any other information which has to do with newspaper releases, television or radio broadcasts, medical journals, or other publications. Although the Hospital will try to avoid errors or inaccuracies with regard to the information divulged, the Hospital will not be responsible for any of the errors that may occur in spite of its due care. Please enumerate any restrictions. _____
_____

2. I also authorize the taking and publication both of still *photos* and films and videos of the patient, of me, and of all members of the patient's family by or under the supervision of the Hospital for use in the newspapers, magazines, television, movies, hospital publications, or medical journals. Please enumerate any restrictions.
_____

3. Because I authorize the Hospital to divulge information, I am also in agreement that neither the Hospital, nor its employees, nor the affiliated physicians will be obligated either to the patient, to me, or to others who may be performing in accordance with this consent, nor will they have to pay either *rights* or compensation or injuries because of any information or photos that may be distributed in accordance with this consent.

4. I can annul this consent upon notifying the Director of Public Affairs at the Hospital. Such revocation will not take effect until or unless it is really received by the aforementioned individual cited by the Hospital.

Name (please print): _____

Signature: _____

Relationship to the patient: _____

Date: _____

CONSENTIMIENTO PARA AUTORIZACION PARA *DIVULGAR INFORMACION*

PACIENTE:_____ CUARTO:_____ EDAD::____
DOMICILIO:_____ TELEFONO:_____

La dedicación del hospital a excelencia de asistencia médica para pacientes, investigación, y enseñanza le ha dado fama nacional de un centro célebre para servicios médicos (pediátricos). Como tal, el Hospital muchas veces recibe solicitudes para información acerca de pacientes de agencias de prensa, otros proveedores médicos, y de investigadores médicos. También el Hospital cree que *es conveniente* compartir esta información por medio de sus propias publicaciones, para educar al público acerca de cuestiones de la salud. Con frecuencia tal instrucción es la clave que le permite comprender ciertas enfermedades de *la niñez* al público. La disponibilidad de tal información del Hospital también puede aliviarles al paciente y su familia de *pedidos* onerosos de la prensa. Para ayudar en estos y otros fines dignos de consideración, el Hospital pide los siguientes consentimientos, descargos, e indemnizaciones. Muchas gracias por su ayuda.

1. *Por la presente* autorizo al Hospital, sus empleados o médicos afiliados con él divulgar información a la prensa e investigadores médicos por lo que se refiere al paciente o su condición o tratamiento, o cualquier tratamiento que se me puede poner o a otros miembros de la familia del paciente, y les autorizo usar tal información en sus propias publicaciones. Tal información puede incluir (pero no se limita a) la edad, nombre, sexo, fecha de ingreso, nombre del médico adscrito así como una descripción de la condición del paciente, la diagnosis, el medicamento, los procedimientos médicos y otra información que tiene que ver con los periódicos, emisiones de televisión o radio, revistas médicas u otras publicaciones. Aunque el Hospital tratará de evitar errores o inexactitudes en cuanto a la información divulgada, el Hospital no será responsable de cualquiera de los errores que ocurran a pesar del debido cuidado. Favor de enumerar cualquier restricción. _____
_____

2. También autorizo sacar y publicar tanto *fotos* inmóviles como películas y videos del paciente, de mí, y de todos los miembros de la familia del paciente por o bajo la supervisión del Hospital para uso en los periódicos, revisitas, televisión, cine, publicaciones del hospital o revistas médicas. Favor de enumerar cualquier restricción.
_____

3. A causa del hecho de que autorizo al Hospital que divulgue información, además me pongo de acuerdo de que ni el Hospital, ni sus empleados, ni los médicos afiliados con el Hospital estará obligado ni al paciente, ni a mí, ni a otros que actúen de acuerdo con este consentimiento, ni tendrán que pagar ni *derechos* ni compensación ni agravios a causa de cualquier información o fotos distribuidas de acuerdo con este consentimiento.

4. Puedo anular este consentimiento al notificar por escrito al Director de Asuntos Públicos al Hospital. Tal revocación no entrará en vigor hasta y a menos que sea recibida en realidad por el individuo anteriormente citado al Hospital.

Nombre (favor de escribir con letras de molde): _____

Firma: _____

Parentesco al paciente: _____

Fecha: _____

REQUEST FOR TRANSFUSION OF *WHOLE BLOOD* OR ANY OF ITS *COMPONENTS*

(Consent and Waiver Form)

I, _____, do *hereby* authorize Dr. _____ (*Attending Physician*) and any of his *assistants* or associates (hereinafter called physician) to administer to me such *blood transfusions* or any *blood components* including, but not limited to, *plasma,* as may be deemed *advisable* in the judgment of any such physician.

It has been explained to me that it is not always possible *to detect* the existence or non-existence of some *elements occasionally* present in blood, such as the *virus* causing *infectious hepatitis* or other unusual blood components, and that there is a possibility of *ill effects,* such as infectious hepatitis resulting from the transmission of its virus or a transfusion *reaction* resulting from the transmission of unusual blood components. I also *understand* that *there* may be the possibility of the transmission of the causative agent of other diseases.

It has also been explained to me that *emergencies* may arise when it is not possible to make adequate *cross-matching* or other *tests* and that immediate need may *require* the use of existing *stocks of blood,* which may include some *incompatible* blood types or substances.

I fully understand that the blood supplied in accordance with this agreement is incidental to the rendition of services and that no requirements, *guarantee* or *warranty* of *fitness,* quality or absence of undetectable substances such as viruses, shall apply.

After *considering* all of the items set forth above and the possibility of *adverse results* from the said blood transfusions, it is still my desire that one or more transfusions of blood or its components be administered to me, if in the opinion of my physician such transfusions are needed.

I hereby *assume* any and all *risks* in connection with any said blood transfusions and *release* physician and _____ Hospital, its personnel and employees, all *blood donors* and all other persons, firms and corporations which in any way handled or processed said blood, from any responsibility whatsoever for any resulting contraction of *viral hepatitis, AIDS,* or any *reaction* from any such transfusion. I further assume any and all risks in connection with said blood transfusions and *agree* that I will never bring *suit* in connection with said transfusions.

Date: _____

Witness: _____

_____ R.N.

_____ M.D.
(Signature of Attending Physician)

_____
(Signature of patient or person authorized
to consent for patient)

_____
(Relationship to patient)

PETICION PARA TRANSFUSION DE *SANGRE PURA* O DE CUALQUIERA DE SUS *PARTES CONSTITUTIVAS*

Por este medio yo _____, *autorizo* al Dr. _____ (*médico asistente*) y a cualquiera de sus *ayudantes* o asociados (más adelante llamados «médico») que me administre tales *transfusiones de sangre o componentes de sangre* incluso, pero no limitado a *plasma*, que según el juicio del médico sean aconsejables.

Se me explicó que no es posible siempre *detectar* la existencia o la falta de existencia de algunos *elementos* presentes *de vez en cuando* en la sangre, como por ejemplo *el virus* que cause *la hepatitis infecciosa*, u otros componentes sanguíneos no muy comunes y que puede haber la posibilidad de *malos efectos*, tal como la hepatitis infecciosa que resulta de la transmisión de su virus o *una reacción* a transfusión que resulta de la transmisión de extraordinarios componentes sanguíneos. Tambien *comprendo* que *haya* la posibilidad de la transmisión de agentes que causan otras enfermedades.

También se me ha explicado que *emergencias* pueden aparecer cuando no sea posible hacer suficientes *pruebas cruzadas* u otras *pruebas* y que la necesidad inmediata pueda *requerir* usar *el depósito de sangre* que incluya algunos tipos o substancias de sangre que sean *incompatibles*.

Comprendo completamente que la sangre provista de acuerdo con este consentimiento es elemento incidental a la rendición de servicios y que nadie me *hace garantías* ni *certificación* de *buena salud*, cualidad ni falta de substancias ocultas como virus.

Después de *considerar* todo lo que se me ha explicado y la posibilidad *de resultados adversos* de las ya citadas transfusiones de sangre, todavía quiero que me sean administradas tantas transfusiones de sangre y sus componentes como mi médico juzgue necesarias.

Por este medio *asumo* cualquiera y todos *los riesgos* con respecto a cualquier citada transfusión de sangre y les *eximo* al médico, al Hospital _____, y a su personal y empleados, a todos *los donantes de sangre* y a todas las personas, firmas y corporaciones que, de cualquier manera hayan manejado o preparado dicha sangre, de cualquier responsabilidad si contraigo *la hepatitis viral*, *SIDA*, o alguna *reacción* de semejante transfusión. Además asumo cualquier y todos los riesgos con respecto a las citadas transfusiones de sangre y *accedo* que nunca seguiré *un pleito* con respecto a tales transfusiones.

Fecha _____

Testigo: _____

_____
(Firma de la *enfermera titulada*)

_____ Médico
(Firma del médico asistente)

_____
(Firma de paciente o de la persona autorizada a dar permiso para el paciente)

_____
(Parentesco al paciente)

AUTHORITY TO PERFORM A *THERAPEUTIC ABORTION*

This is to certify that I, the undersigned, consent to the *administration* of whatever *anesthetic* may be necessary and the *performing* of a therapeutic abortion upon

Name _____

5   Address _____

Signature of Patient _____

Signature of Patient's Husband _____

Witness: _____

Name _____

10   Address _____

AUTORIZACION PARA UN *ABORTO TERAPEUTICO*

Esto es para certificar que yo, la abajo firmada, consiento a *la administración* de cualquier *anestético* que sea necesario y en *la ejecución* de un aborto terapéutico sobre

Nombre _____

<u>5</u>   Dirección _____

Firma de la paciente _____

Firma del esposo de la paciente _____

Testigo: _____

Nombre _____

<u>10</u>   Dirección _____

RELEASE FROM RESPONSIBILITY FOR *ABORTION*

Date, _____ Time: ___A.M./P.M.

This is to certify that I, _____, a patient applying for admission to _____
Hospital, believe that I am in a condition of abortion. I hereby declare that neither the attending physician nor any person employed by or connected with the said hospital has knowingly performed any act

5   that may have contributed to the induction of the abortion, and I do hereby absolve said persons from any
responsibility or liability for my condition.

Witness _____   Signed _____
                                                              (Patient or nearest relative)

Witness _____   _____

10   (Relationship)

Authorization must be signed by the patient, or by the nearest relative when the patient is physically
or mentally incompetent.

EXENCION DE RESPONSABILIDAD PARA UN *ABORTO*

Fecha: _____ ___; Hora: ____

Estos es para *certificar* que yo, ____, una paciente que solicita *admisión* a Hospital ____ , creo estar
en condiciones de aborto. Por la presente declaro que ni el médico que me atiende ni ninguna personal empleada o conectada con este hospital ha realizado ningún acto que haya contribuido a la

5   *inducción del aborto*, y por medio de la presente absuelvo a estas personas de cualquier responsabilidad por mi estado.

Testigo _____   Firma _____
                                                              (Paciente o pariente más cercano)

Testigo _____   _____

10   (Parentesco)

Autorización debe ser firmada por la paciente o por su pariente más cercano cuando la paciente es *incompetente física o mentalmente.*

STERILIZATION PERMIT

We, the *undersigned,* husband and wife, hereby authorize Dr. _____ to perform _____ (name of operation) the sole purpose of which is *to produce permanent sterility,* on _____ (name of patient) which in all likelihood will be the result, but in no case can it be guaranteed. The operation may not *be a success.*

We *voluntarily* request this operation and *understand* that it is intended to result in sterility although this result cannot *be guaranteed.* Sterilization has been explained to us, and we understand that a *sterile person is* not *capable* of *becoming pregnant* and *bearing a child.*

_____
Signed
(Wife)

_____
(Husband)

_____
Date

Witness: _____

Name   _____

Address _____

Date   _____

PERMISO PARA *ESTERLIZACION*

Nosotros, los *abajo firmados,* esposo y esposa, por este medio autorizamos al doctor _____a hacer _____(nombre de la operación) con el propósito único de *producir esterilidad permanente* sobre _____ (Esposa) o_____ (Esposo). Con toda probabilidad la operación *tendrá éxito,* pero existe la posibilidad de que la operación no tenga éxito.

Nosotros solicitamos esta operación por nuestro *libre albedrío* y *comprendemos* que el propósito de la operación es la esterilización, aunque este resultado no puede *ser garantizado.* Se nos explicó lo que es la esterilización, y entendemos que *una persona estéril* no *es capaz* de *quedar encinta (embarazada)* y *tener hijos.*

_____
Firma
(Esposa)

_____
(Esposo)

_____
Fecha

Testigo: _____

Nombre_____

Dirección _____

Fecha   _____

REQUEST FOR POSTMORTEM EXAMINATION

Name _____ Room _____

Age _____ Date _____

Physician _____ Intern _____

   I, _____ , hereby request _____

Hospital to do a postmortem examination on the *body* of my _____ ,
                                                        (relationship)

_____ , with the removal and retention of diseased tissue.
       (name of *deceased*)

_____
   (Special instructions, if any.)

                                    Signed, _____

Witness _____

Witness _____

SOLICITUD PARA AUTOPSIA

Nombre _____ Cuarto _____

Edad _____ Fecha _____

Médico _____ Médico residente_____

   Yo, _____ , por este medio pido al Hospital de _____

_____ que se haga una autopsia del *cadáver* de mi _____ ,
                                                    (Parentesco)

_____ , con el traslado y retención de los tejidos enfermos.
   (Nombre del *difunto*)

_____
         (Instrucciones especiales, si las hay.)

                                   Firma, _____

Testigo _____

Testigo _____

UNDERTAKER'S RELEASE

Date: _____

I hereby grant permission to _____

Undertakers to remove the *body* of _____ from the _____ Hospital.

The *deceased* has been a resident of _____ for years, and has (not) served in the military or naval service of the United States. (If so, what war?)

Social Security Number _____

Signed _____

Relationship _____

Witness _____

DESCARGO PARA LOS *FUNERARIOS*

Fecha _____

Yo, por este medio doy permiso a los funerarios de _____

para que quiten el *cadáver* de _____ del Hospital de _____ . El

difunto ha sido residente de _____ por _____

años, y (no) ha servido en el servicio militar o naval de los Estados Unidos. (Si es así, ¿en qué guerra?)

Número de seguro social _____

Firma _____

Parentesco _____

Testigo _____

Readings for Health Professionals

Lecturas para profesionales médicos, dentales y de asistencia pública

KEY WORDS AND IDIOMS FOR SELECTED READINGS

PALABRAS Y MODISMOS PRINCIPALES PARA LECTURAS SELECTAS

acidosis **acidosis** *f*
acquire (a disease), to **contraer**
acute attack **ataque agudo** *m*
alertness **agudeza mental** *f*
alloy **aleación** *f*
amino acids **aminoácidos** *m, pl*
antibiotic **antibiótico** *m*
assume, to **asumir**
asymptomatic **asintomático** *adj*
auto-immune **autoinmunológico** *adj*
bar of chocolate **chocolatina** *f*
belch, to **eructar**
belching **eructación** *f*; **eructo** *m*
bile **bilis** *f*
bile salt **sal biliar** *f*
bilirubin **bilirrubina** *f*
bite, to **morder [ue]**
bleed excessively, to **desangrarse**
bleeding **sangría** *f*, **hemorragia** *f*;
 flujode sangre *m*
block, to **bloquear, obstruir, tapar**
blockage **obstrucción** *f*
blood pressure **presión sanguíneo** *f*
blood screening **selección de sangre** *f*;
 pruebas selectivas de sangre *f*
bloodstream **corriente sanguínea** *f*
borderline case **caso incierto** *m*, **caso**
 límite *m*, **caso dudoso** *m*
bothersome **incómodo** *adj*
breathing **respiración** *f*
bring about, to **provocar; acarrear**
build up, to **acumular**
bulb **ampolleta** *f*
calcium **calcio** *m*
carbohydrate **carbohidrato** *m*
carbonated **carbonatado** *adj*; **gaseoso**
 adj
catheter **sonda** *f*, **catéter** *m*
cause, to **causar, provocar**
chill **escalofrío** *m*
cholecystogram **colecistograma** *m*
cholesterol **colesterol** *m*
chronically **crónicamente** *adv*
coarse **grueso** *adj*; **áspero** *adj*
complain of, to **quejarse de**
connect, to **juntar**
control, to **controlar, regular**
convert, to **convertir [ie]**
crystal **cristal** *m*
cystoscope **cistoscopio** *m*
daily **cotidiano** *adj*, **diario** *adj*
damage **daño** *m*
deprive, to **privar**
detect, to **descubrir, detectar, rectificar**
diabetic **diabético** *m, adj*
diabetic coma **coma diabético** *m*
diagnose, to **diagnosticar**
digest, to **digerir [ie]**
digestive **digestivo** *adj*
discomfort **aflicción** *f*; **molestia** *f*
discovery **descubrimiento** *m*
disease **enfermedad** *f*
disorder **desorden** *m*
dosage **dosificación** *f*, **dosis** *f*
drop back into, to **caer en**
drowsiness **somnolencia** *f*, **modorra** *f*
duct **conducto** *m*
dye **colorante** *m*, **tinte** *m*
empty, to **vaciar**

endoscope **endoscopio** *m*
energy **energía** *f*
excessive **excesivo** *adj*
exchange list **lista de intercambios** *f*
expect, to **contar [ue] con**
fall, to **caer**
fasting **ayuno** *m*
 fasting blood sugar **glucemia en**
 ayunas *f*
fat **grasa** *f*
fat-like **graso** *adj*
feeding **alimentación** *f*
fill, to **rellenar**
filter, to **filtrar**
flatulence **flatulencia** *f*
flow, to **fluir**
flu **gripe** *f*
fluctuate **oscilar**
flushed **enrojecido** *adj*
frequent **frecuente** *adj*; **habitual** *adj*
fried food **alimento frito** *m*
gallbladder **vesícula biliar** *f*
gallstone **cálculo biliar** *m*
gene **gen** *m*, **gene** *m*
germ **germen** *m*
give birth to, to **dar a luz, parir**
glucagon **glucagón** *m*, **hormona**
 glicética *f*
glucose **glucosa** *f*
glucose tolerance test **prueba de**
 tolerancia a la glucosa *f*
glycogen **glucogeno** *m*; **glicógeno** *m*
goal **meta** *f*, **objetivo** *m*
gradual **gradual** *adj*, **paulatino** *adj*
gravel **arenilla** *f*
groin **ingle** *f*
handle, to **metabolizar, utilizar**
heal, to **curar, sanar**
healing **curación** *f*
heart attack **ataque cardíaco** *m*
heartburn **ardor epigástrico** *m*, **pirosis** *f*
history, (medical) **historial médico**
hormone **hormona** *f*, **hormón** *m*
hyperglycemia **hiperglucemia** *f*;
 hiperglicemia *f*
hypoglycemia **hipoglicemia** *f*;
 hipoglucemia *f*
image **imagen** *f*
imbalance **desequilibrio** *m*
immune system **sistema inmune** *m*
increase **aumento** *m*
indigestion **indigestión** *f*
inflame, to **inflamar**
inject, to **inyectar**
injection **inyección** *f*
insidious **insidioso** *adj*, **engañoso** *adj*
insufficient **insuficiente** *adj*
insulin **insulina** *f*, **insulínico** *adj*
 insulin reaction **reacción insulínica** *f*
interfere, to **interferir [ie]**
interval **intervalo** *m*
intolerance **intolerancia** *f*
intravenous pyelogram [I.V.P.]
 pielograma intravenoso [P.I.V.] *m*
irritate, to **irritar**
itching **comezón** *f*, **escozor** *m*, **picor** *m*,
 prurito *m*
jaundice **ictericia** *f*
juvenile **juvenil** *adj*

keep, to **quedarse**
ketosis **quetosis** *f*
key **llave** *f*
kidney **riñón** *m*
labored **dificultoso** *adj*
liver **hígado** *m*
lower back **espalda inferior** *f*
maturity **madurez** *f*
mental confusion **desorientación**
 mental *f*, **confusión mental** *f*
microbe **microbio** *m*
moist **húmedo** *adj*
move, to **mover(se) [ue]**
neglect, to **descuidar**
nervous system **sistema nervioso** *m*
new born **recién nacido** *m/f*
numbness **adormecimiento** *m*
obstruct, to **obstruir, tapar**
onset **ataque** *m*, **principio** *m*,
 comienzo *m*
oral compound **compuesto oral** *m*,
 compuesto digerible *m*
oral surgeon **cirujano/cirujana oral** *m/f*
overdosage **dosis excesiva** *f*; **sobredosis** *f*
overweight **sobrepeso** *m*, **exceso de**
 peso *m*
painful **doloroso** *adj*; **penoso** *adj*
pale **pálido** *adj*
pancreas **páncreas** *m*
pass over/through, to **pasar por**
passage **paso** *m*
pear-shaped **piriforme** *adj*
persist, to **persistir [en]**
phosphorus **fósforo** *m*
picture **imagen** *m*
potential **potencial** *adj*
precipitate, to **precipitar**
predisposition **predisposición** *f*
rapid heartbeat **ritmo rápido del**
 corazón *m*; **aumento en el ritmo del**
 corazón *m*
recur, to **repetirse [i], volver [ue] a**
 ocurrir
refined **refinado** *adj*
regenerate, to **regenerar**
regurgitation **vómito** *m*, **regurgitación** *f*
release, to **desprender**
relief **alivio** *m*
remove, to **quitar; extirpar; sacar**
renal colic **cólico renal** *m*
responsible for, to be **encargarse de**
rib **costilla** *f*
rinse, to **enjuagar**
rise, to **subir**
sac **saco** *m*
screening **selección** *f*
secrete, to **producir la secreción (de)**;
 secretar
seriousness **gravedad** *f*
shake, to **sacudir**
single out, to **separar**
small intestine **intestino delgado** *m*
source **fuente** *f*
spread, to **extender [ie]**
starch **almidón** *m*
starchy **amiláceo** *adj*, **almidonado** *adj*
store, to **almacenar**
subside, to **calmarse**
sudden **repentino** *adj*, **súbito** *adj*

sugar   azúcar *m*
sugary   que contiene azúcar; azucarado *adj*
suggest, to   sugerir [ie]
swallow, to   tragar
sweaty palm   palma sudorosa *f*, mano sudorosa *f*
symptom   síntoma *m*
syrupy   almibarado *adj*
tasty   de buen gusto
test   prueba *f*; examen *m*
test, to   examinar, poner a prueba
thicken, to   espesar; engrosar

tolerance   tolerancia *f*
too little   muy poco
touch, to   tocar
tract   aparato *m*
trade, to   cambiar
treat   deleite *m*
tube   tubo *m*
ultrasound   onda ultrasónica *f*
underside   superficie inferior *f*
underweight   de peso escaso *adj*, peso escaso *m*
untreated   no tratado *adj*
ureter   uréter *m*

urethra   uretra *f*, caño urinario *m*
uric acid   ácido úrico *m*
urinalysis   urinálisis *f*; análisis de la orina *m*
urinary bladder   vejiga urinaria *f*
urination   urinación *f*
urine   orina *f*, orín *m*
warning sign   signo de advertencia *m*
waste   desecho *m*
well-being   bienestar *m*
with the teeth   a dentelladas
X-ray   radiografía *f*

HOW TO TAKE YOUR CHILD'S TEMPERATURE

Normal temperature *fluctuates* between 97.7°(degrees)F and 98.6°F [36.5°C and 37°C]. It varies greatly in a small child, even as much as 2° per day.[1] Nevertheless, as the child grows, the temperature stabilizes.

5   Among the main causes for the *increase* in temperature are activity, infections, and general excitement. For example, almost all infections produce some increase in temperature—they can cause it to rise up between 102.2°F and 104°F [39°C and 40°C]. Elevation in itself does not indicate the *seriousness* of the illness. As long as it is below 102.2° [39°C], with an absence of other *symptoms,* there is no need to try to reduce it.

In order to read a thermometer, one only need practice. With children a thermometer is neces-
10 sary in order to take a temperature when the child is sick. Sometimes, when touching a child's forehead, it seems that she is burning with fever. When her temperature is taken one sees that it is only 101.3°F [38°C].

A thermometer is the instrument used to take the temperature, which is the measure of the amount of heat. The thermometer consists of a glass tube with a *bulb* at one end. Inside the bulb
15 there is a liquid metal, mercury. This latter expands in heat and contracts in cold. Mercury will rise inside the tube with heat (= fever), and will fall with cold.

The majority of thermometers are marked in the following way:

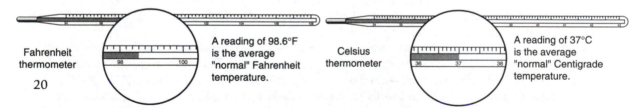

Fahrenheit thermometer

20

A reading of 98.6°F is the average "normal" Fahrenheit temperature.

Celsius thermometer

A reading of 37°C is the average "normal" Centigrade temperature.

The longest and most widely spaced lines indicate whole degrees and the smaller divisions, tenths of a degree. The numbers on the thermometer go from degree to degree, beginning with
25 94°F [35°C]. The little arrow shows the normal temperature limit which is 98.6°F [37°C].

A mercury column is easily seen because one side of the glass tube has a magnifying lens. This permits the best reading of the numbers and the easiest visibility of the mercury. When holding the thermometer between the index finger and the thumb with the numbers and lines in front of
30 the eyes, the mercury (line) is seen as a thick line, and not as a very fine one. In this way it is very easy to see just where the mercury is.

For *newborns* the temperature is taken rectally. A special thermometer is used. It is necessary to lubricate the tip of the rectal thermometer a bit. It is important to recognize that the normal
35 rectal temperature is generally one degree higher than the normal one—that is 99.6°F [37.5°C]. After lubricating the silver tip, spread (open) the (cheeks of the) buttocks in order to be able to see the anus easily. Insert the thermometer slowly and gently until you cannot see the silver tip. Then, hold it in place for two whole minutes. Remove it and read the degree of temperature.

Generally, after three years of age a child refuses to endure the presence of the rectal ther-
40 mometer. Until such a child can hold the oral thermometer under his tongue with his lips carefully closed without biting it, it is best to place the thermometer in the *groin* or under the armpit. (Temperature registers a little bit less in the armpit than in the mouth.) Commonly there is no danger after five years of age, but children vary greatly.

In order to obtain a true indication of the temperature, it is important to clean the thermom-
45 eter well with soap and water or alcohol; to first *shake* the thermometer below 98°F [36.5°C];
and to have the sick child rest and not eat or drink cold or hot liquids immediately before. The
thermometer is usually left in place for three whole minutes, although a very high fever begins to
register after thirty seconds. Afterwards, wash it well in soap and water.

It is not necessary to call the doctor each time that the child has a temperature. However, if,
50 besides the fever, the child *complains* of chest or abdominal pains, vomits or has diarrhea, etc.,
the best thing is to call the physician.

Temperature Variations Considered "Normal"

	ORAL	AXILLARY	RECTAL
Average Normal Temperature	98.6°F (37°C)	97.6°F (36.5°C)	99.6°F (37.5°C)
Range	97.6–99.6°F (36.5–37.5°C)	96.6–98.6°F (36–37°C)	98.6–100.6°F (37–38.1°C)

Questions

1. What is considered to be a normal temperature?
2. Is there any variation?
3. Does an elevated temperature alone, without any other symptoms, indicate a medical problem?
4. What is the purpose of the little arrow on the thermometer?
5. Is there a difference between the normal oral temperature and the rectal one? What is it?
6. Why is it necessary to gently and slowly insert the rectal thermometer into the rectum?
7. How many minutes should the thermometer be kept in the mouth?

COMO TOMAR LA TEMPERATURA DE UNA NIÑA

La temperatura normal *oscila* entre 97.7°(grados)F y 98.6°F [36.5°C y 37°C]. **Varía mucho en una bebé pequeña, incluso hasta 3.6°F [2°C] por día.[2] Sin embargo, al crecer la niña, la temperatura es más estable.**

Entre las causas principales para este *aumento* de temperatura se encuentran la actividad,
5   las infecciones, y la excitación general. Por ejemplo, casi todas las infecciones producen algún aumento de temperatura—pueden hacerla subir hasta los 102.2°F a 104°F [39°C a
40°C]. La elevación en sí no indica *la gravedad* de la enfermedad. Siempre que esté por debajo de los 102.2°F [39°C] y sin otros *síntomas*, no hay necesidad de tratar de rebajarla.

10   Para leer un termómetro, es sólo cuestión de práctica. Con niños es preciso tener un termómetro a fin de tomar la temperatura cuando la niña esté enferma. A veces al tocar la
frente de una niña, parece que arde de fiebre. Cuando le toma la temperatura, se ve que sólo
está en los 101.3°F [38°C].

Un termómetro es el instrumento usado para registrar la temperatura, que es la medida de
15   la cantidad de calor. El termómetro consiste en un tubo de vidrio con una *ampolleta* en un
extremo. Dentro de la ampolleta hay un metal líquido, mercurio. Este se expande en el calor
y se contrae en el frío. El mercurio subirá dentro del tubo con el calor (= fiebre), y bajará
con el frío.

La mayoría de los termómetros están marcados de la manera siguiente:

20

Fahrenheit/ termómetro   Término medio de una temperatura normal rango 98.6°   Celsius/ termómetro   Término medio de una temperatura normal rango 37°

25 Las marcas o rayas más largas y espaciadas señalan grados enteros y las divisiones más pequeñas, las décimas de grado. Los números del termómetro van de grado en grado empezando por los 94°F [35°C]. La flechita muestra el límite de la temperatura normal, que es los 98.6°F [37°C].

En la columna de mercurio se puede ver fácilmente porque un lado del tubo de vidrio tiene cristal de aumento. Esto permite una mejor lectura de los números y la visibilidad más fácil del
30 mercurio. Manteniendo el termómetro entre el índice y el pulgar con los números y las marcas delante de los ojos, la línea de mercurio se ve como una raya gruesa y no una línea delgada. Así, es muy fácil ver donde se encuentra el mercurio.

En *los recién nacidos* la temperatura se toma rectalmente. Se necesita un termómetro espe-
35 cial para esto. Hay que engrasar un poco la ampolleta del termómetro rectal. Es importante darse cuenta de que la temperatura rectal normal generalmente es un grado más alto que la oral normal, es decir, los 99.6°F [37.5°C]. Después de lubricar la punta plateada, separe las nalgas de la bebé para poder ver el recto con facilidad. Inserte el termómetro lenta y suave-
40 mente hasta no poder ver la punta plateada. Entonces, manténgalo en posición unos dos minutos completos. Sáquelo y lea el grado de temperatura.

Generalmente a partir de los tres años una niña se niega a soportar la presencia del termómetro rectal. Hasta que tal niña pueda soportar la presencia del termómetro oral bajo la lengua, con los labios cuidadosamente cerrados, sin morderlo, es mejor colocar el ter-
45 mómetro en *la ingle* o bajo la axila. (La temperatura de la axila marca un poco menos que la de la boca.) Por lo común, no hay peligro después de los cinco años, pero depende de los niños.

A fin de obtener una verdadera indicación de la temperatura, es importante que limpie bien el termómetro con agua y jabón o alcohol; que *sacuda* primero el termómetro bajo los
50 98°F [36.5°C]; que la niña enferma descanse y no coma inmediatamente antes ni beba líquidos fríos ni calientes. El termómetro usualmente se deja en posición durante tres minutos completos aunque una temperatura altísima empieza a registrarse después de treinta segundos. Después, lávelo muy bien con agua y jabón.

55 No es necesario llamar al médico cada vez que la niña tenga fiebre. Pero, si además de fiebre, la niña *se queja de* dolores en el pecho o en el abdomen, o de oído, si vomita o tiene diarrea, etc., lo mejor es llamar al médico.

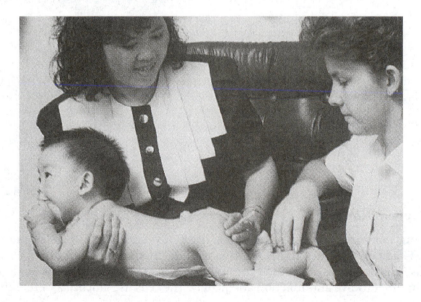

Preguntas

1. ¿Qué se considera como temperatura normal?
2. ¿Hay variación de temperatura?
3. Una elevación de temperatura en sí, sin otros síntomas, ¿es señal de un problema médico?
4. ¿Para qué sirve la flechita del termómetro?

5. ¿Hay diferencia entre la temperatura oral normal y la rectal? ¿Cuál es?
6. ¿Por qué es preciso insertar el termómetro rectal suave y lentamente en el recto?
7. ¿Por cuántos minutos se debe mantener (guardar) el termómetro en la boca?

DIABETES

Diabetes, a common disease, is fairly easy *to detect*. If found early, it can be controlled; if not treated or poorly controlled, it can cause disability or even kill.

There are two major types of diabetes:

1) *insulin dependent diabetes*. Diabetes rarely develops in a child under a year. Insulin depen-
5 dent diabetes is sometimes classified as *type I diabetes* or *juvenile-onset diabetes* because it affects older children and young people under twenty. In this type of diabetes *the pancreas* does not make *insulin*. Those with this type of diabetes *must* take insulin injections daily. Insulin cannot be taken by mouth. About 10 percent of people with diabetes have this type.

10 2) *non-insulin dependent diabetes/diabetes not dependent on insulin*. Non-insulin dependent dia-
betes is also called *type II diabetes* or *adult/maturity-onset diabetes*. In this type of diabetes, the pan-
creas does not make *enough* insulin to control the level of glucose in the blood. Diet, exercise, and medication help some people control their blood *glucose*. Nevertheless, many adults with this type of diabetes are best treated by taking daily insulin shots. About ninety (90) percent
15 of diabetics have this type of diabetes.

Diabetes can be an inherited illness. It can be the result of alcoholism, of obesity, or of any in-
flammatory process of the pancreas.

What Is Diabetes?

20
The full name of this disease is *diabetes mellitus;* a person with it is called a *diabetic*. The origin of the name is from the Greek and Latin—meaning "to pass through" and "honey"—and recognizes a major symptom first described over 1,000 years ago—*sugar* in the *urine*. To understand
25 diabetes, you should know what happens in a person who does *not* have this condition.

30

35

What Happens Normally?

After eating and during the digestive process, the body *digests* food in the stomach and *small*
40 *intestine*. Gradually the body transforms many of the foods consumed into the sugar chemically known as "glucose." This sugar then goes into *the bloodstream*. All the cells of an organism need glucose in order to live and function adequately. The cells use glucose as a fuel in order to produce *energy*.

The body gets its chief source of energy from *carbohydrates* (*sugary* and *starchy* foods) which are
45 changed to glucose. Glucose exists in different foods, especially in the form of carbohydrates [flour, bread, potatoes, etc.]. It is also found in proteins and in *fats* in food. The human body's cells, and especially those of the *nervous system* and those of the brain, need glucose. Without it, they cease functioning. The body transforms carbohydrates into glucose upon digesting them. This

50   change occurs in the *liver*, which *converts* and stores some carbohydrates into *glycogen*, and in the pancreas, which is responsible for the transformation of stored glycogen back into glucose as a readily usable source of energy. The pancreas is an organ found in the abdomen behind the stomach. It is the gland which produces substances and *hormones* which *bring about* many diverse functions in the body. The pancreas does this with two hormones it produces: insulin and *glucagon*. The pancreas *secretes* a quantity of insulin sufficient for the physiological needs of each
55   person. Twenty units is an average normally secreted by the pancreas during the course of a day. The normal level of glucose in the blood is between 70 (seventy) and 120 (one hundred twenty) mg/dL (milligrams of sugar per each deciliter of blood). (Glucagon stimulates the breakdown of glycogen and the release of glucose by the liver.)

 Glucose is normally carried by the *bloodstream* in determined levels. For the cells to utilize glu-
60   cose, they need to absorb it from the blood. The body can neither use nor *store* glucose without the help of the hormone insulin. This hormone assures that glucose enters the cells.

What Happens with Diabetes?

65   When a person has diabetes, the process of *converting* flood into energy does not work as it is supposed to. When a person with diabetes eats, the food is still digested and broken down into glucose. The glucose enters the bloodstream as usual, but because of the diabetes, the pancreas is unable to respond and secrete the insulin needed to process sugar and starches in the proper
70   amounts at the proper times. Thus, the diabetic has a reduced ability to obtain and store energy from the food ingested. As a consequence, glucose is accumulated in the bloodstream until the concentration of sugar in the blood exceeds what is normal. When it exceeds a certain level, the glucose or sugar overflows into the urine. The kidneys must work harder to remove the excess sugar in the urine. When this happens, the person urinates more often and gets very thirsty. Thus,
75   the two typical signs of diabetes are explained: 1) an *excessive* amount of sugar in the blood (*hyperglycemia*); 2) the presence of sugar in the urine (glycosuria).

What Kind of People Get Diabetes?

80   Several distinct factors generally cause type I or insulin-dependent diabetes. The three principal factors are:

1. **HEREDITY:** Some people are born with a greater probability of getting diabetes. They inherit a gene from their parents which permits the development of diabetes more easily than normal. Nevertheless,
85   not everyone who has the gene gets diabetes.
2. **VIRUSES:** Viruses cause certain illnesses, such as colds, *flu*, and mumps. Certain viruses can *cause damage* of the pancreas of those individuals who have inherited the tendency towards diabetes. This damage can *build up* over days, weeks, or even years before bringing about diabetes.
90 3. **IMMUNOLOGICAL REACTION:** The organism or body offers resistance to or protection from viruses and *microbes* or *germs* by means of the *immune system*. The person who acquires insulin-dependent diabetes often has an *auto–immune* reaction. This means that the body's immune system attacks and harms other parts of the body (such as, for instance, the cells of the pancreas which are the producers of in-
95   sulin). Certain genes or viruses can start to bring about a decrease of insulin production, or its abnormal secretion, which is an auto-attack by part of the immune system. Sometimes both special genes and special microbes can lead to this process.

 Anyone may become diabetic, but diabetes, especially in later life—type II diabetes—, is often
100 associated with four groups of people.[3]

1. **FAMILY HISTORY** of diabetes
2. **OVERWEIGHT**
3. **OVER FORTY** (It is primarily a disease of middle and old age. Diabetes rarely occurs in children under a year old. Among older children, up to twenty, diabetes occurs suddenly, and is known as Type I diabetes—juvenile onset diabetes.)
4. **FEMALES** (Two out of three diabetics are women. Between ages fifty-five and sixty-four diabetes is twice
105   as high for women as for men.)
   a. Mothers who have *given birth* to babies who weighed nine pounds or more at birth; and
   b. Women who have shown carbohydrate *intolerance* during pregnancy.

HOW TO RECOGNIZE DIABETES

110
Symptoms of diabetes have to do with the increase in the amount of sugar in the blood and the loss of sugar through the urine. Some manifestations have to do with the excessive production of urine along with great thirst, nycturia, general malaise, lack of appetite, tiredness, lack of energy and recurrent infections of all types.

115   Although not every diabetic has all the potential principal symptoms, the most common are:
- Excessive thirst and/hunger
- Excessive urination
- Loss of weight
120 - Easy tiring, drowsiness
- Slow *healing* of cuts and bruises
- Changes in vision
- Intense itching
- Pain, tingling, or numbness in the feet or hands
125
People who get diabetes at an early age (juvenile diabetics) experience most of these "characteristic" symptoms, but it should be remembered that many diabetic adults are asymptomatic. For them, the *onset* is *insidious.* In mild cases, only one or two of these symptoms may be present; many diabetics are discovered during a periodic physical exam or in a *blood-screening* program.

130
If the amount of sugar in the blood increases to an excessive extreme due to the absence of almost all insulin, the diabetic can suffer serious complications which lead him to *acidosis* (an increase in acidity) and to *diabetic coma* (loss of consciousness). If *not treated,* the coma can be fatal.

135 *Mental confusion* is one alarming manifestation of untreated diabetes. After many years, the diabetic can suffer another group of complications, including diabetic retinopathy which frequently causes blindness if not attended to; renal insufficiency; and circulatory problems which can lead to the loss of the extremities.

Detection and Diagnosis

140
The tests are fairly simple. The most common is a *urinalysis.* A positive urine test is strong but not conclusive evidence that a person has diabetes. The doctor will also test the amount of sugar in the blood. In *borderline cases* (to establish a diagnosis of latent diabetes) the doctor may order a *glucose tolerance* or *fasting blood sugar test* to detect the presence and measure the degree of sever-
145 ity of the disease. The blood glucose tolerance tells how well the body handles a specified amount of sugar (seventy-five–one hundred grams). The patient drinks a *syrupy* liquid, and blood and urine samples are taken following several hours *of fasting,* and at one, two, and three hour intervals after drinking the liquid.

150 ### Treatment

The treatment of diabetes varies with each patient. Nevertheless, it always includes a nourishing regimen which supplies an adequate diet to satisfy the individual's needs. Diet is the primary basis of treatment, especially for those over forty. This includes the elimination of foods rich in
155 carbohydrates and alcoholic beverages.

Other factors of vital importance include physical exercise and weight reduction. Physical activity ought to be part of everyone's daily life. In reality, physical exercise plays an important part in the control of diabetes. When exercising, glucose enters the body's cells more easily, and physical exercise also helps to maintain normal weight.

160
Stress is another factor that can compromise physical well-being because it can affect the control of diabetes. The different ways that stress affects different people is not completely understood. Many times stress will cause high glucose levels; other times glucose levels continue changing. Stress is a part of life and can be hard to control. It is important to recognize that there are times of stress; that people must know how to respond to it by developing defense mecha-
165 nisms against stress which permit them to live and function in a relaxing way; and how this stress affects each individual's control of diabetes.

Severe cases may require daily injections of insulin or an oral compound. The amount of exercise that the diabetic gets plays a part in determining both diet and insulin dosage. Exercise may be

170 enough to diminish the severity of the disease. Successful treatment also depends on mental outlook.

It is up to the physician to decide and determine the necessity to use insulin or oral hypoglycemic agents. Diet should always be the key factor in an adequate control of diabetes, nevertheless. In certain cases, only the loss of weight can resolve the problem of diabetes.

175 **Diet**

A diabetic has the same nutritional needs as anyone else except for difficulty in using starches and sugars. The goal of a diabetic's diet is to completely eliminate refined sugar (that is, sugar that is added to foods) and to limit starches. Diabetics and their families, by utilizing *"Exchange Lists,"* learn how to trade one food for another so that a flexible diet with nutritious, *tasty* meals
180 may be maintained.

The diabetic diet emphasizes good nutrition and healthy eating habits; all family members will benefit by following this diet. The diabetic does not feel singled out as different or deprived, especially if the diabetic is a child; furthermore, the family cook can more easily plan and prepare the family meals.

185

Imminent Complications

HYPOGLYCEMIA: The risk of hypoglycemia [an extreme lowering of the blood sugar] exists
190 whenever medications used to treat diabetes are used. Hypoglycemia can appear as a feeling of hunger, extreme and unexplainable perspiration, trembling of the extremities, mental confusion, or a loss of consciousness. This usually occurs as an *insulin reaction* but may also occur in a person taking an *oral* (sulfonylurea) *compound*. Ordinarily this occurs when the amount of sugar in the blood is too low. It is usually caused by an overdosage of medication; however, too little food
195 or too much exercise may also cause hypoglycemia.

The body sends out *warning signs* before insulin reactions. Symptoms usually involve the nervous system and can include: decrease in or loss of *alertness,* mental confusion, coma, convulsions, rapid pulse, tachycardia (*rapid heartbeat*) and *sweaty palms,* headaches, irritability, blurred vision, nausea, and *drowsiness*/fatigue.
200 Early hypoglycemia responds to concentrated carbohydrate [fruit juice—half (1/2) cup; sugar—five (5) small cubes, two (2) packets, or two (2) teaspoons; a small, little box of raisins; a roll of dried fruit; two (2) teaspoonsful of honey; carbonated beverages—six ounces of pop with sugar; chocolate bar—a quarter (1/4) to a third (1/3) bar]. If the patient does not respond in ten–twenty minutes, repeat the feeding. The symptoms disappear gradually as the pancreas
205 releases glucagon, which causes the liver to release more sugar into the blood. If after the second feeding containing the sugar, there is no improvement, medical assistance is needed. The patient should eat soon after recovering.

DIABETIC COMA: Also known as *acidosis* or *ketosis,* this is caused by insufficient insulin, or when
210 a severely diabetic person neglects his diet. It occurs most commonly in people who have type I diabetics. Occasionally coma is confused with a severe insulin reaction. Coma is the result of too little insulin; a reaction is the result of too much. Both conditions need different treatment. Below is a chart showing the differences of these conditions:

Item	HYPOGLYCEMIA	DIABETIC COMA
1. Onset	Sudden (minutes)	Slow (days)
2. Food	Too little	Too much
3. Skin	Moist, pale	Dry, flushed
4. Hunger	Frequent	Absent
5. Thirst	Absent	Present
6. Insulin	Too much	Too little
7. Vomiting	Absent	Present
8. Urine	Sugar absent or slight	Sugar present in large amounts
9. Breathing	Normal	Deep, labored
10. Blood pressure	Rises	Falls

Situations

You are a health care worker. Explain about the need to lose weight and how to take insulin to a newly diagnosed diabetic middle-aged woman.

You are a dietician. Explain the diabetic dietary requirements to the family of a fifteen-year-old newly diagnosed diabetic.

DIABETES

La diabetes es una enfermedad común que es relativamente fácil de *detectar*. Si se rectifica en su etapa temprana, puede ser controlada; si no se trata o se controla debidamente, puede causar invalideces, y hasta la muerte.

Hay dos tipos principales de diabetes:

5   1) *La diabetes sacarina dependiente de la insulina o diabetes insulino-dependiente.* La diabetes casi nunca ocurre en un niño menor de un año. La diabetes insulino-dependiente a veces es llamada *diabetes de tipo I* o *diabetes (del principio) juvenil o precoz* porque ocurre en muchachos, adolescentes, y jóvenes que tienen menos de veinte años. En este tipo de diabetes, *el páncreas* no produce *insulina*. A la gente que sufre de este tipo de diabetes *hay que* ponerle una

10   inyección de insulina todos los días. No se puede *tomar* la insulina por boca. Aproximadamente diez (10) por ciento de diabéticos que sufre de este tipo de diabetes. 2) *La diabetes sacarina no dependiente de la insulina.* También es llamada *diabetes de tipo II* o *diabetes adquirida durante la madurez,* o *del adulto* o *de comienzo tardío.* Con este tipo de diabetes, el páncrease no produce *suficiente* cantidad de insulina para controlar el nivel de la glucosa en la sangre. Al-

15   gunas personas con este tipo de diabetes pueden controlar el nivel de *la glucosa* en la sangre con dieta, ejercicio, y píldoras. No obstante, muchos adultos con este tipo de diabetes reciben el mejor tratamiento al inyectarse diariamente con insulina. Noventa (90) por ciento de las personas que sufren de diabetes tienen este tipo de diabetes.

20   La diabetes puede ser una enfermedad hereditaria. O puede ser el resultado del alcoholismo, de la obesidad, or de cualquier proceso inflamatorio del páncreas.

¿Qué es la diabetes?

25   El nombre completo de esta enfermedad es *diabetes mellitus;* la persona que sufre de esta enfermedad se conoce como *diabética.* El nombre de la enfermedad tiene sus orígenes en el griego y el latín—significando originalmente "pasar a través de" y "miel"—dando a conocer uno de sus principales síntomas, que fue descrito hace más de 1,000 [mil] años—la presencia de *azúcar* en la *orina.*

30   Para comprender la diabetes, primero usted tiene que saber lo que ocurre en una persona que *NO* tiene esta condición.

35

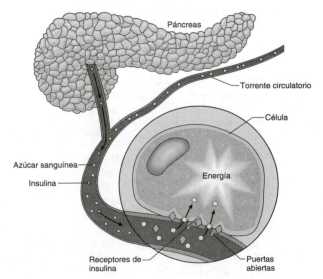

Páncreas

Torrente circulatorio

Célula

Azúcar sanguínea

Insulina

Energía

40

Receptores de insulina

Puertas abiertas

¿Qué ocurre normalmente?

45 Después de comer y durante el proceso digestivo, el cuerpo *digiere* la comida en el estómago y en *el intestino delgado.* Poco a poco el cuerpo transforma muchos de los alimentos consumidos en el azúcar químicamente llamado «glucosa.» Este azúcar entonces entra en *la corriente sanguínea.* A todas las células de un organismo les falta la glucosa para vivir y funcionar adecuadamente. Las células utilizan la glucosa a manera de combustible para
50 producir *energía.*

    La fuente principal de la energía del cuerpo viene de *los carbohidratos* (alimentos *azucarados* y *almidonados*) que se convierten en la glucosa. La glucosa existe en diversos alimentos, sobre todo, en forma de los carbohidratos [harinas, pan, papas, etc.]. También se encuentra en proteínas y en las *grasas* en alimentos. Las células del cuerpo humano, y especialmente
55 las del *sistema nervioso* y las del cerebro, necesitan la glucosa. Sin ella, dejan de funcionar. El cuerpo transforma los carbohidratos en glucosa al digerirlos. Esta conversión tiene lugar en *el hígado,* que *convierte* y almacena algunos carbohidratos en *glicógeno,* y en el páncreas, que *se encarga de* almacenar parte y a la vez controla la conversión del glicógeno en glucosa como
60 una fuente de energía inmediatamente accesible. El páncreas es un órgano encontrado en el abdomen por detrás del estómago. Es la glándula que produce substancias y hormonas que *acarrean* muchas funciones diversas en el cuerpo. Esto lo logra el páncreas por medio de la secreción de dos hormonas que produce: la insulina y *el glucagón.* El páncreas *secreta* una cantidad suficiente de insulina de acuerdo con las necesidades fisiológicas de cada persona.
65 Veinte unidades es un promedio normalmente secretado por el páncreas durante el transcurso de un día. El nivel normal de la glucosa en la sangre varía entre 70 (setenta) y 120 (ciento veinte) miligramos/decilitros (miligramos de azúcar por cada decilitro de sangre). (El glucagón aumenta la concentración de glucosa en la sangre en respuesta a niveles de glucosa sanguínea demasiado bajos o estimula la degradación del glicógeno en el hígado.)
70   Esta glucosa es llevada normalmente por *la corriente sanguínea,* a niveles determinados. Para que las células utilicen la glucosa, necesitan absorberla de la sangre. El cuerpo no puede utilizar *ni almacenar* glucosa sin ayuda de la hormona insulina. Esta hormona asegura que la glucosa entre a las células.

75 ¿Qué ocurre cuando hay diabetes?

Cuando una persona tiene diabetes, el proceso de *convertir* la comida en energía no funciona como es debido. Cuando una persona con diabetes come, los alimentos todavía se digieren y se convierten en glucosa. La glucosa entra en la corriente sanguínea, como siem-
80 pre, pero a causa de la diabetes, el páncreas no responde produciendo la insulina, que se necesita para la conversión de los azúcares y los almidones, en las cantidades suficientes que se requieren al momento. Así, el diabético tiene una abilidad reducida de obtener y almacenar la energía que resulta de ingerir alimentos. Como consecuencia, sin la insulina que sirve
85 a llevar la glucosa a las células del cuerpo, la glucosa se queda en la corriente sanguínea aumentando hasta que la concentración de azúcar en la corriente sanguínea exceda lo normal y pasa a la orina donde los riñones tratan de limpiar la extra glucosa de la sangre. Cuando esto ocurre, la persona orina mucho más de lo común y tiene muchísima sed. Así, se explican dos signos típicos de la diabetes: 1) una cantidad *excesiva* de azúcar en la sangre (*hiperglucemia*);
90 2) la presencia de azúcar en la orina (*glucosuria*).

¿Qué tipos de personas se vuelven diabéticos?

Varios factores distintos causan la diabetes de tipo I, la dependiente de la insulina general-
95 mente. Los tres factores principales son:

1. LA HERENCIA: Algunas personas nacen con mayor posibilidad de contraer la diabetes. Heredan un *gen* (*gene*) de sus padres que permite el desarrollo de la diabetes más fácilmente de lo normal. No obstante, no todo el mundo que tiene el gen desde su nacimiento, contrae la diabetes.
100 2. LOS VIRUS: Los virus causan ciertas enfermedades como un catarro, *la gripe,* y las paperas. Ciertos virus pueden *provocar daño* al páncreas de personas que tienen una tendencia a adquirir la diabetes. Este daño se puede *acumular* por días, semanas, o aun años hantes de que provoque la diabetes.

3. RESPUESTA (REACCIÓN) INMUNOLÓGICA: El organismo o el cuerpo ofrece resistencia a o se
105   protege de los virus y *los microbios* o *gérmenes* por medio del *sistema inmune* (inmunológico). La persona que adquiere la diabetes dependiente de la insulina muchas veces tiene una reacción autoin-
munológica. Esto quiere decir que el sistema inmune del cuerpo ataca y causa daño a otras partes
del cuerpo (como, por ejemplo las células del páncreas que son productoras de la insulina). Ciertos
110   genes o virus pueden empezar a provocar una disminución de la producción de insulina, o su anormal secreción, lo que es un autoataque por parte del sistema inmune. A veces, tanto los genes especiales como los microbios especiales pueden provocar el proceso.

115   Cualquier persona puede resultar con diabetes; pero, la diabetes, especialmente la que
aparece durante la madurez—diabetes de tipo II—, se asocia en muchos casos con cuatro
grupos de personas:

1. Personas en cuya familia hay antecedentes de la diabetes
120   2. Personas que se exceden de peso
3. Personas mayores de cuarenta años de edad (Principalmente se relaciona esta enfermedad con personas en la edad madura y la vejez—aparición en la madurez. La diabetes rara vez se presenta en
niños menores de un año. Entre los niños de más edad, hasta los veinte años, la diabetes
125   aparece súbitamente, y se conoce como la diabetes de tipo I—diabetes de temprana edad).
4. Mujeres (De cada tres diabéticos, hay dos que son mujeres. Entre los cincuenta y cinco y los sesenta
y cuatro años de edad, el número de mujeres diabéticas es dos veces mayor que el número de hombres diabéticos.)
130   A. Madres que hayan *dado luz a* niños que pesaron nueve libras o más al nacer; y
B. Mujeres que han demostrado una *intolerancia* a los carbohidratos durante el embarazo.

¿Cómo se reconoce la diabetes?

135   Los síntomas de la diabetes tienen que ver con el aumento de la cantidad de azúcar en la
sangre y la pérdida de azúcar por la orina. Unas manifestaciones consisten en la producción
excesiva de orina con mucha sed, nicturia, malestar general, falta de apetito, cansancio, falta
de energía e infecciones recurrentes de todos tipos.
140   Aunque no todos los diabéticos presenten todos los síntomas principales posibles, entre
los más comunes se encuentran:

- Sed y/o hambre excesivas
- Micción excesiva (excesiva orina)
- Pérdida de peso
145   - El cansarse fácilmente y la somnolencia
- Lenta *curación* de cortaduras y contusiones
- Cambios en la visión
- Picazones intensivas
- Dolores, hormigueos o entumecimiento, en los pies o las manos

150   Los que sufren de diabetes desde temprana edad presentan la mayoría de estos síntomas
«característicos», pero es necesario recordar que muchas personas maduras que sufren de
diabetes no sufren de ningún síntoma; son asintomáticas. Para ellos, el *comienzo es engañoso*.
En casos leves, es posible que solamente uno o dos de estos síntomas estén presentes;
155   muchos descubren que tienen diabetes durante un periódico reconocimiento físico o durante los programas de *pruebas selectivas de sangre* (un examen de la población en masa para
el diagnóstico de diversas enfermedades, incluyendo la diabetes).

Si la cantidad de azúcar en la sangre aumenta a un extremo excesivo debido a la ausencia
de casi toda la insulina, el diabético puede sufrir complicaciones graves que le llevan a *la*
160   *acidosis* (aumento de la acidez) y al *coma diabético* (pérdida del conocimiento). Si no se trata, el
coma puede ser fatal. *La confusión mental* es una manifestación alarmante de la diabetes *no
tratada*. Después de muchos años, el diabético puede sufrir de otro grupo de complicaciones, incluyendo la retinopatía diabética que con frecuencia causa la ceguera si no es atendida; la insufi-
165   ciencia renal; y los problemas circulatorios que pueden llevar a la pérdida de las extremidades.

Detección y diagnóstico

Las pruebas son bastante sencillas. La más común es *el análisis de la orina*. Indicios muy
170   buenos, pero no evidencia decisiva, que una persona sufre de la diabetes son un resultado

positivo en la urinálisis. También el médico tendrá que mandar a hacer otras pruebas para determinar la cantidad de azúcar en la sangre. En *casos inciertos* (para establecer un diagnóstico de diabetes latente) el médico puede pedir una *prueba de tolerancia a la glucosa* o una
175 prueba de glucemia/glicemia/en ayunas (una prueba al ayunar del azúcar sanguínea) a fin de descubrir la presencia y medir la gravedad de la enfermedad. La tolerancia de azúcar sanguínea indica el grado en que el cuerpo puede utilizar una cantidad designada de azúcar (de setenta y cinco a cien gramos). La (el) paciente toma un líquido *almibarado* y luego se le sacan muestras de sangre y orina después de permanecer varias horas *en ayunas* antes de comenzar
180 la prueba, y a intervalos de una, dos, y tres horas después de beber el líquido.

Tratamiento

El tratamiento de la diabetes varía con cada paciente. Sin embargo, siempre incluye un régi-
185 men alimenticio que proporciona una dieta adecuada para satisfacer las necesidades del individuo. El régimen es la base principal del tratamiento, especialmente para los que tienen más de cuarenta años de edad. Esto incluye el evitar los alimentos ricos en carbohidratos y las bebidas alcohólicas.
Otros factores de vital importancia incluyen el ejercicio físico y la reducción de peso. La
190 actividad física debe ser parte de la vida diaria de todo el mundo. Los muchachos con la diabetes deben ser tan activos como sus amigos. En realidad, el ejercicio físico es una parte importante en el control de la diabetes. Al hacer ejercicios físicos, la glucosa entra en las células del cuerpo más fácilmente, y el ejercicio físico también ayuda a bajar el nivel de grasa (el colesterol y los triglicéridos) en la sangre. El ejercicio físico también ayuda a
195 mantener normal el peso.
El estrés es otro factor que puede comprometer el bienestar físico porque tiene relación con el control de la diabetes. No se sabe exactamente cómo cada tensión en la vida diaria le afecte a cada individuo. Muchas veces el estrés causará altos niveles de glucosa; otras veces los niveles de glucosa cambian constantemente así que están tanto elevados como disminui-
200 dos [altos y bajos]. El estrés es una parte de la vida; no puede ser siempre evitado y puede ser difícil controlarlo. Es importante reconocer que hay períodos de tensiones en la vida diaria conocidos por el nombre de estrés; al que se debe responder desarrollando mecanismos de defensa contra el estrés que permiten vivir y actuar en una manera relajada; y como el
205 estrés afecta el control de la diabetes de cada individuo.
En casos severos, quizás se requieran inyecciones diarias de insulina o la ingestión de un compuesto en forma digerible. El ejercicio total que hace el diabético es un factor en la determinación tanto del régimen alimenticio como de las dosis de insulina. Con esto quizás se logre reducir el grado de severidad de la enfermedad.
210 El médico debe decidir y determinar la necesidad del uso de insulina o los hipoglicemiantes orales. La dieta siempre debe ser el factor primordial en un control adecuado de la diabetes, no obstante. En ciertos casos, la sola reducción de peso puede resolver el problema de la diabetes.
215
Régimen alimenticio

Las necesidades nutritivas de los diabéticos son iguales a las de las demás personas, a
220 diferencia de que tienen dificultades en la utilización de los almidones y azúcares. La meta que propone el régimen alimenticio para diabéticos es la de eliminar por completo el azúcar refinado (es decir, el azúcar que se utiliza en las comidas), y limitar el uso de almidones. Los diabéticos y sus familias aprenden a sustituir un tipo de comida por otro al usar «*Listas de intercambios*» a fin de mantener una dieta flexible que sea a la vez nutritiva y *de buen gusto*.
225 En el régimen alimenticio del diabético se acentúan la buena nutrición y las costumbres saludables en el comer; todos los miembros del hogar se beneficiarían siguiendo este régimen alimenticio. El diabético no se sentirá distinto de los demás, especialmente si es niño; además, se le facilitará el trabajo a la persona encargada de planear y preparar las comidas en el hogar.
230

Complicaciones inminentes

235 HIPOGLICEMIA: El riesgo de la hipoglicemia [baja extrema de glucosa en la sangre] existe siempre que se utilicen medicamentos para el tratamiento de la diabetes. Hipoglicemia puede manifestarse a manera de sensación de hambre, sudoración extrema e inexplicable, temblor de las extremidades, confusión mental, o pérdida del conocimiento. Normalmente
240 ocurre como una *reacción a la insulina*, pero también se da en casos donde se ingiere *un compuesto digerible* (es decir, sulfonilurea). Generalmente ocurre cuando la cantidad de azúcar en la sangre es insuficiente—demasiado baja. Se debe por regla general a sobredosis de medicamentos; sin embargo, la hipoglicemia también puede ser causada por insuficiencia nutritiva o hacer demasiado ejercicio.

El cuerpo da *signos de advertencia* antes de la reacción a la insulina. Los síntomas general-
245 mente se relacionan con el sistema nervioso, y pueden incluir: disminución o pérdida de *agudeza mental*, desorientación mental, coma, convulsiones, pulso acelerado, taquicardia (*aumento en el ritmo del corazón*) y *palmas sudorosas*, dolores de cabeza, irritabilidad, visión borrosa, náusea, y *somnolencia*/fatiga.

En sus comienzos la hipoglicemia responde a tratamiento con carbohidratos concentrados
250 [jugos de frutas como jugo de naranja—media (1/2) taza; azúcar—cinco (5) terrones, dos (2) bolsitas, o dos (2) cucharaditas; una cajita pequeña de pasas; un rollo de fruta seca; dos (2) cucharaditas de miel; bebidas *gaseosas*—seis (6) onzas de gaseosa «regular» con azúcar; *chocolatina*—la cuarta parte (1/4) a la tercera parte (1/3) de una barra]. Si el paciente no
255 responde en diez o veinte minutos, se debe repetir la comida anterior. Los síntomas desaparecen paulatinamente a medida que el páncreas produzca la secreción de glucagón, lo cual hace a su vez que el hígado produzca la secreción de más azúcar en la sangre. Si, después de la segunda ingestión de azúcar, no hay mejoría, se necesita asistencia médica. El paciente debe comer inmediatamente después de recuperarse.

260 COMA DIABETICO: Conocido también como *acidosis* o *quetosis*, es causado por una insuficiencia de insulina o por descuido en el cumplimiento del régimen alimenticio por parte de una persona gravemente diabética. Ocurre con más frecuencia en los diabéticos de tipo I. De vez en cuando el coma se confunde con una reacción grave a la insulina. El coma es el resultado de no tener <u>bastante</u> insulina; la reacción es el resultado de tener <u>demasiado</u>. Las dos condiciones requieren tratamiento diferente. Abajo está una gráfica que deja ver las diferencias de estas dos condiciones.

Rasgo	HYPOGLICEMIA	COMA DIABETICO
1. Comienzo	Repentino (minutos)	Lento (días)
2. Alimentos	Muy poco	Demasiado
3. Piel	Húmeda, pálida	Seca, rubefacción facial
4. Hambre	Frecuente	Ausente
5. Sed	Ausente	Presente
6. Insulina	Demasiado	Muy poca
7. Vómitos	Ausente	Presente
8. Orina	Azúcar ausente o insignificante	Azúcar presente en grandes cantidades
9. Respiración	Normal	Profunda, penosa
10. Presión arterial	Sube	Cae

Preguntas

1. ¿Qué puede ocurrir si no se trata la diabetes?
2. ¿Cuáles son las maneras de tratar la diabetes?
3. ¿Cuáles son las diferencias entre la diabetes de tipo I (de temprana edad) y la de tipo II (de aparición en la madurez)?
4. ¿Qué complicaciones inminentes puede resultar de una cantidad inestable de insulina?

GALLSTONES

Gallstones are a problem for many people who have a *predisposition* to digestive disorders. More women than men have them, as do more overweight people than those of average or underweight.

5 How do they occur? The liver *secretes* a fluid called bile. Small crystals precipitate out of bile and are stored and concentrated in the *gallbladder.* These are gallstones. They may range in size from an inch or more in diameter down to a collection of what looks like *gravel.*

The gallbladder is a *pear-shaped* sac that is attached to the underside of the liver, beneath the ribs. The gallbladder releases bile to help digest fats and fat-like substances. *Cholesterol, bile salts* 10 and *bilirubin* make up bile.

Early *symptoms* of gallbladder trouble can include indigestion or *heartburn* after eating *fried foods, coarse* vegetables, or raw fruits. *Flatulence,* nausea and *belching,* or *regurgitation* can occur. *Gradual* pain which then intensifies and later slowly *subsides* is common. *Sudden* and severe 15 pain will occur if a gallstone blocks one of the ducts that leads to the small intestine. Such pain usually begins in the middle or right upper part of the upper abdomen, and may spread to the right shoulder and around to the back. The pain may be severe enough to suggest a heart attack.

If the stone *passes through the duct* or if it drops back into the gallbladder, the symptoms and pain 20 may stop. If the stones *persist,* severe infection can occur along with fever and chills. If the bile does not flow because the duct is obstructed, *jaundice* [a yellow discoloration of the skin] results.

How are gallstones *diagnosed?* Previous *medical history,* pain, and tenderness are signs. A special gallbladder X-ray, a *cholecystogram,* makes the problem evident. The X-ray requires *swallowing* a *dye.* Gallstones can also *be detected* by *ultrasound.* Here a special instrument is passed over a part 25 of the body and registers *a picture* on a film.

If the gallstones that produce problems are not *removed,* the gallbladder may become *chronically* inflamed and thickened so that it does not fill or empty properly. Surgery is usually performed after acute attacks subside. It is common to *remove* the entire gallbladder. In this case 30 other organs *assume* the function of the gallbladder. Most people get complete and total relief.

If gallstones are present but *asymptomatic,* doctors tend to be more conservative in their treatment. Often an *endoscope,* a special instrument, is enough to *remove* small stones located at the end of the gallbladder duct.

Ask your own physician to help you select the proper diet for you, based on your own health 35 problems.

Questions

1. What are the symptoms of gallbladder problems?
2. How are gallstones diagnosed?
3. What treatment may be prescribed for gallstones?

Situation:

You are a patient suffering from gallstones. Describe your symptoms to your doctor.

LOS CALCULOS BILIARES

Los cálculos biliares son un problema para los que tienen una tendencia a padecer de desórdenes del aparato digestivo. Las que suelen sufrir de cálculos biliares con frecuencia son las mujeres y las personas de peso excesivo. No ocurre tanto en los varones o en las personas de peso normal o escaso.

5 ¿Cómo ocurren? El hígado *produce una secreción* llamada bilis. Esta produce un precipitado de pequeños cristales, los que se almacenan y se concentran en *la vesícula biliar.* Son los cálculos biliares los que varían de tamaño de una pulgada o más en diámetro hasta convertirse en lo que parece ser una colección de *arenilla.*

La vesícula biliar es un saco *piriforme* ligado a la superficie inferior del hígado, debajo de 10 las costillas. La vesícula biliar deja salir la bilis, lo que ayuda a digerir las grasas y sustancias grasas. La bilis se compone de *colesterol, sales biliares,* y *bilirrubina.*

Los primeros *síntomas* de la enfermedad de la vesícula biliar pueden incluir la indigestión, o *ardor epigástrico,* después de comer *alimentos fritos,* legumbres *ásperas,* o fruta cruda. Otros 15 síntomas que pueden ocurrir son: *flatulencia,* náusea y *eructos,* o *vómitos.* Es común tener un dolor *paulatino* que primero se intensifica y luego, poco a poco, *se calma.* Si un cálculo biliar

obstruye uno de los conductos que va al intestino delgado, ocurrirá un dolor *repentino* y severo. Generalmente tal dolor empieza en medio de o en la parte superior derecha del abdomen superior, y puede extenderse hacia el hombro derecho y alrededor de la espalda. El
20 dolor puede ser tan severo que parece un ataque cardíaco.

Si el cálculo biliar *pasa por el conducto* o si cae nuevamente en la vesícula biliar, los síntomas y el dolor pueden cesar. Si los cálculos *persisten,* tanto una infección aguda como fiebre y escalofríos pueden ocurrir. Si la bilis no fluye porque el conducto está obstruido, ocurre *la ictericia* [la piel amarilla].
25 ¿Cómo se *diagnostican* los cálculos biliares? Los signos más comunes son previo *historial médico,* dolor, y sensibilidad. Una radiografía especial de la vesícula biliar, un *colecistograma,* hace evidente la enfermedad. Para la radiografía es necesario *tragar* un *colorante.* Se pueden *detectar* los cálculos biliares también por medio de *ondas ultrasónicas.* En este caso un instrumento especial se pasa a lo largo de una parte del cuerpo el cual registra una *imagen* en una
30 foto.

Si no se le *remueven* los cálculos biliares que producen la enfermedad, la vesícula biliar puede inflamarse *crónicamente* y *engrosarse* tanto que ni se *rellena* ni se *vacía* adecuadamente. Después de que un ataque agudo pasa, se hace la operación. Es común *extirpar* toda la vesícula biliar. Si ocurre esto, los otros órganos *asumen* su funcionamiento. Para la mayoría
35 de estos pacientes, hay un alivio completo y total.

Si existen cálculos biliares, pero no molestan (es decir, si son *asintomáticos*), los médicos se inclinan a ser más conservadores en cuanto a su tratamiento. Muchas veces un *endoscopio,* un instrumento especial, basta para *sacar* los pequeños cálculos que se hallan al final del conducto de la vesícula biliar.
40 Pida ayuda a su médico para que le seleccione un régimen alimenticio adecuado basado en su propio problema de salud.

Preguntas

1. ¿Cuáles son los síntomas de la enfermedad de la vesícula biliar?
2. ¿Cómo se diagnostican los cálculos biliares?
3. ¿Cuál es el tratamiento para los cálculos biliares?

KIDNEY STONES

These stones are more *bothersome* than gallstones. They cause *sudden,* intense pain. Each individual is born with two *kidneys,* located on each side of the vertebral column in the lower back. The kidneys, which are constantly working, filter the blood and remove unnecessary products from the body. These *wastes* leave in the form of *urine.*
5 No one knows exactly what causes kidney stones. It is known that kidney stones may contain *calcium, phosphorus,* or *uric acids,* as well as *amino acids.* Chemical *imbalances* in the body may play a role, as may obstructions of the urinary tract.

Kidney stones, when large, cause great *discomfort.* If infection or bleeding occurs prior to the discovery and treatment of the problem, serious *damage* may occur to the kidneys.
10 If the kidney stones are small, they *may* cause no problems. They either remain in the kidney or flow with the urine through the *ureter,* eventually leaving the body. The ureter is a thin muscular tube that connects the kidney with the *urinary bladder.* Urine is temporarily stored in this bladder, as well as possible kidney stones. The waste passes out of the bladder through the *urethra.*
15 If the kidney stone does not stay in the kidney, and if it is large enough to irritate the ureter, or *block* the flow of urine from the kidney to the urinary bladder, trouble results. A *blockage* may produce blood in the urine and a horrible, intense pain, which begins beneath the *ribs* in the back and travels around to the abdomen into the groin. This pain is called *renal colic,* and may come and go. It is an important *symptom* of the *passage* of a stone.
20 If the urine does not *flow* because of a block, an infection may occur. Fever, violent *chills,* nausea, vomiting, and frequent or painful urination are often present. Pain medication helps the patient. *Antibiotics* or other drugs are commonly prescribed to control infection. In some cases a *catheter* is used *to empty* the kidney.

25 Positive diagnosis of kidney stones is made with a special X-ray of the kidney, an *IVP—intra-venous pyelogram.* If the stone does not pass on its own, a special instrument is used to help move it. The thin instrument is called a *cystoscope,* and is inserted through the urethra, giving the doctor a visual examination of both the bladder and the ureter.

If the stone obstructs the flow of urine for a prolonged period, surgery becomes necessary to prevent kidney damage. (The kidney is an organ which cannot *regenerate itself* and whose func-
30 tions cannot be assumed by other organs.) After the surgery the ureter is sutured in order to assure its proper size in the future.

Occasionally kidney stones do *recur.* People who are prone to kidney stones should consult a physician for the appropriate diet and drugs to help prevent stones.

Questions

1. What is the function of the kidneys?
2. What problems may result from kidney stones?
3. How may kidney stones be treated?

LOS CALCULOS RENALES [NEFRITICOS]

Estos cálculos molestan más que los cálculos biliares. Causan un dolor *repentino* e intenso.

Cada individuo tiene dos *riñones* al nacer, los cuales se hallan a cada lado de la columna vertebral en la parte inferior de la espalda. Los riñones, los cuales funcionan constante-
5 mente, filtran la sangre y quitan del cuerpo todos los elementos que no sean necesarios. Estos *desechos* salen en forma de *orina.*

Nadie sabe exactamente cuál sea la causa de los cálculos renales. Se sabe que los cálculos renales pueden contener tanto *calcio, fósforo* o *ácidos úricos* como *aminoácidos. Desequilibrios* químicos del cuerpo al igual que obstrucciones del aparato urinario pueden ser causantes de
10 cálculos renales.

Cuando son grandes, los cálculos renales causan mucha molestia. Si ocurriese infección o derrame de sangre antes de que se descubra y trate la enfermedad, el *daño* causado a los riñones puede ser muy serio.

Si los cálculos renales son pequeños, es posible que no causen daño alguno. Se quedan en
15 el riñón o pasan con la orina por *el uréter,* saliendo del cuerpo eventualmente. El uréter es un delgado tubo muscular que une el riñón con *la vejiga urinaria.* La orina es almacenada temporalmente en esta vejiga así como posibles cálculos renales. El desecho sale de la vejiga por medio de *la uretra* (*el caño urinario*).

Si el cálculo renal no se queda en el riñón, y si es lo suficientemente grande o para irritar
20 el uréter o para *obstruir* el flujo de la orina del riñón a la vejiga urinaria, puede causar problemas. Una *obstrucción* puede producir sangre en la orina y un dolor horrible e intenso empezando debajo de las *costillas* cerca de la columna vertebral que va en dirección del abdomen hacia la ingle. Este dolor se llama *cólico renal,* y puede aparecer y desaparecer. Es un *síntoma* importante del *paso* de un cálculo.

25 Si la orina no *fluye* a causa de una obstrucción, el resultado puede ser una infección. Con frecuencia hay fiebre, *escalofríos* violentos, náusea, vómitos, y dolor habitual y penoso al orinar. Medicamentos para el dolor ayudan al paciente. *Antibióticos* u otros medicamentos son recetados frecuentemente para controlar la infección. En algunos casos se usa *un catéter* para *vaciar* el riñón de orina.

30 Se hace un diagnóstico positivo de cálculos renales por medio de una radiografía especial del riñón, el cual se llama *un pielograma intravenoso—PIV.* Si el cálculo no es expulsado por sí mismo, se usa un instrumento especial para moverlo. Este instrumento delgado se llama *un cistoscopio* y se inserta por la uretra, dándole al médico una vista tanto de la vejiga como del uréter.

35 Si el cálculo obstruye la vía urinaria por mucho tiempo, es necesario hacer una operación para prevenir daño a los riñones. (El riñón es un órgano que no puede *regenerarse* el mismo, y cuyo funcionamiento no puede ser asumido por otros órganos.) Al final de la operación, se sutura el uréter para que su tamaño sea el correcto en el futuro.

40   A veces los cálculos renales vuelven. Las personas que estén predispuestas a tales cálculos, deben consultar a un médico para un régimen dietético y medicinas adecuadas que puedan ayudar a prevenir otros cálculos.

Preguntas

1. ¿Que función tienen los riñones?
2. ¿Qué tipo de problemas pueden traer como consecuencia de los cálculos renales?
3. ¿Cómo se pueden tratar los cálculos renales?

M.R.I. INSTRUCTIONS

A member of the MRI (Magnetic Resonance *Images*) Center staff will ask you a series of questions about your *medical history.*

Metal objects, such as *keys* and jewelry, could *interfere* with your MRI and could be *dangerous* to you during the exam. You should even remove your makeup, since it is possible that it may contain metallic *alloys.* You will be asked to put on a hospital gown. The staff will put your personal effects in a safe place and will return them to you after the test.

Before the *test* begins, the technician will answer any questions that you may have.

During the test you will hear tapping sounds which are the result of the normal operation of the machine. You will be able to communicate with the technician during the test.

Occasionally an injection which contains an *enhancing agent* is given. This assists the radiologist to better see the images during your test and he will discuss the results with your physician.

Your doctor will speak to you about the results and will answer any questions that you may have.

INSTRUCCIONES PARA LA PRODUCCION DE IMAGENES POR RESONANCIA MAGNETICA

Un miembro del personal del centro de MRI (Producción de *Imágenes* por Resonancia Magnética) le hará una serie de preguntas sobre su *historial médico.*

Los objetos de metal, tales como las *llaves* y joyas, podrían *interferir* con su examen de MRI y podrían ser *peligrosos* para Vd. durante el examen. Se debe quitar hasta el maquillaje, ya que es posible que contenga *aleaciones* metálicas. Le pedirán que se ponga una bata de hospital. El personal pondrá sus efectos personales en un lugar seguro y se los devolverá después del examen.

Antes de que comience *el examen*, el técnico contestará a cualquier pregunta que Vd. tenga.

Durante el examen Vd. escuchará sonidos como golpes que son el resultado de la operación normal de la máquina. Vd. se podrá comunicar con el técnico durante el examen.

Algunas veces se pone una inyección que contiene *un agente intensificador.* Esto puede ayudar a que el radiólogo vea mejor las imágenes de su examen y examinará los resultados con el médico de Vd.

Su médico hablará con Vd. sobre los resultados y contestará a cualquier pregunta que Vd. tenga.

POST-OPERATIVE ORAL SURGERY INSTRUCTIONS

1. *HEALING*—Do not disturb the wound by touching it with your fingers, tongue, or a toothpick. The blood clot which forms over the area is nature's way of healing and should not be disturbed.
2. *BLEEDING*—Bite on your gauze one hour WITHOUT moving it. Very slight bleeding will be noticed as streaks of blood in your saliva for one to two days. If this is troublesome, place fresh gauze over the area and bite steadily on the compress. For the maximum effect, keep the compress still under biting pressure for 1 hour. Rest when you do this. If bleeding is excessive, call NOW!
3. *DIET*—Liquids today or as directed by your doctor. Do not use straws. Eat frequently and in increased amounts. Eat a soft diet beginning tomorrow and progress to a regular diet as tolerated.
4. *RINSING*—Do not rinse your mouth at all for the first 24 (twenty-four) hours. Clean your mouth beginning tomorrow; use PLAIN water. Clean immediately after eating. Your doctor may recommend the use of saline (salt water) rinses instead. Follow his/her instructions exactly.
5. *PAIN*—Expect some pain in the form of soreness around the operated area. This usually lasts a few days. Take medication exactly as directed. Do not change the dose or frequency of medication unless you are directed by your doctor. Report any reaction or upset that seems to come from taking your medication properly. At that time, cease all medications.
6. *SWELLING*—Expect some swelling for about three days; this is normal. The swelling begins to go away after the fourth day. Mild skin bruising may accompany this.
7. *USE OF COLD*—Begin as soon as possible after surgery. Place an ice bag over the area nearest the surgery. Keep it in place continuously for 30 (thirty) minutes, then remove it for 30 minutes. Alternate like this for the first 24 hours after the surgery. If the swelling continues after the first 24 hours, apply warm, moist compresses to the outside of your face for 30 minutes at a time.
8. Do not hesitate to call if you have any questions or problems pertaining to your surgery.

INSTRUCCIONES PARA LA CIRUGIA ORAL POST-OPERATORIA

1. *LA CICATRIZACION*—Se ruega no tocarla con los dedos, la lengua o el mondadientes. El coágulo de sangre que se forma allí es el método natural de cicatrización. Se ruega no tocarla.
2. *EL FLUJO DE SANGRE*—*Muerda a dentelladas* una gasa SIN moverla. Por uno o dos días se observará por medio de rayos de sangre en la saliva un pequeñito flujo de sangre. Si le molesta, ponga Vd. una gasa nueva encima de la herida oral y muerda la compresa sin cesar. Lo mejor es morderla fijamente por una hora. Descanse Vd. mientras la muerde. Si *se desangra*, llame inmediatamente.
3. *LA DIETA*—Hoy coma Vd. líquidos o lo que indique su *cirujano oral*. No use Vd. pajas. Coma frecuentemente y en cantidades cada vez mayores. Empezando mañana, siga una dieta blanda (al tacto). Vuelva poco a poco a su dieta normal dependiendo de su *tolerancia*.
4. *EL ENJUAGUE*—No enjuague Vd. la boca para nada durante las primeras 24 (veinticuatro) horas. Limpie Vd. la boca empezando mañana. Use agua SIMPLE/CLARA. Inmediatamente después de comer, limpie la boca. Puede ser que su cirujano oral le recomiende el uso de enjuagues salinos (agua salada) en vez de agua clara. Siga sus instrucciones exactamente.
5. *EL DOLOR*—*Cuente* Vd. *con* padecer un poco, en la forma de una parte adolorida por toda la superficie afectada. Este dolor dura por lo regular unos pocos días. Tome Vd. su medicina exactamente como sea recetada. No cambie la dosis ni la frecuencia de la medicina a menos que su cirujano oral lo indique. Informe al doctor inmediatamente de cualquier reacción o malestar que, en su opinión, es originada por su medicina. En el momento que tal cosa ocurra, deje de tomar la medicina.
6. *LA HINCHAZON*—Cuente Vd. con alguna hinchazón durante tres días, más o menos. Es normal. La hinchazón empieza a disminuir después del cuarto día. Es posible que ocurra, además, una contusión ligera de la piel.
7. *EL EMPLEO DE COMPRESAS FRÍAS*—Empiece Vd. tan pronto como le sea posible después de la cirugía. Ponga Vd. una bolsa de hielo sobre la superficie más cercana a la cirugía. *Quédese* con el hielo sin moverlo nada por 30 (treinta) minutos; entonces, quítelo por 30 minutos. Alterne de esta manera durante las primeras veinticuatro horas después de la cirugía. Si la hinchazón continúa después de 24 horas, aplique compresas calientes y húmedas al exterior de la cara por 30 minutos a la vez.
8. No vacile Vd. en telefonear cuando quiera si tiene preguntas o problemas tocante a su cirugía.

Situations

You're the oral surgeon. Tell your patient about post-operative care of your mouth.
You are the patient. You have just had two lower wisdom teeth extracted. Ask about the diet that you should follow, and what you should take for pain.

CARE OF THE MOUTH AFTER A PULPOTOMY

A pulpotomy procedure consists of removing (all or) part of the nerve and blood vessels (pulp) of a tooth.

1. If there is discomfort, give your child a Tylenol or other type of over-the-counter pain reliever. The pain should subside within 24 (twenty-four) hours.
2. Medication is sealed in the tooth for a maximum of two weeks. Your child must return within this period to have the medication removed. If this is not done, the tooth may have to be extracted.
3. There is a temporary filling sealing the medication into the tooth; therefore, it is very important that no gum or candy be eaten during this period.

If you have any questions or problems, please call our office.

CUIDADO BUCAL DESPUES DE UNA PULPOTOMIA

Una pulpotomía es un procedimiento que consiste en la extirpación (total o) parcial del nervio y los vasos sanguíneos (la pulpa) de un diente.

1. Si hay molestia, déle a su hijo/hija un Tylenol u otro tipo de medicamento que se vende sin receta para el control de dolor. El dolor debe disminuir dentro de 24 (veinticuatro) horas.
2. Se pone un medicamento dentro del diente por un máximo de dos semanas. Su hijo/hija tiene que volver dentro de este período de tiempo para que podamos quitarle el medicamento. Si no lo hace, quizás será necesario sacarle el diente.
3. Hay un empaste provisional que encierra el medicamiento dentro del diente. Por eso, es urgente que no coma ni chicle ni dulces durante el período del tratamiento.

Si hay cualquier pregunta o problema, por favor, llame a nuestro consultorio dental.

Notes *Notas*

1. In order to convert from F to C, a formula is used: $C = (F - 32°)/1.8$.
2. **Para hacer la conversión de F a C, se usa una fórmula: $C = (F - 32°)/1.8$. Vea Capítulo 4, pág. 92.**
3. The incidence of diabetes among Mexican-Americans is as much as 2.8 times greater than among white, non-Hispanic adults, according to the American Association of Diabetes Educators. Obesity, a key risk factor for the onset of diabetes in adults, is also higher for Mexican-Americans than for the white, non-Hispanic adult population. More than 30% of the former are overweight. Research documents that Mexican-American women are as likely as black women to be overweight, and that Mexican-American men are more likely than black or white men to be overweight.

The Hispanic population is expected to continue its current growth pattern in the coming decades. By the year 2080, 17 percent of the Hispanic population will be 65 years and older, a significant increase from the 1985 3.1 percent figure in this age bracket. One result will be larger numbers of Hispanics in this age group more prone to diabetes. Diabetes, already one of the three main health care concerns of Hispanics along with drugs and alcoholism, will have a dramatic increase among Hispanics. Professionals treating Hispanics with the disease will have to consider and educate all family members. *Chicago Tribune*, September 10, 1987, Section 5, p. 2.

Crucial Vocabulary for Health Professionals

Vocabulario crucial para profesionales médicos, dentales y de asistencia pública

CONTENTS

INDICES

MAJOR CLINICS

CLINICAS PRINCIPALES

Acute Care **primeros auxilios** *m, pl*
Admitting **ingresos** *m, pl*
Allergy **alergia**
Audiology **audiología**
Bronchology **broncología**
Cardiology **cardiología**
  Congenital Cardiology
    cardiología congénita
  Rheumatic Cardiology
    cardiología reumática
Central Testing Laboratory
    laboratorio central
Chest **pulmonar** *adj*
Dental **dental** *adj*
  Dentistry **dentistería;**
    odontología; estomatología
Dermatology **dermatología**
Diabetic **diabética** *adj*
ECG—Electrocardiogram
    electrocardiograma *m*
EEG—Electroencephalogram (Brain
    Wave Test) **laboratorio para**
    encefalogramas
Emergency Room **sala de**
    urgencia/emergencia

Employees' Health Service
    dispensario de empleados
Endocrinology **endocrinología**
ENT—Ear, Nose, and Throat **GNO-**
    garganta, nariz, oídos
Eyes **ojos**
Genetics **genética**
Gerontology **gerontología**
Gynecology **ginecología**
Hematology **hematología**
Immunology **inmunología**
Kidneys—**nephritic**
    riñonesnefrítica
Maternity **maternidad** *f*
Medicine **medicina; médica** *adj*
MRI—Magnetic Resonance Images
    IRM—Imágenes por Resonancia
    Magnética *f*
Nephrology **nefrología**
Neurology **neurología**
Obstetrics **obstétrica**
Occupational Therapy **terapia**
    ocupacional
Oncology **oncología**
Operating Room **sala de**
    operaciones; quirófano

Ophthalmology **oftalmología**
Optics **óptica**
Orthopedics **ortopedia**
  Special Orthopedics **ortopedia**
    especial
Outpatient Clinic **clínica para**
    pacientes ambulatorios
Pediatrics **pediatría**
Pharmacy **farmacia**
Physical Therapy **fisioterapia**
Psychiatry **psiquiatría**
Pulmonary Disease **enfermedad**
    respiratoria *f*
Rheumatology **reumatología**
Social Service **servicio social**
Special Seizure **convulsiones** *f*
Speech **del habla** *m*
  Voice, Articulation **voz,**
    articulación *f*
Surgery **cirugía**
  Plastic Surgery **cirugía plástica**
  Special Surgery **cirugía especial**
Urology **urología**
X-rays **radiografía; rayos x (equis)**
    m

KEY DISEASES, SYMPTOMS, AND INJURIES

ENFERMEDADES, SINTOMAS, Y HERIDAS PRINCIPALES

abrasion **razpón** *m;* **rozadura**
abscess **absceso; hinchazón** *f, fam*
accident **accidente** *m*
acne **acné** *f;* **espinillas; cácara** *Chicano*
Acquired Immune Deficiency Syndrome
    Síndrome de inmuno[logía]
    deficiencia adquirida *m*
"acute abdomen" **abdomen agudo** *m*[1]
addicted **adicto** *adj*
AIDS **SIDA** *m*
ailment **dolencia**
alcoholism **alcoholismo**
allergic reaction **trastorno alérgico;**
    reacción alérgica *f*
allergy **alergia**
amblyopia **ambliopia**
anemia **anemia; sangre clara** *f, fam;*
    sangre débil *f, fam;* **sangre pobre** *f,*
    fam
  aplastic anemia **anemia aplástica**
  iron deficiency anemia **deficiencia**
    de hierro
  pernicious anemia **anemia**
    perniciosa
  sickle cell anemia **anemia**
    drepanocítica; drepanocitemia
  thalassemia **talasemia**
aneurysm **aneurisma**
angina **angina**
  angina pectoris **angina del pecho**
angioma **angioma** *m;* **cabecita de vena**
    Chicano
anxiety **ansiedad** *f*
aortic insufficiency **insuficiencia**
    aórtica
aphasia **afasia**

aphonia (hoarseness) **afonia; ronquera**
apoplexy, stroke **apoplejía**
appendicitis **apendicitis** *f;* **panza**
    peligrosa *slang*[2]
ARC/AIDS related complex—CRS
    complejo relacionado al SIDA
arrhythmia, cardiac **arritmia cardíaca**
arteriosclerosis **arteriosclerosis** *f*
arthritis **artritis** *f*
  rheumatoid arthritis **artritis**
    reumatoidea
asthma **asma; fatiga** *slang;* **ahoguío**
    fam, Mex.
  asthmatic attack, seizure **ataque**
    asmático *m*
  asthmatic wheeze **resuello asmático**
  bronchial asthma **asma bronquial**
astigmatism **astigmatismo**
athlete's foot **pie de atleta** *m;* **infección**
    de serpigo *f*
atrial fibrillation **fibrilación auricular**
    f
atrophy **atrofia**
attack **ataque** *m*
bacterium **bacteria**
bald **calvo** *adj*
  baldness **calvicie** *f*
bearing **porte** *m*
bedbug **chinche** *f*
bedsore **úlcera por decúbito; llaga de**
    cama
Bell's palsy **parálisis facial** *f*
bite (animal) **mordedura**
  cat bite **mordedura de gato**
  dog bite **mordedura de perro**
  human bite **mordedura humana**

scorpion bite[3] **mordedura de**
    escorpión
snake bite **mordedura de serpiente**
bite (insect), sting[4] **picadura**
bite (toothmark) **dentellada**
black and blue **amoratado** *adj*
blackeye **ojo morado**
blackhead, shin **espinilla**
bleed excessively, to **desangrar**
bleeding **pérdida de sangre (de poca**
    intensidad); sangría; hemorragia
  bleeding tendencies **tendencias a**
    sangrar
  internal bleeding **hemorragia**
    interna
blemish **lunar** *m;* **mancha**
blepharitis **blefaritis** *f*
blind **ciego** *adj*
  blind in one eye **tuerto** *adj*
blindness **ceguera; ceguedad** *f*
  color blindness **daltonismo;**
    acromatopsia; ceguera para los
    colores
  night blindness (nyctalopia)
    nictalopía; ceguera nocturna
  river blindness (oncocerciasis)[5]
    oncocercosis *f;* **oncocerciasis** *f;*
    cerguera del río
blisters **ampolla; vesícula; bulla**
  blister on sole of foot **sietecueros** *inv*
blocked intestine **intestino obstruido/**
    tripa ida
blood clot **coágulo de sangre;**
    cuajarón *m*
blood poisoning **envenenamiento de la**
    sangre; toxemia; septicemia; sepsis *f*

blood pressure **presión arterial** *f;* **tensión arterial** *f;* **presión de la sangre** *f;* **presión sanguínea** *f*
  high blood pressure **presión arterial alta; hipertensión arterial; presión sanguínea alta** *f*
  low blood pressure **presión arterial baja; hipotensión arterial**
boil **furúnculo; nacido; sisote** *m;* **tacotillo** *Chicano*
bowel obstruction **obstrucción de la tripa** *f;* **tripa ida** *fam;* **panza peligrosa**[6] *slang;* **abdomen agudo**[6] *m, slang*
bronchitis **bronquitis** *f*
bruise **contusión** *f;* **magulladura; moretón** *m, Mex., Hond.;* **lastimadura**
  bruised **moreteado** *adj, Chicano*
bubo **búa; ganglio; incordio; seca** *fam*
bubonic plague **peste bubónica** *f*
bulging eyes **ojos saltones; ojos capotudos** *Chicano*
bullet **bala**
  bullet wound **balazo**
bunion **juanete** *m*
burn **quemadura; quemazón** *m*
  acid burn **quemadura por ácido**
  alkali burn **quemadura por álcali**
  chemical burn **quemadura química**
  dry heat burn **quemadura por calor seco**
  scald **escaldadura**
  sunburn **quemadura solar; solanera; eritema solar** *m*
bursitis **bursitis** *f*
buzzing in the ears **zumbido en los oídos**
callus **callo**
cancer **cáncer** *m*[7]
  cancerous **canceroso** *adj*
canker **úlcera; llaga ulcerosa; ulceración** *f*
carcinoma **carcinoma** *m*
cardiac arrest **fallo cardíaco; paro cardíaco**
caries **caries** *finv;* **cavidad dental** *f;* **diente podrido** *m*
case **caso**
cataract **catarata**
catch a disease, to **contraer una enfermedad; agarrar; pegarle**
celiac disease **celíaca**
cerebral paralysis **parálisis cerebral** *f*
cerebrospinal meningitis **meningitis cerebroespinal** *f*
chafing **irritación** *f;* **rozadura**
Chagas's disease **enfermedad de Chagas** *f*
chancre **chancro**
  soft chancre **chancro blando**
change of life **cambio de vida**
chapped **cuarteado** *adj;* **rozado** *adj*
chap skin, to **cuartearse rozarse**
cheilosis (sore at corner of mouth) **boquilla**
chicken pox **varicela; viruelas locas** *slang;* **bobas; tecunda** *Mex.*
chilblain **sabañón** *m*
chills **escalofríos**
choking **asfixia**
cholera **cólera** *m*
chorea **corea; mal o baile de San Guido o de San Vito** *m*

chronic **crónico** *adj;* **duradero** *adj*
cirrhosis of the liver **cirrosis del hígado** *f;* **cirrosis hepática** *f*
cleft palate **paladar partido** *m;* **fisura palatina; paladar hendido** *m;* **grietas en el paladar; boquineta** *m, Chicano*
club foot **pie deforme** *m;* **pie zambo** *m;* **talipes** *m*
coated tongue **lengua saburrosa; lengua sucia**
cold **catarro; resfriado**
  common cold **resfriado común "stopped-up" head; head cold constipado**
colic **cólico**
colitis **colitis** *f*
collapse **colapso**
colostomy **colostomía**
coma **coma** *m*
complaint, chronic **alifafe** *m, slang*
complication **complicación** *f;* **accidente** *m*
concussion **concusión** *f;* **golpe** *m*
congenital **congénito** *adj*
  congenital anomaly **anomalía congénita**
congestion of the chest **ahoguijo; ahoguío** *fam*
conjunctivitis (pinkeye) **conjunctivitis** *f;* **mal de ojo** *m, fam;* **tracoma** *m;* **oftalmia contagiosa; catarral aguda** *f*
constipation **constipación** *f;* **estreñimiento; entablazón** *f, Chicano*
contagious **contagioso** *adj;* **pegadizo** *adj*
contusion **contusión** *f*
convalescence **convalecencia**
convulsion **convulsión** *f;* **ataque** *m*
corn **callo**
coronary thrombosis **trombosis coronaria** *f*
corpse **cadáver** *m*
cough **tos** *f*
  smoker's cough **tos por fumar**
  cough, to **toser**
  cough up phlegm, to **esgarrar; desgarrar** *Chicano*
cramps **calambres** *m*
  abdominal cramps **retortijón** *m;* **torsón** *m*
  cane-cutter's cramps **calambres de los cortadores de caña**
  charley horse **rampa**
  heat cramps **calambres térmicos**
  menstrual **dolores del período** *m*
  postpartum **entuertos**
  stomach **retortijón de tripas; torcijón cólico** *m, Mex.*
cretinism **cretinismo**
cripple **tullido** *adj, m;* **inválido** *adj, m*
crippled **lisiado** *adj;* **cojo** *adj;* **empedido** *adj*
  crippled hand **manco** *adj*
cross-eyed **bizco** *adj:* **bisojo** *adj;* **turnio** *adj*
cross-eyes **bizquera**
croup **crup** *f;* **ronquera**
cut **cortada** *Sp. Am.;* **cortadura**
cyst **quiste** *m*
  cystic fibrosis **fibrosis quística** *f*
cystitis **cistitis** *f;* **infección de la vejiga** *f*
dacryocystitis **dacriocistitis** *f* **infección de la bolsa de lágrimas** *f*

dandruff **caspa**
dead **muerto** *adj, m*
deaf **sordo** *adj*
  deaf mute **sordomudo**
  deafness **sordera; ensordecimiento**
death **muerte** *f;* **fallecimiento**
  death rattle **estertor agónico** *m*
defect **defecto**
deficiency **carencia; deficiencia**
deformed **deforme** *adj;* **eclipsado** *adj, fam, Sp. Am.;* **inocente** *adj, Mex.*
deformity **deformidad** *f*
dehydration **deshidratación** *f;* **desecación** *f*
delirium **delirio**
delouse, to **espulgar**
dementia **demencia**
dengue **dengue** *m;* **fiebre rompehuesos** *f*
depressed **deprimido** *adj*
depression **depresión** *f;* **abatimiento**
dermatitis **dermatitis** *f*
detached retina **retina desprendida**
diabetes **diabetes** *f*
  diabetes insipidus **diabetes insípida**
  diabetes mellitus **diabetes mellitus; diabetes sacarina**
diabetic **diabético** *m, adj*
diagnosis **diagnóstico; diagnosis** *f/inv*
diarrhea **diarrea; cursera** *slang;* **turista** *slang;* **chorro** *slang;* **asientos** *slang;* **chorrillo** *slang;* **cámara** *slang;* **soltura** *Chicano;* **corredera** *Chicano;* **cagadera** *vulgar, Chicano*
diphtheria **difteria; garrotillo**
disability **inhabilidad** *f;* **incapacidad** *f;* **invalidez** *f*
disc, calcified **disco calcificado**
disc, slipped **disco desplazado; disco intervertebral luxado**
discharge **secreción** *f;* **flujo; supuración** *f;* **descarga**
  bloody discharge **derrame** *m*
  vaginal discharge **flujo vaginal**
  white discharge **flores blancas** *f, fam;* **flujo blanco**
discomfort **malestar** *m*
disease **enfermedad** *f;* **mal** *m;* **dolencia**
  disease due to an act of witchcraft **enfermedad endañada** *Chicano, Mex.*
  disease that is "going around" **enfermedad de andancia** *Chicano*
  notifiable disease **enfermedad de notificación**
  reportable disease **enfermedad obligatoria**
dislocated **dislocado** *adj;* **zafado** *adj, Sp. Am.*
dislocation **dislocación** *f;* **luxación** *f*
diverticulitis **diverticulitis** *f;* **colitis ulcerosa** *f*
dizziness **vértigo; vahido; tarantas** *Mex. Hond.*
Down's syndrome **mal de Down** *m;* **mongolismo**
drainage **supuración** *f;* **drenaje** *m*
  draining, dripping **escurrimiento**
dropsy **ahogamiento; hidropesía**
drowsiness **modorra**
drug addict[8] **drogadicto; adicto a las drogas**
drug addiction[8] **narcomanía; dependencia farmacológica**

drug overdose[8] sobredosis de
drogas f/inv
drunk borracho adj; pisto adj;
tacuache adj; tlacuache adj;
tronado adj; alumbrado adj,
slang, Chicano; rascado adj, Ven.
to be/get drunk emborracharse
andar bombo; andar eléctrico;
andar en la línea; andar loco;
estar mediagua; ponerse alto
fam; rascar Sp. Am.
drunkenness borrachera
dwarf enano m/f
dysentery disentería
ameobic dysentery disentería
amebiana
bacillary dysentery disentería
bacilar
dysmenorrhea dismenorrea;
menstruación dolorosa f
dyspnea dificultad al respirar f
dysuria dolor al orinar m
earache dolor de oído m
earwax, impacted tapón de cera m
eczema eccema m/f;
rezumamiento
edema edema m
emaciation enflaquecimiento;
demacración f
embolism embolismo; embolia
emergency emergencia; urgencia;
caso urgente
emphysema enfisema m
encephalitis encefalitis f
enlargement ensanchamiento;
ampliación f, agrandamiento
epidemic epidémico adj; epidemia
epilepsy epilepsia; ataque (de
epilepsia) m
epileptic attack ataque
epiléptico m; convulsión f
eruption erupción f
erysipelas erisipela; dicipela Chicano
exhaustion agotamiento; fatiga
fainting spell desmayo; mareo
fam; vértigo; desvanecimiento;
desfallecimiento
fallen fontanel[9] caída de la
mollera
farsighted présbita adj
farsightedness presbicia;
hipermetropía, presbiopía
fatigue fatiga
fear[10] miedo
fever[10] fiebre f; calentura
acute infectious adenitis fiebre
ganglionar
breakbone fever fiebre
rompehuesos; dengue m
Colorado tick fever fiebre de
Colorado; fiebre tra(n)smitida
por garrapatas
enteric fever fiebre entérica
fever blister llaga de fiebre;
herpe febril m/f
glandular fever fiebre glandular
hay fever fiebre de(l) heno;
alergia; jey fíver m/f; catarro
constipado Chicano
intermittent fever fiebre
intermitente
malarial fever fiebre palúdica;
chucho Arg., Chile

Malta fever fiebre de Malta;
fiebre ondulante;
brucelosis f
paratyphoid fever fiebre
paratifoidea; fiebre paratífica
parrot fever fiebre de las
cotorras
rabbit fever fiebre de conejo
rat-bite fever fiebre por
mordedura de rata
rheumatic fever fiebre
reumática
Rocky Mountain fever fiebre de
las Montañas Rocosas;
maculosa de las Montañas
Rocosas
scarlet fever fiebre escarlatina
spotted fever fiebre purpúrea
(de las Montañas Rocosas);
tifus exantemático m; fiebre
manchada
thermic fever fiebre térmica
typhoid fever fiebre tifoidea;
tifus abdominal m
typhus tifus m; tifo; tifus
exantemático; úrzula Chicano
undulant fever fiebre ondulante
valley fever (coccidioidomycosis)
fiebre del valle
yellow fever fiebre amarilla;
tifus icteroides m; fiebre
tropical; tifo de América;
vómito negro
fibroma fibroma m
fissure fisura; grieta; partidura
fistula fístula
fit convulsión; arrebato;
paroxismo
flat foot pie plano m; planovegus m
flatus flato; ventosidad f; pedo
slang
flea pulga
floater mosca volante; mancha
volante
flu influenza f; gripe f; gripa f;
monga P.R.[1]
Asiatic flu influenza asiática
folk illness[11] enfermedad casera f
foul-smelling apestoso adj
fracture fractura; quebradura de
huesos
complicated fracture fractura
complicada
compound fracture fractura
compuesta
green stick fracture fractura en
tallo verde
multiple fracture fractura
múltiple
open fracture fractura abierta
pathologic fracture fractura
patológica
serious fracture fractura mayor
simple fracture fractura simple
spontaneous fracture fractura
espontánea
freckle peca
frigidity frigidez f
frostbite congelación f; daño
sufrido por causa de la helada
fungus hongo
athlete's foot pie de atleta m;
infección de serpigo f

moniliasis candidiasis f;
boquera; muguet m/f;
moniliasis f
ringworm/tinea culebrilla; tiña;
empeine m; serpigo; sisote m,
Chicano
tinea corporis jiotes f, fam
furuncle furúnculo
gait marcha
gallbladder attack ataque vesicular
m; dolor de la vesícula m
gallstone cálculo en la vejiga;
cálculo biliar; piedra en la
vejiga
gangrene gangrena; cangrena
gash cuchillada
gastritis gastritis f
germ germen m; microbio
German measles rubéola;
sarampión alemán m; fiebre de
tres días f; alfombría Chicano;
alfombrilla Chicano; sarampión
bastardo m
glaucoma glaucoma m
goiter bocio; buche m, slang;
güegüecho
gonorrhea gonorrea; purgación f,
slang; blenorragia; chorro fam
gout gota
hallucination alucinación f
hammertoe dedo gordo en
martillo
handicap impedimento
hangnail padrastro fam; cutícula
desgarrada
hangover malestar post-
alcohólico m
hard of hearing duro de oído;
corto de oído
harelip labio leporino; cheuto adj,
Chile; jane adj, Hond.; labio
cucho Chicano; boquineta m,
Chicano
harsh, raucous sound ronquido
headache dolor de cabeza m;
jaqueca; cajetuda Chicano
heart attack ataque al corazón m;
ataque cardíaco m; ataque del
corazón m; infarto
heartbeat latido (cardíaco);
palpitación f
irregular heartbeat (arrhythmia)
latido irregular; palpitación
irregular; arritemia
rhythmical heartbeat
palpitación rítmica
slow heartbeat palpitación
lenta
tachycardia (rapid heartbeat)
taquicardia f; palpitación
rápida
heartburn acedía; agriera Sp. Am.;
agruras; cardialgia; pirosis f;
ardor de estómago m
heart disease enfermedad del
corazón f; enfermedad cardíaca f;
cardiopatías f
heart failure insuficiencia
cardíaca; fallo del corazón; paro
del corazón
heart murmur soplo; murmullo
heat exhaustion agotamiento por
calor

heat stroke **golpe de calor** *m;* **insolación** *f*

hematuria **hematuria; sangre en la orina** *f*

hemophilia **hemofilia**

hemorrhage **hemorragia; desangramiento; morragia** *Chicano*

hemorrhoids **almorranas; hemorroides** *f, pl*

hepatitis **hepatitis** *f;* **inflamación del hígado** *f;* **fiebre** *f, fam, Mex.*

hernia **hernia; quebradura; desaldillado** *Mex.;* **destripado** *slang*

femoral hernia **hernia femoral**

inguinal hernia **hernia inguinal; quebradura en la ingle**

umbilical hernia **hernia del ombligo; ombligo salido** *slang;* **ombligón** *m, slang*

herpes **herpes** *m/f*

hiccough, hiccup **hipo; hipsus** *m*

high arched foot **pie hueco** *m*

high cholesterol **colesterol elevado** *m*

high triglycerides **triglicéridos elevados** *m*

hives **urticaria; ronchas**

hoarse **afónico** *adj;* **ronco** *adj*

hoarseness **ronquera; carraspera** *fam*

hot flashes **calores** *m;* **llamaradas; calofrío** *Chicano*

hunchback **jorobado** *m, adj*

hydrocele **hidrocele** *m/f*

hyperlipidemia **hiperlipidemia**

hypertension (high blood pressure) **presión arterial alta** *f;* **hipertensión arterial** *f*

hyperventilation **hiperventilación** *f;* **susto con resuello duro** *fam*

hyphemia **hifemia; hemorragia detrás de la córnea**

hypochondria **hipocondría; hipocondria**

hypochondriac **hipocóndrico** *m, adj;* **adolorado** *adj, Chicano;* **adolorido** *adj, Chicano*

hypopyon **pus detrás de la córnea** *m*

hypotension (low blood pressure) **hipotensión arterial** *f;* **presión arterial baja** *f*

hysteria **histeria**

ill **malo** *adj;* **enfermo** *adj*

illness **mal** *m;* **enfermedad** *f;* **padecimiento**

acute illness **enfermedad aguda**

chronic illness **enfermedad crónica**

contagious illness (disease) **enfermedad contagiosa; enfermedad trasmisible**

mental illness **enfermedad mental**

minor illness **enfermedad leve**

organic illness (disease) **enfermedad orgánica**

serious illness **enfermedad grave**

tropical illness (disease) **enfermedad tropical**

immune **inmune** *adj*

immunization **inmunización** *f;* **vacuna**

impetigo **impétigo** *m;* **erupción cutánea**

impotence **impotencia**

indigestion **indigestión** *f;* **mala digestión** *f;* **dispepsia estómago sucio**[12] *Chicano;* **insulto** *Chicano*

infantile paralysis—polio (myelitis) **parálisis infantil** *f;* **polio (mielitis)** *f*

infarct **infarto**

infection **infección** *f;* **pasmo**

infectious **infeccioso** *adj*

inflammation **inflamación** *f;* **encono**

inflammation of the throat **garrotillo**

influenza **influenza; gripe** *f;* **gripa**

ingrown nail **uña encarnada; uña enterrada; uñero**

injured **herido** *adj;* **lisiado** *adj*

injury **herida; lesión; lastimadura**

insanity **locura; demencia**

manic-depressive **locura de doble forma; mania-melancolía; sicosis maníaco-depresiva** *f*

insomnia **insomnio; pérdida del sueño**

intoxication **embriaguez** *f*

intussusception **intususcepción** *f*

irritability **bilis**[13] *f*

irritation **irritación** *f*

itch **picazón** *f;* **comezón** *f;* **sarna** *f*

jaundice **derrame biliar** *m;* **ictericia; piel amarilla** *f, fam*

kidney disease **mal del riñón** *m*

kidney stone **cálculo en el riñón; ataque vesicular** *m;* **dolor de la vesícula** *m;* **cálculo renal; piedra en los riñones**

knot (type of tissue swelling) **bolas** *pl, Chicano;* **nudo**

laceration **laceración** *f;* **desgarradura; cortada**

lame **lisiado** *adj;* **cojo** *adj;* **rengo** *adj*

lameness **cojera**

laryngitis **laringitis** *f*

leishmaniasis **roncha mala; roncha hulera**

leprosy **lepra; lazarin** *m;* **mal de San Lázaro** *m;* **mal de Hansen** *m*

lesion **lesión** *f*

oral lesion **pupa; afta; perleche** *f;* **boquera**

leukemia **leucemia** *f;* **cáncer de la sangre** *m*

limp, to **cojear; renguear** *Sp. Am.*

lisp (stutter) **tartamudeo** *m;* **ceceo** *m*

lockjaw **tétanos; trismo**

lump **dureza; protuberancia; hinchazón** *f/m;* **borujo**

large lump **borujón** *m*

lump or bump on head **chichón** *m;* **pisporr(i)a** *Chicano*

mad (insane) **loco** *adj*

madness **locura; manía**

malaise **malestar** *m*

malaria **malaria; paludismo; fríos** *Sp. Am.*

malignancy **malignidad** *f*

malignant **maligno** *adj*

malnourished **desnutrido** *adj;* **mal nutrido** *adj*

malnutrition **malnutrición** *f;* **desnutrición** *f;* **mala alimentación** *f*

kwashiorkor **kwashiorkor** *m;* **mala alimentación mojada** *f*

marasmus **marasmo; mala alimentación seca** *f*

mania **manía**

maniac **maníaco** *adj*

masturbation **masturbación** *f;* **casqueta** *Chicano*

measles **sarampión** *m;* **morbilia; tapetillo de los niños** *fam,* **granuja** *slang*

melancholia **melancolía**

membrane **membrana; tela**

Ménière's disease **enfermedad de Ménière** *f*

meningitis **meningitis** *f*

menopause **menopausia; cambio de vida; período climatérico**

mental retardation **retraso mental**

metastasis **metástasis** *f*

migraine **migraña; jaqueca**

mild **leve** *adj*

mirror writing **escritura como en un espejo**

mold **moho**

mononucleosis **mononucleosis infecciosa** *f*

mucus **moco; frío** *slang, Mex.*

multiple sclerosis **esclerosis múltiple** *f;* **esclerosis en placa** *f*

mumps **paperas; parótidas** *pl;* **farfallota** *P.R.;* **bolas** *Chicano;* **coquetas** *Mex.;* **buche** *m, Mex.;* **mompes** *m, pl, Chicano*

muscular dystrophy **distrofia muscular progresiva**

mute **mudo** *adj*

myocardial infarct **infarto miocardíaco**

myopia **miopía**

myopic **miope** *adj*

nasal drip **goteo nasal; moqueadera** *Chicano*

nausea **náusea; basca**

morning nausea **malestares de la mañana** *m;* **asqueo; enfermedad matutina** *f*

nearsighted **miope** *adj;* **corto de vista** *adj*

nearsightedness **miopía**

nephritis **nefritis** *f*

nervous breakdown **desarreglo nervioso; colapso; neurastenia**

nervous disorder **desorden nervioso** *m*

nervousness **nerviosidad** *f*

neuralgia **neuralgia**

neurasthenia **neurastenia**

neurasthenic **neurasténico** *adj*

neuritis **neuritis** *f*

neurosis **neurosis** *f*

neurotic **neurótico** *adj*

nightmare **pesadilla**

noninfectious **no infeccioso** *adj*

nosebleed **hemorragia nasal**

nose bleeding **epistaxis** *f*

numb **adormecimiento**

obese **obeso** *adj;* **gordo** *adj*

obeseness **obesidad** *f;* **gordura**

obstruction **obstrucción** *f;* **impedimento**

nasal obstruction **mormación** *f, Chicano*

stomach obstruction **entablazón** *f, Chicano*

old age **senectud; vejez** *f*

one-eyed **tuerto** *adj;* **virulo** *adj, Chicano*

ophthalmia (inflammation of the eye) **oftalmía; inflamación de los ojos** *f*

osteomyelitis **osteomielitis** *f;* **inflamación de la médula del hueso** *f*

otitis **otitis** *f*
overdose **dosis excesiva** *f, inv*
overweight **sobrepeso; exceso de peso**
overweight (adj) **excesivamente gordo**
   adj; **excesivamente grueso** *adj*
pain, ache **dolor** *m*
   boring pain **dolor penetrante**
   burning pain **dolor ardiente; dolor**
      quemante
   colicky pain **dolor cólico**
   constant pain **dolor constante**
   dull pain **dolor sordo**
   growing pain **dolor de crecimiento**
   labor pain **dolor de parto**
   mild pain **dolor leve**
   moderate pain **dolor moderado**
   phantom limb pain **dolor de**
      miembro fantasma
   pressure-like pain **dolor opresivo**
   referred pain **dolor referido**
   root pain **dolor radicular**
   severe pain **dolor severo**
   sharp pain **punzada** *f;* **dolor agudo**
   sharp intestinal pain **torzón** *m*
   shooting pain **dolor fulgurante**
   steady pain **dolor continuo**
   thoracic pain **dolor torácico**
   twinge **latido**[14] *m*
palpitation **palpitación** *f;* **latido**[14]
palsy **parálisis** *f;* **paralización** *f*
   Bell's palsy **parálisis facial**
   cerebral palsy **parálisis cerebral**
   shaking palsy (Parkinson's disease)
      enfermedad de Parkinson *f;*
      parálisis agitante
pancreatitis **pancreatitis** *f*
paralysis **parálisis** *f;* **paralización** *f*
paranoia **paranoia**
paraplegia **paraplejía; parálisis de la**
   mitad inferior del cuerpo
parasite **parásito**
   amoeba **ameba; amiba**
   ascaris (roundworm) **ascaris** *f;*
      lombriz grande redonda *f;* **ascáride** *f*
   chigger flea **nigua; garrapata; guina**
      Mex.
   common name **nombre común** *m*
   cysticercus (bladderworm) **cisticerco**
   distribution **distribución** *f*
   flea **pulga**
   focus of infection **foco de infección**
   form of parasite in feces **forma de**
      los parásitos en heces
   giardia **giardia**
   gnat **jején** *m, Sp. Am.;* **bobito** *Chicano*
   louse **piojo**
      crab louse **ladilla**
      nit **liendre**
   metazoos **metazoos**
   mite **ácaro**
   parasitic cyst **quiste** *m;* **ladilla**
   pediculosis **pediculosis** *f;* **piojería**
   protozoa **protozoarios**
      flagellates **flagelados**
   route of entry **vía de entrada**
   schistosoma **esquistosoma** *f;*
      bilharzia
   sporozoa **esporozoarios**
   tapeworm **solitaria; lombriz**
      solitaria; tenia
      solium **solitaria; gusano tableado**
   threadworms **tricocéfalos** *f;* **oxiuro;**
      lombriz chiquita afilada *f*

trichinosis **triquinosis** *f*
trichocephalus **tricocéfalo; lombriz**
   de látigo *f*
uncinaria (hookworm) **uncinaria;**
   lombriz de gancho *f*
   worm **gusano; lombriz** *f*
      intestinal worm **verme** *m*
pellagra **pelagra**
perforated eardrum **tímpano perforado**
pericarditis **pericarditis** *f*
peritonitis **peritonitis** *f;* **panza**
   peligrosa[15] *slang;* **abdomen agudo**[15]
   m, slang
pertussis **tos convulsiva** *f;* **tosferina;**
   coqueluche *f;* **tos ferina** *f;* **tos**
   ahogana *f*
pharyngitis **faringitis** *f*
phlebitis **flebitis** *f;* **tromboflebitis** *f*
phlegm **flema**
phthisis **tisis** *f;* **consunción** *f*
pigeon-toed **patizambo** *adj*
pile **almorrana; hemorroides** *f, pl*
pimple **grano de la cara, barrillo;**
   butón *m;* **pústula; buba**
   blackhead pimple **espinilla; barro**
pinched nerve **nervio aplastado**
plague **peste** *f;* **plaga**
   bubonic plague **peste bubónica; tifo**
      de oriente
pleurisy **pleuresía**
pneumonia **pulmonía; neumonía**
pock **viruela; postilla; cacaraña** *Guat.,*
   Mex.
poison **veneno** *manmade;* **ponzoña**
   natural
   poison ivy **hiedra venenosa;**
      chechén *m;* **zumaque venenoso** *m*
poisoning **envenenamiento;**
   intoxicación *f*
   botulism poisoning **intoxicación**
      botulínica
   carbon monoxide poisoning
      intoxicación por monóxido de
      carbono
   food poisoning **envenenamiento**
      por comestibles; intoxicación con
      alimentos
   lead poisoning **envenenamiento del**
      plomo; saturnismo;
      envenenamiento plúmbico
   salmonella poisoning **intoxicación**
      por salmonellas
   staphylococcal poisoning
      intoxicación por estafilococos
polyp **pólipo**
poor health, in **en mala salud**
presbyopia **presbiopía; presbicia;**
   hipermetropía
prickly heat **salpullido; picazón** *f;*
   erupción debido al calor *f*
proctitis **proctitis** *f*
prostatitis **prostatitis** *f;* **tapado de orín** *m*
prostration **postración** *f*
   heat prostration **postración del calor**
psoriasis **soríasis** *f;* **mal de pintas** *m*
psychosis **sicosis** *f*
psychosomatic **sicosomático** *adj*
psychotic **sicótico** *adj*
pterygium **pterigión** *m;* **carnosidad** *f,*
   fam
pus **pus** *m*
pustule **pústula; grano; bubón** *m*
pyorrhea **piorrea; mal de las encías** *m*

quinsy (sore throat) **esquinancia;**
   amigdalitis supurativa *f*
rabies **rabia; hidrofobia**
rape **violación** *f;* **rapto** *Chicano*
rash **salpullido; erupción** *f;* **alfombra**
   P.R., Cuba; **sarpullido**
   diaper rash **pañalitis** *f;* **chincual** *m,*
      Mex.
   wheals (hives) **ronchas**
redness **rubor** *m*
relapse **recidiva; recaída; atrasado** *adj*
renal **renal** *adj*
rheum **reuma** *m*
rheumatism **reumatismo; reumas** *m*
rhinitis **rinitis** *f;* **escurrimiento de la**
   nariz
rickets **raquitis** *m;* **raquitismo**
risk **riesgo**
roseola **roséola; rubéola**
rubella **sarampión alemán** *m;* **rubéola;**
   roséola epidémica; fiebre de tres días
   f; **peluza** *Mex.;* **alfombría** *Chicano;*
   alfombrilla *Chicano;* **sarampión**
   bastardo *m*
rupture (hernia) **hernia; ruptura;**
   relajación *f;* **rotura; reventón** *m;*
   quebradura; rotadura *Chicano*
sarcoma **sarcoma**
   Kaposi's sarcoma **sarcoma de Kaposi**
scab **postilla; costra** *m;* **cuerín** *m,*
   Chicano; **cuerito** *Chicano*
scabies **sarna; guaguana** *slang;* **gusto**
   slang
scale **escama** *f*
scar **cicatriz** *f*
schizophrenia **esquizofrenia**
schizophrenic **esquizofrénico** *adj*
sciatica **ciática**
scotoma (spots before the eyes)
   escotoma *m;* **manchas frente a los ojos**
scratch **rasguño; rascado; raspón** *m,*
   Sp. Am.
   to scratch (relieve hurt) **rascar(se)**
   to scratch (hurt) **rasguñar**
scurvy **escorbuto**
seasickness **mareo; mal de mar** *m*
seborrhea **seborrea**
seizure **ataque** *m;* **convulsión** *f*
senile **senil** *adj*
senility **senilidad** *f;* **senectud** *f;*
   caduquez *f*
septicemia **septicemia; bacteriemia;**
   toxemia; piemia; infección en la
   sangre *f, fam*
serious **grave** *adj;* **serio** *adj*
severe **agudo** *adj;* **severo** *adj;* **fuerte** *adj*
shingles **zona; herpes** *m;* **zoster** *f*
shock **choque** *m;* **sobresalto;**
   commoción nerviosa *f;* **susto**
   anaphylactic shock **choque alérgico**
      fam; **choque anafiláctico**
sick **enfermo** *adj;* **malo** *adj*
short of breath **ahoguío** *fam;* **ahoguijo**
   fam
shortsighted **miope** *adj;* **cegato** *adj, fam*
sickliness **achaque** *m*
sickly **enfermizo** *adj;* **pálido** *adj;*
   demacrado *adj;* **cholenco** *adj, Chicano*
sickness **enfermedad** *f;* **padecimiento;**
   mal *m;* **dolencia**
simulation **fingimiento**
sinus congestion **congestión** *f;*
   sinusitis *f*

sleeping sickness **enfermedad del sueño** *f*

smallpox **viruela**

smegma **esmegma** *m*; **queso** *slang*

sore **pena; dolor** *m*; **aflicción** *f*
  sore ears **mal o dolor de oídos** *m*
  sore eyes **dolor de ojos** *m*
  sore throat **mal o dolor de garganta** *m*; **garganta inflamada**

sore (wound) **llaga; úlcera; grano**

souffle **silbido** *Mex.*

spasm **espasmo; contracción muscular** *f*; **latido** *Chicano*

spasmodic **espasmódico** *adj*; **intermitente** *adj*; **irregular** *adj*

spastic **espástico** *adj*; **espasmódico** *adj*

splinter (in the eye) **esquirla** *f*; **astilla (en el ojo)**

spot **mancha**

spotted sickness **mal de pinto** *m*; **pinta**

sprain **torcedura; dislocación** *f*; **esguince** *f*; **falseo** *Chicano*

squint-eyed **ojituerto** *adj*; **bizco** *adj*; **bisojo** *adj*

stammering **tartamudeo; balbucencia**

stiff **tieso** *adj*
  stiff ("frozen") joint **articulación envarada** *f*; **articulación trabada** *f*
  stiff neck **nuca tiesa** *fam*; **torticolis** *m*; **tortícolis** *m*

sting (of an insect) **picadura; piquete** *m*; **punzada**
  ant sting **picadura de hormiga**
  bee sting **picadura de abeja**
  blackwidow spider sting **picadura de viuda negra; picadura de ubar** *fam*
  botfly sting **picadura de moscardón**
  chigoe/jigger/sandflea sting **picadura de nigua**
  flea bite **picadura de pulga**
  hornet sting **picadura de avispón**
  mosquito sting (bite) **picadura de mosquito**
  scorpion sting (bite) **picadura de alacrán**
  spider sting **picadura de araña**
  tick **picadura de garrapata**
  wasp sting **picadura de avispa**

stomachache **dolor de estómago** *m*

strabismus **estrabismo; bizco** *C.A.*

strain **tensión** *f*; **torcedura**
  straining (tenesmus) **pujos** *fam*

strep throat **estreptococia; mal o dolor de garganta por estreptococo** *m, fam*

stress **tensión** *f*

stricture **constricción** *f*; **estrictura; estenosis** *f*; **estrechez** *f*

stroke **derrame cerebral** *m*; **embolia cerebral; parálisis** *f*; **hemorragia vascular; ataque fulminante** *m*; **apoplejía; estroc** *m, Chicano*; **embolio** *Chicano*

stuffed-up head **constipado**

stuttering **tartamudez** *f*; **balbucencia**

sty **orzuelo; perrilla** *fam*

suffocation **sofocación** *f*; **asfixia**

suicide **suicidio**

sunstroke **insolación** *f*; **soleada** *Am.*

suntanned **bronceado** *adj*; **tostado** *adj*

suppuration **supuración** *f*

swelling **hinchazón** *f*; **tumor** *m*; **tumefacción** *f*

bump on the head **chichón** *m*

swollen **hinchado** *adj*

symptom **síntoma** *m*

syndrome **síndrome** *m*

syphilis **sífilis** *f*; **sangre mala** *f, slang*; **mal francés** *m, slang*; **mal de bubas** *m, slang*; **infección de la sangre** *f, euph*; **lúes** *f*; **avariosis** *f, Sp. Am.*

tachycardia **taquicardia**

tantrum **berrinche** *m, fam*
  temper tantrum **pataletas**

tartar, dental **sarro; saburra; tártaro**

tattoo(ing) **tatuaje** *m*

tetanus **tétanos; mal de arco** *m, slang*; **trimo**
  infantum tetanus **moto** *slang, Mex.*; **siete (7) días** *m*; **mozusuelo** *Mex.*

thrombophlebitis **tromboflebitis** *f*; **flebitis** *f*

thrombosis **trombosis** *f*
  coronary thrombosis **trombosis coronaria** *f*

thrush **afta; algodoncillo** *fam*

tic **tic** *m*; **tirón** *m*; **sacudida**
  tic douloureux **tic doloroso de la cara** *m*

tonsillitis **amigdalitis** *f*; **tonsilitis** *f*

toothache **dolor de muelas** *m*; **dolor de dientes** *m*; **odontalgia** *f*

tooth decay **caries** *f*; **dientes podridos** *m*

toxemia **toxemia**

tracheostomy **traqueostomía**

trauma **traumatismo; trauma** *m*

tremor **tremor** *m*; **tremblor** *m*

tubercular **tuberculoso** *adj*; **afectado** *adj, Chicano*

tuberculosis **tuberculosis** *f*; **tisis** *f*; **manchado del pulmón** *Mex.*; **afectado del pulmón** *Chicano, Mex.*; **peste blanca** *f*
  scrophula (scrofula) **escrófula**
  skin TB **tuberculosis de la piel** *f*

tumor **tumor** *m*; **neoplasma** *m*; **neoformación** *f*; **tacotillo** *Chicano*

tumor on the head **chiporra** *Guat., Hond.*

twisted **torcido** *adj*; **zambo** *adj*

ulcer **úlcera**
  gastric ulcer **úlcera gástrica**
  peptic ulcer **úlcera péptica**

unconscious **inconsciente** *adj*; **naqueado** *adj, Chicano*

unconsciousness **insensibilidad** *f*; **inconsciencia**

underweight **peso escaso; falta de peso**

uremia **uremia; intoxicación de orín** *f*

urinary problem **mal de orín** *m*; **problema de las vías urinarias** *m*

urticaria **urticaria**

uterus prolapse **prolapso de la matriz; caída de la matriz; prolapso del útero**

varicose vein **várice** *f*; **vena varicosa; variz** *m*

venereal disease (VD) **enfermedad venérea** *f*; **secreta** *slang*; **EV** *f*
  canker sore **postemilla; úlcera gangrenosa**
  chancre **chancro; grano**
    hard **chancro duro; chancro sifilítico**
    noninfecting **chancro simple; chancro blando**

chlamidia **clamidia**

cold sore **fuegos en la boca no los labios; herpes labial** *m*

condyloma **condiloma** *m*

genital wart **verruga genital; verruga venérea**

gonorrhea **gonorrea; blenorragia** *f*; **purgaciones** *f, pl, slang*; **gota** *slang*; **mal de orín** *m, slang*; **chorro** *euph, Chicano*

herpes **herpe(s)** *m/f*
  genitalis **herpes genitalis** *m*
  menstrualis **herpes menstrual** *m*
  zoster **herpes zoster** *m*

lymphogranuloma venereum **linfogranuloma venéreo** *m*; **bubones** *m*

moniliasis **moniliasis** *f*; **algodoncillo; boquera; candidiasis** *f*; **muguet** *m/f*

nongonoccocal urethritis **uretritis no gonococal** *f*

nonspecific urethritis **uretritis no específica** *f*; **uretritis inespecífica** *f*

sexually transmitted diseases **enfermedades pasadas sexualmente** *f*

syphilis **sífilis** *f*; **sangre mala** *f, slang*; **infección de la sangre** *f, euph*

trichomonas **tricomonas**

venereal lesion **úlcera; chancro; grano**

vesicular eruption **erupción vesicular** *f*

victim **víctima**

virus **virus** *m*

vision, blurred **vista borrosa**

vision, double **vista doble**

vitiligo **vitíligo; ciricua** *fam*; **jiricua** *slang*

vomit **vómito**

wart **verruga; mezquino** *Mex.*
  plantar wart **ojo de pescado** *fam*

weak **débil** *adj*

weakness **debilidad** *f*

weal (large welt) **verdugón** *m*; **cardenal** *m*

wen **lobanillo; lupia**

wheal **roncha; pápula**

whiplash **lesión de latigazo** *f*; **contusión de la columna vertebral** *f*; **latigazo** *fam*

whooping cough **tos convulsiva** *f*; **tos ferina** *f*; **coqueluche** *f*; **tosferina** *f*; **tos ahogona** *m, Mex.*

wound **herida; llaga; lastimadura; coco**
  abrasion **abrasión** *f*; **escoriación** *f*
  chafe **rozadura**
  cut **cortadura; cortante** *f*
  incised wound **herida incisa**
  incision **incisión** *f*; **cisura**
  knife wound **filorazo** *Chicano*
  laceration **laceración** *f*
  open skin wound **grano**
  puncture **herida penetrante; herida punzante**
  scrape **raspadura**
  tear (torn wound) **desgarro**

xerosis **xerosis** *f*; **resequedad de los ojos** *f*

PRINCIPAL MEDICAL ABBREVIATIONS

PRINCIPALES ABREVIATURAS MEDICAS

The following are selected medical abbreviations of Latin or Greek origin that are frequently used in prescription writing.

a a (ana—Greek)	of each	de cada uno (una)
aa	equal parts	a partes iguales
a.c. (ante cibos)	before meals	antes de comer
alt. dieb. (alternis diebus)	every other day	cada dos días
alt. hor. (alternis horis)	every other hour	cada dos horas
alt. noc. (alternis noctus)	every other night	cada dos noches
aq. (aqua)	water	agua
aq. dest. (aqua destillata)	distilled water	agua destilada
bib (bibe)	drink	beba
b.i.d. (bis in die)	twice a day	dos veces al (por) día
b.i.n. (bis in noctus)	twice a night	dos veces a la (por) noche
c̄ (cum)	with	con
cap. (capsula)	capsule	cápsula
et (et)	and	y
Gtt., gtt. (guttae)	drops	gotas
H. (hora)	hour	hora
h.n. (hac nocte)	tonight	esta noche
h.s. (hora somni)	at bedtime	al acostarse
liq. (liquor)	liquid; fluid	líquido; flúido
no. (numero)	number	número
non rep. (non repetatur)	do not refill; do not repeat	no se repita
noxt. (nocte; noxte)	at night	a la (por la) noche
omn. hor. (omni hora)	every hour	cada hora
omn. noct. (omni nocte)	every night	cada noche
os. (os; ora)	mouth	boca
p.c. (post cibum)	after meals	después de comer
p.r.n. (pro re nata)	as needed	cada vez que sea necesario
q.d. (quaque die)	every day	cada día
q.h. (quaque hora)	every hour	cada hora
q.i.d. (quarter in die)	four times a day	cuatro veces al (por) día
q. 2h.	every 2 hours	cada dos horas
q. 3h.	every 3 hours	cada tres horas
q. 4h.	every 4 hours	cada cuatro horas
q.l.; q.v.	as necessary	tanto como desee, a voluntad
q.m. (quaque mãne)	every morning	cada mañana
q.n. (quaque nocte)	every night	cada noche
q.s.; q. suff. (quantum sufficiat)	a sufficient quantity	cantidad suficiente
quotid. (quotidie)	every day	cada día
℞ (recipe)	take	tome
rep. (repetatur)	repeat; refill	repítase
S. (signa)	mark	indique
s (sans)	without	sin
Sig. (signetur)	directions	método
s.o.s. (si opus sit)	if necessary	si es necesario
stat. (statim)	immediately	inmediatamente
tab. (tabella)	tablet	tableta
t.i.d. (ter in die)	three times a day	tres veces al (por) día
t.i.n. (ter in nocte)	three times a night	tres veces a la (por la) noche

COMMON MEDICATIONS AND TREATMENTS

MEDICINAS Y TRATAMIENTOS COMUNES

acetaminophen **acetaminofén** m
acid **ácido**
  acetylsalicylic acid **ácido acetilsalicílico**
  ascorbic acid **ácido ascórbico**
  boric acid **ácido bórico**
  folic acid **ácido fólico**
  p-aminosalicylic acid (PAS) **ácido paraminosalicílico**
activated charcoal **carbón activado** m

adhesive plaster **emplasto adhesivo**
adhesive tape **esparadrapo; tela adhesiva; cinta adhesiva**
adrenalin **adrenalina**
alcohol **alcohol** m
  rubbing alcohol **alcohol para fricciones**
ammonia **amoníaco**
amphetamine **anfetamina**[16]
ampicillin **ampicilina**

ampule **ampolleta**
analgesic **analgésico** m, adj
anesthesia **anestesia**
anesthetic **anestético** m, adj; **anestésico** m, adj.
ankle support **tobillera**
antacid **antiácido** m, adj
antibiotic **antibiótico** m, adj
  broad-spectrum **de alcance amplio; de espectro amplio**

limited-scope   **de alcance reducido;
de espectro reducido**
antibody   **anticuerpo**
anticholinergic   **anticolinérgico** *m, adj*
anticoagulant   **anticoagulante** *m, adj*
antidote   **antídoto**
antiemetic   **antiemético** *m, adj*
antigen   **antígeno**
antihemorrhagic   **antihemorrágico** *adj*
antihistamine   **antihistamínico** *m, adj;*
droga antihistamínica
antimalarial   **antipalúdico** *m, adj*
antipyretic   **febrífugo; antipirético**
antiseptic   **antiséptico** *m, adj*
antispasmodic   **antiespasmódico** *m, adj*
antitetanic/anti-tetanus   **antitetánico** *adj*
antitoxin   **antitoxina; contraveneno**
application   **aplicación** *f*
arch supports   **soportes para el arco del
pie** *m*
arsenic   **arsénico**
artificial   **artificial** *adj;* **postizo** *adj*
artificial limb   **miembro artificial**
artificial respiration   **respiración
artificial** *f*
aspirin   **aspirina**[17]
children's aspirin   **aspirina para
niños**[17]
astringent   **astringente** *m, adj*
atropine   **atropina**
balsam   **bálsamo; ungüento**
band   **cinta; faja**
Band-Aid   **curita; venda; parchecito**
bandage   **vendaje** *m;* **venda**
elastic bandage   **vendaje elástico**
swathing bandage   **faja abdominal**
barbiturate   **barbiturato**[18]
bath   **baño**
bran bath   **baño de salvado**
emollient bath   **baño emoliente**
mustard bath   **baño de mostaza**
oatmeal bath   **baño de harina de avena**
potassium permanganate bath   **baño
de permanganato de potasio**
saline bath   **baño salino**
shower bath   **baño de regadera**
Chicano; **ducha**
sitz bath   **baño de asiento; semicupio**
sodium bath   **baño de sodio**
sponge bath   **baño de esponja; baño
de toalla** *Chicano*
starch bath   **baño de almidón**
sulfur bath   **baño de azufre**
tar bath   **baño de brea**
belladonna   **belladona**
benzedrine   **bencedrina**
benzoin   **benjuí** *m;* **benzoína**
bicarbonate of soda   **bicarbonato de soda**
binder   **vendaje abdominal** *m;* **cintura;
faja**
bleach   **cloro; blanqueo**
blood   **sangre** *f*[19]
blood count   **hematimetría**
blood plasma   **plasma sanguíneo** *m*
blood sugar   **azúcar sanguínea** *f*
blood transfusion   **transfusión de
sangre** *f*
booster shot   **inyección secundaria** *f;*
búster *m; Chicano* **inyección de
refuerzo** *f;* **reactivación** *f*
borax   **bórax** *m*
bottle   **botella; envase** *m;* **frasco**
brace   **braguero; aparato ortopédico**

Brewer's yeast   **levadura de cerveza**
bromide   **bromuro**
calamine   **calamina**
calcium   **calcio**
calcium sulfate   **escayola; sulfato de
calcio**
cane   **bastón** *m;* **báculo**
walking cane   **bastón de paseo**
capsule   **cápsula**
carbon tetrachloride   **tetracloruro de
carbono**
cast   **yeso; calote** *m;* **enyesadura;
vendaje enyesado** *m*
gypsum cast   **vendaje de yeso**
walking cast   **enyesadura para caminar**
cataplasm   **cataplasma**
cathartic   **purgante** *m*
catheter   **catéter** *m;* **sonda; tubo;
drenaje** *m, Chicano*
cauterization   **cauterización** *f*
camomile tea   **té de manzanilla** *m;* **agua
de manzanilla** *f*
chloramphenicol   **cloranfenicol** *m*
chloride   **cloruro**
chlorine   **cloro**
chloromycetin   **cloromicetín** *m;*
chloromycetin *m*
chlorophyll   **clorofila**
chloroquinine   **cloroquina**
cleanliness   **limpieza; aseo**
coagulant   **coagulante** *m, adj*
coal tar   **brea de hulla**
cocaine   **cocaína; nieve** *f, slang*[20]
cocoa butter   **manteca de cacao**
codeine   **codeína**[20]
cold pack   **emplasto frío; compresa fría**
comb, fine-tooth   **chino** *Mex.*
compress   **compresa; cabezal** *m*
contact lens   **lente de contacto** *m;*
pupilente *m;* **lentilla** *Spain*
contamination   **contaminación** *f*
contraceptive   **contraceptivo;
anticonceptivo**[21]
contraceptive pills   **pastillas
anticonceptivas**[21]
Coramine   **coramina**
corn plaster   **emplasto para callos;
parches para callos** *m*
corticosteroid   **corticosteroide** *m*
cortisone   **cortisona**
cotton   **algodón** *m*
absorbent cotton   **algodón absorbente**
cotton swab   **hisopillo; escobillón** *m*
sterile cotton   **algodón estéril**
cough drops   **gotas para la tos; pastillas
para la tos**
cough lozenges   **pastillas para la tos**
cough suppressant   **béquico; calmante
para la tos** *m*
cough syrup   **jarabe para la tos** *m*
crutch   **muleta**
cure   **cura; método curativo**
curettage   **curetaje** *m;* **raspado**
decongestant   **descongestionante** *m, adj*
dental floss   **hilo dental; cordón dental**
m; **seda encerada**
dentifrice   **dentífrico** *m, adj*
deodorant   **desodorante** *m, adj.*
depilatory   **depilatorio** *m, adj*
dextrose   **dextrosa; azúcar de uva** *m*
dialysis   **en diálisis**
diaphragm   **diafragma** *m;* **diafragma
anticonceptivo** *m*

digitalin   **digitalina**
diphenhydramine   **difenhidramina**
disinfectant   **desinfectante** *m, adj*
diuretic   **diurético** *m, adj;* **píldora
diurética**
dose   **dosis** *f, inv;* **medida**
douche   **ducha; ducha interna; lavado
vaginal; lavado interno; ducha
vaginal; irrigación** *f*
DPT   **vacuna triple**
drainage   **desagüe** *m*
drainage (surgical)   **drenaje** *m*
dram   **dracma** *m*
dressing   **cura** *f;* **curación** *f;* **apósito;
emplaste** *m;* **parche** *m;* **vendaje** *m*
dropper   **cuentagotas** *m, sg*
eye dropper   **gotero (para los ojos)**
Sp. Am. **cuentagotas** *m, sg*
drops   **gotas**
drug   **droga; medicina**
drug store   **farmacia** *f, Spain, Sp. Am.;*
droguería *f, Sp. Am.;* **botica**
electricity   **electricidad** *f*
current   **corriente** *adj*
ground(ing)   **a tierra**
lead wire   **alambre de contacto** *m*
outlet   **salida**
plug   **enchufe** *m;* **clavija de contacto**
polarity   **polaridad** *f*
socket   **enchufe** *m;* **tomacorriente** *f,
Sp. Am.*
electrocardiogram   **electrocardiograma**
m
electroencephalogram
electroencefalograma *m*
emetic   **emético** *m, adj;* **vomitivo** *m, adj*
emollient   **emoliente** *m, adj*
emulsion   **emulsión** *f*
enema   **enema** *f/m;* **lavativa; ayuda;
lavado**
enema bag   **bolsa para enema**
cleansing enema   **(enema) de
limpieza**
retention enema   **(enema) de
retención**
soapsuds enema   **(enema) jabonosa**
ephedrine   **efedrina**
epidemic   **epidemia**
Epsom salt   **sal de higuera** *f;* **sal de
Epsom** *f*
erythromycin   **eritromicina**
estrogen   **estrógeno**
eucalyptus leaves   **hojas de eucalipto**
expectorant   **expectorante** *m, adj*
expiration date   **fecha de caducidad**
external   **externo** *adj*
extract   **extracto**
eyecup   **copa ocular; ojera; lavaojos** *m,
inv*
eyeglasses   **anteojos** *m, pl;* **lentes** *m, pl;*
gafas *f, pl;* **espejuelos** *m, pl;* **quevedos**
m, pl
eye salve   **ungüento para los ojos**
first aid   **primeros auxilios** *m, pl;*
primera ayuda
flask   **frasco**
fluoride   **flúor** *m*
foam   **espuma**
forceps   **pinzas; fórceps** *m;* **gatillo** *m,
dental;* **tenazas** *f*
frozen section   **corte por congelación** *m*
fumigation   **fumigación** *f*
fungicide   **fungicida** *m, adj*

gargle   **gárgara**

gargle, to   **hacer gárgaras; hacer buches** *fam*

gauze   **gasa**

gentian violet   **violeta de genciana**

germicide   **germicida** *m, adj*

glass eye   **ojo de vidrio**

glucose   **glucosa**

glue   **goma; cola**

glycerine   **glicerina**

graft   **injerto**

guaiacol   **guayacol** *m*

hearing aid   **aparato para la sordera; prótesis auditiva** *f;* **prótesis acústica** *f;* **audífono; aparato auditivo; audiófono**

heat   **calor** *m*

heat therapy   **termoterapia; tratamiento térmico**

hemostat   **hemostato**

herbicides   **herbicidas** *m;* **matayerbas** *f*

heroin   **heroína**

home cure   **curación casera** *f*

home remedy   **remedio casero**

hormone   **hormón** *m;* **hormona**

hot water bag   **bolsa de agua caliente**

hydrogen peroxide   **agua oxigenada; peróxido de hidrógeno**

hypodermic injection   **inyección hipodérmica** *f*

hypodermic needle   **aguja hipodérmica**

hypodermic syringe   **jeringuilla hipodérmica**

ice   **hielo**

ice(bag) pack   **bolsa de hielo; bolsa de caucho para hielo**

ichthyol   **ictiol** *m*

immunization (vaccine)   **inmunización** *f;* **vacuna**

booster dose   **dosis de refuerzo** *f, inv*

schick test   **prueba de schick**

ingredient   **ingrediente** *m*

injection   **inyección** *f;* **indección** *f, Chicano;* **chot** *m, Chicano*

intracutaneous injection   **inyección intracutánea**

intradermic injection   **inyección intradérmica**

intramuscular injection   **inyección intramuscular**

intravenous injection   **inyección intravenosa**

subcutaneous injection   **inyección subcutánea**

inoculation   **inoculación** *f*

insecticide   **insecticida** *m, adj*

insect repellant   **repelente de insectos** *m*

instrument, sharp-edged   **instrumento afilado**

insulin   **insulina**

internally   **internamente** *adv*

intrauterine device   **dispositivo intrauterino; aparato intrauterino**

intrauterine loop   **espiral intrauterino** *m*

iodine   **yodo**

iron   **hierro**

isolation   **aislamiento por cuarentena**

IV (intravenous) solution   **solución endovenosa** *f;* **suero por la vena**

jelly   **jalea**

kilogram   **kilogramo**

kit   **estuche** *m;* **botiquín** *m*

emergency kit   **botiquín de emergencia** *m*

first aid kit   **botiquín de primeros auxilios; equipo de urgencia**

knife   **cuchillo**

knot   **nudo**

label   **etiqueta**

laboratory   **laboratorio**

laboratory findings   **hallazgos de laboratorio**

laboratory test   **análisis de laboratorio** *m, inv*

laryngoscope   **laringoscopio**

lavage   **lavado**

lavatory   **lavamanos** *m, inv*

laxative   **laxativo; laxante** *m;* **purgante** *m*

lens   **lente** *m*

level   **al ras**

lindane   **lindano**

liniment   **linimento**

liquid   **líquido**

liter   **litro**

liver extract   **extracto de hígado**

loop (IUD)   **lazo**

lotion   **loción** *f;* **crema**

lozenge   **pastilla; trocisco; pastilla de chupar**

LSD   **drogas alucinantes; DAL** *f*

lubricant   **lubricante** *m;* **lubricativo** *adj*

lukewarm   **templado** *adj;* **tibio** *adj*

lye   **lejía**

magnesia   **magnesia**

milk of magnesia   **leche de magnesia**

magnifying glass   **lupa**

marijuana   **mariguana;**[25] **yerba; grifa**

mask   **máscara**

massage   **masaje** *m*

mattress   **colchón** *m*

measure   **medida**

measuring cup   **taza de medir**

medication   **medicación** *f;* **medicamento; medicina**

medicine   **medicina; medicamento; droga**

medicine cabinet (medicine chest)   **botiquín** *m;* **despensa** *Chicano*

patent medicine   **medicina de la farmacia; medicina de la botica; medicina patentada** *f;* **medicina registrada**

menthol   **mentol** *m*

mentholatum   **mentolato** *Chicano*

Mercurochrome   **mercurocromo**

Merthiolate   **mertiolato**

methadone   **metadona**

milligram   **miligramo**

milliliter   **mililitro**

mineral   **mineral** *m*

mineral water   **agua mineral**

mint leaves   **hojas de yerbabuena**

mixture   **mezcla**

moderate   **moderado** *adj*

moist   **húmedo** *adj*

morphine   **morfina**

mouthwash   **lavado bucal; enjuagatorio; listerina** *fam*

mouthpiece   **bocal** *m;* **boquilla**

mustard   **mostaza**

mustard bath   **baño de mostaza**

mustard plaster   **cataplasma de mostaza; sinapismo**

narcotic   **narcótico; droga somnífera; droga estupefaciente; estupefaciente** *m*

needle   **aguja**

hypodermic needle   **aguja hipodérmica; jeringa; jaipo** *slang*

nitro(glycerin)   **nitro(glicerina)** *f*

novocaine   **novocaína**

oil   **aceite** *m*

baby oil   **aceite para niños**

castor oil   **aceite de ricino**

cod liver oil   **aceite de hígado de bacalao**

mineral oil   **aceite mineral**

ointment   **ungüento; crema; pomada; unto**

operation   **operación** *f*

ophthalmic   **oftálmico** *adj*

ophthalmoscope   **oftalmoscopio**

opium   **opio; chinaloa** *slang*

oxygen   **oxígeno**

pacemaker   **aparato cardiocinético; marcador de paso** *m;* **marcapaso; monitor cardíaco** *m;* **marcador de ritmo** *m;* **seno auricular**

pain killer   **calmante** *m;* **analgésico**

palliative   **paliativo** *m, adj*

Pap smear   **test de Pap** *m;* **prueba de Papanicolaou; untos de Papanicolaou; frotis de Papanicolaou** *m*

paregoric   **paregórico**

patch   **parche** *m*

penicillin   **penicilina**

pennyroyal leaves   **hojas de poleo**

peroxide   **peróxido**

hydrogen peroxide   **agua oxigenada; peróxido de hidrógeno**

sodium peroxide   **peróxido de sodio**

pesticide   **pesticida** *m;* **plaguicida** *m*

pharmacy   **farmacia; botica**

phenobarbital   **fenobarbital** *m*

pill   **píldora; pastilla**

birth control pill   **píldoras para control de embarazo**[21]; **pastillas para no tener niños**[21]; **píldora anticonceptiva**[21]

sleeping pill   **píldora para dormir; sedativo; píldora somnífera; somnífero; soporífera**

thyroid pill   **medicación tiroides** *f*

pillow   **almohadilla**

inflatable rubber "doughnut"   **almohadilla neumática en forma de anillo**

piperazine   **piperazina; piperawitt** *m/f;* **piperidol** *m;* **anterobius** *m*

plasma   **plasma** *m*

plaster of Paris   **yeso mate**

pleural tap   **toracentesis** *f;* **toracocentesis** *f;* **punción quirúrgica de la pared torácica** *f*

poison   **veneno; ponzoña; intoxicación** *f*

poisonous   **venenoso** *adj;* **ponzoñoso** *adj*

pomade   **pomada**

potassium   **potasio**

potassium iodide   **yoduro de potasio**

potassium permanganate   **permanganato de potasio**

potion   **poción** *f;* **dosis** *f, inv*

poultice   **cataplasma; emplasto**

powder   polvo

powdered   en polvo *adj*

powdery   polvoriento *adj;* polvoroso *adj;* empolvado *adj*

prescribe, to   recetar; prescribir (un remedio)

prescription   receta; prescripción *f*

prick   pinchazo; punzada; afilerazo

prick, to   pinchar; punzar

probe   estilete *m;* sonda; tienta

prophylactic   profiláctico *m, adj*

prosthesis   prótesis *f;* miembro artificial

purgation   purgación *f*

purgative   purgante *m;* catártico *m, adj*

purge   purga; purgante *m;* lavado; lavativo

quart   cuarto

quinine   quinina

radiation shield   blindaje contra la radiación *m*

radiation therapy   radioterapia

radiation treatment   radiaciones *f*

relief   alivio

relieve, to   aliviar

remedy   remedio; medicamento

restraining device   coercitivo; medio de restricción

restroom   baño; cuarto de baño; servicios; WC[22] *m* excusado

resuscitation   resucitación *f*
   cardiopulmonary resuscitation (CPR)   resuscitación cardiopulmonar (RCP)
   mouth-to-mouth resuscitation   resucitación boca a boca

rhythm method   método del ritmo; ritmo

ring (IUD)   anillo

rub   fricción *f;* frotación *f*

rub, to   frotar; restregar

rubber (condom)   goma; condón *m;* preservativo

rubber bulb, syringe   pera de goma

rubber gloves   guantes de goma *m, pl*

saccharine   sacarina

saline solution   agua con sal *f;* agua salina *f*

salt   sal *f*
   salt water   agua salada
   iodized salt   sal yodada
   noniodized salt   sal corriente
   smelling salts   sales aromáticas *pl;* sales perfumadas *pl*

salve   pomada; ungüento

sample   muestra

sanitary napkin   kotex *m;* servilleta sanitaria; almohadilla higiénica; absorbente higiénico *m*

scalpel   escalpelo; bisturí *m*

sedative   sedante *m;* sedativo; calmante *m*

serum   suero
   antivenin serum   suero antiviperino
   black widow spider antivenin serum   suero antialacrán

shield (IUD)   escudo

shot   inyección *f;* chot *m, Chicano*

silver nitrate   nitrato de plata

size   tamaño
   assorted size   tamaño surtido
   large size   tamaño grande
   small size   tamaño pequeño

sling   cabestrillo; honda

soap   jabón *m*

sodium pentothal   pentotal de sodio *m;* pentotal sódico *m*

solution   solución *f*

soporific   soporífico; narcótico

specimen   muestra; espécimen *m*

spectacles   anteojos *pl, general term;* lentes *m, pl, Mex.;* espejuelos *pl, Cuba;* gafas *pl; (quevedos pl, wire-rimmed)*

spermaticide, vaginal   espermaticida vaginal

spinal puncture (spinal tap)   punción lumbar *f*

spiral (IUD)   espiral *m*

splint   tablilla; férula
   in a splint   entablillado *adj*

spoonful   cucharada

spray   rociador *m;* pulverizador *m;* pulverización *f*

stain (staining)   coloración *f;* colorante *m*
   acid-fast stain   coloración acidorresistente
   Giemsa's stain   coloración de Giemsa
   Gram's stain   coloración de Gram
   methylene blue stain   coloración de azul de metileno
   Wright's stain   coloración de Wright
   Ziehl-Neelsen stain   colorante de Ziehl-Neelsen

steam   vapor *m*

sterile   estéril *adj;* infecundo *adj*

sterility   esterilidad *f;* infecundidad *f*

sterilization   esterilización *f*

sterilized   esterilizado *adj*

sterilizer   esterilizador *m*

stethoscope   estetoscopio; fonendoscopio

stimulant   estimulante *m*

stitch   sutura; punto; puntada

stocking, elastic   calceta elástica

stomach pump   bomba estomacal

streptomycin   estreptomicina

stylet   estilete *m*

substitute   substituto

sugar   azúcar *m/f*

sulfathiazole   sulfatiazol *m*

sulphur   azufre *m*
   sulphur powder   polvo de azufre

sunglasses   gafas de sol *f, pl;* anteojos oscuros *m, pl*

suntan lotion   crema para el sol; loción bronceadora *f*

support   apoyo; soporte *m;* sostén *m*

supporter, athletic   suspensorio

suppository   supositorio; cala; calilla
   vaginal suppository   óvulos *pl*

suture   sutura; puntada

sweetener   dulcificante *m*

sweets   dulces *m, pl;* golosinas *f, pl*

syringe   jeringa; jeringuilla
   disposable syringe   jeringa descartable; jeringa desechable
   glass cylinder syringe   jeringa con cilindro de cristal
     hollow needle syringe   jeringa con aguja hueca
   hypodermic syringe   jeringuilla hipodérmica; jaipo *slang*
   piston, plunger of syringe   émbolo

syrup of ipecac   jarabe de ipeca *m;* jarabe de ipecacuana *m*

tablespoonful   cucharada

tablet   comprimido; tableta; pastilla

tampon   tampón *m;* tapón *m*

tea   té[23] *m*
   chamomile tea   té de manzanilla;[23] agua de manzanilla[23] *f*
   croton tea   té de pionillo[23]
   damiana tea   té de damiana[23]
   desert milkweed tea   té de hierba del indio[23]
   elderberry and lavender tea   té de flor de sauz y hojas de alhucema[23]
   herb rose tea   té de rosa de castilla[23]
   "Mormon" tea   té de cañutillo (del campo)[23]
   parsley tea   té de oshá[23]
   sarsaparilla tea   té de cocolmeca;[23] té de zarzaparrilla[23]
   spasm herb tea   té de hierba del pasmo[23]
   spearmint tea   té de yerbabuena;[23] té de menta verde[23]
   spider milkweed tea   té de inmortal[23]
   swamp root tea   té de hierba del manzo[23]
   tansy mustard herb tea   té de pamita[23]
   wild marjoram tea   té de orégano[23]
   wormseed tea   té de epazote;[23] té de México;[23] té borde[23]

teaspoonful   cucharadita
   level teaspoonful   cucharadita llena al ras

tepid   tibio *adj*

Terramycin   terramicina

test   examen *m;* prueba; análisis *m, inv*
   serology test   prueba serológica
   skin test   reacción cutánea *f*
   sputum test   análisis de esputos
   test tube   tubo de ensayo
   tuberculin test   tuberculina
   urinalysis   urinálisis *m, inv;* análisis de la orina *m, inv*

tetanus   tétano(s); mal de arco *m;* pasmo seco

tetracycline   tetraciclina

therapeutic   terapéutico *adj*

therapy   terapia; tratamiento

thermomenter   termómetro
   oral   oral *adj*
   rectal   rectal *adj*

tongue-depressor   pisa-lengua *f;* abatelengua *f;* depresor de la lengua *m*

tonic   tónico

tourniquet   torniquete *m;* liga

traction   tracción *f*

tranquilizer   tranquilizante *m;* calmante *m;* apaciguador *m*

transfusion   transfusión *f*

transmission   transmisión *f*
   droplet transmission   transmisión por gotillas
   transmission by contact   transmisión mediante contacto
   vector transmission   transmisión mediante vector

vehicle   vehículo

treatment   tratamiento

truss   braguero; faja

turpentine   trementina

ultraviolet lamp   lámpara de rayos ultravioletas

unguent   pomada; ungüento

urinalysis   urinálisis *m, inv;* análisis de la orina *m, inv*
   midstream urinalysis   orina recogida a mitad de la micción; uricultivo

vaccination **vacunación** *f;* **inoculación** *f*
  booster **refuerzo**
  DPT **triple** *f*
vaccine, immunization **vacuna;**
  inmunización *f*
  oral polio vaccine **vacuna oral**
    contra polio; gotas para polio
Vaseline **vaselina**
vermifuge **vermífugo** *m, adj;*
  antihelmíntico *m, adj*
vial **vial** *m;* **botella; frasco** *m;* **ampolla**

vinegar **vinagre**
vitamin **vitamina**
  calcium **calcio**
  iron **hierro; sulfato ferroso**
  niacin **niacina**
  vitamin B_1 **tiamina**
  vitamin B_2 **riboflavina**
  vitamin B_6 **piridoxina**
  vitamin C **ácido ascórbico**
vomitive **vomitivo** *m, adj;* **emético** *m,*
adj

walker **andador** *m*
warm **tibio** *adj*
warmer **más caliente** *adj;* **calentador**
weight **peso**
wheelchair **silla de ruedas**
wrapping in a cold (wet) sheet
  empacamiento en sábana fría
  (mojada)
x-ray **radiografía** *f;* **rayos equis; retrato**
  del x-ray *Chicano*
x-ray therapy **radioterapia**

COMMON POISONS

VENENOS COMUNES

INHALED POISONS *VENENOS ASPIRADOS*

gas **gas** *m*

smoke **humo**

vapor **vapor** *m*

INJECTED POISONS *VENENOS INYECTADOS*

rat bites **picadas de ratas**
scorpion bites **picadas de escorpión**

snake bite **mordedura de culebra**

snake bite, poisonous **mordedura de**
  víbora venenosa

ORAL POISONS *VENENOS TOMADOS POR LA BOCA*

acetic acid **ácido acético (puro)**
ammonia **amoníaco**
arsenic acid **ácido arsénico**
ascorbic acid **ácido ascórbico**
bichloride of mercury **cloruro mercúrico**
camphor **alcanfor** *m*
carbolic acid **ácido carbólico**
carbon tetrachloride **tetracloruro de**
  carbono
cyanic acid **ácido cianótico**
detergents **detergentes** *m*
disinfectant **desinfectante** *m*
furniture polish **pulimento para**
  muebles

hydrochloric acid **ácido clorhídrico**
hydrofluoric acid **ácido fluorhídrico**
iodine **yodo**
kerosene **keroseno; querosén** *m;*
  queroseno
lye **lejía**
mushrooms **hongos**
nitric acid **ácido nítrico**
oil of wintergreen **aceite de gaulteria** *m*
oxalic acid **ácido oxálico**
phosphoric acid **ácido fosfórico**
pine oil **aceite de pino** *m*
rubbing alcohol **alcohol para**
  fricciones *m*

silver nitrate **nitrato de plata**
sodium carbonate **carbonato de sodio**
sodium hydroxide **hidróxido de sodio**
sodium hypochlorite (bleach)
  hipoclorito de sodio (blanqueador
  de ropa, *m***)**
sodium sulfate (in toilet cleaners)
  sulfato de sodio (en limpiadores de
  inodoros)
strychnine **estricnina**
sulfuric acid **ácido sulfúrico**
turpentine **esencia de trementina**

ANTIDOTES

ANTIDOTOS

cause vomiting, to **provocarse el vómito**
drink plenty of, to **beber mucho (mucha)**
egg white **clara de huevo**
flour **harina**
ground chalk in water **creta**
  pulverizada en agua
hot coffee **café caliente** *m*
milk **leche** *f;* **milque** *f, Chicano*
mustard water **agua con mostaza**

salt water **agua salada**
soapy water **agua jabonosa**
starch **almidón** *m*
stomach pump **bomba estomacal**
strong tea **té cargado** *m;* **té fuerte** *m*
syrup of ipecac **jarabe de ipecacuana** *m*
universal antidote **antídoto universal**
  animal carbon—2 parts **carbón**
    animal—dos partes

calcined magnesia—1 part **magnesia**
  calcinada—una parte
tannic acid—1 part **ácido tánico—**
  una parte
vomit, to **vomitar; dompear** *Chicano;*
  arrojar *fam*

SELECTED DRUG ABUSE TERMINOLOGY

TERMINOLOGIA ESCOGIDA PARA EL ABUSO DE DROGAS—PARA LOS ESTUPEFACIENTES[24]

Acapulco gold (Marijuana)
  colombiana; grifa; grifo; Juana;
  Juanita; lucas; mariguana[25]**, monte;**
  mota; yerba; yesca; zacate; sinsemilla

acid (LSD) **ácido; aceite; azúcar; LSD**[22]
addict (drug) **adicto; adicto a**
  droga(s); adicto a las drogas
  narcóticas; drogadicto;

morfinómano; tecato; toxicómano;
  yeso
addict in search of a fix **buscatoques**
  m/f, inv

addiction (drug)   **adicción; drogadicción; farmacodependencia; hábito; toxicomania**

administer marijuana to someone, to   **amarihuanar; engrifar; enmarihuanar**

amphetamine   **anfetamina; ácido; a; bombido; estimulante; naranjas**
amphetamine + heroin + barbiturates + IV amphetamines   **bombita**

ampule   **pomo**

angel dust (PCP)   **cucuy; fencycladina; líquido; PCP[22]; polvo**

artillery   **equipo hipodérmico; estuche; herramienta; herre; R**

bad trip   **mal viaje; experiencia mala en el uso de drogas**

bag   **bolsita; paquete** *m*

balloon (of heroin)   **cimbomba; globo**

bang, to   **clavarse; componerse; curarse; filerearse; jincarse; picarse; rayarse; shootear**

barbiturate (pill)   **barbitúrico; barbiturato; cacahuate** *m*; **colorada; globo**

barrels (green)/(the) beast   **aceite** *m*; **ácido; azúcar; LSD[22]**

be carrying narcotic drugs, to   **andar carga; andar cargado; cargar; traer carga**

be (non-)habit forming, to   **(no) crear vicio**

bennies (benz, benzies—amphetamines)   **anfetaminas; benzedrinas; blancas**

be on the nod, to (be under the influence of heroin)   **cotorear**

big C (cocaine)   **carga; coca; cocaína; nieve** *f*; **perico** *Cuba*; **talco** *Texas, Cuba*

bindle (quantity of marijuana or narcotics)   **bolsita, paquete** *m*

blasted, to be   **andar botando; andar hypo; andar loco; andar locote; andar pasado; andar prendido; andar servido; andar hasta las manitas; hasta las manos; elevado a-mil; subido a-mil**

blow snow, to   **aspirar cocaína**

blue angels (blue devils, blue dolls, blue heavens, blues—amobarbital sodium)   **amital; cápsulas azules**

blue star (morning-glory seeds)   **dompedro; semillas de dondiego de día**

boy (heroin)   **azúcar** *Arizona, Texas*; **caballo; carga; chiva; cohete** *m*; **heroína**

brick (usually a kilogram of marijuana or narcotics)   **ladrillo**

burn out, to   **doblar(se)**

busted, to be   **ser arrestado; ser torcido**

buzz, to get a   **agarrar onda**

buzz, to have a (effect of a drug)   **sonarse**

buzzed, to be   see "high, to be," "blasted, to be"

caffeine   **cafeína**

candy (barbiturates)   **barbitúricos**
(cocaine)   **carga; coca; cocaína; nieve** *f*; **perico** *Cuba*; **talco** *Texas, Cuba*

cap (capsule)   **cachucha; cápsula; deque** *m*; **gorra**

charged up, to be   see "high, to be," "blasted, to be"

chip, to (to use narcotics infrequently)   **chipiar, chipear**

cigarette butt   **bachica** *esp. marijuana*; **tecolota; tecla**

clean, to be   **andar derecho; andar limpio**

clear up, to   **cortarse el vicio; kikear; quitear**

coast, to   see "high, to be," "blasted, to be"

cocaine[26]   **acelere; aliviane; alucine; arponazo; azúcar; blanca nieves; carga; chutazo; coca; cocacola; cocada; cocazo; coco; coka; cotorra; cucharazo; doña blanca; glacis** *m*; **knife** *m*; **marizazo; nice, nieve** *f*; **nose; pase** *m*; **pepsicola; pericazo; perico** *Cuba*; **polvo; polvito; talco** *Texas, Cuba*; **tecata**

crack cocaine   **crac** *m*; **crack** *m*

codeine[27]   **codeína**

cold turkey   **a la brava; a lo bronco**

croaker, hungry[28]   **matasanos avaricioso**

deal in drugs, to   **dilear; diliar**

depressant   **deprimente; debilitante**

devils (seconal, barbiturates)   **coloradas; diablos; rojas**

dexedrine (dexies—dextroamphetamine)   **dexedrina; dextroanfetamina**

dime   **diez dólares; diez años de prisión;** *sinónimo para diez*

dime bag (envelope of heroin, cocaine, or marijuana)   **paquete de drogas**

dope   **droga; estupefaciente; fármaco; narcótico; nombre inglés para mariguan (see below)**

dope pusher   **narcotraficante; burro; madre; pusheador**

doper   **mariguano; moto; quemón; yesco**

downer (downs—barbiturate)   **calmante; sedativo; tranquilizante**

drag (puff of marijuana cigarette)   **toque** *m*

drop(n)   **entrega; lugar donde se deja o se esconde una droga**

drug   **droga; estupefaciente** *m*; **fármaco; narcótico**

drug, to   **endrogar**

drug abuse   **abuso de las drogas, de los estupefacientes**

drugged   **endrogado; prendido**

drug habit   **morfinomanía**

drug supply   **cachucha**

drug traffic   **venta y tráfico de drogas**

dump, to (to get rid of)   **dompear**

dust (cocaine, PCP)   **cucuy; fencycladina; líquido; PCP[22]; polvo**

falling out (overdose of narcotics or sedatives)   **durmiéndose; durmiéndose a medias**

fit (outfit—tools necessary for injection of drugs: needle, syringe [eyedropper and rubber bulb] cooker, cotton and matches, tie off)   **equipo hipodérmico; estuche** *m*; **herramienta; herre** *f*; **R[22]** *f*

fix (an IV injection of drugs)   **abuja; abujazo; cura; filerazo; gallazo**

fix, to (to inject drugs)   **clavarse; componerse; curarse; filerearse; jincarse; picarse; rayarse; shootear**

fix up, to (to heat and mix heroin)   **arreglar; cuquear**

flashing, to be[29]   **oler cola**

flip, to   **volverse(ue) loco**

floating, to be   see "high, to be," "blasted, to be"

flying saucers (morning-glory seeds)   **dompedro; semillas de dondiego de día**

freak out, to   see "high, to be," "blasted, to be"

gallery (place to take drugs)   **galería**

gas (nitrous oxide)   **gas exhilarante; gas hilarante; óxido nitroso**

get down, to (to acquire drugs)   **tomar drogas; usar drogas**

get in the groove, to   **ponerse al tanto**

glass eyes (drug addict)   see "addict (drug)"

glue   **cola; goma**

glue sniffer   **glufo**

gluey   **drogadicto a cola**

goofballs (sedatives, especially barbiturates)   **cápsulas de drogas**

gravy (a mixture of blood and heroin)   **salsa**

gun   **equipo hipodérmico; estuche; herramienta; herre, R[22]**

H (heroin)   **azúcar** *Arizona, Texas*; **caballo; carga; chiva; cohete; heroína**

habit   **adicción; drogadicción; farmacodependencia; hábito; habituación; toxicomanía**

hallucinogen   **alucinante; alucinógeno**

hangover, to have a   **andar crudo**

hash (hashish)   **hachís; hachich; haschich** *m*

heroin[30]   **achivia; adormidera; amor; ardor; arpon; arponazo; azúcar, azufre, banderilla; blanca; blanco; borra blanca; ca-ca; caballo; cagada** *vulgar*; **carga; cáscara; chiva; chutazo; cohete; cristales; cura; dama blanca; gato; golpe; goma; H[22]; helena; heroica; heroína; la cosa; la duna; lenguazo; manteca; nieve; papel; papelito; pasta; pericazo; piquete; polvo; polvo amargo; polvo blanco; stufa; tecata**

heroin capsule   **cachucha; capa; gorra; timba**

heroin user (addict)   **tecato**

high, to be   **andar botando; andar hypo; andar loco; andar locote; andar pasado; andar prendido; andar servido; andar hasta las manitas; hasta las manos; elevado a-mil; subido a-mil**

high, to get   **agarrar onda; andar botando; andar hipo; andar loco; andar locote; andar pasado; andar prendido; andar servido; sonarse**

high from glue sniffing   **glufo** *adj*

high from sniffing paint thinner   **tiniado** *adj*

high on (marijuana) (turned on)   **moteado** *adj*; **motiado** *adj*

high on (narcotics)   **alivianado; caballón; loco; locote; sonámbulo; sonado**

high on pills   **píldoro**

hit up, to   **clavarse; componerse; curarse; filerearse; jincarse; picarse; rayarse; shootear**

hooked on drugs   **prendido**

hook on narcotics, to   **prender**

hot shot ([often fatal]) overdose   **dosis excesiva; sobredosis; sobredosis tóxica**

hype (an addict who uses subcutaneous injections)   **adicto; adicto a drogas; drogadicto; tecato** hypo, to lay the   see "bang, to"

hypodermic needle used to inject drugs   **jaipo**

ingest narcotic pills, to   **pildorear(se); pildoriar(se)**

inhalant   **inhalante**

inhale glue, to   **aspirar cola; inhalar cola; respirar cola**

injection (of a narcotic substance)   **abuja; abujazo; inyección; piquete** *m*

inject oneself with drugs, to   **clavarse; componerse; curarse; darse un piquete; filerearse; inyectarse; jincarse; picarse; rayarse; shootear**

in need, to be   **andar enfermo**

in transit   **tripeando**

jab, to jack off, to   "inject oneself with drugs, to," see "inject oneself with drugs, to"

jagged up, to be (under the influence of drugs)   "blasted, to be"

jerk off, to   see "inject onself with drugs, to"

jive stick (marijuana cigarette)   **charuto; cigarro de mariguana; frajo; frajo de seda; leño; leñito; pito**

joint (marijuana cigarette)   **abuja; charuto; cigarro de mariguana; frajo; frajo de seda; leño; pito**

jolly pop, to (to use drugs infrequently)   **chipear; chipiar**

joy pop, to (to use drugs infrequently)   **chipear; chipiar**

junkie (narcotic addict)   **adicto; adicto a drogas; drogadicto; morfinómano; tecato; toxicómano; yeso**

kick   **patada**

kick the habit, to   **cortarse el vicio, kikear, quitear**

kit   see "fit"

lactose (used to cut heroin)   **lactosa**

layout   see "fit"

letdown   **bajón**

loaded, to be   see "blasted, to be"

loaded, to get   **agarrar onda; sonarse**

load of narcotics   **carga**

LSD[31]   **aceite; aceitunas; acelide; ácido(s); alucinantes; avándaro; azúcar; blanco de España; bomba; café; cápsulas; chochos; cohete; colorines; cristales; diablos; divina; droga alucinante; dulces; elefante blanco; en onda; gis; grasas; la salud; lluvia de estrellas; mica; mureler; nave; orange; papel; paper; piedrita de la luna; pit; purple haze; saturnos; sugar; sunshine; tacatosa; terrones; trip; viaje; viaje en las nubes; white; ácido; lisérgico; droga LSD; ALD**

machinery   see "fit"

magic mushrooms (psilocybin)   **hongos**

mainline, to   **inyectar drogas directamente en la vena principal del brazo**

mainliner   **jaipa; jaipo**

maincure, to (clean and prepare marijuana for rolling into cigarettes)   **limpiar (mariguana)**

marijuana[32]   **achicalada; alfalfa; bacha; bailarina; café; campechana verde; canabis; cáñamo; carrujo; cartucho; chara; chester; chiclona; chichara;** chira; chupe; churus; cochornis; coffee; colombiana; cosa; cris; de la buena; diosa verde; doña Juanita; epazote; fitoca; flauta; flor de Juana; frajo; ganga; ganja; gavos; golden; griefo; grifa; grifo; grilla; grass; guato; güera; habanita; hashi; hierba; hoja verde; huato; índico; jani; Jefferson; joint; Juana; Juanita; Kris Kras; la verde; lucas; macoña; mafufa; mani; Margarita; mari; María; Maria Juanita; Mariana; mariguana; marihuana; marijuana; marinola; mariola; marquita; Mary Jane; Mary Poppins; meserole; monstruo verde; monte; mora; mostaza; mota; oro verde, panetela; pasto; pastura; pepita verde; petate; petate del soldado; pitillo; pito; pochola; pod; polillo; pot; queta; rollo; té; toque; tronadora; verdosa; yedo; yerba; yerba verde; yerba de oro; yerba del diablo; yerba santa; yerbabuena; yesca; zacate *low-grade variety*

marijuana smoker   **yesco**

marijuana user   **grifo; mariguano; marihuano; marijuano; moto; quemón; yesco**

marks   see "tracks"

member of police narcotics squad   **narco**

mescaline[33]   **mescalina**

morning glory seeds[34]   **semillas de dondiego del día; dompedro**

morphine[35]   **morfi; morfina**

nail (needle for drug injection)   **abuja; aguja; filero; hierro; jeringuilla; punta**

narcotic   **narcótico; droga; estupefaciente; fármaco**

narcotic pills   **pinguas**

narcotic substitute   **la otra cosa**

nebbis[36] (barbiturates)   **amarillas; gorras amarillas**

need, to be in   **andar enfermo**

needle   **abuja; aguja; filero; hierro; jeringuilla; punta**

OD, to (to overdose)   **doblar(se); dar una dosis excesiva**

opiate   **opiáceo; opiado**

opium[37]   **goma; material negro; opio**

outift   see "fit"

overdose   **dosis excesiva; sobredosis; sobredosis tóxica**

overdosed   **sobredosado**

packet of heroin   **gramo**

paraphernalia   see "fit"

paregoric   **paregórico**

PCP[38]   **cucuy; fencycladina; líquido; PCP[22]; polvo**

peddler (drug dealer)[39]   **burro; madre; narcotraficante; pusheador; traficante; vendedor de drogas**

person high on drugs   **cócono**

pill freak   **píldoro**

pill head   **píldoro**

pill popper   **píldoro**

pop, to (to inject with a needle)   see "inject onself with drugs, to"

poppy   **amapola**

Product IV   **combinación de PCP y LSD**

provide an addict with a fix, to   **curar** psilocybin[40]   **las mujercitas; los niños; hombrecitos; hongos**

psychedelic   **droga psicodélica; sicodélico**

push, to   **pushar**

put heroin in capsules, to   **capear; capiar**

roach (butt of a marijuana cigarette)   **bacha; bachilla; colilla; cucaracha; tecla; tecolota; tocola**

runner (carrier of drugs)[41]   **caballo; mula**

scoff, to   **ingerir/injerir (ie) narcóticos**

scoop, to   **aspirar narcóticos**

score, to   see "inject oneself with drugs, to"

seconal[42]   **seconal; colorada; diablo; roja**

sedative   **calmante; sedativo**

shoot (up), to   see "inject onself with drugs, to"

shoot oneself, to   see "inject oneself with drugs, to"

skin, to   **inyectar narcóticos**

sleep walker (heroin addict)   **tecato; adicto a heroína**

smoke marijuana, to   **motear; motiar; tronar(se); quemar**

sniff glue, to   **aspirar cola; hacer(se) a la glu(fa); inhalar cola; respirar cola; sesonar**

snort, to (to sniff residue of powdered narcotics)   **estufear; estufiar; aspirar narcóticos por la nariz**

snow bird   **adicto a cocaína**

soaring, to be   see "blasted, to be"

spaced (out), to be   see "blasted, to be"

spike (a hypodermic needle)   **abuja; aguja; filero; hierro; jeringuilla; punta**

stash, to (to hide supply of drugs)   **clavar; plantar**

stimulant   **estimulante; exitante**

stoned, to be   see "blasted, to be"

strung out, to be   see "blasted, to be"

syringe   see "spike"

take (drugs), to   **ingerir (ie); injerir (ie); adminstrarse; tomar**

take a hit, to (to take a puff from a joint)   **quemar; tronarse; tronársela**

take marijuana, to   **amarihuanarse, enmarihuanarse, engrifarse**

take up, to   see "take a hit, to"

tolerance   **tolerancia**

track marks   see "tracks"

tracks (marks and scars caused by use of hypodermic needle)   **marcas; trakes, traques**

traffic in drugs, to   **dilear; diliar; traficar**

tranquilizer   **ansilítico; tranquilizante**

trip, to   **tripear**

trip out, to   **agarrar onda; sonarse**

user   **adicto; adicto a drogas; drogadicto; tecato; toxicómano; yeso**
   of marijuana, cocaine and morphine   **maricocaimorfi**
   of morphine   **morfiniento**
   of pills   **pildoriento**

weed, to blow (to smoke marijuana)   **motear; motiar; tronar**

wired, to be   see "inject oneself with drugs, to"

yage[43]   **ayahuasca**

zonked, to be   see "blasted, to be"

EXCRETIONS

EXCRECIONES

excretion   excreción *f;* miércoles *m, inv, euph*

feces   "aguas mayores" *f;* caca *slang;* cámara; deposiciones *f;* evacuación del vientre *f;* excrementos; heces fecales *f, pl;* materia fecal; miércoles *m, inv, euph;* mierda *vulgar;* pase del cuerpo *m*

stool   see "feces"
   stool specimen   muestra de excremento; muestra de heces fecales

sweat   sudor *m*

urine   "aguas menores" *f;* chi *f, vulgar;* orina *f;* orines *m*

collection of the specimen   acumulación de la muestra *f;* toma de la muestra; recolección de la muestra *f*

color of the urine   color de la orina *m*
   straw   de paja
   yellow   amarillo

urine constituents   componentes de orina *m*
   acetone   acetona
   albumin   albúmina
   ammonia   amoníaco
   bile   bilis *f*

bilirubin   bilirrubina
blood   sangre *f*
calcium   calcio
chlorides   cloruro
creatine   creatina
crystal(s)   cristal(es) *m*
glucose   glucosa
phosphate   fosfato
solids   sólidos
total nitrogen   nitrógeno total
total sulphur   azufre total *m*
urea   urea
urobilin   urobilina
urobilirubin   urobilirrubina

BLOOD

SANGRE

antibody   anticuerpo

antigen   antígeno

bleeding   pérdida de sangre de poca intensidad; sangría; flujo de sangre
   bleeding tendencies   tendencias a sangrar
   bleeding time   tiempo de hemorragia; tiempo de sangría

blood   sangre *f;* colorada *slang, Chicano*
   blood, cord   sangre umbilical
   blood, occult   sangre oculta
   blood, whole   sangre entera; sangre pura

blood bank   banco de sangre

blood chemistry (analysis of blood)   análisis de sangre *m, inv*

blood clot   coágulo de sangre; cuajarón de sangre *m*

blood component   componente de sangre *m;* componente sanguíneo *m*
   dessicated red blood cells   hematíes desecados *m*
   fresh blood   sangre fresca *f*
   oxalated blood   sangre oxalatada *f*
   platelet enriched blood   sangre enriquecida en plaquetas *f*
   stored blood   sangre conservada *f*
   whole blood   sangre pura *f*

blood corpuscles   corpúsculos de la sangre; glóbulos
   blood corpuscles, red   eritrocitos; glóbulos rojos
   blood corpuscles, white   glóbulos blancos; leucocitos

blood count   biometría hemática; recuento hemático; recuento sanguíneo; cifra de los elementos figurados de la sangre; hematimetría

blood culture   hemocultivo

blood donor   donante de sangre *m/f;* donador(a) de sangre *m/f*
   plasmapheresis donor   donante para plasmaféresis

blood exchange   exanguino-transfusión *f*

blood flow   corriente sanguínea *f*

blood formula   fórmula hemática

blood group   grupo sanguíneo
   universal donor   donante universal *m/f*
   universal recipient   receptor *(a)* universal *m/f*

blood-grouping   determinación de los grupos sanguíneos *f*

blood lavage   lavado de la sangre

blood oxygen analyzer   analizador del oxígeno de la sangre *m*

blood path   vía sanguínea

blood picture   cuadro hemático; fórmula hematológica

blood pigment   pigmento sanguíneo

blood plasma   plasma sanguíneo *m*

blood platelet (blood plaque)   plaqueta sanguínea; trombocito

blood poisoning   intoxicación de la sangre *f;* toxemia; septicemia; sepsis *f;* envenenamiento de la sangre

blood pressure   presión de la sangre *f;* presión arterial *f;* tensión arterial *f*
   blood pressure cuff (sphygmoma-nometer)   esfigmomanómetro; manguito de presión sanguínea
   blood pressure gauge   hemodinamómetro

blood serum   suero sanguíneo

blood smear   frotis sanguíneo *m;* extensión de sangre *f*

bloodstained   sanguinolento *adj*

blood stock   depósito de sangre

bloodstream   corriente sanguínea *f;* torrente circulatorio *m*

blood studies   exámenes hematológicos *m*

blood sugar   azúcar sanguíneo *m;* glucemia

blood supply   aporte de sangre *m;* irrigación *f*

blood test   examen de la sangre *m;* análisis de sangre *m, inv*

SMA analisis   múltiple secuencial *m, inv*

blood transfusion   transfusión sanguínea *f*

blood type   grupo sanguíneo

blood typing   determinación del grupo sanguíneo *f*

blood urea   urea

blood vessel   vaso sanguíneo

clot reaction time   tiempo de retracción del coágulo

coagulation time   tiempo de coagulación

cross match   pruebas cruzadas

determination of circulation time   determinación del tiempo de circulación *f*

erythrocytes (red blood cells)   eritrocitos; glóbulos rojos; hematíes *m*

fibrin   fibrina

hemoglobin   hemoglobina

leukocytes (white blood cells)   leucocitos; glóbulos blancos
   nucleated leukocytes   leucocitos nucleados
   acidophiles   acidófilos
   basophiles   basófilos
   blood platelets   plaquetas sanguíneas
   eosinophiles   eosinófilos
   lymphocytes   linfocitos
   monocytes   monocitos
   polymorphonuclear neutrophiles   neutrófilos polimorfonucleares
   "polymorphs"   "polimorfos"
   reticulocytes   reticulocitos
   thrombocytes   trombocitos

plasmapheresis   plasmaféresis *f*

prothrombin time   tiempo de protrombina

RBC (red blood count)   numeración de glóbulos rojos *f;* NGR *f*

sedimentation   sedimentación *f*
   erythrosedimentation   eritrosedimentación *f*

unit of blood   unidad de sangre *f*

WBC (white blood count)   numeración de glóbulos blancos *f;* NGB *f*

PREGNANCY, CHILDBIRTH, CONTRACEPTION, POSTNATAL CARE OF THE MOTHER

▌ *EMBARAZO, PARTO, CONTRACEPCION, CUIDADO POSNATAL DE LA MADRE*

abortion   **aborto**
  induced abortion   **aborto inducido; aborto provocado**
  spontaneous abortion   **aborto espontáneo**
  therapeutic abortion   **aborto terapéutico**
  threatened abortion   **amenaza de aborto**
abscess   **absceso**
abscessed (adj)   **apostemado** *adj*
abstain from sexual relations, to   **abstenerse de las relaciones sexuales**
add, to   **añadir; agregar**
afterbirth   **secundinas** *f, pl, Mex.;* **placenta; segundo parto** *Chicano*
alcohol   **alcohol** *m*
  rubbing alcohol   **alcohol para fricciones**
amenorrhea   **amenorrea**
amniocentesis   **amniocentesis** *f;* **prueba del saco amniótico**
amniotic sac   **saco amniótico**
amniotic fluid   **agua del amnios**
anesthesia   **anestesia**
  block   **anestesia de bloque**
  caudal   **anestesia caudal**
  epidural   **anestesia epidural**
  general   **anestesia total**
  inhalation   **anestesia por inhalación**
  local   **anestesia local**
  regional   **anestesia regional**
  saddle block   **anestesia en silla de montar**
  spinal   **anestesia espinal; anestesia raquídea**
  twilight sleep   **sueño crepuscular**
apron   **delantal** *m*
baby, infant   **criatura; bebé** *m;* **nene** *m;* **nena; guagua** *m/f, Chile, Ec., Peru, Bol., Ur.;* **tierno** *C.A.*
bag of waters   **fuente** *f, fam;* **bolsa de las aguas; bolsa membranosa; aguas** *f, pl*
bathe, to   **bañar**
bear down, to   **pujar; hacer bajar por fuerza**
become bloated, to   **abotagar**
bed   **cama; lecho**
bilirubin   **bilirrubina**
bind, to   **atar; amarrar**
binder   **cintura; faja**
  "belly" binder   **ombliguero**
birth   **nacimiento**
  at term   **a término**
  multiple birth   **nacimiento múltiple**
  post-term   **nacimiento tardío**
  premature   **nacimiento prematuro**
birth, to give   **dar a luz; parir; alumbrar; sanar** *euph;* **salir de su cuidado** *Chicano;* **aliviarse** *Chicano*
birth canal   **canal del parto** *m*
birth certificate   **certificado de nacimiento; partida de nacimiento**
birth control   **control de la natalidad**
  Billing's method   **método de Billing**

cervical cap   **gorro cervical**
coil   **coil** *m, Chicano*
coitus interruptus   **interrupción de coito** *f;* **retirarse** *m;* **salirse** *m, slang*
condom   **condón** *m;* **hule** *m, slang;* **forro** *vulgar, Arg.;* **preservativo** *slang;* **goma**
diaphragm   **diafragma (anticonceptivo)** *m*
IUD   **DIU** *m;* **dispositivo intrauterino; aparato intrauterino; aparatito** *Chicano*
loop   **alambrito; lupo; asa**
pill   **píldora; pastilla**
rhythm   **ritmo; método de ritmo**
rubber   **goma; forro** *vulgar, Arg.;* **hule** *m, slang*
sterilization   **esterilización** *f*
tubal ligation   **ligadura de (las) trompas**
vaginal cream   **crema vaginal**
vaginal foam   **espuma vaginal**
vaginal jelly   **jalea vaginal**
vasectomy   **vasectomía**
birthmark   **lunar** *m*
birth weight   **peso del nacimiento**
bladder   **vejiga**
blanket   **frazada**
bleed in excess, to   **desangrar**
bleeding   **flujo de sangre; pérdida de sangre de poca intensidad; hemorragia;** (hemorrhage); **sangría**
bleeding (adj)   **sangrante** *adj*
bleeding, breakthrough   **hemorragia inesperada; flujo de sangre por la vagina inesperadamente**
bleeding to excess   **desangramiento**
bloated   **hinchado** *adj;* **abotagado** *adj*
blood   **sangre** *f*
  blood circulation   **circulación sanguínea** *f*
  blood clot   **coágulo sanguíneo; cuajarón** *m*
  blood count   **hematimetría; recuento sanguíneo**
  blood donor   **donante de sangre** *m/f*
  blood group   **grupo sanguíneo**
  blood plasma   **plasma sanguíneo** *m*
  bloodstain   **mancha de sangre**
  bloodstained   **manchado de sangre** *adj*
  blood transfusion   **transfusión de sangre** *f*
  blood, whole   **sangre entera; sangre pura**
bloody   **cruento** *adj;* **sangriento** *adj*
bloody show   **muestra de sangre; tapón de moco** *m, Mex.;* **secreción mucosa mezclada con sangre** *f;* **mucosidad teñida de sangre** *f*
blotches, skin   **manchas oscuras en la piel**
boil the bottles, to   **hervir (ie) las botellas**

bottle, baby   **biberón** *m;* **bote** *m, slang, Chicano;* **botella; mamadera** *Sp. Am.;* **pacha** *Chicano;* **tele** *f, Chicano*
breast   **seno; pecho; teta; chichas** *pl, C.R.;* **chiche** *m, Sp. Am.;* **chichi** *f, Mex.;* **tele** *f, Chicano*
  breast of a wet nurse   **chiche** *m, Mex. Guat.*
  caked breast   **mastitis por estasis** *f*
  painful breasts   **senos dolorosos**
breastfeed, to   **dar el pecho; dar de mamar; dar chiche; criar con pecho** *Chicano*
breastfeeding   **lactancia maternal**
breast pump   **mamadera; bomba de ordeñar; tiraleches** *f, inv*
breechbirth (frank breech)   **presentación trasera** *f;* **presentación de nalgas** *f*
burp   **eructo; regüeldo**
burp, to   **eructar; repetir (i); sacar aire** *Chicano;* **urutar** *Chicano*
buttock[44]   **nalga; salvohonor** *m, fam;* **bombo** *Ur.*
caeserean delivery   **parto cesáreo; parto por operación**
caesarean section   **operación cesárea** *f;* **sección cesárea** *f*
can opener   **abrelatas** *m, inv*
catheter   **catéter** *m;* **sonda**
catheterize   **cateterizar**
cervix   **cerviz** *f;* **cuello de la matriz; cuello del útero; cérvix** *f*
childbirth   **parto; alumbramiento**
chloasma (facial discoloration) (mask of pregnancy)   **paño; mancha del embarazo; mancha de la preñez; cloasma** *m*
circumcise, to   **circuncidar**
circumcision   **circuncisión** *f*
clitoris   **clítoris** *m;* **bolita** *slang;* **pelotita** *slang*
coitus   **coito**
colic   **cólico** *adj*
colostrum   **calostro**
conceive, to   **concebir (i)**
conception   **concepción** *f;* **fecundación del huevo** *f*
confinement   **puerperio; cuarentena;[45] riesgo; alumbramiento**
congenital malformations   **malformaciones congénitas** *f*
constipation   **estreñimiento**
continue working, to   **seguir (i) trabajando**
contraceptive   **anticonceptivo** *m, adj;* **contraceptivo** *m, adj*
contractions   **contracciones de la matriz** *f;* **dolores de parto** *m*
cord   **cordón** *m*
  umbilical cord   **cordón umbilical; cordón del ombligo**
cotton   **algodón** *m*
  cotton swab   **hisopo de algodón**
crack, to   **agrietar; rajar**

cramps (menstrual) **calambres** m; **dolores del período** m
  (muscular) **calambres** m
  (postpartum pains) **entuertos**
crib **camilla de niño; cuna**
  warming crib **camilla calentadora de niño; incubadora; estufa; armazón de calentamiento** f
crown, to **coronarse; estar coronando**
crowning **coronamiento**
curettage **curetaje** m; **raspado**
D&C **raspa** fam; **legrado** fam
dangle one's legs, to **colgar (ue) las piernas**
deliver, to **dar a luz; parir; tener el niño; aliviarse** Chicano
delivery **parto**
  abdominal **parto abdominal**
  breech **extracción de nalgas**
  delivery room **sala de partos**
  forceps **extracción con fórceps** f
  premature **parto prematuro**
diaper **pañal** m; **braga; zapeta** Mex.; **pavico** Chicano
diaper, to **cambiar el pañal; renovar (ue) el pañal; proveer con pañal**
diaper rash **salpullido; escaldadura (en los bebés); chincual** m, Mex., Chicano
diet **dieta; régimen** m
  be on a diet, to **estar a dieta**
  put on a diet, to **poner a dieta**
dilation (of cervix) **dilatación del cuello de la matriz** f
dirty, to be **estar caquis maquis** euph
discharge **flujo; secreción** f; **supuración** f; **desecho; descarga**
discharge (bloody) **derrame** m
discharge (from the hospital), to **dar de alta**
dissolve, to **disolver (ue)**
douche **lavado vaginal; ducha vaginal**
drop **gota**
dry, to **secar**
duct **conducto**
eclampsia **eclampsia**
edema **edema** m; **hinchazón** f
ejaculate, to **eyacular; venirse** slang
elbow **codo**
embryo **embrión** m
enema **enema** f/m
  barium **enema de bario; enema opaca**
  soapsuds **enema jabonosa**
engorgement **estancamiento**
episiotomy **corte de las partes** m; **episiotomía; tajo** slang
estrogen **estrógeno**
exercise moderately, to **hacer ejercicios moderados**
expulsion **expulsión** f
eyepads **paños en los ojos; toallas en los ojos**
eye shield **escudo ocular**
fainting spell **desvanecimiento**
  during pregnancy **achaque** m, C.R.
family **familia**
  family planning **planificación de la familia** f; **planificación familiar** f
feed, to **alimentar**
fetal heart tone **latido del corazón fetal**
fetoscope **estetoscopio fetal; fetoscopio**
fetus **feto**

fever **fiebre** f; **calentura** Mex., Chicano
fill, to **llenar**
fissure **fisura; cisura**
fontanel **fontanela; mollera**
forceps (obs.) **fórceps** m
formula **fórmula**
forty days following parturition **cuarentena**[46]
fundus **fondo del útero**
funnel **embudo**
gestation **gestación** f; **gravidez** f
glass (drinking) **vaso**
glucose water **agua con azúcar**
go down in the birth canal, to **encajarse**
gynecologist **ginecólogo**
hair **pelo; cabello(s)**
  pubic hair **vello púbico; pelo púbico; pendejo** slang
heartbeat **latido cardíaco**
heartburn **acedía; agriera** Sp. Am.; **agruras; pirosis** f; **acidez** f
heating pad, electric **almohadilla caliente eléctrica**
hemorrhoids **hemorroides** f; **almorranas**
hormone **hormona; hormón** m
hymen **himen** m
ice **hielo**
  ice bag **bolsa de hielo**
  ice pack **aplicación de hielo empaquetado** f
inch **pulgada**
incision **incisión** f; **cortada**
incubator **incubadora; estufa**
infant **bebé** m; **criatura; nene** m; **nena**
infection **infección** f
infertile **infértil** adj; **estéril** adj; **capón** adj, Chicano
intercourse **relación sexual** f
jar **frasco; envase** m
labor **parto; trabajo de parto**
  artificial **parto artificial**
  be in labor, to **estar de parto; enfermarse** Chicano
  complicated **parto complicado**
  dry **parto seco**
  false **parto falso**
  first stage of **primer período del parto**
  immature **parto inmaturo**
  induced **parto inducido**
  instrumental **parto instrumental**
  multiple **parto múltiple**
  pains **dolores de parto** m
  premature **parto prematuro**
  prolonged **parto prolongado**
  room, labor **sala de partos; sala prenatal**
  second stage of **segundo período del parto**
  spontaneous **parto espontáneo**
  third stage of **tercer período del parto**
lactation **lactancia**
length of pregnancy (LOP) **duración del embarazo** f
lump **tumorcito; bola; bulto; protuberancia**
lying-in after childbirth **sobreparto**
massage **masaje** m
massage, to **sobar; dar masaje**
masturbate, to **masturbar(se); puñetear** vulgar; **hacerse la casqueta** Chicano

maternity **maternidad** f; **de maternidad** adj
  maternity clothes **ropa de maternidad**
  maternity floor **piso de maternidad**
  maternity hospital **casa de maternidad**
measure, to **medir (i)**
  measuring cup **taza de medir**
menarche **primera regla menarquia**
menstruate, to **menstruar; perder (ie) sangre; estar mala; estar indispuesta; tener el mes; estar mala de la luna; estar mala de la garra; tener/traer la garra**
menstruation **menstruación** f, general term; **mes** m; **período** fam; **administración** f, Mex.; **regla** Mex., P.R.; **costumbre** f; **luna** Chicano; **enferma** euph; **tiempo del mes** fam
mentally retarded **retardado** adj; **simple** adj, euph; **inocente** adj, euph
mental retardation **retardo mental; retraso mental**
midwife (quack) **rinconera**
  (trained) **partera**
  (untrained) **comadrona**
miscarriage **malparto; parto malogrado**
mix, to **mezclar**
morning sickness **vómitos del embarazo; enfermedad matutina** f; **mal de madre** m; **ansias matutinas**
navel **ombligo**
nipple (breast) **pezón** m; **chichi** f, Arg.
  nipple, cracked **grieta del pezón**
  nipple, engorged (caked) **pezón enlechado**
  (of a baby nursing bottle) **tetilla; chupón** m; **mamadera; tetina; tetera** Mex. Cuba, P.R.
  nipple shield **escudo para el pezón; pezonera**
nurse **enfermera**
  baby nurse **nodriza; ama de cría; niñera**
  nursemaid **niñera**
  wet nurse **nodriza; chichi** f, fam, Mex., Guat.; **chichigua** vulgar, Sp. Am.
nurse, to **amamantar; dar el pecho al niño; criar a los pechos; dar de mamar**
nursery **cuarto de los niños**
  newborn nursery **sala de los recién nacidos**
nursing **amamantamiento; crianza; lactante** adj; **de crianza** adj
  nursing bottle **biberón** m; **mamadera; tetera**
  nursing bra **sostén de maternidad** m
  nursing pad **almohadita**
obstetric **obstétrico** adj
obstetrical **obstétrico** adj
obstetrician **obstétrico** m/f; **médico partero** m/f; **tocólogo** m/f
obstetrics **obstetricia; tocología**
oil **aceite** m
ointment **ungüento; pomada**
orgasm **orgasmo**
ounce **onza**
outpatient **paciente externo** m/f; **paciente ambulatorio** m/f
ovary **ovario**
overdue **atrasado** adj

ovulate, to **ovular**
ovulation **ovulación** *f*
ovum **óvulo; huevo**
oxytocic **oxitócico**
oxytocin **oxitocina**
pacifier **chupete** *m;* **mamón** *m, Chicano*
pain **dolor** *m*
  bearing-down **sensación de pesantez en el perineo** *f*
  expulsive **dolores expulsivos**
  false **dolores falsos**
  hunger **dolores de hambre**
  intermenstrual **dolores intermenstruales**
  labor **dolores de parto**
  premonitory **dolores premonitorios**
  shooting **dolor fulgurante**
  wandering **dolor errante**
pant, to **jadear; resollar (ue)**
panting **jadeante** *adj;* **jadeo**
pediatric **pediátrico** *adj*
pediatrician **pediátra** *m/f*
pediatrics **pediatría** *f, inv*
pelvic **pelviano** *adj;* **pélvico** *adj*
pelvimeter **pelvímetro**
pelvis **pelvis** *f*
perforation **perforación** *f*
perineal **perineal** *adj*
perineum **perineo**
physician **médico; doctor (doctora)** *m/f*
  attending physician **médico de cabecera; médico a cargo; médico asistente**
  consulting physician **médico consultor; médico de apelación**
  resident physician (house) **médico residente**
pitocin **pitocin** *m;* **pitocina**
PKU (phenylketonuria) **prueba del pañal; fenilcetonuria; fenilquetonuria**
placenta **placenta; secundinas; segundo parto** *Chicano;* **lo demás** *slang*
  placenta previa **placenta previa**
placental **placentario** *adj*
planned parenthood **procreación planeada** *f;* **natalidad dirigida** *f*
postnatal care **cuidado postnatal**
pounds **libras**
pregnancy **preñez** *f;* **embarazo; gravidez** *f;* **estado interesante** *euph*
  ectopic pregnancy **embarazo ectópico; embarazo fuera de la matriz**
  false **embarazo falso**
  hysteria **embarazo histérico**
  incomplete **embarazo incompleto**
  tubal pregnancy **embarazo tubárico; embarazo en los tubos**
pregnant **preñada** *adj;* **gruesa** *adj, fam;* **embarazada** *adj;* **encinta** *adj;* **grávida** *adj;* **panzona** *vulgar*
premature **prematuro** *adj;* **sietemesino** (literally "seven months")
prenatal **prenatal** *adj*

prenatal care **cuidado prenatal**
prescribe, to **recetar; prescribir**
prescription **receta médica; prescripción** *f*
presentation **presentación** *f*
procreate **procrear**
progeny **prole** *f;* **progenie** *f*
progesterone **progesterona**
prolapse **prolapso; caída de la matriz**
prophylactic **profiláctico** *adj*
puerile **pueril** *adj*
puerperal **puerperal** *adj*
puerperal fever **fiebre puerperal** *f*
puerperium **puerperio; riesgo**
pull back foreskin of penis, to **pelársela** *fam*
pull up (one's) knees, to **encoger las rodillas**
pump, to **sacar (leche) por medio de una bomba**
push, to **pujar**
quadruplet **cuatrillizo; cuadrúpleto**
quintuplet **quintillizo; quíntuplo**
rabbit test **examen de conejo** *m*
recessive **recesivo** *adj*
  recessive character **carácter recesivo** *m*
rectal **rectal** *adj*
rectocele **rectocele** *m*
rectum **recto**
reddish **rojizo** *adj;* **bermejizo** *adj, hair*
red-haired **pelirrojo** *adj*
reduce, to **reducir(se)**
reducing exercises **ejercicios físicos para adelgazar**
relation **pariente** *f;* **parentesco; relación** *f*
relations, to have sexual **tener relaciones sexuales; dormir (ue) con alguien; estar con alguien; chingar** *vulgar;* **cojer/coger** *vulgar, P.R., Mex. Arg.;* **conocer; hacer cositas** *euph, Chicano;* **dar una atascada** *vulgar;* **echar un palito** *Chicano;* **chopetear** *slang;* **dar pa' dentro** *vulgar;* **tumbar**
relationship **relación** *f;* **parentesco**
relax, to **relajar; aflojarse; relajar el cuerpo**
relaxation **relajación** *f;* **descanso**
relaxation of tension **disminución de la tirantez** *f*
Rh factor **factor Rh** *m;* **factor Rhesus** *m*
  Rh negative **Rh-negativo** *adj*
  Rh positive **Rh-positivo** *adj*
rinse, to **enjuagar**
rub, to **frotarse; pasar la mano sobre la superficie de**
rubbing alcohol **alcohol para fricciones** *m*
sanitary pad **kotex** *m;* **servilleta sanitaria**
shave, to **rasurar; afeitar**
sitz bath **baño de asiento; semicupio**
soap **jabón** *m*
soft **suave** *adj*

specimen, urine **muestra de la orina**
speculum **espejo vaginal; espéculo**
sperm **semen** *m;* **espermatozoide** *m;* **semilla** *Mex. slang;* **mecos** *m, slang;* **esperma**
spotting **manchado; manchas de sangre**
squat, to **acuclillarse; ponerse de cuclillas**
sterility, female **frío de la matriz**
sterilize, to **castrar; esterilizar**
  sterilize the bottles, to **esterilizar botellas**
sterilizer **esterilizador** *m*
stillbirth **parto muerto; natimuerto**
stillborn **nacido muerto** *adj;* **mortinato** *adj*
stir, to **revolver (ue)**
stretch marks (strias) **estrías**
subtract, to **sustraer; deducir**
suck, to **mamar; chupar**
supplementary feedings **alimentación suplementaria** *f*
suture **sutura**
  dissolving suture **sutura absorbible**
swallow, to **tragar**
tampax **tampax** *m*
tampon **ta(m)pón** *m*
tear **desgarramiento**
tie the tubes, to **ligar trompas; ligar los tubos de Falopio; ligar los tubos uterinos**
toxemia **toxemia**
  of pregnancy **toxemia del embarazo**
triplet **trillizo**
tub **tina de baño; bañera**
tube **tubo**
  Fallopian tube **trompa de Falopio; tubo de Falopio**
  (for feeding) **sonda**
twin **gemelo; mellizo; jimagua** *m/f;* **cuate** *m/f, Mex.*
umbilical cord **cordón umbilical** *m;* **cordón del ombligo** *m*
umbilicus **ombligo**
urine specimen **muestra de la orina**
uterus **útero; matriz** *f*
vagina **vagina**[47]
vaginal **vaginal** *adj*
vaginitis **vaginitis** *f*
varicose **varicoso** *adj*
varicose vein **várice** *f;* **variz** *m;* **vena varicosa**
varicosity **varicosidad** *f*
vulva **vulva**
wash, to **lavar**
wean, to **destetar**
weigh, to **pesar**
well-being **bienestar** *m*
wet **mojado** *adj*
womb **matriz** *f;* **útero**
x-ray, chest **radiografía del tórax; rayos X del pecho**

MEDICAL SPECIALISTS

ESPECIALISTAS MEDICOS

anesthesiologist **anestesiólogo**
attending physician **médico de cabecera; médico a cargo**

bacteriologist **bacteriólogo**
biologist **biólogo**
cardiologist **cardiólogo**

charge nurse **enfermera de cargo**
chiropodist **quiropodista; pedicuro; callista**

chiropractor **quiropráctico; quiropractor**
consulting physician **médico consultor; médico de apelación**
cytologist **citólogo**
day nurse **enfermera de día**
dentist **dentista**
dermatologist **dermatólogo**
dietician **dietista**
doctor **médico, doctor**
druggist **farmacéutico; boticario**
ear, nose and throat specialist (otorhinolaryngologist) **otorrinolaringólogo**
embryologist **embriólogo**
endocrinologist **endocrinólogo**
endodontist **endodontista**
general duty nurse **enfermera general**
general practitioner **médico general**
gynecologist **ginecólogo**
head nurse **jefa de enfermeras**
hematologist **hematólogo**
histologist **histólogo**
homeopathist **homeópata**
house staff **personal médico**
house surgeon **cirujano asistente; médico interno**
hygienist **higienista**
intern **interno; médico practicante**

internist **internista**
midwife (trained) **partera** (untrained) **comadrona**
neurologist **neurólogo**
neuropsychiatrist **neuro(p)siquiatra**
neurosurgeon **neurocirujano**
night nurse **enfermera de noche**
nurse **enfermero, enfermera**
nurse on duty **enfermera de guardia**
nurse's aide **ayudante de enfermera**
obstetrician **obstétrico, médico partero, tocólogo**
occulist **oculista**
ophthalmologist **oftalmólogo**
optician **óptico**
optometrist **optometrista**
oral surgeon **cirujano oral**
orderly **ayudante (de hospital)**
orthodontist **ortodontista**
orthopedist **ortopedista**
orthoptist **ortóptico**
osteopath **osteópata**
otolaryngologist **otolaringólogo**
otologist **otólogo**
paramedic **paramédico**
pathologist **patólogo**
pediatrician **pediatra; pedíatra**
pedodontist **pedodontista**
periodontist **periodontista**

pharmacist **farmacéutico; boticario**
pharmacologist **farmacólogo**
physician **médico; doctor**
physiotherapist **fisioterapeuta**
plastic surgeon **cirujano plástico**
podiatrist **podiatra**
practical nurse **enfermera no diplomada; enfermera práctica**
private nurse **enfermera privada**
psychiatrist **psiquiatra**
psychoanalyst **psicoanalista**
psychologist **psicólogo**
public health nurse **enfermera de salud pública**
radiologist **radiólogo**
registered nurse **enfermera diplomada**
social worker **trabajador(-a) social**
stretcher bearer **camillero**
surgeon **cirujano, quirurgo**
therapist **terapeuta**
tocologist **tocólogo**
traumatologist **traumatólogo**
urologist **urólogo**
venereologist **especialista en enfermedades venéreas**
veterinarian **veterinario**
visiting nurse **enfermera ambulante**

PLACES IN THE HOSPITAL

LUGARES EN EL HOSPITAL

basement **sótano**
cafeteria **cafetería; cafetín** m, fam; **lonchería** Chicano
cashier **departamento de caja**
chapel **capilla**
department of welfare **departamento de bienestar**
doctor's office **consultorio**
elevator **elevador** m; **ascensor** m
emergency room **sala de emergencia; sala de urgencia**
floor **piso**
front desk **recepción** f

home health agency **agencia de salud doméstica**
hospital care **cuidado en el hospital**
infirmary **enfermería**
laboratory **laboratorio**
lobby **salón principal** m; **vestibulo; zaguán** m
lounge **salón de entrada** m
medical records **departamento de archivo clínico**
mental health department **departamento de enfermedades mentales**
nursery **guardería**

nursing home care **cuidado en los asilos; cuidado en un hospicio para ancianos**
operating room **sala de operaciones; quirófano**
personnel department **departamento de personal**
pharmacy **farmacia**
snack shop **tienda de refrescos**
stairway **escalera**
tomography **tomografía**
waiting room **sala de espera; cuarto de estar**
ward **crujía; pabellón** m

THE FAMILY[48]

LA FAMILIA

Many nouns of relationship ending in -o change it to -a to form the feminine.

the bachelor **el soltero**
the boy **el muchacho**
the brother **el hermano**
the brother-in-law **el cuñado**
the cousin m **el primo**
the father-in-law **el suegro**
the fiancé **el novio**
first cousin **el primo hermano**
the foster son **el hijo de leche**
the friend **el amigo**
the godson **el ahijado**
the grandfather **el abuelo; el abue** Chicano
the grandson **el nieto**
the great grandfather **el bisabuelo**
the great grandson **el biznieto**

the bachelorette **la soltera**
the girl **la muchacha**
the sister **la hermana**
the sister-in-law **la cuñada**
the cousin f **la prima**
the mother-in-law **la suegra**
the fiancée **la novia**
the first cousin **la prima hermana**
the foster daughter **la hija de leche**
the friend **la amiga**
the goddaughter **la ahijada**
the grandmother **la abuela; la abue** Chicano
the granddaughter **la nieta**
the great grandmother **la bisabuela**
the great granddaughter **la biznieta**

the great great grandfather   **el tatarabuelo**   the great great grandmother   **la tatarabuela**
the great great grandson   **el tataranieto**   the great great granddaughter   **la tataranieta**
the half brother   **el medio hermano**   the half sister   **la media hermana**
the husband   **el esposo**   the wife   **la esposa**
the little boy   **el niño**   the little girl   **la niña**
the nephew   **el sobrino**   the niece   **la sobrina**
the newlywed   **el recién casado**   the newlywed   **la recién casada**
the older son   **el hijo mayor**   the older daughter   **la hija mayor**
the orphan   **el huérfano**   the orphan   **la huérfana**
the son   **el hijo**   the daughter   **la hija**
the son-in-law   **el yerno**   the daughter-in-law   **la nuera**
the stepbrother   **el hermanastro**   the stepsister   **la hermanastra**
the stepson   **el hijastro**   the stepdaughter   **la hijastra**
the uncle   **el tío**   the aunt   **la tía**
the widower   **el viudo**   the widow   **la viuda**

Other nouns of relationship must be memorized.

adult   **el adulto**
ancestor   **el antepasado**
baby   **el bebé; la criatura; el(la) nene**
   (-a); el(la) guagua *Chile, Ec., Peru, Bol.*
dad   **el papá; el tata**
daddy   **papí** *m*
deceased   **difunto**
dependent   **dependiente** *m/f*
descendant   **descendiente** *m/f*
divorced   **divorciado** *adj*
family name   **apellido**
father   **el padre**
female   **la hembra**
first name   **el (primer) nombre**
foster mother   **ama de leche**
godfather   **el padrino**

godmother   **la madrina**
guardian   **el guardián; la guardiana**
lover   **amante**
maiden name   **el nombre de soltera**
male   **el varón**
man   **el hombre**
marital status   **el estado civil**
marriage   **el casamiento; el**
   matrimonio
middle name   **el segundo nombre**
mom   **mamá**
mommy   **mamita; mami** *f*
mother   **la madre**
nickname   **el mote; el apodo**
parenthood   **paternidad** *f*
puberty   **la pubertad**

quadruplets   **cuadrúpletos**
quintuplets   **quintillizos; quíntuplos**
race   **la raza**
relationship (family)   **el parentesco**
relatives   **los parientes; los familiares**[49]
stepfather   **el padrastro**
stepmother   **la madrastra**
surname   **el apellido**
survivor   **sobreviviente** *m/f*
triplets   **trillizos**
twins   **mellizos; gemelos**
under age   **menor de edad**
virgin   **la virgen**
woman   **la mujer**
young person   **joven** *m/f*
youth   **la juventud**

NOTE: Nouns designating relationship are used in the masculine plural to denote individuals of both sexes.

the parents, the fathers   **los padres**
the brothers, the brother and sister, the brothers and sisters   **los hermanos**

BATHROOM, TOILET ARTICLES, AND PERSONAL EFFECTS

ARTICULOS PARA EL BAÑO, EL TOCADOR Y OBJETOS PERSONALES

ashtray   **cenicero**
bag   **bolsa; cartera; saco**
bath powder   **polvos de baño** *pl*
beautify oneself, to   **embellecerse**
bedpan   **bacín** *m;* **bidet** *m;* **chata;**
   cómodo *Mex.;* **cuña; paleta, pato;**
   silleta; taza
billfold   **cartera; billetera**
bleach, to   **blanquear**
bobby pin   **horquilla; clip** *m*
book   **libro**
bracelet   **brazalete** *m;* **pulsera**
brush one's teeth, to   **cepillarse los**
   dientes
checkbook   **talonario (de cheques);**
   chequera; libreta de cheques
cigar   **cigarro; puro; tabaco; habano**
cigarette   **cigarrillo; pitillo** *Spain;*
   cigarro *Sp. Am.* **cigarro de papel**
cigarettes, carton of   **caja de cigarrillos**
cleansing cream   **crema limpiadora**
clippers   **maquinilla para cortar**
coat hanger   **percha; gancho** *Mex.*
cold cream   **crema facial**
cologne   **agua de colonia; colonia**
comb   **peine** *m*
comb, to   **peinar(se)**
compact   **polvera**

contact lenses   **lentes de contacto** *m;*
   pupilentes *m;* **lentillas** *f, Spain*
   gas permeable   **poroso** *adj*
   hard   **duro** *adj*
   soft   **suave** *adj*
contact lens case   **estuche** *m*
cosmetic   **cosmético** *adj*
cosmetics   **cosméticos** *pl;* **productos de**
   belleza *pl*
cream   **crema**
curlers   **rizadores** *m;* **rollos; rulos; tubos**
cut hair, to   **cortar el pelo**
dental floss   **hilo dental**
denture cup   **recipiente para guardar la**
   dentadura *m*
deodorant   **desodorante** *m*
depilatory   **depilatorio**
drug   **droga**
drugstore   **farmacia** *Spain Sp. Am.;*
   droguería *Sp. Am.;* **botica**
dry, to   **secar**
dye   **tintura; tinte** *m*
dye, to   **teñir (i)**
earring   **arete** *m;* **zarcillo; pantalla** *P.R.*
   earring, drop   **pendiente** *m;* **arracada**
emery board   **lima para las uñas**
emesis bowl   **riñonera; vasija para**
   vomitar

envelope   **sobre** *m*
face powder   **polvo facial**
facial tissues   **servilletas faciales;**
   pañuelos faciales; kleenex *m*
flowers   **flores** *f*
foot powder   **polvos para los pies**
glasses   **anteojos** *m, pl;* **gafas** *f, pl;*
   lentes *m, pl, Mex.;* **espejuelos** *m, pl,*
   Cuba
   glass case   **estuche** *m;* **funda de gafas**
   sunglasses   **gafas de sol** *f, pl*
hairbrush   **cepillo para el pelo; cepillo**
   de cabeza
haircut   **corte de pelo** *m*
hairdresser   **peluquero (-a)** *m/f*
hair dye   **tinte para el pelo** *m*
hair net   **redecilla**
hairpin   **horquilla; gancho para el**
   pelo; sujetador *m*
hair spray   **fijador para el pelo** *m*
hair tonic   **tónico para el pelo**
handbag   **saquito de mano**
hand cream   **crema para las manos**
hankie, handkerchief   **pañuelo**
jewelry   **joyas** *f, pl*
key   **llave** *f*
Kleenex   **kleenex** *m;* **pañuelo de papel**
lather   **espuma**

lather the face, to **enjabonar la cara; dar jabón en la cara**
letter **carta**
lipstick **lápiz labial** *m;* **pintura de labios; lápiz para los labios** *m*
lotion **loción** *f;* **crema** *Mex.*
magazine **revista**
makeup **maquillaje** *m*
makeup, to put on **maquillarse**
manicure **manicura; arreglo de uñas**
mascara **rimel** *m*
match **fósforo; cerilla** *Spain;* **cerillo** *Mex.*
medicated soap **jabón medicinal** *m*
medicine **medicina**
mirror **espejo**
mouthwash **lavado bucal; enjuague** *m*
nail file **lima para las uñas**
nail polish **esmalte de uñas** *m;* **pintura de uñas; barniz** *m;* **laca de uñas**
nail polish remover **quitador de esmalte de uñas** *m*
necklace **collar** *m;* **gargantilla**
needle **aguja**
newspaper **periódico; diario**
package **paquete** *m;* **cajetilla**
perfume **perfume** *m*
permanent wave **ondulación permanente** *f;* **ondulado permanente**
pin **alfiler** *m;* **prendedero**
pipe **pipa; cachimba** *Sp. Am.*
pitcher **jarra**
pocketbook **cartera; portamonedas** *f, inv;* **bolsa; bolso**
postcard **tarjeta postal**
powder **polvo**
powder puff **mota para empolvarse; borla; bellota**

purse **monedero; bolso; bolsa**
put up one's hair, to **ponerse los rulos**
razor **navaja de afeitar; cuchilla de afeitar**
razor, safety **máquina de afeitar; maquinilla de afeitar; maquinilla de seguridad**
razor blade **hoja de afeitar; navajita; gillette** *m, C.A.*
ring **anillo; sortija; argolla** *parts of Sp. Am.*
  engagement ring **anillo de prometida; anillo de compromiso** *Mex.*
  wedding ring **alianza; anillo (o sortija) de matrimonio, de boda, de casamiento**
rinse **enjuague** *m*
rinse, to **enjuagar; aclarar**
rouge **colorete** *m*
rubber gloves **guantes de goma** *m*
safety pin **imperdible** *m;* **alfiler de seguridad** *m*
sanitary napkin **servilleta sanitaria; kotex** *m;* **almohadilla higiénica; absorbente higiénico** *m*
scissors **tijeras** *f, pl*
set (setting) **peinado**
set, to **marcar**
shampoo **champú** *m;* **shampoo** *m*
shave **afeitada; rasuración** *f*
shave (oneself), to **afeitar(se); rasurar(se)**
shaving cream **crema de afeitar**
shower **ducha; regadera** *Mex.;* **baño de China** *Arg.*
shower, to **ducharse**
smoke, to **fumar; pitar** *Arg., Chile*

smoke a pipe, to **fumar en pipa; pipar**
soap **jabón** *m*
stamp (postage) **timbre** *m, Mex.;* **estampilla** *Sp. Am.;* **sello** *Spain*
stationery **papel de escribir** *m*
suitcase **maleta; velís** *m, Mex.*
suntan lotion **loción/crema para el sol** *f;* **loción bronceadora** *f*
talcum powder **talco**
tampon **tampón** *m;* **tapón** *m*
thread **hilo**
tie clasp **alfiler de corbata** *m*
toilet paper **papel de baño** *m;* **papel de inodoro** *m;* **papel higiénico**
toothbrush **cepillo de dientes**
toothpaste **pasta dental; dentífrico; pasta dentífrica**
tooth powder **polvo dental**
towel **toalla**
  clean **toalla limpia**
  dirty **toalla sucia**
truss **braguero**
tube **tubo**
tweezer **pinzas**
urinal **orinal** *m*
vaseline **vaselina**
wallet **cartera; billetera; portamonedas** *m, inv*
wash, to **lavar(se)**
washbasin **basija; jofaina; ponchera** *C.A.;* **palangana** *f, Mex.;* **lavabo**
washcloth **paño de lavarse; toallita**
waste basket **papelera**
watch **reloj** *m*
  wristwatch **reloj de pulsera**
wig **peluca**

BEDDING

ROPA DE CAMA

bed **cama**
bedboard **tabla para la cama**
bed pad **colchoncillo para la cama**
blanket **frazada; manta; cobija** *Mex.*
  electric blanket **frazada eléctrica**
cot **catre** *m*
cover **cubierta**
covers **cobertores** *m, pl;* **cobijas** *pl, Mex. and elsewhere*
crib **cuna; camita de niño**
hammock **hamaca**

mattress **colchón** *m*
  air mattress **colchón de aire; colchón de viento**
  (inner)spring mattress **colchón de muelles**
mosquito net **mosquitero**
pad **cojincillo; almohadilla**
pillow **almohada**
  feather pillow **edredón** *m*

pillowcase **funda (de almohada); almohada**
quilt **colcha; sobrecama acolchada; edredón** *m*
sheepskin **zalea**
sheet **sábana**
  plastic sheet **sábana de plástico**
side rail **riel del costado** *m;* **baranda protectora**

CLOTHING

ROPA

apron **delantal** *m*
bathing suit **traje de baño** *m;* **bañador** *m, Spain*
bathrobe **bata (de baño); salto** *Arg.* (terrycloth) **albornoz** *m*
bedclothes **ropa de cama; tendido** *Col Ec. Mex.*
belt **cinto; cinturón** *m*
blouse **blusa**

blue jeans **pantalones vaqueros** *m, pl;* **mezclillas** *Mex.*
boot **bota**
bra (brassiere) **sostén** *m;* **sostenedor** *m;* **portabustos; corpiño** *Arg.;* **ajustador** *m;* **justillo**
buckle **hebilla**
button **botón** *m*
button, to **abotonar; abrochar**

cap **gorra; montera; cachucha** *Mex.*
change clothes, to **mudarse de ropa; cambiarse la ropa**
cloth **tela; paño; tejido**
  batiste **batista**
  calfskin **becerro**
  cotton **algodón** *m*
  dark **oscuro** *adj*
  heavyweight **grueso** *adj*

light   claro *adj*
lightweight   delgado *adj*
linen   lienzo; lino; hilo
satin   raso
silk   seda
wool   lana
woolen   de lana *adj*
clothes, apparel   ropa *sg*; vestimenta
coat   abrigo
   fur   abrigo de piel
   jacket   chaqueta
   lightweight   abrigo de entretiempo
   overcoat   abrigo; sobretodo
   rain   impermeable *m*
collar   cuello
corset   corsé *m*
diaper   pañal *m*
dress   vestido; traje *m*, *Perú, Pan.*
   dress, house   vestido para la casa
   maternity   vestido de maternidad
   wash   vestido que puede lavarse
dress, to   vestir(se) (i)
dry clean, to   limpiar en seco
fade, to   desteñir (i)
fur   piel *f*
galoshes   galochas; chanclo *Spain*
garter   liga
garter belt   portaligas *m, inv*
girdle   ceñidor *m*; cinturón *m*; faja
gloves   guantes *m*
handkerchief   pañuelo
hat   sombrero
heel   tacón *m*; taco *Arg.*
hook   gancho
hose   medias *pl*
   pantyhose   medias; medias
      pantalón; pantimedias *pl*

jacket   chaqueta; saco; americana
   ski   gamberro; anorak *m*
jeans   pantalones vaqueros *m, pl*;
   mesclillas *Mex.*; pantalones de
   mesclilla *m, pl*
leather   cuero
light (color)   claro *adj*
   (weight)   delgado *adj*
lingerie   ropa interior de mujer
necktie (tie)   corbata
nightgown   camisón de dormir *m*;
   camisa de noche; bata
nylon   nilón *m*
overalls   guardapolvo
oxfords   zapatos bajos *pl*; zapatos de
   estilo Oxford
pair   par *m*
pajama   pijama *f/m*; piyama *f/m*
panties   bragas; calzones *m, pl*;
   pantalones interiores de mujer *m*;
   pantaleta
pants (men's)   pantalones *m*
rubber heel   tacón de goma *m*
rubber overshoe   chanclo *m, Spain*;
   zapato de goma *m, Sp. Am.*, zapato de
   hule *m, Mex.*
rubber pants   pantalones de goma *m,
   pl*; pantalones plásticos *m, pl*
sandals   sandalia; guaraches *m, Mex.*;
   caites *m, C.A.* ojotas *Chile, Ec., Perú,
   Bol.*
scarf   bufanda
shawl   chal *m*; rebozo *Mex.*
shirt   camisa
   sweatshirt   camisa enguatada

under   camiseta
   (T-shirt)   polera *Sp. Am.*
shoe   zapato
   high-heeled shoes   zapatos de
      tacones altos
   low-heeled shoes   zapatos de tacones
      bajos
shorts   calzones cortos *m*
shorts, under   calzoncillos
skirt   falda; saya; sayuela; pollera *Arg.,
   Chile*
sleeve   manga
slip   combinación *f*; enagua; refajo;
   fondo *Spain*
slipper   zapatilla; chinela; chancleta
sneaker   zapato de goma; zapato de
   gimnasio; tenis *m, Mex.*
sock   calcetín *m*; media *Arg.*
sole (of shoe)   suela
stockings   medias
suit   traje *m*; vestido *Perú, Pan.*
sweater   sweater *m*; suéter *m*; jersey *m*
trousers   pantalones *m*
trunks   calzones de baño *m*; shorts *m*
unbutton, to   desabotonar;
   desabrochar
underpants   calzoncillos
undershirt   camiseta
underwear   ropa interior
uniform   uniforme *m*
wash, to   lavar
wrinkle   arruga
zipper   cierre automático *m*; cierre
   relámpago *m*

COLORS

COLORES

beige   beige
black   negro
blonde   rubio; chelo *Mex.*
blue   azul
brown   moreno; pardo; carmelita
   Cuba, Chile; marrón
brunette   moreno; trigueño
chestnut   castaño; pardo
clear   incoloro
color   color *m*

cranberry   arándano
dark   oscuro
gold   dorado
gray   gris
green   verde
light (color)   claro
maroon   rojo obscuro
opaque   opaco
orange   anaranjado
pale   pálido

pink   rosado
purple   púrpura; morado
red   rojo
ruby   rubí
silver   plateado
transparent   transparente
violet   violeta
white   blanco
yellow   amarillo

PRACTITIONERS OF THE MAJOR RELIGIONS

PRACTICANTES DE LAS RELIGIONES PRINCIPALES

Agnostic   agnóstico
Anglican   anglicano
Atheist   ateo
Baptist   bautista
Born-again Christian   cristiano
   renacido
Buddhist   budista
Catholic   católico
   Greek Catholic (Greek Orthodox)
      católico de rito griego

Roman Catholic   católico romano
Christian   cristiano
Christian Scientist   miembro de la
   ciencia cristiana
Congregationalist   congregacionalista
Covenanter   covenantario; pactante
   Evangelical Convenanter
      covenantario evangélico; miembro
      del Pacto
Episcopalian   episcopalista

Evangelist   evangelista
Hindu   hindú
Jehovah's Witness   testigo de Jehová
Jew   judío
Lutheran   luterano
Methodist   metodista
Mormon   mormón
Moslem   mahometano, musulmán,
   islámico
Presbyterian   presbiteriano

Protestant **protestante**
Quaker **cuáquero, cuákero**
Seventh-Day Adventist **adventista del**
séptimo día
Shintoist **sinoísta**
Taoist **taoísta**
Unitarian **unitario**
Zoroastrian **zoroástrico**

COUNTRIES AND NATIONALITIES

PAISES Y NACIONALIDADES

PAISES[50]	HABITANTES[51]	CAPITALES	HABITANTES
México ⎱ Méjico ⎰	mexicano ⎱ mejicano ⎰	México ⎱ Méjico ⎰	mexicano ⎱ mejicano ⎰
Cuba	cubano	La Habana	habanero
Puerto Rico	puertorriqueño	San Juan	sanjuanero
La República Dominicana	dominicano	Santo Domingo	santodominicano
Guatemala	guatemalteco	Guatemala	guatemalteco
El Salvador	salvadoreño	San Salvador	sansalvadoreño
Honduras	hondureño	Tegucigalpa	tegucigalpense
Nicaragua	nicaragüense	Managua	managüense
Costa Rica	costarricense	San José	(san)josefino
Panamá	panameño	Panamá	panameño
Colombia	colombiano	Bogotá	bogotano
Venezuela	venezolano	Caracas	caragueño
El Ecuador	ecuatoriano	Quito	quiteño
El Perú	peruano	Lima	limeño
Bolivia	boliviano	La Paz	paceño
Chile	chileno	Santiago	santiaguino
(La) Argentina	argentino	Buenos Aires	bonaerense
El Uruguay	uruguayo	Montevideo	montevideano
El Paraguay	paraguayo	Asunción	asunceño
El Brasil	brasileño	Brasilia	brasileño
España	español	Madrid	madrileño
Estados Unidos (EEUU)[52]	estadounidense	Washington, D.C.	Washington, D.C.

OCCUPATIONS[53]

PROFESIONES

actor **actor**
actress **actriz**
administrator **administrator; gobernante**
advertiser **anunciador; anunciante**
adviser, advisor **consejero; consultor**
agent **agente; representante**
architect **arquitecto**
artist **artista**
assistant **asistente; ayudante**
athlete **atleta**
attorney **abogado; procurador**
author **autor**
babysitter **niñera por horas**
baker **panadero; hornero**
ballplayer **pelotero; beisbolista**
banker **banquero**
barber **barbero; peluquero**
bartender **cantinero; tabernero**
beautician **cosmetólogo**
biologist **biólogo**
bookkeeper **tenedor de libros; contable**
bookseller **librero; vendedor de libros**
broker **agente de negocios; intermediario**
builder **constructor; arquitecto**
bullfighter **torero; matador**
bus driver **conductor de ómnibus**

businessman **hombre de negocios; comerciante; negociante**
businesswoman **mujer de negocios; mujer de empresa**
butcher **carnicero**
cab driver **taxista; cochero**
carpenter **carpintero**
cashier **cajero**
chauffeur **chófer; chofer** *Sp. Am.*
chef **cocinero; jefe de cocina**
chemist **químico; farmacéutico**
civil servant **funcionario público; empleado del estado**
cleaner **tintorero; lavandero**
cleaning woman **criada que limpia la casa**
clergyman **clérigo; sacerdote; ministro; pastor; rabí; rabino**
clerk **oficinista, empleado de oficina, secretario** *offices;* **dependiente, empleado de tienda, vendedor** *stores;* **escribano** *law*
coach **maestro particular** *tutor;* **entrenador** *sports*
coal miner **minero de carbón**
conductor **conductor, guía, director** *music;* **recogedor de billetes** *train*
construction worker **obrero de edificación construcción**

cook **cocinero**
correspondent **correspondiente; corresponsal**
counselor **consejero; abogado consultor**
dancer **bailador; danzante**
day laborer **jornalero; bracero**
dental technician **técnico dental**
detective **detective; investigador**
diagnostician **experto en hacer diagnósticos**
dietician **dietista**
director **director; administrador; dirigente**
dishwasher **lavaplatos; lavador(a) de platos**
dockhand **estibador; cargador**
doctor **doctor; médico**
domestic **doméstico; criado; sirviente**
draftsman **dibujante; diseñador; bosquejador**
dressmaker **modista; costurera**
driver **piloto; conductor; cochero; maquinista**
druggist **farmacéutico; boticario**
editor **redactor titular** *newspaper;* **editor** *literary*
educator **educador; maestro; pedagogo; instructor**
electrician **electricista**

engineer **ingeniero**
engraver **grabador**
exporter **exportador**
farmer **agricultor; hacendado**
farmhand **labrador; campesino**
fireman **bombero**
fisherman **pescador**
florist **florista**
garbage collector **basurero**
gardener **jardinero**
guide **guía**
handyman **hacelotodo; factótum**
hard-hat **operario de construcción**
helper **ayudante; asistente**
hired hand **mozo de campo**
housekeeper **ama de llaves; ama de gobierno; casera**
housewife **ama de casa; madre de familia**
houseworker **doméstico; criado; sirviente**
husband **esposo; marido**
industrialist **industrialista**
inspector **inspector; supervisor**
instructor **instructor; profesor; maestro**
insurance agent **agente de seguros**
interior decorator **decorador de interiores**
interpreter **intérprete**
inventor **inventor; creador**
investigator **investigador; indagador**
ironworker **herrero**
janitor **portero; conserje**
jeweler **joyero**
journalist **periodista; cronista**
junk dealer **chatarrero**
laboratory technician **técnico de laboratorio**
laborer **obrero; trabajador; jornalero; bracero**
lathe operator **tornero**
laundress **lavandera**
lawman **agente de policía; alguacil**
lawyer **abogado; letrado; licenciado**
librarian **bibliotecario**
lifeguard **salvavidas**
longshoreman **estibador; cargador**
machinist **mecánico; maquinista**
maid **criada; sirvienta**
mail carrier **cartero**
manager **gerente; director; administrador; superintendente**
manicurist **manicuro; manicura**
manual laborer **obrero de mano**
mason **albañil**
masseur **masajista**
mathematician **matemático**
mechanic **mecánico**
merchant **mercader; comerciante; negociante**
messenger **mensajero; mandadero; recadero**
metalworker **metalario; metalista**
minister (religion) **ministro; clérigo; pastor; sacerdote; cura; rabí** (diplomat) **ministro; enviado**
motorcyclist **motociclista**
motorman **motorista; conductor**
mover **empleado de una casa de mudanzas**
musician **músico**
navigator **navegador; navegante**

newsboy **vendedor de periódicos; diariero**
newscaster **cronista de noticiarios; comentarista radiofónico**
newsman **reportero; periodista**
notary (public) **escribano (público); notario (público)**
nun **monja; religiosa**
nursemaid **niñera; aya; ama**
occupational therapist **terapeuta ocupacional; ergoterapeuta**
office boy **mandadero; mensajero**
office clerk **oficinista; escribano**
office manager **jefe de oficina**
officer **funcionario; oficial; policía; agente**
oil field worker **obrero petrolero**
oilman **petrolero**
operator **operador; telefonista**
painter **pintor**
patrolman **policía; guardia**
peddler **buhonero; mercachifle**
pharmacist **farmacéutico; boticario; farmaceuta** Sp. Am.
photographer **fotógrafo; fotógrafa**
physical therapist **fisioterapeuta**
physicist **físico**
pilot **piloto; guía**
plasterer **enlucidor; revocador**
plowman **arador; labrador; yuguero**
plumber **plomero; cañero**
policeman **policía** m; **vigilante** Ven.; **guardia; gendarme** Mex.
policewoman **mujer policía**
politician **político; estadista**
porter **portero; conserje**
presser **planchador**
priest **sacerdote; presbítero; clérigo; cura**
principal **director; rector**
printer **impresor; tipógrafo**
publisher **editor; publicador**
rabbi **rabí; rabino**
ranchman **hacendado; ganadero**
ranger **vigilante**
reader **lector**
realtor **corredor de bienes raíces**
receptionist **recibidor(a); recepcionista**
registrar **registrador; archivista; jefe de registros civiles**
repairman **reparador; mecánico de reparaciones**
reporter **repórter; reportero; noticiero**
retailer **menorista** Sp. Am.; **comerciante al por menor**
retired **jubilado** adj
road worker **peón caminero**
sailor **marinero**
salesclerk **vendedor(a); dependiente; dependienta**
saloonkeeper **tabernero; cantinero**
scavenger **basurero**
schoolteacher **maestro (-a) de escuela**
scientist **científico**
scrubwoman **fregona**
seamstress **costurera; modistilla**
secretary **secretario (-a)**
serviceman **mecánico; reparador; militar**
sheriff **alguacil de policía**
shipping clerk **dependiente encargado del envío de mercaderías**
shoemaker **zapatero**
shopkeeper **tendero; almacenista**
singer **cantante; cantatriz**

social worker **asistente social; trabajador social**
soldier **soldado**
solicitor **solicitador**
steelworker **obrero en una fábrica de acero**
stenographer **estenógrafo; taquígrafo**
stevedore **estibador**
stockbroker **bolsista; corredor de bolsa**
street cleaner **barredor de calles**
supervisor **superintendente**
surveyor **topógrafo**
switchman **guardagujas**
tailor **sastre**
taxi driver **taxista, chofer de taxi** Sp. Am.
teacher **maestro (-a); profesor; instructor**
teamster **carretero**
technician **técnico; especialista; experto técnico**
telephone operator **telefonista**
teller **pagador; cajero**
therapist **terapeuta**
ticket agent **agente de viajes; taquillero**
timekeeper **cronometrador (-a)**
toreador **torero**
trackman **guardavía**
tradesman **tendero; comerciante al por menor**
train dispatcher **despachador de trenes**
translator **traductor**
travel agent **agente de viajes**
treasurer **tesorero (-a)**
truck driver **camionero; conductor de camión**
trunk dealer **baulero; cofrero**
trustee **consignatario; fiduciario**
tutor **preceptor; maestro particular**
typesetter **compositor; tipógrafo**
typist **mecanógrafo (-a); dactilógrafo (-a); tipiadora**
undertaker **funerario; agente de entierros**
unemployed **cesante** adj
unskilled laborer **peón de pico y pala**
unskilled workman **obrero no especializado**
upholsterer **tapicero**
valet **asistente personal; valet**
varnisher **barnizador; charolista**
vendor **vendedor; buhonero**
vocalist **cantante; vocalista**
waiter **mozo; camarero; mesero** Mex.
waitress **moza de restaurante; camarera**
warden **carcelero**
warehouse keeper **guardalmacén**
washer **lavandero (-a)**
watchmaker **relojero**
watchman **sereno; guardián**
weatherman **meteorologista**
weaver **tejedor (-a)**
welder **soldador**
wet nurse **nodriza; ama de crianza**
white-collar worker **oficinista profesional**
wholesaler **mayorista** Sp. Am.; **comerciante al por mayor**
wigmaker **fabricante de pelucas**

FOODS AND MEALS

ALIMENTOS Y COMIDAS

SPECIAL DIETS   *DIETAS ESPECIALES*

absolute diet   **dieta absoluta**
acid-ash diet   **dieta de residuo ácido**
alkali-ash diet   **dieta de residuos alcalinos**
balanced diet   **dieta balanceada**
bedtime snack, feeding   **colación** *f*
bland diet   **dieta blanda**
diabetic diet   **dieta para los diabéticos**
diet to control weight   **dieta para controlar el peso**
diet to gain weight   **dieta para aumentar de peso**
diet to lose weight   **dieta para perder peso; adelgazar**
elimination diet   **dieta de eliminación**
fat-free diet   **dieta sin grasa**
gallbladder diet   **dieta para la vesícula**
gluten-free diet   **dieta libre de gluten**
high-carbohydrate diet   **dieta rica en carbohidratos**

high-fat diet   **dieta rica en grasas**
high-protein diet   **dieta de elevado contenido proteico; dieta rica en proteína**
high-residue diet   **dieta de elevado residuo**
iron-enriched diet   **dieta rica en hierro**
light diet   **dieta ligera**
liquid diet   **dieta de líquidos; dieta líquida**
   clear liquid diet   **dieta de líquidos claros**
   full (nourishing) liquid diet   **dieta de líquidos nutritivos; dieta de líquidos espesos**
low-calorie diet   **dieta de pocas calorías**
low-carbohydrate diet   **dieta baja en carbohidratos**
low-fat diet   **dieta de escaso contenido graso**

low-protein diet   **dieta de escaso contenido proteico; dieta baja en proteína**
low-residue diet   **dieta de escaso residuo; dieta gástrica**
low-salt diet   **dieta con escaso contenido de sal**
mineral enriched diet   **dieta rica en minerales**
nutritional diet   **dieta alimenticia**
purine-free diet   **dieta sin purinas**
restricted diet   **dieta rigurosa**
salt-free diet   **dieta sin sal; dieta desc1orurada**
smooth diet   **dieta pobre en celulosa**
ulcer diet   **dieta para las úlceras**
vitamin-enriched diet   **dieta rica en vitaminas**

See Food Guide Pyramid on page 248.

COOKING TERMS   *TERMINOLOGIA DE COCINA*

appetite   **apetito**
appetizing   **apetitoso** *adj*
aversion   **aversión** *f*; **repugnancia**
bake, to   **asar al horno; hornear; cocer en horno**
baked   **al horno; horneado** *adj*
beaten   **batido** *adj*
bitter   **amargo** *adj*
boil, to   **hervir (ie)**
boiled   **cocido** *adj*; **hervido** *adj*
boil in water, to   **cocer; hervir (ie)**
breaded   **empanado** *adj*
breakfast   **desayuno**
breakfast, to have, to eat   **desayunar (se)**
broiled   **asado; asado a parrilla** *adj*
browned   **dorado** *adj*
calorie   **caloría**
can   **lata**
canned   **enlatado** *adj*; **en conserva** *prep*
chew, to   **masticar**
chop, to   **picar**
cold   **frío** *adj*
cook, to   **guisar; cocinar**
cookbook   **libro (manual) de cocina**
cooked   **cocinado** *adj*
crush, to   **machacar**
crushed   **machacado** *adj*
cut, to   **cortar**
defrost, to   **deshelar (ie)**
delicious   **delicioso** *adj*
diced   **cortado en cuadritos**
diet   **dieta; régimen** *m*
diet, to   **estar a dieta**
dinner   **cena; comida**
dinner, to have   **cenar**
dish   **plato**
dry, dried   **seco** *adj*
eat, to   **comer**
eat heartily, to   **comer por cuatro**
enjoy eating or drinking, to   **saborear**

enriched   **enriquecido** *adj*
entrée   **principio; entrada**
feed, to   **alimentar; dar de comer**
feeding   **alimentación** *f*
flavor   **sabor** *m*
food   **alimento; comestibles** *m, pl*; **vianda**
food stamps   **cupones de comida** *m*
fortify   **fortalecer**
freeze, to   **congelar; helar (ie)**
fresh   **fresco** *adj*
fried   **frito** *adj*
frosted sugary   **azucarado** *adj*
frozen   **helado; congelado** *adj*
fry, to   **freír (i)**
grated   **rallado** *adj*
gravy (au jus)   **salsa**
greasy   **grasiento** *adj*; **con grasa** *prep*
grilled   **asado a la parrilla** *adj*
grind, to   **moler (ue)**
ground   **molido** *adj*
heat, to   **calentar (ie)**
hot   **caliente** *adj*
juicy   **jugoso** *adj*
kosher   **cácher** *adj*; **kosher** *adj*
larded   **mechado** *adj*
lean   **magro** *adj*
lunch   **almuerzo**
lunch, to eat   **almorzar (ue)**
marinate, to   **marinar; escabechar**
mashed   **amasado** *adj*; **majado** *adj*
measure   **medir (i)**
medium   **medio** *adj*
mince, to   **desmenuzar**
mix, to   **mezclar**
mixed   **mezclado** *adj*
not agree, to   **caer mal**
nourish, to   **alimentar**
nourishment   **alimentación** *f*; **alimento**
nutriment   **alimento**
nutritious   **alimenticio; nutritivo** *adj*

pat   **cuadrado**
peel, to   **pelar**
pickled   **encurtido; en escabeche** *adj*
poach   **escalfar**
poached   **escalfado** *adj*
pour, to   **verter (ie)**
precooked   **precocinado** *adj*
protein   **proteína**
puree   **puré** *m*
put on weight, to   **engordar**
rare (meat)   **poco asado; poco frito; poco hecho; medio crudo; poco cocido** *adj*
raw   **crudo** *adj*
relish   **entremés** *m*
rind   **cáscara**
rinse, to   **enjuagar**
ripe   **maduro** *adj*
roast, to   **asar**
roasted   **asado** *adj*
rough   **áspero** *adj*
round slice   **rueda**
salty   **salado** *adj*
sauce   **salsa**
sauté   **salteado** *adj*
scrape, to   **raspar**
scrub, to   **restregar**
season, to   **condimentar; sazonar**
shred, to   **desmenuzar**
sip   **trago; sorbo**
sip, to   **sorber**
slice   **rebanada; tajado**
slice, to   **rebanar; tajar**
smoke, to (food)   **ahumar**
smoked   **ahumado** *adj*
smooth   **blando** *adj*
snack   **merienda**
soak, to   **remojar**
soft   **blando** *adj*
solid   **sólido** *adj*
sour   **agrio** *adj*

spicy   **picante; condimentado** *adj*
starch   **almidón** *m*
steamed   **cocido** *adj*
stew, to   **estofar; guisar**
stewed   **guisado** *adj*
strain, to   **colar**
strip   **lonja**
stuffing   **relleno**
supper   **cena**
supper, to eat   **cenar**

swallow, to   **tragar**
sweet   **dulce** *m, adj*
sweetness   **dulzura**
taste, to   **saborear**
tasteless   **sin sabor; insípido** *adj*
temperature, at room   **al tiempo** *adj*;
    natural *adj*
tender   **tierno** *adj*
thaw, to   **deshelar (ie)**
thick (liquid)   **espeso** *adj*

toast, to   **tostar**
toasted   **tostado** *adj*
victuals   **viandas**
wash, to   **lavar**
wean, to   **destetar**
well cooked   **bien cocinado** *adj*
well done (steak)   **bien frito** *adj*; **bien
    asado** *adj*; **bien cocida** *adj*
whipped   **batido** *adj*
wrap, to   **envolver (ue)**

SEASONING   *CONDIMENTOS*

anise seed   **anís** *m*
basil   **albahaca**
bay leaves   **hojas de laurel**
black pepper   **pimienta**
butter   **mantequilla**
catsup   **salsa de tomate**
chile   **ají** *m;* **chile** *m*
chile powder   **polvo de chile**
cinnamon   **canela**
cloves   **clavos**
condiment   **condimento**
corn oil   **aceite de maíz** *m*
cornstarch   **maicena**
cottonseed oil   **aceite de semillas de
    algodón** *m*
cumin seed   **comino**
fat   **manteca; grasa**
garlic   **ajo**
ginger   **jengibre** *m*

grease   **grasa; manteca**
honey   **miel** *f*
horseradish   **rábano picante**
hot sauce   **salsa picante; picante** *m*
jelly   **jalea**
lard   **manteca**
lemon   **limón** *m*
margarine   **margarina**
marjoram   **orégano**
marmalade   **mermelada**
mayonnaise   **mayonesa; salsa
    mayonesa**
MSG   **glutamato monosódico**
mushroom   **seta; hongo**
mustard   **mostaza**
nutmeg   **nuez moscada** *f*
oil   **aceite** *m*
    olive oil   **aceite de oliva**

paprika   **pimentón** *m*
red pepper   **pimiento**
red pepper sauce *Mex.*   **mole** *m*
saccharine   **sacarina**
saffron   **azafrán** *m*
salt   **sal** *f*
    iodized   **sal yodada**
    noniodized   **sal corriente**
sauce   **salsa**
sesame oil   **aceite de sésame** *m;* **aceite
    de ajonjolí** *m*
spice   **especia**
sugar   **azúcar** *m*
    brown sugar   **panocha** *Mex.*
tarragon   **tarrago**
thyme   **tomillo**
vinegar   **vinagre** *m*
Worcestershire sauce   **salsa inglesa**

SOUPS   *SOPAS*

broth   **caldo**
chicken soup (with noodles)   **sopa de
    gallina (con fideos); caldo de pollo
    (con fideos)**
consomme   **consomé** *m*

cream of tomato soup   **crema de
    jitomate**
onion soup   **sopa de cebollas**
oyster soup   **caldo de ostras; sopa de
    ostiones**

tomato soup   **sopa de tomate**
vegetable soup   **sopa de vegetales;
    caldo de vegetales**

SALADS   *ENSALADAS*

cucumber and tomato   **pepinos con
    tomates**
fruit salad   **ensalada de frutas**

lettuce with mayonnaise   **lechuga con
    mayonesa**

mixed green salad   **ensalada mixta**

EGGS AND CEREALS   *HUEVOS Y CEREALES*

barley   **cebada**
bran   **acemite** *m;* **salvado**
cooked cereal   **cereal cocido** *m*
cornflakes   **copos de maíz**
corn flour   **maicena**
cream of wheat   **crema de trigo**
dry cereal   **cereal seco** *m*
egg   **huevo; blanquillo** *Mex.*
    egg shell   **cáscara de huevo**
    egg white   **clara de huevo**

egg yolk   **yema de huevo**
fresh egg   **huevo fresco**
fried eggs   **huevos fritos**
hard-boiled eggs   **huevos duros;
    huevos hervidos; huevos cocidos**
omelette with ham   **tortilla con
    jamón**
poached eggs   **huevos escalfados;
    huevos blandos**
rotten eggs   **huevos podridos**

scrambled eggs   **huevos revueltos**
soft-boiled eggs   **huevos pasados por
    agua; huevos tibios**
grits   **sémola**
hot cereal   **cereal caliente** *m*
millet   **mijo**
oatmeal   **avena**
rice   **arroz** *m*
sorghum   **sorgo**
wheat   **trigo**

BREADS AND NOODLES   *PANES Y PASTAS*

biscuit   **bizcocho; galleta; rosca**
bread   **pan** *m*
    bran bread   **acemita**
    cassava bread (or cake)   **cazabe** *m, Sp.
        Am.*
    corn bread   **pan de maíz**
    dark bread   **pan negro; pan moreno**
    French bread   **pan francés**
    fresh bread   **pan del día; pan tierno**
    home-made bread   **pan casero**

rye bread   **pan de centeno**
stale bread   **pan duro; pan sentado**
white bread   **pan blanco**
whole wheat bread   **pan de trigo
    entero; pan de grano integral**
cracker   **galleta; galletica**
    soda cracker   **galleta salada**
crumb   **miga(ja)**
crust   **corteza**
fiber (natural)   **fibra (natural)**

hot cakes   **queques** *m, pl, Mex.;*
    panqueques *m, pl, Sp. Am.;* **tortitas
    calientes** *pl*
macaroni   **macarrones** *m, pl*
nixtamal (corn processed for making
    tortillas)   **nixtamal** *m, Mex.*
noodle   **fideo; tallarín** *m*
pancake, cornmeal and cheese   **panocha**
    Col., C.R., Chile
pasta   **pasta**

roll   **panecillo; bollo de pan; bolillo** *Mex.*
sandwich   **sandwich** *m;* **emparedado; bocadillo** *Spain*

slice   **rebanada; tajada**
spaghetti   **espaguetis** *m, pl;* **tallarín** *m*
sweet roll   **pan dulce** *m, Mex.*

toast   **tostada de pan; pan tostado** *m;* **tostadas** *f, pl, Spain*
French toast   **tostada al estilo francés**
waffles   **queques** *m, pl, Mex.;* **wafles** *m*

BUTTER AND CHEESE   *MANTEQUILLA Y QUESO*

butter   **mantequilla; manteca de vaca** *Spain*
cheese   **queso**
   cottage cheese   **requesón** *m;* **naterón** *m;* **názula**
   cream cheese   **queso crema**

goat's cheese   **queso de cabra**
headcheese   **queso de cerdo**
cooking fat   **grasa de cocinar; aceite de comer** *m*
dairy products   **productos lácteos**
fat   **manteca; grasa**

lard   **manteca (de puerco)**
margarine   **margarina; mantequilla artificial**
peanut butter   **mantequilla de maní; crema de cacahuete**
vegetable oil   **aceite vegetal** *m*

VEGETABLES   *LEGUMBRES Y VERDURAS*

artichoke   **alcachofa**
asparagus   **espárragos** *m, pl*
avocado   **aguacate** *m*
bean   **haba; judía; habichuela; frijol** *m*
   dried beans   **habichuelas secas**
   French beans   **habichuela**
   green beans   **habichuelas verdes; ejotes** *m*
   kidney beans   **habichuela; frijol** *m*
   lima beans   **habas**
   navy beans   **frijol blanco común** *m*
   soy bean   **soya; soja**
   string beans   **habichuelas verdes; judías verdes; ejotes** *m, pl, Mex.;* **chauchas** *f, pl, Arg.*
beet   **remolacha; betabel** *m*
broccoli   **brécol** *m*
brussels sprouts   **col de Bruselas** *m*
cabbage   **col** *m;* **repollo**
carrot   **zanahoria**
cauliflower   **coliflor** *f*
celery   **apio**
chard   **acelga**
chick pea   **garbanzo**
collards   **berzas**
corn   **maíz** *m*

corn on the cob (sweet corn)   **elote** *m, Mex.*
green corn   **maíz tierno**
sweet corn   **choclo** *Sp. Am.*
cucumber   **pepino**
dandelion   **amargón** *m*
eggplant   **berenjena**
endive   **escarola**
green pepper   **pimiento verde**
greens   **verduras**
green vegetables   **hortalizas de hoja verde**
   dark green vegetables   **verduras de hojas verdes oscuras**
kale   **berza; col rizada** *f*
legumes   **legumbres** *f*
lentil   **lenteja**
lettuce   **lechuga**
maize   **maíz** *m*
mushroom   **hongo; seta; champiñón** *m*
okra   **quimbombó; quinbombó**
onion   **cebolla**
parsley   **perejil** *m*
pea   **guisante** *m;* **alverjas** *f, pl, Sp. Am.;* **chícharo; arveja** *Sp. Am.*

green pea   **guisante** *m;* **chícharo**
split pea   **arveja seca**
pickle   **pepinillo; encurtido; picles** *m*
potato   **patata; papa** *Sp. Am.*
   baked potatoes   **papas asadas**
   fried (French fried)   **papas fritas**
   mashed potatoes   **puré de papas** *m;* **puré de patata** *m*
   sweet potato   **camote** *m, Mex.;* **batata; buniato**
radish   **rábano; rabanito**
rutabaga(s)   **nabo de Suecia**
sauerkraut   **berza; col agria** *f*
spinach   **espinaca**
squash   **calabaza**
tomato   **tomate** *m;* **jitomate** *m, Mex.*
   stewed tomatoes   **puré de tomates** *m*
turnip   **nabo**
turnip greens   **hojas de nabo**
vegetables   **vegetales** *m;* **hortalizas; legumbres** *f;* **verduras**
   yellow vegetables   **vegetales de pulpa amarilla**
watercress   **berro**
yam   **batata; buniato**

MEAT   *CARNE*

bacon   **tocino**
barbecue   **barbacoa**
beef   **carne de vaca** *f;* **carne de res** *f*
   beefsteak   **bistec** *m;* **biftec** *m;* **filete** *m;* **bife** *m, Arg.*
   broiled (beef)steak   **churrasco** *Arg., Chile*
   roast beef   **rosbif** *m;* **carne asada**
brains   **sesos** *m, pl*
chop, cutlet   **chuleta; costilla**
cold cuts   **fiambres** *m, pl*
frankfurter   **salchicha**
giblets   **menudillo**
ground meat   **carne molida** *f*
ham   **jamón** *m*
hamburger   **hamburguesa**
hot dog   **perro caliente**
kid   **cabrito**

kidneys   **riñones** *m, pl*
lamb   **cordero; borrego** *Chicano*
   lamb meat   **carne de cordero** *f*
liver   **hígado**
meatballs   **albóndigas** *pl*
meatpie   **empanada**
meat stew and ají (*Chile*)   **ajiaco**
mutton   **carnero**
   leg of mutton   **pierna de carnero**
pork   **cerdo; carne de puerco** *f;* **chancho** *Sp. Am.*
   pork rind (roast pork)   **chicharrón** *m, Perú*
   stew of pork, corn and chile   **pozole** *m, Mex.*
   young pig   **lechón** *m;* **lechoncillo**
ribs   **costillas asadas**

baked ribs   **costillas al horno**
barbecued ribs   **costillas a la parrilla**
roast   **asado** *m, adj*
sausage   **salchicha**
   blood sausage   **morcilla**
   bologna   **salchichón** *m*
   pork sausage   **chorizo**
sirloin   **solomillo**
stew   **cocido; estofado; guisado**
sweetbreads   **mollejas**
tenderloin   **filete** *m*
   tenderloin tips   **puntas de filete**
tongue   **lengua**
tripe   **mondongo; callos**
veal   **carne de ternera** *f*
   breaded veal cutlet   **milanesa; ternera apanada**

POULTRY AND GAME   *AVES Y CAZA*

capon   **capón** *m*
chicken   **pollo**
   boiled chicken   **pollo cocido**
   breast of chicken   **pechuga de pollo**
   broiled chicken   **pollo a la parrilla**
   fried chicken   **pollo frito**
   roast chicken   **pollo asado**

stuffed chicken   **pollo relleno**
duck   **pato**
   wild duck   **pato silvestre**
fowl   **ave** *f*
goose   **ganso**
hare   **liebre** *f*

hen   **gallina**
partridge   **perdiz** *f*
pheasant   **faisán** *m*
rabbit   **conejo**
turkey   **pavo; guajolote** *m, Mex.;* **guanajo** *Cuba*

FISH AND SEAFOOD   *PESCADO Y MARISCOS*

anchovies   **anchoas**
bass   **mero; lobina**
bluepoint   **ostra pequeña**
caviar   **caviar** *m*
clam   **almeja**
cod (fish)   **bacalao**
crab   **cangrejo; jaiba** *Sp. Am.*
eel   **anguila**
fish (living)   **pez** *m*
fish (already caught)   **pescado**
   pickled fish   **escabeche** *m*
fishbone   **espina**
flounder   **lenguado**

haddock   **róbalo**
hake (a type of bass)   **merluza**
herring (smoked)   **arenque (ahumado)**
   m
lobster   **langosta**
mackerel   **pejerrey** *m;* **caballa**
octopus   **pulpo**
oyster   **ostra; ostión** *m, Mex.*
perch   **percha**
prawn   **langostino**
red snapper   **huachinango** *Mex.;* **pargo**
   Cuba
roe   **hueva**

salmon   **salmón** *m*
sardines   **sardinas**
scallop   **escalope** *m*
shellfish   **marisco**
shrimps   **camarones** *m;* **gambas**
snapper   **pargo**
sole   **lenguado**
squid   **calamar** *m*
trout   **trucha**
tuna   **atún** *m*
turtle   **tortuga**
white fish   **corégono**

FRUITS   *FRUTAS*

apple   **manzana**
apricot   **albaricoque** *m;* **chabacano**
avocado   **aguacate** *m, Mex., C.A.;* **palta**
   Sp. Am.
banana   **banana; plátano; guineo**
berry, wild   **baya silvestre**
blackberry   **zarza**
blueberry   **vaccinio**
cherry   **cereza**
citrus fruit   **fruta cítrica**
currant   **grosella**
date   **dátil** *m*
fig   **higo**
gooseberry   **grosella silvestre**
grape   **uva**

grapefruit   **toronja; pomelo** *Sp. Am.*
guava   **guayaba**
lemon   **limón** *m*
lime   **lima**
mango   **mango**
melon   **melón** *m*
nut   **nuez** *f*
orange   **naranja; china** *P.R.*
papaya   **papaya; fruta boma** (Cuba—
   Avoid use of *papaya* in this country!)
peach   **melocotón** *m;* **durazno**
pear   **pera**
   prickly pear   **tuna**
pineapple   **piña** *f;* **ananá** *m/f*
pit   **hueso**

plantain   **plátano; banana** *m*
plum   **ciruela**
pomegranate   **granada**
prune   **ciruela seca; ciruela pasa; pruna**
   Chicano
pumpkin   **calabaza**
quince   **membrillo**
raisin   **pasa**
raspberry   **frambuesa**
seed   **pepita**
skin (of fruit)   **cáscara**
strawberry   **fresa; frutilla** *Sp. Am.*
tangerine   **mandarina**
watermelon   **sandía**

DESSERTS   *POSTRES*

bonbon   **bombón** *m*
cake   **torta; bizcocho; queque** *m*
   cheese cake   **quesadilla**
   small pastry cake   **bollo**
candy   **dulces** *m, pl;* **confites** *m, pl*
chewing gum   **chicle** *m*
chocolate bar   **barra de chocolate**
cookie   **galleta; galletica; pasta** *f*
custard   **flan** *m;* **natillas**
dessert   **postre** *m*

doughnut   **rosquilla; donut** *m, Chicano;*
   buñuelo
eclair   **pastelillo de crema**
ice cream   **helado; mantecado; nieve** *f*
jello   **gelatina**
lollipop   **caramelo en un palito; paleta;**
   pirulí *m*
meringue   **merengue** *m*
nut   **nuez** *f*
pastry   **pasta; pastel** *m*

sweet pastry   **quesadilla**
pie   **pastel** *m*
pudding   **budín** *m;* **pudín** *m*
rice pudding   **arroz con leche** *m*
sherbet   **sorbete** *m;* **nieve** *f, Mex.*
sweet   **dulce** *m*
syrup   **jarabe** *m*
tapioca   **tapioca**
whipped cream   **nata batida**

BEVERAGES   *BEBIDAS*

alcohol   **alcohol** *m*
ale   **cerveza inglesa**
atole (drink made with cornmeal gruel)
   atole *m, Sp. Am.*
beer   **cerveza; helada** *Chicano*
beverage   **bebida**
   cold beverage   **refresco**
brandy   **coñac** *m;* **aguardiente** *m*
champagne   **champaña**
chocolate   **chocolate** *m*
   chocolate milk   **leche con chocolate** *f*
   cocoa   **cacao**
   hot chocolate   **chocolate caliente** *m*
cider   **sidra**
   can cider   **guarapo**
   fruit cider, fermented maize   **chicha**
   Sp. Am.
cocktail   **coctel** *m*
coffee   **café** *m*
   black coffee   **café solo; café puro;**
     café tinto *Col.*
   coffee with cream   **café con crema**
   coffee with cream and sugar   **café con**
     azúcar y crema

coffee with milk   **café con leche**
coffee with sugar   **café con azúcar**
decaffeinated coffee   **café**
   descafeinado
instant coffee   **café instantáneo;**
   nescafé *m*
strong coffee   **café fuerte; café**
   cargado
weak coffee   **café débil; café claro;**
   café simple; café suave; café ralo
cream   **crema**
drink   **bebida; trago** (usually alcoholic)
   carbonated drink   **gaseosa**
   cold drink   **bebida fría**
   hot drink   **bebida caliente**
gin   **ginebra**
juice   **jugo**
   apple juice   **jugo de manzana**
   cranberry juice   **jugo de arándano**
   grape juice   **jugo de uvas**
   grapefruit juice   **jugo de toronja**
   lemon juice   **jugo de limón**
   lime juice   **jugo de lima**
   orange juice   **jugo de naranja**

pineapple juice   **jugo de piña**
prunce juice   **jugo de ciruela**
tomato juice   **jugo de tomate**
lemonade   **limonada**
liqueur   **licor** *m*
milk   **leche** *f*
   buttermilk   **leche agria; suero de**
     leche
   condensed milk   **leche condensada**
   cow's milk   **leche de vaca**
   dry milk   **leche en polvo**
   evaporated milk   **leche evaporada**
   malted milk   **leche malteada**
   pasteurized milk   **leche pasteurizada**
   skim milk   **leche desnatada; leche**
     sin crema; leche descremada
   orangeade   **naranjada**
pop   **soda; gaseosa; coca cola**
punch   **ponche** *m*
refreshment   **refresco**
rum   **ron** *m*
tea   **té** *m*
   iced tea   **té helado**
   Paraguay tea   **yerba mate** *Sp. Am.*

strong tea **té fuerte; té cargado**	drinking water **agua potable**	whiskey **whiskey** *m*
weak tea **té débil; té claro; té simple; té suave; té ralo**	mineral water **agua mineral**	wine **vino**
	seltzer water **agua de Seltz**	claret, red wine **vino tinto**
water **agua**	soda water **agua de soda; soda**	white wine **vino blanco**
carbonated water **agua gaseosa**		

DISHES AND UTENSILS *LOZA Y UTENSILIOS*

bowl **escudilla; tazón** *m, Mex*	knife **cuchillo**	saucer **platico; platillo**
china **loza; porcelana**	ladle **cucharón** *m*	spoon **cuchara**
coffeepot **cafetera**	lid **tapa**	straw **pajiza; popote** *m*
cup **taza**	napkin **servilleta**	tablespoon **cuchara grande; cuchara de sopa**
dish **plato; platico**	pepper shaker **pimentero**	
fork **tenedor** *m*	plate **plato**	teapot **tetera**
frying pan **sartén** *f*	platter **fuente** *f*	teaspoon **cucharita; cucharilla; cuchara de café**
glass **vaso**	pot **caldera; olla; puchero; pote** *m*	
jar **jarra; frasco,** *Mex*	salt shaker **salero**	tray **bandeja; charola; charo/m,** *Sp.*
jug **jarra**	saucepan **cacerola**	*Am.*

Notes *Notas*

1. This may refer to appendicitis, peritonitis, or a bowel obstruction.
2. See note 1.
3. In northwestern Mexico a poisonous lizard is called a scorpion.
4. See "sting," page 338.
5. This illness is found in southern Mexico, the high plateaus of Guatemala, and eastern Venezuela.
6. This may also refer to appendicitis or peritonitis.
7. In rural areas, especially of Mexico and Puerto Rico, peasants often call any serious skin disease, especially infected wounds or gangrene, **cancer.**
8. See **Selected Drug Abuse Vocabulary,** pages 343–345.
9. See Chapter 1, pages 22–23 for a discussion of this.
10. See page 24 for a discussion of "fever."
11. For a fuller discussion of folk illnesses, see Chapter 1, pages 17–25.
12. See page 24.
13. This "disease" has nothing to do with bile.
14. See Chapter 1, page 24.
15. See above, note 1.
16. See **Selected Drug Abuse Vocabulary** below, page 344.
17. A common brand of aspirin in Latin America is **mejoral** or **mejoralito,** for children.
18. See **Selected Drug Abuse Vocabulary** below, page 344.
19. See page 346.
20. See **Selected Drug Abuse Vocabulary** below, page 344.
21. See **Pregnancy, Childbirth, Contraception, Postnatal Care of the Mother,** pages 347–349; and Chapter 12, pages 267–272.
22. Use the Spanish pronunciation of these letters.
23. See Chapter 1, Table 1.1, pages 20–21.
24. This is new vocabulary, not necessarily listed nor yet recognized by the Royal Academy of Spanish Grammar. It is understood that this vocabulary is primarily slang. Unless otherwise indicated, the gender of nouns is assumed to be obvious.
25. I have followed the spelling given in the *Diccionario de la lengua española,* RAE, 21st edition, 1990. Spanish does recognize variations using **j** and **h.**
26. The English street terminology for *cocaine* includes: angel dust, Bernice gold dust, bernies, big C, blow, burese, C, candy, c-game, C & H, carrie, Cecil, Charlie, cholly, coca, coke, Corine, dream, dust, dynamite, flake, gin, girl, gold dust, happy dust, heaven dust, her, jelly, joy powder, King's habit, killer stuff, lady, lady snow, leaf, love affairs, M & C, Merck, nose, nose candy, nose powder, one & one, paradise, rich man's heroin, rock, schmeck, schoolboy code, sleigh ride, snow, snowbird, speedball, star dust, thing, white lady, white stuff, whiz bang.
27. Street terminology generally uses "syrup" (terpinhydrate) and terps for codeine.
28. A croaker is a physician who dispenses prescriptions for drugs.
29. A flash is the euphoric initial reaction to IV narcotics.
30. The English street terminology for *heroin* includes: a-bomb, big H, blanks, boss, boy, brother, brown, ca-ca, caballo, carga, C & H, China white, Chinese red, chiva, cobics, crap, dogie, doojee, doojie, dope, duji, dynamite, dyno, eighth, Frisco speedball, girl, goods, gravy, H, hairy, hard stuff, harry, H-caps, Henry, him, hochs, horse, joy powder, junk, ka-ka, killer stuff, lemonade, love affairs, Mexican brown, Mexican horse, Mexican mud, noise, peg, poison, scag, scar, schmeck, shit, skag, smack, smeck, snow, speedball, stuff, sugar, tecata, thing, TNT, white junk, white lady, white stuff, whiz bang.
31. The English street terminology for *LSD* includes: acid, barrels, (the) beast, big D, blue acid, blue cheer, blue heavens, blue mist, blue sky, blue tab, blue wedge, brown dots, California sunshine, cherry dome, cherry top, (the) chief, chocolate chips, Christmas acid, clear-light, coffee, contact lens, crackers, crystals, cube, cupcakes, deeda, dome, dots, double dimples, electric kool-aid, fifty, flats, gammon, (the) Ghost, grape parfait, grays, green barrels, (the) hawk, haze, heavenly blue, hit, instant Zen, L, LSD 25, Lucy in the sky (with diamonds), lysergide, mellow yellows, micro dots, mikes, mind detergent, oranges, orange mushrooms, orange sunshine, orange wedge, Owsley's acid, Ozzie's stuff, paper acid, peace, peace acid, peace pills, pearly gates, pellets, pink wedge, product IV, psychedelic, purple barrels, purple dome, purple dots, purple haze, purple microdots, purple ozoline, purple wedge, royal blue, smears, squirrels, Stanley's stuff, strawberry field, sunshine, tabs, ticket, trips, turtle, twenty-five, wedge, white lightning, window pane (paine) yellow dimples.
32. The English street terminology for *marijuana* includes: a-bomb, a-stick, Acapulco gold, ace, African black, Alice B. Toklas, baby, bale, bar, bhang, black gunion, boo, brick, broccoli, buddha sticks, bush, butter flower, can, Canadian black, cannabis, cannabis

sativa, charge, cocktail, colombo, Colombian, Colombian red, C.S. dagga, dawamesk, doobee, dope, dry high, dube, duby, fatty, finger lid, flower tops, fuma d'Angola, funny stuff, gage, Gainesville green, ganga, gangster, ganja, giggle weed, giggles-smoke, goblet of jam, gold, gold Colombian, golden leaf, gold star, goof but, grass, grasshopper, green, grefa, greta, griefo, griefs, grifa, griffo, gunga, gungeon, gunja, haircut, has, Hawaiian, hay, hemp, herb, hooch, Indian hay, Indian hemp, intsaga, intsagu, J, Jane, jay, jay smoke, jive, jive stick, Juana, Juanita, Juanita weed, juja, kaif, Kansas grass, kauii, kee, key, ki, kick sticks, kif, killer weed, kilter, light stuff, loaf, loco, locoweed, loveweed, mach, macon, maconha, marihuana, mariguana, Mary, Mary Anne, Mary Jane, Mary Warner, Mary Werner, Mary Wearver, Mary Weaver, Mary Worner, match box, mauii, Mex, Mexican, Mexican brown, Mexican green, Mexican locoweed, M.J., mohasky, moocah, moota, mooters, mootie, mor a grifa, mota, moto, mu, muggles, muta(h), nail, nigra, number, Panama gold, Panama red, panatella, pin, pod, pot, potlikker, P.R. (Panama red), Puff the Dragon, rainy day woman, red dirt marijuana, reefer, righteous bush, roach, root, rope, Rose Maria, rough stuff, sativa, seeds, shit, skinny, smoke, smoke Canada, snop, stack, stems, stick, super pot, Sweet Lucy, T, tea, Texas tea, thrupence bag, thumb, tustin, twist, weed, wheat, yesca.

33. The English street terminology for *mescaline* includes: anhalonium, beans, big chief, blue caps, blue devils, buttons, cactus, full moon, hikori, huatari, mesc, mescal, mescal buttons, moon, plants, seni.

34. The English street terminology for *morning glory seeds* includes: badoh negro, blue star, flying saucers, glory seeds, heavenly blues, pearly gates, pearly whites, seeds.

35. The English street terminology for *morphine* includes: cobies, dope, emsel, first line, goods, hard stuff, hocus, junk, M, morf, morphie, morpho, morphy, mud, sister, Miss Emma, mojo, cube.

36. Also known as nembutol, nimbies, nemish, nimby.

37. The English street terminology for *opium* includes: black, black stuff, gow, gum, hop, leaf, Mash Allah.

38. The English street terminology for PCP includes: amoeba, angel dust, angel hair, animal tranquilizer, cadillac, C.J., crystal, crystal joints, cyclones, dead on arrival, D.O.A., dust, elephant tranquilizer, goon, hog, horse tranquilizer, killer weed, K.J., mist, peace pill, pig tranquilizer, rocket fuel, scuffle, sheets, snorts, soma.

39. Other slang terms include: dealer, mother, pusher.

40. The English street terminology for *psilocybin* includes: hombrecitos, little children, little men, little women, magic mushroom, las mujercitas, mushrooms, los niños, noble princess of the waters.

41. Another slang term is mule.

42. The English street terminology for *seconals* include: bullets, devils, M & M, red devils, reds.

43. The English street terminology for *yage* includes: ayahuasca, caapi, drug, jungle drug.

44. For a more complete listing, see **Anatomical Vocabulary**, page 69.

45. This is the forty-day period following delivery during which there is a prolonged period in bed, much freedom from household responsibilities, and abstention from sexual intercourse.

46. See note 45.

47. See **Anatomical Vocabulary** (page 69) for slang terminology.

48. All of the words in this vocabulary belong to "standard" Spanish, understood by all who know Spanish. Yet many variants exist for all of these nouns, depending upon the influence of the many distinct and unrelated Indian dialects that have entered the language. An example of this is seen in the different forms Hispanic America has for *little boy*: Argentina—**pibe**; Chile—**cabro**; Colombia—**pelado**; Cuba—**chico**; El Salvador—**cipote**; Guatemala—**patojo**; Mexico—**chamaco**; Panamá—**chico.**

49. In the Spanish-speaking world, it is common to have relatives living in a household—grandparents, aunts, and uncles—along with the nuclear family. The typical Hispanic attitude is that older people are happiest when with their children. An elderly parent *or* relative who is chronically sick will be cared for at home as long as possible.

For most Hispanics family gatherings are a very important part of their social life. The extended family members often live within a few blocks of each other. Family members usually stick together, but especially in times of trouble.

50. See Maps on pages 358–360.

51. Some nouns or adjectives of nationality—like **nicaragüense**—have only one form; others—like **boliviano**—change the masculine *-o* to *-a* for the feminine; those ending in a consonant add *-a* for feminine; **español/española.**

52. Spanish-speaking countries refer to people from the United States in a number of different ways. People from Colombia, Perú, Chile, and Venezuela call them *gringos.* That term in Mexico, however, is derogatory. People from Mexico, along with Spain and Argentina, use *norteamericano.* (*Estadounidense* is considered more correct, but is difficult to say. It is used in formal writing, when filling out forms, or in formal speeches.)

The term *norteño* is used to refer to someone of Mexican descent who resides in *el Norte,* meaning in the United States. When used in Mexico, the term refers to someone living in the northern states of Mexico. It is important to remember in any case, that all people who live in the Western Hemisphere consider themselves *americanos,* not just those from the United States.

53. There is a tendency to differentiate gender of nouns of occupation. New feminine forms are rapidly being incorporated into the Spanish language (e.g., **abogada, arquitecta, presidenta**). Nouns of occupation are presented here in one gender. Nouns referring to "masculine" occupations are usually masculine (**el químico** the chemist, **el médico** the physician).

As a rule, nouns of occupation ending in o can be made feminine by changing the o to **a.** Masculine nouns of occupation that end in **or** can be made feminine by adding an **a** (el trabajador, la trabajadora).

The Americas *Las Américas*

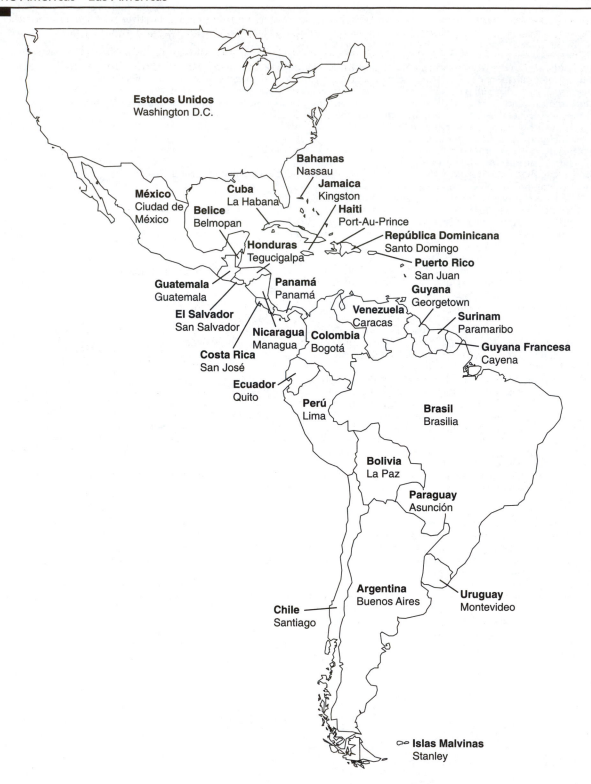

Estados Unidos
Washington D.C.

Bahamas
Nassau

México
Ciudad de
México

Cuba
La Habana

Jamaica
Kingston

Belice
Belmopan

Haiti
Port-Au-Prince

Honduras
Tegucigalpa

República Dominicana
Santo Domingo

Puerto Rico
San Juan

Guatemala
Guatemala

Panamá
Panamá

Guyana
Georgetown

El Salvador
San Salvador

Venezuela
Caracas

Surinam
Paramaribo

Nicaragua
Managua

Colombia
Bogotá

Guyana Francesa
Cayena

Costa Rica
San José

Ecuador
Quito

Perú
Lima

Brasil
Brasilia

Bolivia
La Paz

Paraguay
Asunción

Argentina
Buenos Aires

Uruguay
Montevideo

Chile
Santiago

Islas Malvinas
Stanley

LOS ESTADOS DE MEXICO

Mexico, like the United States, is a republic made up of states and a Federal District (*el Distrito Federal*, which is abbreviated "D.F."). There are 31 states in the Mexican Republic, six of which border on the United States. Mexicans introduce themselves by their city and state of origin, rather than say they are Mexican i.e., *Soy de Guadalajara, estado de Jalisco*. When Mexicans say, *Soy de México*, they usually mean they are from the capital of the state of Mexico.

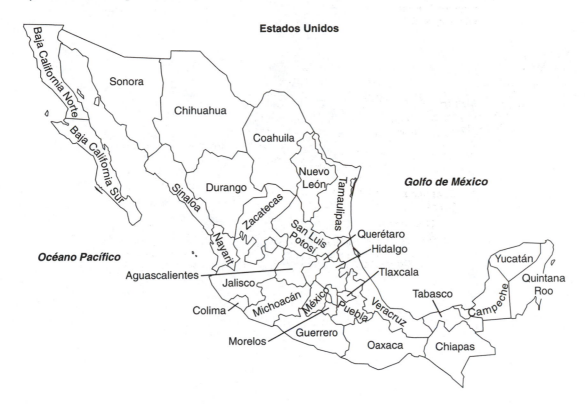

¿Dónde Está . . . ?

Señala en el mapa.

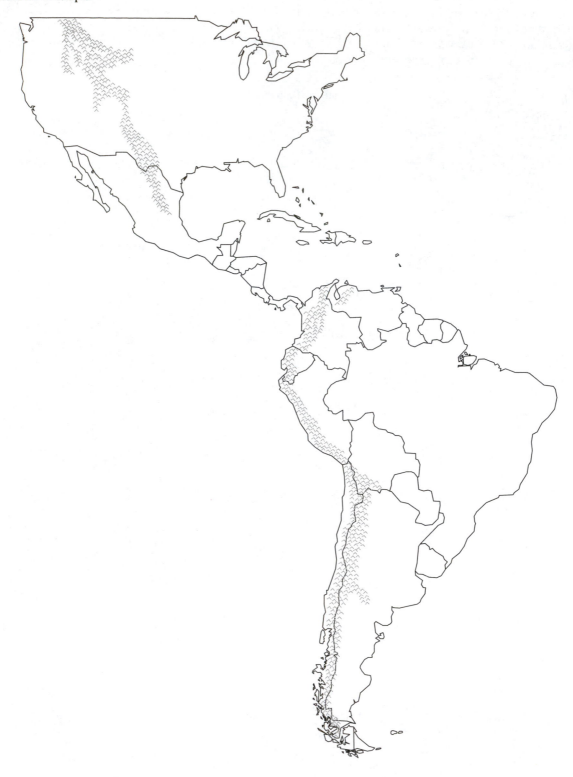

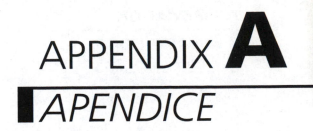

APPENDIX **A**
APENDICE

English-Spanish Vocabulary

Vocabulario inglés-español

ABBREVIATIONS
ABBREVIATURAS

adj	adjective	**adjetivo**
adv	adverb	**adverbio**
euph	euphemism	**eufemismo**
f	feminine noun	**sustantivo feminino**
fam	familiar/colloquial	**familiar/coloquial**
inv	invariable	**invariable**
m	masculine noun	**sustantivo masculino**
m/f	masculine or feminine noun	**sustantivo masculino** o **feminino**
pl	plural	**plural**
sg	singular	**singular**

Unless specified, words ending with **a** are feminine, words ending with **o** are masculine

SPECIAL WORDS USED TO INDICATE REGIONAL OCCURRENCES
PALABRAS ESPECIALES USADAS PARA INDICACION REGIONAL

Arg.	Argentina	**la Argentina**
Bol.	Bolivia	**Bolivia**
C.A.	Central America (Guatemala, El Salvador, Honduras, Costa Rica, Nicaragua)	**Centroamérica (Guatemala, el Salvador, Honduras, Costa Rica, Nicaragua)**
Carrib.	(Cuba, Puerto Rico, Dominican Republic)	**(Cuba, Puerto Rico, la República Dominicana)**
Chicano	Chicano (southwestern U.S.)	**Chicano**
Chile		
Col.	Columbia	**Colombia**
C.R.	Costa Rica	**Costa Rica**
Cuba		
Ec.	Ecuador	**el Ecuador**
Guat.	Guatemala	**Guatemala**
Hond.	Honduras	**Honduras**
Mex.	Mexico	**México**
Nic.	Nicaragua	**Nicaragua**
Pan.	Panama	**Panamá**
Para.	Paraguay	**Paraguay**
Peru		**Perú**
P.R.	Puerto Rico	**Puerto Rico**
Riopl.	Rio de la Plata region (Eastern Argentina, Uruguay)	**Río de la Plata (la Argentina oriental, el Uruguay)**
Sal.	El Salvador	**el Salvador**
Sp.Am.	Spanish America	**América del Sur**
Spain		**España**
Ur.	Uruguay	**el Uruguay**
Ven.	Venezuela	**Venezuela**

VOCABULARY
VOCABULARIO

abdomen abdomen *m;* panza *fam;* vientre *m*
abortion aborto
  abortion, induced aborto inducido; aborto provocado
  abortion, spontaneous aborto espontáneo
  abortion, therapeutic aborto terapéutico
  abortion, threatened amenaza de aborto
abrasion razpón *m;* rozadura

abscess absceso; hinchazón *f*
abscessed apostemado *adj*
abstain from sexual relations, to abstenerse de las relaciones sexuales
accident accidente *m*
acetaminophen acetaminofén *m*
acid ácido
  acetic acid ácido acético (puro)
  acetylsalicylic acid ácido acetilsalicílico
  acid, arsenic ácido arsénico
  acid, ascorbic ácido ascórbico

  acid, boric ácido bórico
  acid, cyanic ácido ciánico
  acid, folic ácido fólico
  acid, p-aminosalicylic (PAS) ácido paramino salicílico
acne acné *f;* cácara *Chicano;* espinillas *f*
Acquired Immune Deficiency Syndrome/AIDS Síndrome de Inmuno(logía) Deficiencia Adquirida/SIDA *m*
acrylic acrílico *adj*

activated charcoal carbón activado *m*
acupunture acupuntura
acute abdomen abdomen agudo *m*
Adam's apple bocado de Adán; manzana *Mex*; nuez de Adán *f*
add, to agregar; añadir
addict (drug) adicto; adicto a droga(s); adicto a las drogas narcóticas; drogadicto; morfinómano; toxicómano; yeso
addict in search of a fix buscatoques *m/f, inv*
addicted adicto *adj*; prendido *adj*
addiction (drug) toxicomanía
adenoids vegetaciones adenoideas *f*
adhesive adhesivo *adj*
  adhesive plaster emplasto adhesivo
  adhesive tape cinta adhesiva; esparadrapo; tela adhesiva
administer marijuana to someone, to engrifar; enmarihuanar; marihuanar
adrenalin adrenalina
advantage ventaja
adverse result resultado adverso
afterbirth placenta; secundinas *f, pl, Mex.*; segundo parto *Chicano*
AIDS SIDA *m*
ailment dolencia
albumen albúmina; albumen *m*
alcohol alcohol *m*
  alcohol, rubbing alcohol para fricciones *m*
alcoholism alcoholismo
alertness viveza
allergic reaction reacción alérgica *f*; trastorno alérgico
allergy alergia
alveoli alvéolos
amalgam amalgama
amenorrhea amenorrea
amino acids aminoácidos
ammonia amoníaco
amniocentesis prueba del saco amniótico
amniotic sac saco amniótico
amniotic fluid agua del amnios
amoebic dysentery disentería amibiana
amphetamine anfetamina
  amphetamine, heroin, and barbiturate——Class IV bombita
  amphetamines, a; ácido *sg* bombido; naranjas; pepas *slang*
ampicillin ampicilina
ampoule ampolleta
amuse oneself, to have a good time divertirse (ie)
analgesic analgésico
anemia anemia; sangre clara *fam*; sangre débil *f, fam*; sangre pobre *f, fam*
  anemia, aplastic anemia aplástica
  anemia, iron deficiency deficiencia de hierro
  anemia, pernicious anemia perniciosa
  anemia, sickle cell anemia drepanocítica; drepanocitemia
  anemia—thalassemia talasemia
anesthesia anestesia
  anesthesia, block anestesia de bloque
  anesthesia, caudal anestesia caudal
  anesthesia, epidural anestesia epidural
  anesthesia, general anestesia total
  anesthesia, inhalation anestesia por inhalación

anesthesia, local anestesia local
anesthesia, regional anestesia regional
anesthesia, saddle block anestesia en silla de montar
anestesia, spinal anestesia espinal; anestesia raquídea
anesthesia—twilight sleep sueño crepuscular
anesthetic anestético *m, adj*; anestésico *m, adj*
aneurysm aneurisma *m*
anger cólera; coraje *m*; rabia
angina angina
  angina pectoris angina del pecho
angiomate angioma *m*; cabecita de vena *Chicano*
anguish angustia; congoja
ankle tobillo
  ankle support tobillera
antacid antiácido *m, adj*
antibiotic antibiótico *m, adj*
  antibiotic, broad-spectrum antibiótico de alcance amplio; antibiótico de espectro amplio
  antibiotic, limited-spectrum antibiótico de alcance reducido; antibiótico de espectro reducido
antibody anticuerpo
anticholinergic anticolinérgico *m, adj*
anticoagulant anticoagulante *m, adj*
antidote antidoto
  antidote, universal antidoto universal
antiemetic antiemético *m, adj*
antigen antígeno
antihemorrhagic antihemorrágico *adj*
antihistamine antihistamínico *m, adj*; droga antihistamínica
antimalarial antipalúdico *m, adj*
antipyretic antipirético *m, adj*; febrífugo *m, adj*
antiseptic antiséptico *m, adj*
antispasmodic antiespasmódico *m, adj*
antitetanic; anti-tetanus antitetánico *adj*
antitoxin antitoxina; contraveneno
anus ano; agujero *vulgar, Chicano*; chicloso *vulgar, Chicano*; chiquito *vulgar, Chicano*; fundillo *Mex.*; istantino *fam*
anxiety ansiedad *f*
aortic insufficiency insuficiencia aórtica
aphasia afasia
aphonia (hoarseness) afonia; ronquera
apoplexy (stroke) apoplejía
apparatus aparato
  apparatus, prosthetic aparato prostético; prótesis *f*
appendicitis apendicitis *f*; panza peligrosa *slang*; abdomen agudo *m, slang*
appendix apéndice *m*; apendix *f*; tripita *fam*
appetite apetito *m*
application aplicación *f*; *(request)* solicitud *f*; petición *f*
apply for admission, to solicitar admisión a
appointment cita; turno
apron delantal *m*
aqueous humor humor acuoso *m*
ARC/AIDS Related Complex CRS Complejo Relacionado al SIDA

arch supports soportes para el arco del pie *m*
arm brazo
  arm, bend of the flexura del brazo
armpit axila; sobaco; arca *Mex.*
arrhythmia, cardiac arritmia cardíaca
arsenic arsénico
arteriosclerosis arteriosclerosis *f*
arthritis artritis *f*
articulation articulación *f*; coyuntura
artificial artificial *adj*; postizo *adj*
  artificial limb miembro artificial
  artificial respiration respiración artificial *f*
Asiatic flu influenza asiática
ask (for) (to request) pedir (i)
aspirin aspirina
  aspirin, children's aspirina para niños
assume asumir
asthma ahoguío *fam, Mex.*; asma; fatiga *slang*
  asthma, bronchial asma bronquial
asthmatic asmático *adj*
  asthmatic attack (seizure) ataque asmático *m*
  asthmatic wheeze resuello asmático
astigmatism astigmatismo
astringent astringente *m, adj*
asymptomatic asintomático *adj*
atrial fibrillation fibrilación auricular *f*
atropy atrofia
atropine atropina
attack ataque *m*
authorization autorización *f*, permiso
authorize, to autorizar
baby (infant) bebé *m*; criatura; guagua *m/f, Bol, Chile, Ec., Perú*; nene *m*; nena
back dorso; espalda
backbone columna vertebral
bacteremia bacteriemia
bacterium bacteria
bag of waters aguas *f*; bolsa de las aguas; bolsa membranosa; fuente *f, fam*
bald calvo *adj*
baldness calvicie *f*
balloon (of heroin) globo
balsam bálsamo; ungüento
band cinta; faja
bandage venda; vendaje *m*
  bandage, elastic vendaje elástico
  bandage, swathing faja abdominal
  bandage, to fajar; vendar
Bandaid curita; parchecito; venda
barbiturate barbiturato
barbiturate (pill) barbiturato; barbitúrico; cacahuate *m*; colorada; globo
base of the cranium base del cráneo *f*
bath baño
  bath, bran baño de salvado
  bath, emollient baño emoliente
  bath, mustard baño de mostaza
  bath, oatmeal baño de harina de avena
  bath, potassium permanganate baño de permanganato de potasio
  bath, saline baño salino
  bath, shower ducha; baño de regadera *Chicano*
  bath, stiz baño de asiento; semicupio
  bath, sodium baño de sodio
  bath, sponge baño de esponja; baño de toalla *Chicano*

bath, starch   baño de almidón
bath, sulfur   baño de azufre
bath, tar   baño de brea
bathe, to *(someone)* bañar; *(take a bath, to)* bañarse
be, to   estar; ser
  be—years old, to   tener—años
  be afraid, to   tener miedo
  be ashamed, to   tener vergüenza
  be blue, to   tener murria
  be called, to *(be named, to)* llamarse
  be careful, to   tener cuidado
  be carrying narcotic drugs, to   andar carga; andar cargado (cargada); traer carga
  be cold, to   tener frío
  be gowned, to   vestirse (i) de bata de hospital
  be guaranteed, to   ser garantizado (garantizada)
  be guilty, to *(be at fault, to)* tener la culpa
  be (non)habit forming, to   (no) crear vicio
  be high, to   andar/ponerse + *adj* (see "high")
  be hungry, to   tener hambre *f*
  be in a hurry, to   tener prisa
  be in the habit of, to   soler (ue)
  be late, to   tener retraso
  be on the road to recovery, to   estar recuperándose
  be quiet, to   callarse
  be right, to   tener razón
  be sleepy, to   tener sueño
  be successful, to   tener éxito
  be thirsty, to   tener sed *f*
  be under the weather, to   estar pachucho (pachucha) *Spain*
  be up and about after an illness, to   estar pachucho (pachucha) *Spain*
  be warm, to   tener calor *m*
  be wrong, to   no tener razón
beard   barba
bear down, to   hacer bajar por fuerza; pujar
bearing   porte *m*
become, to *(something)* hacerse + *something*
become *(turn)* **+ adj, to**   ponerse + *adj of emotional/mental state*
become bloated, to   abotagar
bed   cama; lecho
bedbug   chinche *f*
bedpan   bacín *m*; bacinilla; chata; vasín de cama *m*
bedsore   llaga de cama; úlcera por decúbito
beg, to   rogar (ue)
begin, to   comenzar (ie); empezar (ie)
belch, to   eructar; regoldar (ue); regurgitar
belladonna   belladona
Bell's palsy   parálisis facial *f*
belly   barriga; panza *fam*
  "belly" binder   fajero; ombliguero
bend over, to   agacharparse; agachar(se); doblarse
benzedrine   bencedrina
benzoin   benzoína; benjuí *m*
bewitch, to   aojar; embrujar; hechizar
bicarbonate of soda   bicarbonato de soda; salarete *m*
biceps   bíceps *m*; conejo *slang, Chicano*; mollero *fam*

bichloride of mercury   cloruro mercúrico
bicuspid   bicúspide *m, adj*; diente premolar *m*
bile   bilis *f*; hiel *f*; biliar *adj*
  bile salt   sal biliar *f*
bilirubin   bilirrubina
bind, to   amarrar; atar
binder   cintura; faja; vendaje abdominal *m*
birth *(childbirth)* alumbramiento; nacimiento; parto
  birth, at term   a término
  birth canal   canal del parto *m*
  birth certificate   certificado de nacimiento; partida de nacimiento
  birth control   control de la natalidad *m*
    Billings' method   método de Billings
    cervical cap   gorro cervical
    coil   coil *m, Chicano*
    coitus interruptus   interrupción de coito *f*; retirarse *m*; salirse *m, slang*
    condom   condón *m*; forro *vulgar, Arg.*; goma; hule *m, slang*; preservativo; profiláctico
    diaphragm   diafragma (anticonceptivo) *m*
    IUD   aparatito *Chicano*; aparato intrauterino; DIU *m*; dispositivo intrauterino
    loop   alambrito; asa; lupo
    pill   pastilla; píldora
    rhythm   método de ritmo; ritmo
    rubber   forro *vulgar, Arg.*; goma; hule *m, slang*
    sterilization   esterilización *f*
    tubal ligation   ligadura de trompas
    vaginal cream   crema vaginal
    vaginal foam   espuma vaginal
    vaginal jelly   jalea vaginal
    vasectomy   vasectomía
  birth, multiple   nacimiento múltiple
  birth, post-term   nacimiento tardío
  birth, premature   nacimiento prematuro
  birth, to give   alumbrar; dar a luz; parir; salir due su cuidado *Chicano*; sanar *euph*
birthmark   lunar *m*
birthweight   peso del nacimiento
bite *(animal)* mordedura
  bite, cat   mordedura de gato
  bite, dog   mordedura de perro
  bite, human   mordedura humana
  bite, scorpion   mordedura de escorpión
  bite, snake   mordedura de serpiente
bite *(toothmark)* dentellada
bite *(insect)*, **sting**   picadura
  spider   picadura de araña
bite, to   morder (ue); picar
black and blue   amoratado *adj*
blackeye   ojo morado
blackhead   espinilla
bladder   vejiga; vesícula
blanket   cobija; frazada; manta
bleach   blanqueo; cloro
bleed, to   sangrar
  bleed excessively, to *(bleed in excess, to)* desangrar
bleeding *adj* sangrante *adj*; *n* flujo de sangre; hemorragia

bleeding, breakthrough   flujo de sangre por la vagina inesperadamente; hemorragia inesperada
bleeding, internal   hemorragia interna
bleeding tendencies   tendencias a sangrar
bleeding time   tiempo de hemorragia
bleeding to excess   desangramiento
blemish   lunar *m*; mancha
blepharitis   blefaritis *f*
blind   ciego *adj*
  blind in one eye   tuerto *adj*
blindness   ceguedad *f*; ceguera
  blindness, color   acromatopsia; ceguera para los colores; daltonismo
  blindness, night *(nyctalopia)* ceguera nocturna; nictalopía
  blindness, river *(onchocerciasis)* ceguera del río; oncocercosis *f*
blink, to   parpadear
blister   ampolla; bulla; vesícula
  blister on sole of foot   sietecueros *m, inv*
bloated   abotagado *adj*; hinchado *adj*
block   bloqueo
  block nerve   bloqueo nervioso
block, to   bloquear; obstruir
  block the nerve, to   obstruir el nervio
blockage   obstrucción *f*
blocked intestine   intestino obstruido; tripa obstruida
blood   sangre *f*; colorada *slang, Chicano*; sanguíneo *adj*
  blood bank   banco de sangre
  blood chemistry *(analysis of blood)* análisis de sangre *m, inv*
  blood circulation   circulación sanguínea *f*
  blood clot   coágulo de sangre; coágulo sanguíneo; cuajarón *m*, cuajarón de sangre *m*
  clot reaction time   tiempo de coagulación
  blood coagulation time   tiempo de coagulación
  blood component   componente de sangre *m*; componente sanguíneo *m*
  blood count   biometría hemática; hematimetría; recuento sanguíneo
  blood culture   hemocultivo
  blood donor   donante de sangre *m/f*
  blood group   grupo sanguíneo
    universal donor   donante universal *m/f*
    universal recipient   receptor (receptora) universal *m/f*
  blood, occult   sangre oculta
  blood, oxalated   sangre oxalatada
  blood oxygen analyzer   analizador del oxígeno de la sangre *m*
  blood plasma   plasma sanguíneo *m*
  blood poisoning   envenenamiento de la sangre; intoxicación de la sangre *f*; sepsis *f*; septicemia; toxemia
  blood pressure   presión arterial *f*; presión sanguínea *f*
    high b.p.   hipertensión arterial *f*; presión sanguínea alta *f*
    low b.p.   hipotensión arterial *f*; presión arterial baja
  blood, screening   prueba selecta de sangre

blood smear   frotis sanguíneo *m*; extensión de sangre *f*

bloodstain   mancha de sangre

bloodstained   manchado de sangre *adj*

bloodstock   depósito de sangre

bloodstream   corriente sanguínea *f*; torrente sanguíneo *m*; torrente circulatorio *m*

blood sugar   azúcar sanguínea *f*; glicemia; glucemia

blood test   examen de la sangre *m*

blood transfusion   transfusión de sangre *f*

blood type   grupo sanguíneo; tipo de sangre

blood vessel   vaso sanguíneo

blood, whole   sangre entera; sangre pura

bloody   cruento *adj*; sanguíneo *adj*

   bloody show   muestra de sangre; tapón de moco *m, Mex.*; secreción mucosa mezclada con sangre *f*

blotches, skin   manchas oscuras en la piel

blow one's nose, to   sonarse la nariz

body   cuerpo

   body, ciliary   cuerpo ciliar

boil   furúnculo; nacido; sisote *m*; tacotillo *Chicano*

boil the bottles, to   hervir (ie) las botellas

bone   hueso

booster shot   búster *m, Chicano*; inyección de refuerzo *f*; reactivación *f*

borax   bórax *m*

borderline case   caso dudoso; caso incierto; caso límite

bosom   senos *m, pl*

bothersome   incómodo *adj*

bottle   botella; envase *m*; frasco

   bottle baby   biberón *m*; bote *m, slang, Chicano*; botella; mamadera *Sp.Am.*; pacha *Chicano*; tele *Chicano*

bowel   intestino inferior

   bowel obstruction   abdomen agudo *m, slang*; obstrucción de la tripa *f*; panza peligrosa *slang*

bowels   entrañas; tripa *fam*

brace   braguero

braces   aparato ortodóntico; frenos *Arg., Mex.*

brain   cerebro

brains   sesos

breast   agarraderas *f, Chicano*; busto; chichas *f, pl, C.R.*; chiche *f*; chichi *f, Mex.*; pecho, seno, tele *f*; teta *slang*

   breast, caked   mastitis por estasis *f*

   breast, of a wet nurse   chiche *m, Mex., Guat.*

   breast, painful   seno doloroso

breastbone   esternón *m*

breastfeed, to   criar con pecho *Chicano*; dar chiche; dar de mamar; dar el pecho

breastfeeding   lactania maternal

breast pump   bomba de ordeñar; bomba para mamar; mamadera; tiraleches *f, inv*

breast self-examination (BSE)   auto exploración de las mamas *f*; autoexamen mensual de los senos *m*

breath   aliento

breathe, to   resollar (ue); respirar

   breathe hard, to   exhalarse

breathing   respiración *f*; resuello

breechbirth (*frank breech*)   presentación de nalgas *f*; presentación trasera *f*

brewer's yeast   levadura de cerveza

bridge (*dental*)   puente *m*

   bridge, fixed   puente fijo

   bridge, removable   puente movible

bromide   bromuro

bronchia   bronquios *m*

bronchitis   bronquitis *f*

bruise   contusión *f*; lastimadura; magulladura; morete *m, Mex., Hond.*; moretón *m*

bruised   moreteado *adj, Chicano*

brush one's teeth, to   cepillarse los dientes

bubo   búa; ganglio; incordio; seca *fam*

bubonic plague   peste bubónica *f*

bulging eyes   ojos saltones; ojos capotudos *Chicano*

bullet   bala

   bullet wound   balazo

bunion   juanete *m*

burn (oneself), to   quemar(se)

burn   quemadura; quemazón *m*

   burn, acid   quemadura por ácido

   burn, alkali   quemadura por álcali

   burn, chemical   quemadura química

   burn, dry heat   quemadura por calor seco

   burn, scald   escaldadura

   burn, sun   eritema solar *m*; bronceado; quemadura solar; solanera

burp   eructo; regüeldo

burp, to   eructar; repetir (i); sacar aire *Chicano*; urutar *Chicano*

burr   fresa

bursitis   bursitis *f*

buttock   anca; aparato *Chicano*; bombo *Ur.*; buche *m, vulgar, Chicano*; común *m, Mex.*; culo *fam, Arg.*; fondillo *Cuba*; fondongo *slang*; fundillo *Mex.*; nalga; olla *slang, Chicano*; pellín *m, Chicano*; salvohonor *m, fam*; sentadera

buzzing in the ears   zumbido en los oídos

caffeine   cafeína

calamine   calamina

calcium   calcio

calcium sulfate   escayola; sulfato de calcio

calloused   calloso *adj*

callus   callo

calm down, to   calmar(se)

camphor   alcanfor *m*

cancer   cáncer *m*

cancerous   canceroso *adj*

cane   báculo; bastón *m*

canker   llaga ulcerosa; úlcera; ulceración *f*

   canker sore   postemilla; ulceración *f*

can opener   abrelatas *m, inv*

capillary   capilar *m*; vaso capilar

capsule   cápsula

   homemade drug capsule   encachucha

carbohydrate   carbohidrato

carbolic acid   ácido carbólico

carbon tetrachloride   tetracloruro de carbono

carcinoma   carcinoma *m*

cardiac   cardíaco *adj*

   cardiac arrest   fallo cardíaco; paro cardíaco

   cardiac arrythmia   arritmia cardíaca

   cardiac care   cuidado cardíaco

cardiopulmonary resuscitation   resucitación cardiopulmonar *f*

cardiopulmonary resuscitator   resucitador cardiopulmonar *m*

cardioscope   cardioscopio

careless (*neglected*)   descuidado *adj*

caries   caries *f, inv*; cavidad dental *f*; diente cariado *m*; diente picado *m*; diente podrido *m*; picadura

carrier   portador (portadora) de enfermedad *m/f*

cartilage   cartílago

case   caso

cast   calote *m*; yeso; enyesadura

   cast, gypsum   vendaje de yeso *m*

cataplasm   cataplasma

cataract   catarata; granizo

catch, to (*come down with a disease*)   caer con algo

   catch a cold, to   constiparse *Spain*; coger (un) catarro; pescar un catarro; acatarrarse; agriparse; resfriarse

   catch a disease, to   contraer una enfermedad; agarrar; pegarle

cathartic   purgante *m*

catheter   catéter *m*; drenaje *m, Chicano*; sonda; tubo

catheterize, to   cateterizar

caucasian   caucasiano *adj*

cause vomiting, to   provocarse el vómito

cauterization   cauterización *f*

cavity   cavidad *f*; hueco; (*dental*) caries *f, inv*; diente cariado *m*; diente picado *m*; diente podrido *m*; picadura; neguijón *m*

celiac disease   enfermedad celíaca *f*

cell   célula

   cell, ciliated   célula ciliada

   cell, sickle   célula falciforme

cementum   cemento

cerebral   cerebral *adj*

   cerebral cortex   corteza cerebral; materia gris *fam*

   cerebral hemisphere   hemisferio cerebral

   cerebral paralysis   parálisis cerebral *f*

cerebrospinal meningitis   meningitis cerebroespinal *f*

cerebrum   cerebro

   cerebrum, anterior chamber of   cámara anterior del cerebro

   cerebrum, posterior chamber of   cámara posterior del cerebro

certify, to   certificar

cervix   cérvix *f*; cerviz *f*; cuello de la matriz; cuello del útero

cesarean delivery   parto cesáreo; parto por operación

cesarean section   operación cesárea *f*; sección cesárea *f*

chafing   irritación *f*; rozadura

Chagas' disease   enfermedad de Chagas *f*

chancre   chancro

   chancre, soft   chancro blando

change of life   cambio de vida; menopausia

change (oneself), to   cambiar(se)

chapped   cuarteado *adj*; rozado *adj*

chap skin, to   cuartearse; rozarse

chart   diagrama *m*

checkup   chequeo *Chicano*

cheek (*buttocks*):   cacha; (*part of the face*): cachete *m*; mejilla; (*side wall of mouth*): carrillo

cheekbone   pómulo

cheilosis (*sore at corner of mouth*)   boquilla

chest   pecho; tórax *m*
chew, to   mascar; masticar
chicken pox   bobas; tecunda *Mex.*; varicela; viruelas locas *slang*
chigger flea   garrapata; güina *Mex.*; nigua
chilblain   sabañón *m*
childbirth   alumbramiento; parto
chill   escalofrío
chin   barba; barbilla; mentón *m*; piocha; talache *m*
chloasma *(facial discoloration, mask of pregnancy)*   cloasma *m*; mancha de la preñez; mancha del embarazo; paño
chloramphenicol   cloranfenicol *m*
chloride   cloruro
chlorine   cloro
chloromycetin   chloromicetín *m*; cloromicetina
chlorophyll   clorofila
chloroquinine   cloroquina
choke, to   ahogarse; atorarse; atragantarse
choking   asfixia
cholecystogram   colecistograma *m*
cholera   cólera *m*
cholesterol   colesterol *m*; grasa en las venas
choose, to   elegir (i)
chorea   corea; mal/baile de San Guido/de San Vito *m*
chor(i)oid   coroides *f, inv*; corioide *f*
chronic   crónico *adj*; duradero *adj*
cigarette butt   bachica *(esp. marijuana)*; tecla; tecolota
circulation   circulación *f*
circumcise, to   circuncidar
circumcision   circuncisión *f*
cirrhosis of the liver   cirrosis del hígado *f*; cirrosis hepática *f*
clasp   gancho
cleaning   limpieza
cleanliness   aseo
clean, to   limpiar
clean oneself, to   limpiarse
cleft palate   boquineta *m, Chicano*; fisura palatina; grietas en el paladar; paladar hendido *m*; paladar partido *m*
climb up, to   subirse
clitoris   bolita *slang*; clítoris *m*; pelotita *slang*; pepa *slang*
close, to   cerrar (ie)
clot, to   cuajar
club foot   pie deforme *m*; pie zambo *m*; talipes *m*
coagulant   coagulante *m, adj*
coal tar   brea de hulla
coarse   grueso *adj*
coated tongue   lengua saburrosa; lengua sucia
cocaine   acelere; aliviane; alucine; arponazo; azúcar; blanca nieves; carga; coca; cocacola; cocada; cocaína; cocazo; coco; coka; cotorra; cucharazo; chutazo; doña blanca; glacis; knife; marizazo; nice; nieve; nose; pase; pericazo; pepsicola; perico *slang, Cuba*; polvito; polvo; talco *Texas, Cuba*; tecata
crack cocaine   crac *m*; crack *m*
coccyx   cóccix *m, Chicano*; colita; coxis *m*; rabadilla
cocoa butter   manteca de cacao
codeine   codeína
coitus   coito

cold *n*   catarro; resfriado; resfrío *Chile adj* frío *adj*
cold, common   resfriado común
cold, "stuffed-up" head   constipado
cold pack   compresa fría; emplasto frío
colic   cólico
colitis   colitis *f*
collapse   colapso
collapse, physical   colapso físico
collar bone *(clavicle)*   clavícula; cuenca
colon   colon *m*
colon, sigmoid   colon sigmoide(o)
colostomy   colostomía
colostrum   calostro
coma   coma *m*
comb   peine *m*
comb, fine-tooth   chino *Mex.*
comb one's hair, to   peinarse
come, to   venir
comfortable   cómodo *adj*
communicate a disease, to   contagiar
compete, to   competir (i)
complain, to   quejarse
complication   accidente *m*; complicación *f*
compress   cabezal *m*; compresa
conceive, to   concebir (i)
conception   concepción *f*; fecundación del huevo *f*
concussion   concusión *f*; golpe *m*
confess, to   confesar (ie)
confinement   alumbramiento; cuarentena; puerperio; riesgo
congenital   congénito *adj*
congenital anomaly   anomalía congénita
congenital malformations   malformaciones congénitas *f*
congested *(stuffed up)*   constipado *adj*
congestion   congestión *f*
congestion of the chest   ahoguijo; ahoguío
conjunctiva   conjuntiva
conjunctivitis   conjuntivitis *f*; mal de ojo *m, fam*; tracoma *m*
connect, to   conectar
consent, to   consentir (ie)
constipated   estreñido *adj*
constipation   constipación *f*; entablazón *f, Chicano*; estreñimiento
contact   contacto
contact lens   lente de contacto *m*; microlentilla; pupilente *m*
contagious   contagioso *adj*; pegadizo *adj*; pegajoso *adj, fam*
contamination   contaminación *f*
continue, to   continuar; seguir (i)
continue working, to   seguir (i) trabajando
contraceptive   anticonceptivo *adj*; contraceptivo *m, adj*
contraceptive pills   pastillas anticonceptivas
contraction   contracción de la matriz *f*; contracción uterina *f*; dolor de parto *m*
control, to   controlar; regular
contusion   contusión *f*
convalescence   convalecencia
convalescent   convalecente *m/f, adj*
convert, to   convertir (ie)
convulsion   ataque *m*; convulsión *f*
coramine   coramina
cord   cordón *m*
cord blood   sangre umbilical *f*

cord, umbilical   cordón del ombligo; cordón umbilical
corn   callo
corn plaster   emplasto para callos; parches para callos *m*
cornea   córnea
coronary   coronario *adj*
coronary thrombosis   trombosis coronaria *f*
corpse   cadáver *m*
corticosteriod   corticoesteroide *m*
cortisone   cortisona
cost, to   costar (ue)
cotton   algodón *m*
cotton, absorbent   algodón absorbente
cotton, sterile   algodón estéril
cotton swab   escobillón *m*; hisopillo; hisopo de algodón
cough   tos *f*
cough drops   gotas para la tos; pastillas para la tos
cough lozenges   pastillas para la tos
cough, non-productive   tos seca
cough, productive   tos productiva; tos húmeda
cough suppressant   calmante para la tos *m*
cough syrup   jarabe para la tos *m*
cough, smoker's   tos por fumar
cough, whooping   tos ferina; coqueluche *f*; tos convulsiva; tosferina
cough, to   toser
cough up phlegm, to   desgarrar *Chicano*; esgarrar
Coumadin   Cumadina
count, to   contar (ue)
crack *(drug)*   crac *m*; crack *m*
crack, to   agrietar; rajar
cramps   calambres *m*
charleyhorse   rampa
cramps, abdominal   retortijón *m*; torcijón *m*
cramps, cane-cutters'   calambres de los cortadores de caña
cramps, heat   calambres térmicos
cramps, menstrual   dolores del período *m*; calambres
cramps, muscular   calambres
cramps *(postpartum pains)*   entuertos
cramps, stomach   retortijón de tripas *m*; torcijón cólico *m, Mex.*
cretinism   cretinismo
crib   camilla de niño; cuna
crib, warming   armazón de calentamiento *f*; camilla calentadora de niño; estufa; incubadora
cripple   inválido *m, adj*; tullido *m, adj*
crippled   cojo *adj*; empedido *adj*; lisiado *adj*
crippled hand   manco *adj*
cross-eyed   bisojo *adj*; bizco *adj*; turnio *adj*
cross-eyes   bizquera
cross match   pruebas cruzadas
crotch   entrepiernas *f, pl*
croup   crup *f*; garrotillo
crown   corona
crown of the head   mollera
crown of tooth   corona; filet *m*
crown, acrylic jacket   corona acrílica
crown, porcelain jacket   corona de porcelana

crown, to coronar; estar coronando
crowning coronamiento
crow's feet patas de gallo
crush, to machucar
crutch muleta; sobaquera *fam*
cry, to llorar
crystalline cristalino
cure cura; método curativo
cure-all sanalotodo *Chicano*
cure, to aliviar
  cure from the evil eye, to desaojar
curettage curetaje *m*; raspado
cuspid cúspide *m*; colmillo; canino
cut cortada *Sp.Am.*; cortadura
cut (oneself), to cortar(se)
cut teeth, to dentar (ie); echar dientes;
  endentecer
cuticle cutícula
cyst quiste *m*
cystic fibrosis fibrosis quística *f*
cystitis cistitis *f*; infección de la vejiga *f*
cystoscope cistoscopio
dacryocystitis daciocistitis *f*; infección
  de la bolsa de lágrimas *f*
daily cotidiano *adj*; diario *adj*; por día
damage daño
D&C legrado *fam*; raspa *fam*
dandruff caspa
dangerous peligroso *adj*
dangle one's legs, to colgar (ue) las
  piernas
dazed atarantado *adj*
dead muerto *m, adj*
deaden the nerve, to adormecer el nervio
deaf sordo *adj*
deaf-mute sordomudo
deafness ensordecimiento; sordera
deal in drugs, to dilear; diliar; puchar
  deal heroin, to llevar carga; llevar
  mula
death fallecimiento; muerte *f*
death rattle estertor agónico *m*
decongestant descongestionante *m, adj*
deep profundo *adj*
defecate, to andar el cuerpo; hacer caca;
  hacer el cuerpo; ir al inodoro *fam*;
  obrar *Mex.*
defect defecto
defibrillator defibrilador *m*
deficiency carencia; deficiencia
deformed deforme *adj*; eclipsado *adj*;
  inocente *adj, Mex.*
deformity deformidad *f*
dehydrate, to deshidratar; perder (ie)
  flúidos del cuerpo
dehydration desecación *f*;
  deshidratación *f*
delirium delirio
deliver, to dar a luz; parir; tener el
  niño; aliviarse *Chicano*
delivery parto
  delivery, abdominal parto abdominal
  delivery, breech extracción de nalgas
  f
  delivery, forceps extracción con
  fórceps *f*
  delivery, premature parto prematuro
  delivery room sala de partos
  delivery table mesa del parto
delouse, to espulgar
dementia demencia
demonstrate, to *(show, to)* demostrar
  (ue)
dengue dengue *m*; fiebre rompehuesos *f*

dental dental *adj*
  dental artery arteria dental
  dental drill taladro; torno; trépano
  dental floss cordón dental *m*; hilo
  dental; seda encerada
  dental forceps gatillo; pinzas;
  tenazas de extracción
  dental hygienist higienista dental
  m/f
  dental impression mordisco
  dental nerve nervio dental
  dental office clínica dental
  dental vein vena dental
dentifrice dentífrico *m, adj*
dentine dentina
dentition dentición *f*; dentadura
denture dentadura (postiza)
  denture, full dentadura completa
  denture, partial dentadura parcial
deny, to negar (ie)
deodorant desodorante *m, adj*
depilatory depilatorio *m, adj*
depressed deprimido *adj*
depression abatimiento; depresión *f*
deprive, to privar
dermatitis dermatitis *f*
desire (to), to tener deseos (de)
destroyed destruido *adj*
detached retina retina desprendida
detect, to descubrir; detectar
detergents detergentes *m*
determination of circulation time
  determinación del tiempo de
  circulación *f*
detox, to desintoxicarse
detoxification program programa de
  destoxificación *m*
dextrose azúcar de uva *m*; dextrosa
diabetes diabetes *f*
  diabetes insipidus diabetes insipida
  diabetes, insulin-dependent
  diabetes insulino-dependiente;
  diabetes sacarina dependiente de la
  insulina
  diabetes, juvenile onset diabetes
  (del principio) juvenil; diabetes
  precoz
  diabetes mellitus diabetes mellitus;
  diabetes sacarina
  diabetes, non-insulin-dependent
  diabetes sacarina no dependiente de
  la insulina
diabetic diabético *m, adj*
diagnose, to diagnosticar
diagnosis diagnosis *f, inv*; diagnóstico
dialysis en diálisis
diaper braga; pañal *m*; pavico *Chicano*;
  zapeta *Mex.*
  diaper rash chincual *m*; escaldadura
  (en los bebés); pañalitis *f*;
  salpullido
diaper, to cambiar el pañal; proveer con
  pañal; renovar (ue) el pañal
diaphragm diafragma anticonceptivo *m*
diarrhea asientos *m, slang*; cagadera
  vulgar, Chicano; cámara; chorrillo *slang*;
  chorro *slang*; corredera *Chicano*;
  cursera *slang*; diarrea; soltura *Chicano*;
  turista *slang*
diastole diástole *f*
die, to morir (ue) *(impersonal)*; morirse
  (ue) *(personal)*
  die of old age, to morir (ue) de viejo
diet dieta; régimen *m*

diet, liquid dieta de líquidos
diet, be on a -, to estar a dieta
diet, put on a -, to poner a dieta
digest, to digerir (ie)
digestion digestión *f*
digestive system aparato digestivo
digitalin digitalina
dilation (of cervix) dilatación del
  cuello de la matriz *f*
diphenhydramine difenhidramina
diphtheria difteria; garrotillo
disability incapacidad *f*; inhabilidad *f*;
  invalidez *f*
disc disco
  disc, calcified disco calcificado
discern, to discernir (ie)
discharge flujo; secreción *f*; supuración
  f; descarga
  discharge, bloody derrame *m*
  discharge, vaginal flujo vaginal
  discharge, white flores blancas *f*;
  flujo blanco
discharge (from the hospital), to dar
  de alta
discomfort incomodidad *f*; malestar *m*
discovery descubrimiento
disease dolencia; enfermedad *f*; mal *m*
  disease due to act of witchcraft
  enfermedad endañada *Chicano*
  disease, notifiable enfermedad de
  notificación
  disease, reportable enfermedad
  obligatoria
  disease that is "going around"
  enfermedad de andancia *f, Chicano*
disinfectant desinfectante *m, adj*
disorder desorden *m*
dissolve, to disolver (ue)
  dissolve heroin in a spoon over a
  flame, to cukear; cuquear
diuretic diurético *m, adj*
diverticulitis colitis ulcerosa *f*;
  diverticulitis *f*
dizziness tarantas *f, Mex., Hond.*;
  vahido; vértigo
dizzy vertiginoso *adj*
doctor's bag maletín *m*
dope pusher narcotraficante *m/f*
dosage dosificación *f*; dosis *f, inv*
dose dosis *f, inv*, medida
douche ducha interna; ducha vaginal;
  irrigación *f*; lavado interno; lavado
  vaginal
down *(soft hair on human body)* vello
Down's syndrome mal de Down *m*;
  mongolismo
DPT vacuna triple
drag *(puff of [marijuana] cigarette)*
  toque *m*
drainage desagüe *m*; drenaje *m*;
  supuración *f*
  drainage (surgical) drenaje *m*
draining (dripping) escurrimiento
dram dracma *m*
dream (of), to soñar (con) (ue)
dress (oneself), to vestir(se) (i)
dressing apósito; cura; curación *f*;
  emplaste *m*; parche *m*; vendaje *m*
drill, to perforar; taladrar
drink plenty of . . . beber mucho . . .
drop gota
drop back into to retroceder
dropper cuentagotas *m, inv*
dropsy ahogamiento; hidropesía

drowsiness   mordorra; somnolencia
drug   droga; medicina
   drug abuse   abuso de (las) drogas
   drug addict   adicto (adicta) a las drogas; drogadicto
   drug addiction   dependencia farmacológica; narcomanía
   drugs, bag of   clavo de drogas; talega de drogas
   drug habit   morfinomanía
   drug hallucinogenic   alucinógeno; droga alucinadora
   drug overdose   sobredosis de drogas *f, inv*
   drugstore   botica; droguería *Sp.Am.;* farmacia *Spain*
   drug supply   cachucha
drunk   alumbrado *adj, slang, Chicano;* bolo *adj, C.A.;* borracho *adj;* caneco *adj, Bol, Ven;* intoxicado *adj;* pisto *adj;* rascado *adj, Ven.;* tacuache *adj;* tlacuache *adj;* tronado *adj*
drunk, to be *(to get)*   andar bombo; andar eléctrico (eléctrica); emborracharse; estar borracho; estar mediagua; ponerse alto *fam;* rascar *Sp.Am.*
drunkenness   borrachera
dry, to   secar
duct   conducto
duodenum   duodeno
dwarf   enano *m/f*
dye   tinte *m*
dying   moribundo *adj*
dysentery   disentería
   dysentery, amoebic   disentería amibiana
   dysentery, bacillary   disentería bacilar
dysmenorrhea   dismenorrea; menstruación dolorosa *f*
dyspnea   dificultad al respirar *f*
dysuria   dolor al orinar *m*
ear   oreja
ear *(organ of hearing)*   oído
   auditory   auditivo *adj*
   earlobe   lóbulo
      external ear   aurícola; oído externo; pabellón externo de la oreja *m*
      eardrum *(tympanic membrane)*   tímpano
      external ear canal   canal de le oreja *m, fam;* conducto auditivo externo
   inner ear   oído interno
      cochlea   caracol *m;* cóclea
      earwax   cera de los oídos; cerilla; cerumen *m*
      earwax, impacted   tapón de cera *m*
      Eustachian tube   trompa de Eustaquio
      saccule   sáculo
      semicircular canal   conducto semicircular
   middle ear   oído medio
      anvil *(incus)*   yunque *m*
      hammer *(malleus)*   martillo
      stirrup *(stapes)*   estribo
earache   dolor de oído *m*
eat breakfast, to   desayunarse
eclampsia   eclampsia
eczema   eccema *m/f;* rezumamiento; lepra *fam*
edema   edema *m;* hinchazón *f*
egg white   clara de huevo

ejaculate, to   eyacular; venirse *slang*
elbow   codo
electricity   electricidad *f*
electrical   eléctrico *adj*
   electrical current   corriente *f, adj*
   electrical ground(ing)   polaridad *f*
   electrical lead wire   alambre de contacto *m*
   electrical outlet   salida
   electrical plug   clavija de contacto; enchufe *m*
   electric polarity   polaridad *f*
   electric socket   enchufe *m;* tomacorriente *m/f;* tomada *Sp.Am.*
electrocardiogram   electrocardiograma *m*
electroencephalogram   electroencefalograma *m*
emaciation   demacración *f;* enflaquecimiento
embolism   embolia; embolismo
embryo   embrión *m*
emergency   caso urgente; emergencia; urgencia
emesis basis   riñonera
emetic   emético *m, adj;* vomitivo *m, adj*
emollient   emoliente *m, adj*
emphysema   enfisema *m*
empty, to   vaciar
emulsion   emulsión *f*
enamel   esmalte *m*
encephalitis   encefalitis *f*
endometrium   endometrio
endoscope   endoscopio
enema   ayuda; enema *m/f;* lavado; lavativa
   enema bag   bolsa para enema
   enema, barium   enema de bario; enema opaca
   enema, cleansing   enema de limpieza
   enema, nutritive   enema nutritiva
   enema, retention   enema de retención
   enema, soapsuds   enema jabonosa
energy   energía
engorgement   estancamiento
enlargement   agrandamiento; ampliación *f;* ensanchamiento
enzyme   enzima; jugo digestivo
ephedrine   efedrina
epidemic   epidemia; epidémico *adj*
epidermis   epidermis *f*
epilepsy   ataque (de epilepsia) *m;* epilepsia
epileptic attack   ataque epilético *m;* convulsión *f*
episiotomy   corte de las partes *m;* episiotomía; tajo *slang*
epsom salt   sal de epsom *f;* sal de higuera *f*
erysipelas   dicipela *Chicano;* erisipela
erythrocytes *(red blood cells)*   eritrocitos; glóbulos rojos; hematíes *m*
erythromycin   eritromicina
esophagus   esófago; tragante *m, Chicano*
estrogen   estrógeno
   estrogen replacement therapy   terapia sustitutoria con estrógeno
eucalyptus leaves   hojas de eucalipto
every   cada *adj*
exam, medical   examen médico *m*
examination   examinación *f;* reconocimiento; chequeo *Chicano*

examine, to   examinar
excessive   excesivo *adj*
exchange list   lista de intercambios
excretion   excreción *f;* excremento; miércoles *m, slang*
exempt, to *(release, to)*   eximir
exercise moderately, to   hacer ejercicios moderados
exhale, to   exhalar; espirar
exhaustion   agotamiento; fatiga
expectorant   expectorante *m, adj*
expel anal gas, to   tirarse flato; tirarse un pedo
expiration date   fecha de caducidad
expulsion   expulsión *f*
external   externo *adj*
extract   extracto
extraction   extracción *f*
eye   ojo
   chorioid   corioide *f;* coroides *f, inv*
   cone   cono
   conjunctiva   conjuntiva
   cornea   córnea
   dropper *(medicine dropper)*   cuentagotas *m, inv;* goteador *m;* gotero (para los ojos) *Sp.Am.*
   eyeball   globo del ojo; globo ocular; tomate *m, slang, Chicano*
   eyebrow   ceja
   eye cup   copa ocular; lavaojos *m, inv;* ojera
   eyelash   pestaña
   eyelid   párpado
   eyepads   paños en los ojos; toallas en los ojos
   glasses   anteojos *pl;* espejuelos *pl;* gafas *pl;* lentes *pl;* quevedos *pl*
   iris   iris *m*
   lachrymal   lacrimal *adj;* lagrimal *adj*
   lens   cristalino
   pupil   niña del ojo; pupila
   retina   retina
   rod   bastoncillo
   salve   ungüento para los ojos
   sclera   esclerótica; esclera; córnea opaca
   shield   escudo ocular
   tear duct   conducto largrimal
   tear sac   bolsa de lágrimas
face   cara; carátula *slang; Chicano;* rostro
faint, to   desmayarse
fainting spell   desfallecimiento; desmayo; desvanecimiento; mareo *fam;* vértigo
   fainting spell during pregnancy   achaque *m, C.R.*
fall, to   caer
   fall asleep, to *(doze off, to)*   dormirse(ue)
   fall down, to   caerse
fallen fontanel   caída de la mollera
Fallopian tubes   trompas de Falopio; tubos
family   familia
   family planning   planificación de la familia *f;* planificación familiar *f*
farsighted   hiperópico *adj;* présbita *adj*
farsightedness   hipermetropía; presbicia; presbiopía
fasting   ayuno *m, adj;* en ayunas
   fasting blood sugar   glucemia en ayunas
fat   gordo *adj;* grasa
fatigue   fatiga
fauces   fauces *f, pl*

fear   miedo

features   facciones *f*

feces *(stool)*   «aguas mayores» *f, euph;* caca *slang;* cagada *vulgar;* cámara; deposiciones *f;* evacuación del vientre *f;* excrementos *m;* heces fecales *f, pl;* materia fecal; pase del cuerpo *m*

feeble   enfermizo *adj*

feed, to   alimentar

feeding   alimentación *f*

feel, to *(regret, to)*   sentir (ie)
  feel (emotion/pain), to   sentirse (ie)
  feel *(touch)*, to   tocar
  feel like, to   tener ganas (de)
  feel nothing, to   no sentir (ie) nada

femur   fémur *m*

fester, to   enconarse

fetal heart tone   latido del corazón fetal

fetoscope   estetoscopio fetal; fetoscopio

fetus   feto

fever   calentura; fiebre *f*
  fever, acute infectious adentitis   fiebre ganglionar
  fever blister   herpe febril *m/f;* llaga de fiebre
  fever, breakbone   fiebre rompehuesos
  fever, Colorado tick   fiebre de Colorado; fiebre tra(n)smitida por garrapatas
  fever, enteric   fiebre entérica
  fever, glandular   fiebre glandular
  fever, hay   alergia; catarro constipado *Chicano;* fiebre de(l) heno; jey fíver *m/f*
  fever, intermittent   fiebre intermitente
  fever, malarial   chucho *Chile, Arg.;* fiebre palúdica
  fever, Malta   brucelosis *f;* fiebre de Malta; fiebre ondulante
  fever, paratyphoid   fiebre paratífica; fiebre paratifoidea
  fever, parrot   fiebre de las cotorras
  fever, rabbit   fiebre de conejo
  fever, rat bite   fiebre por mordedura de rata
  fever, rheumatic   fiebre reumática
  fever, Rocky Mountain spotted   fiebre de las Montañas Rocosas; maculosa de las Montañas Rocosas
  fever, scarlet   fiebre escarlatina
  fever, spotted   fiebre manchada; tifus exantemático
  fever, thermic   fiebre térmica
  fever, typhoid   fiebre tifoidea; tifo abdominal
  fever, typhus   tifo; tifus *m;* tifus exantemático *m;* úrzula *Chicano*
  fever, undulant   fiebre ondulante
  fever, valley *(coccidiodoimycosis)*   fiebre del valle
  fever, yellow   fiebre amarilla; fiebre tropical; tifo de América; tifus icterodes *m;* vómito negro

fibrin   fibrina

fibroid   fibroideo *adj*

fibroma   fibroma *m*

fibula   peroné *m*

file down, to   limar

fill, to   calzar; empastar; emplomar *Arg.;* llenar; rellenar; tapar
  fill prescriptions, to   hacer recetas
  fill with gold, to   orificar

filling   empastadura; empaste *m;* emplomadura *Arg.;* relleno; tapadura
  filling, temporary   empaque *m, Chicano;* empaste provisional
  lose a filling, to   caérsele un empaste a alguien

filter, to   filtrar

find, to   encontrar (ue)

finger   dedo
  finger, fleshy tip of the   yema
  finger, index   índice *m*
  knuckle   nudillo
  finger, little   meñique *m*
  finger, middle   dedo del corazón; dedo del medio
  finger, ring   dedo anular
  finger, thumb   dedo gordo; pulgar *m*
  ball of thumb   pulpejo

first aid   primera ayuda; primeros auxilios *m, pl*

fissure   cisura; fisura; grieta; partidura

fist   puño

fistula   fístula

fit   arrebato; convulsión *f*

fitness *(good health)*   buena salud *f*

fix *slang*   abuja; abujazo; cura; filerazo; gallazo

flank   costado

flap of skin   colgajo

flask   frasco

flat foot   pie plano *m;* planovegus *m*

flatulence   flatulencia; ventosidad *f*

flatus   aire *m;* flato; pedo *slang;* ventosidad *f;* viento

flea   pulga

flesh   carne *f*

floater   mancha volante; mosco volante

flour   harina

flow, to   fluir

flu   gripa; gripe *f;* influenza

fluoride   fluoruro

fluorine   flúor *m*

flushed   enrojecido *adj*

foam   espuma

folk illness   enfermedad casera *f*

follicle   folícula

follow, to   seguir (i)

fontanel   fontanela; mollera

foot   pie *m*
  foot, sole of the   planta del pie

foramen   agujero; foramen *m*

forceps *(obstetric)*   fórceps *m;* *(dental)* gatillo; tenazas

forearm   antebrazo

forehead   frente *f*

foreskin   prepucio

formula   fórmula

forty days following parturition   cuarentena

fossa   fosa

foul-smelling   apestoso *adj*

fovea centralis   fóvea central

fracture   fractura; quebradura de huesos
  fracture, avulsion   fractura por arrancamiento
  fracture, closed   fractura simple; fractura cerrada
  fracture, comminuted   fractura conminuta
  fracture, complicated   fractura complicada
  fracture, compound   fractura compuesta

fracture, green stick   fractura en tallo verde

fracture, impacted   fractura impactada

fracture, multiple   fractura múltiple

fracture, oblique   fractura oblicua

fracture, open   fractura abierta; fractura complicada

fracture, serious   fractura grave; fractura mayor

fracture, simple   fractura simple

fracture, skull   fractura del cráneo

fracture, spontaneous   fractura espontánea

fracture, transverse   fractura transversa

fracture, to   fracturar; quebrarse

freckle   peca

free   gratis *adv;* libre *adj*
  free will   libre albedrío

frenum of the tongue   frenillo

frigidity   frigidez *f*

frontal   frontal *adj*

frostbite   congelación *f;* daño

frozen section   corte por congelación *m*

fumigation   fumigación *f*

fundus   fondo del útero

funeral   entierro

funeral home   funeraria

fungicide   fungicida *m, adj*

fungus   hongo
  athlete's foot   infección de serpigo *f;* pie de atleta *m*
  moniliasis   boquero; candidiasis *f* moniliasis *f;* muguet *m*
  ringworm *(tinea)*   culebrilla; empeine *m;* serpigo; sisote *m Chicano;* tiña
  tinea corporis   jiotes *f, fam*

funnel   embudo

furniture polish   pulimento para muebles

gain weight, to   engordar

gait   marcha

gallbladder   vejiga de la bilis; vesícula biliar

gallbladder attack   ataque vesicular *m;* dolor de la vesícula *m*

gallstone   cálculo biliar; cálculo en la vejiga; piedra en la vejiga

ganglion   ganglio

gangrene   cangrena; gangrena

gargle *(act)*   gárgara; *(liquid)* gargarismo

gargle, to   hacer buches (de sal) *fam;* hacer gárgaras

gas   gas *m*

gash   cuchillada

gastric juice   jugo gástrico

gastritis   gastritis *f*

gastrointestinal system   aparato/sistema gastrointestinal *m*

gauze   gasa

genitals   órganos genitales; partes *f, slang;* partes ocultas *f, slang;* verijas

genitourinary system   aparato/sistema genito-urinario *m*

gentian violet   violeta de genciana

germ   germen *m,* microbio

German measles   alfombría *Chicano;* alfombrilla *Chicano;* fiebre de tres días *f;* peluza *Mex.;* rubéola; sarampión alemán *m;* sarampión bastardo *m*

germicide   germicida *m*

gestation   gestación *f*; gravidez *f*
get, to   obtener; *(a disease)* coger
   get angry, to   enfadarse; enojarse
   get close, to   acercarse
   get drunk, to   jalarse *Sp.Am.*
   get frightened, to   asustarse
   get goose bumps, to   enchinarse la piel; ponerse chinito; ponérsele la piel de gallina
   get high on drugs, to   ponerse loco
   get high on speed, to   poner blancas
   get married, to *(marry)*   casarse con
   get old, to   envejecer(se)
   get sick, to   enfermarse
   get tired, to   cansarse; fatigarse
   get undressed, to   desvestirse (i)
   get up, to *(from bed)*   levantarse; *(stand up, to)* levantarse; ponerse de pie; *(wake up, to)* despertarse (ie)
   get wet, to   mojarse
gingiva   encías
give up (a claim), to   ceder
gland   glándula
   gland, adrenal   glándula suprarrenal
   gland, carotid   glándula carotídea; carótida
   gland, endocrine   glándula endocrina
   gland, lymph   glándula linfática
   gland, mammary   glándula mamaria
   gland, parathyroid   glándula paratiroides
   gland, pineal   glándula pineal
   gland, pituitary   glándula pituitaria
   gland, prostrate   glándula de la próstata; glándula prostática; próstata
   gland, sebaceous   glándula sebácea
   gland, sweat   glándula sudorípara
   gland, thyroid   glándula tiroides
glans, (penis)   bálano; cabeza *slang*; glande *m*
glass *(drinking)*   vaso
glass eye   ojo de vidrio
glaucoma   glaucoma *m*
glucagon   glucagón *m*; hormona glicética
glucose   glucosa
   glucose water   agua con azúcar
glue   cola; goma
glue sniffer   glufo
gluteal region   glúteo; región glútea *f*
glycerine   glicerina
glycogen   glicógeno; glucógeno
gnat   bobito *Chicano*; jején *m, Sp.Am.*
goal   meta; objetivo
go, to   ir
   go away, to   irse; marcharse
   go down in the birth canal, to   encajarse
   go to bed, to   acostar(se) (ue)
goiter   bocio; buche *m, slang*; gueguecho
gold   oro
gonorrhea   blenorragia; chorro *fam*; gonorrea; purgación *f, slang*
gout   gota
gown   bata; camisón *m*
graft   injerto
green card *(migration card)*   mica
groin   empeine *m*; ingle *f*; aldilla
ground chalk in water   creta pulverizada en agua
guaiacol   guayacol *m*
guarantee, to   hacer garantías

gums   encías
gynecological floor   piso ginecológico
gynecologist   ginecólogo
hair   cabello(s); chimpa *Chicano*; pelo
   hair, curly   pelo chino *Mex*; pelo rizado
   hair, kinky   pelo grifo
   hair, prematurely gray   canas verdes
   hair, pubic   pelo púbico; vello púbico; pelitos *m, pl, Chicano*
   hair, straight   pelo liso
   hair, wavy   pelo ondulado
hairy   peludo *adj*; tarántula *Chicano*
hallucination   alucinación *f*
hallucinogen   alucinógeno; droga alucinadora
hammertoe   dedo en martillo
hand   mano *f*
   hand, back of the   dorso de la mano
   hand, palm of the   palma de la mano
handicap   impedimento
hang, to   colgar (ue)
hangnail   cutícula desgarrada; padrastro *fam*
hangover   malestar post-alcohólico *m*
hangover, to have   andar crudo (cruda)
hard of hearing   corto de oído; duro de oído
harelip   boquineta *m, Chicano*; cheuto *adj. Chile*; jane *adj, Hond.*; labio cucho *Chicano*; labio leporino
harsh, raucous sound   ronquido
hash *(hashish)*   hachich *m*; hachís *m*; haschich *m*
have, to   tener; haber *auxiliary*
   have to, to *(must)*   tener que + *infinitive*
   have a cold, to   tener catarro; estar resfriado; estar acatarrado; estar agripado
headache   cajetuda *Chicano*; dolor de cabeza *m*; jaqueca
headrest   apoyo para la cabeza
heal, to   curar; sanar
healing   curación *f*
hearing aid   aparato auditivo; aparato para la sordera; audífono; prótesis acústica *f*; prótesis auditiva *f*
heart   corazón *m*
   heart, apex of   punta del corazón
   heart attack   ataque al corazón *m*; ataque cardíaco *m*; ataque del corazón *m*; infarto
   heartbeat   latido cardíaco; palpitación *f*
   heartbeat, irregular *(arrhythmia)*   arritmia; latido irregular; palpitación irregular
   heartbeat, rapid *(tachycardia)*   palpitación rápida; taquicardia
   heartbeat, rhythmical   palpitación rítmica
   heartbeat, slow   palpitación lenta
heartburn   acedía; agriera *Sp.Am.*; agruras *f*; ardor de estómago *m*; cardialgia; pirosis *f*
heart disease   cardiopatías *f*; enfermedad cardíaca *f*; enfermedad del corazón *f*
heart failure   fallo del corazón; insuficiencia cardíaca; paro del corazón
heart murmur   murmullo; soplo
heart valve   válvula del corazón

heat   calor *m*
   heat exhaustion   agotamiento por calor
   heat stroke   insolación *f*; golpe de calor *m*
   heat therapy   termoterapia; tratamiento térmico
heating pad, electric   almohadilla caliente eléctrica
heel   calcañar *m*; talón *m*
hematuria   hematuria; sangre en la orina *f*
hemoglobin   hemoglobina
hemophilia   hemofilia
hemorrhage   desangramiento; hemorragia; morragia *Chicano*
hemorrhoids   almorranas; hemorroides *f, pl*
hemostat   hemostato
hepatitis   fiebre *f, fam, Mex.*; hepatitis *f*; inflamación del hígado *f*
   hepatitis, infectious   hepatitis infecciosa
   hepatitis, viral   hepatitis viral
herbicides   herbicidas *m*; matayerbas *m, inv*
hernia   desaldillado *Mex.*; hernia; quebradura
   hernia, femoral   hernia femoral
   hernia, inguinal   hernia inguinal; quebradura en la ingle
   hernia, umbilical   hernia del ombligo; ombligón *m, slang*; ombligo salido *slang*; desombligado *adj, fam*
heroin   achivia; adormidera; amor; ardor; arpon; arponazo; azúcar; azufre; banderilla; blanco (blanca); borra blanca; caballo; ca-ca; cagada *vulgar*; carga; cáscara; chiva; chutazo; cohete; cura; cristales; dama blanca; golpe; goma; gato; H; helena; heróica; heroína; la cosa; la duna; lenguazo; manteca; nieve; papel; papelito; pasta; pericazo; piquete; polvo; polvo amargo; polvo blanco; stufa; tecata
   heroin capsule   cachucha; capa; gorra
   heroin user   heroínomania; tecato
herpes   herpes *m/f*
hiccough *(hiccup)*   hipo; hipsus *m*
hide, to   esconder(se)
high   alto *adj*
   high arched foot   pie hueco *m*
   high cholesterol   colesterol elevado *m*
   high from glue sniffing   tiniado *adj*
   high from sniffing paint thinner   tiniado *adj*
   high *(turned on)* **on marijuana**   motiado *adj*
   high on narcotics *(turned on)*   alivianado *adj*; caballón *adj*; loco *adj*; locote *adj*; sonado *adj*; sonámbulo *adj*
   high on pills   píldoro *adj*
   high triglycerides   triglicéridos elevados *m*
hip   cadera; cuadril *m, Mex., Chicano*
hit oneself, to   golpearse
hives   ronchas; urticaria
hoarse   afónico *adj*; ronco *adj*
   hoarse, chronically   carrasposo *adj*
   hoarse, to be   carraspear
hoarseness   carraspera *fam*; ronquera

home remedy remedio casero
hooked on drugs prendido *adj*
hook on narcotics, to prender
hormone hormón *m*; hormona
hospital hospital *m*; nosocomio *Chicano*
hot caliente *adj*
  hot coffee café caliente *m*
  hot flashes bochornos; calofrío *Chicano*; calores *m*; fogajes *m, P.R.*; llamaradas; sofocones *m*
  hot water bag bolsa de agua caliente
humerus húmero
hunchback jorobado *m, adj*
hurt, to *(ache, to)* doler (ue)
hydrocele hidrocele *f*
hydrochloric acid ácido clorhídrico
hydrofluoric acid ácido fluorhídrico
hymen himen *m*
hyperglycemia hiperglucemia; hiperglicemia
hyperlipidemia hiperlipidemia
hypertension hipertensión *f*
hyperventilation hiperventilación *f*; susto con resuello duro *fam*
hyphemia hemorragia detrás de la córnea; hifemia
hypochondria hipocondría/hipocondria *f*
hypochondriac adolorado *m, adj, Chicano*; adolorido *m, adj, Chicano*; hipocondríaco *m, adj*
hypodermic needle jaipo
hypoglycemia hipoglucemia; hipoglicemia
hypopyon pus detrás de la córnea *m*
hypotension hipotensión *f*
hysteria histeria
ice hielo
  ice bag *(ice pack)* aplicación de hielo empaquetado *f*; bolsa de caucho para hielo; bolsa de hielo
ice cream helado; nieve *f, Sp.*
ichthyol ictiol *m*
ileum íleon *m*
ilium ilion *m*
ill enfermo *adj*; malo *adj*
illness enfermedad *f*; mal *m*; padecimiento
  illness, acute enfermedad aguda
  illness, chronic enfermedad crónica
  illness *(disease)*, **contagious** enfermedad contagiosa; enfermedad trasmisible
  illness, mental enfermedad mental
  illness, minor enfermedad leve
  illness *(disease)*, **organic** enfermedad orgánica
  illness, serious enfermedad grave
  illness, *(disease)*, **tropical** enfermedad tropical
imbalance desequilibrio
immobilization inmovilización *f*
immune inmune *adj*
immunization inmunización *f*; vacuna
  immunization—booster dose dósis de refuerzo *f, inv*
  immunization—Schick test prueba de Schick
impaction impacción *f*
impetigo erupción cutánea *f*; impétigo
impotence impotencia
impression impresión *f*

improve, to *(get better, to)* mejorarse
inch pulgada
incision cortada; incisión *f*
incompatible incompatible *adj*
increase *(persist)*, **to** *(fever)* cargar la calentura *Chicano*
incubator estufa; incubadora
indigestion dispepsia; estómago sucio *Chicano*; indigestión *f*; insulto *Chicano*; mala digestión *f*
infant bebé *m*, criatura; nena; nene *m*
infantile paralysis parálisis infantil *f*
infarct infarto
infect, to contagiar infectar
infection infección *f*; pasmo
infectious infeccioso *adj*
infertile capón *adj, Chicano*; estéril *adj*; infértil *adj*
inflame, to inflamar
inflammation encono; inflamación *f*
  inflammation of the throat garrotillo
influenza gripa; gripe *f*; influenza
ingest narcotic pills, to pildorear(se); pildoriar(se)
ingredient ingrediente *m*
ingrown toenail uña encarnada; uña enterrada; uñero
inhale, to aspirar; inspirar; *med* inhalar; *med* sorber por la nariz; *(smoke)* tragar el humo
inject (oneself), to inyectar(se)
  inject oneself with drugs, to darse un piquete; inyectarse; picarse
injection inyección *f*; indección *f, Chicano*; chot *m, Chicano*
  injection *(of a narcotic substance)* abuja; abujado; piquete *m*
  injection, hypodermic inyección hipodérmica
  injection, intracutaneous inyección intracutánea
  injection intradermic inyección intradérmica
  injection, intramuscular inyección intramuscular
  injection, intravenous inyección endovenosa; inyección intravenosa
  injection, subcutaneous inyección subcutánea
injure, to hace daño; lastimar; herir (ie); lesionar
injured herido *adj*; lisiado *adj*
injury herida; lastimadura; lesión *f*
inlay incrustación *f*; orificación *f*
inoculation inoculación *f*
insanity demencia; locura
  insanity, manic-depressive locura de doble forma; maniamelancolía; sicosis maníacodepresiva *f*
insecticide insecticida *m*
insect repellent repelente de insectos *m*
insidious insidioso *adj*
insomnia insomnio; pérdida del sueño
instep empeine *m*
instrument, sharp-edged instrumento afilado
insulin insulina; insulínico *adj*
intensive care cuidado intensivo
intercourse relación sexual *f*
internally internamente *adv*
interval intervalo
intestine intestino

intestine, large intestino grueso
intestine, small intestino delgado
intolerance intolerancia
intoxication embriaguez *f*
intrauterine device *(IUD)* aparato intrauterino; DIU *m*; dispositivo intrauterino
intrauterine loop espiral intrauterino *m*
intussusception intususcepción *f*
iodine yodo
iron hierro
irritability *(not related to bile)* bilis *f*
irritate, to irritar
irritation irritación *f*
isolate, to aislar; apartar
isolation aislamiento por cuarentena
itch comezón *f*; picazón *f*; sarna
itching escozar *m*; picor *m*; prurito
IV *(intravenous solution)* solución endovenosa *f*; suero por la vena
IVP *(intravenous pyleogram)* PIV *(pielograma intravenoso)* *m*
jar frasco
jaundice derrame biliar *m*; ictericia; piel amarilla *f, fam*
jaw mandíbula; quijada
  jaw bone mandíbula
  jaw, broken quijada/mandíbula rota
jejunum yeyuno
jelly jalea
jog, to trotar
jogger trotador (trotadora) *m/f*
joint articulación *f*; coyuntura; *(of knuckle)* nudillo; (of a narcotic cigarette) abuja; griga; hierba; leño
junkie tecato
kerosene keroseno; querosén *m*
ketosis quetosis *f*
kick patada
kidney riñón *m*
  kidney disease mal de riñón *m*
  kidney stone cálculo en el riñón; cálculo renal; cálculo urinario; piedra en los riñones
kilogram kilogramo
kilometer kilómetro
kit botiquín *m*; estuche *m*
  kit, emergency botiquín de emergencia
  kit, first aid botiquín de primeros auxilios; equipo de urgencia
knee rodilla
  knee, back of the corva; flexura de la pierna
  kneecap choquezuela; rótula
knife cuchillo
knot nudo; *(type of tissue swelling)* bolas *f, pl, Chicano*
knuckle nudillo
label etiqueta
labor parto; trabajo de parto
  labor, artificial parto artificial
  labor, complicated parto complicado
  labor, dry parto seco
  labor, false parto falso
  labor, first stage of primer período del parto
  labor, immature parto inmaturo
  labor, induced parto inducido
  labor, instrumental parto instrumental
  labor, multiple parto múltiple

labor pains dolores de parto *m*

labor, premature parto prematuro

labor, prolonged parto prolongado

labor room sala de partos; sala prenatal

labor, second stage of segundo período del parto

labor, spontaneous parto espontáneo

labor, third stage of tercer período del parto

labor, to be in enfermarse *Chicano*; estar de parto

laboratory laboratorio

laboratory findings hallazgos de laboratorio

laboratory test análisis de laboratorio *m, inv*

labored dificultoso *adj*

laceration cortado; desgarradura; laceración *f*

lactation lactancia

lame cojo *adj*; lisiado *adj*; rengo *adj*

lameness cojera

lap regazo

laryngitis laringitis *f*

laryngoscope laringoscopio

larynx laringe *f*

laugh, to reír (i)

lavage lavado

lavatory lavamanos *m, inv*

lawsuit pleito

laxative laxante *m*; laxativo; purgante *m*

lazy (indolent) indolente *adj*

leave, to (go away, to) irse; jalarse *P.R.*; salir

leg pierna

leg, calf of the pantorrilla; chamorro *Chicano*

leishmaniasis roncha hulera; roncha mala

length of pregnancy (LOP) duración del embarazo *f*

lens lente *m*

leprosy lepra; lazarín *m*; mal de Hansen *m*; mal de San Lázaro *m*

leprous leproso *adj*; lazarino *adj*

lesion lesión *f*

lesion, oral afta; perleche *f*; pupa

let go of, to soltar (ue)

leukemia cáncer de la sangre *m*; leucemia

leukocytes (white blood cells) glóbulos blancos; leucocitos

level al ras

lie, to mentir (ie)

lie down, to acostarse (ue)

lift, to levantar

ligament ligamento

light, to (turn on, to) encender (ie)

limb extremidad *f*; miembro

limp (floppy) flác(c)ido *adj*; (lameness) cojera

limp, to (hobble, to) cojear; renguear *Sp.Am.*

lindane lindano

lingual lingual *adj*

liniment linimento

lip labio

liquid líquido

lisp (stutter) ceceo; tartamudeo

listen (to), to escuchar

liter litro

liver hígado

liver extract extracto de hígado

load of narcotics carga

lockjaw tétanos *m*; trismo

loin lomo

look (appear) well, to tener buena cara

loop (IUD) lazo

lose, to perder (ie)

lose weight, to adelgazar; perder (ie) peso

lotion loción *f*

lower the cholesterol count, to bajar el nivel del colesterol

lozenge pastilla; pastilla de chupar; trocisco

LSD aceite; aceitunas; acelide; ácido; ácido lisérgico; ácidos; alucinantes; avándaro; azúcar; blanco de España; bomba; café; cápsulas; chochos; cohete; colorines; cristales; diablos; divina; droga alucinante; droga LSD; dulces; elefante blanco; en onda; gis; grasas; la salud; lluvia de estrella; mica; mureler; nave; orange; papel; paper; piedrita de la luna; pit; purple haze; saturnos; sugar; sunshine; tacatosa; terrones; trip; viaje; viaje en las nubes; white

lubricant lubricante *m*; lubricativo *adj*

lukewarm templado *adj*; tibio *adj*

lump bola; borujo; bulto; dureza; hinchazón *f*; protuberancia; tumorcito

lump, large borujón *m*

lump (bump) on the head chichón *m*; pisporr(i)a *Chicano*

lunch, to have almorzar (ue)

lung pulmón *m*; bofe *m, Chicano, Sp.Am.*

lye lejía

lying-in after childbirth sobreparto

lymph linfa; linfático *adj*

lymph glands glándulas linfáticas

lymph node nódulo linfático; nudo linfático *fam*

mad (insane) loco *adj*

madness locura; manía

magnesia magnesia

magnesia, milk of leche de magnesia *f*

Magnetic Resonance Images/MRI Imagenes por Resonancia Magnética/IRM

magnifying glass lupa

mainline drugs, to chutear; inyectarse

"mainliner" jaipa; jaipo

make better, to aliviar

make-up, to put on maquillarse

make worse, to empeorar

malaise malestar *m*

malaria malaria; paludismo; fríos *Sp.Am.*

malignancy malignidad *f*

malignant maligno *adj*

malnourished desnutrido *adj*; mal nutrido *adj*

malnutrition desnutrición *f*; mala alimentación *f*; malnutrición *f*

malnutrition—kwashiorkor kwashiorkor *m*; mala alimentación mojada

malnutrition—marasmus mala alimentación seca; marasmo

malpractice impericia; malpraxis *f*; práctica impropia (inhábil)

mammogram mamografía; mamograma *m*

mania manía

maniac maníaco *adj*

marijuana achicalada; alfalfa; bacha; bailarina; café; campechana verde; canabis; cáñamo; carrujo; cartucho; chara; chester; chícara; chiclona; chira; chupe; churus; cochornis; coffee; colombiana; cosa; cris; de la buena; diosa verde; doña Juanita; epazote; fitoca; flauta; flor de Juana; frajo; ganga; ganja; gavos; golden; griefo; grifa; grifo; grilla; grass; guato; güera; habanita; hashi; hierba; hoja verde; huato; índice; jani; Jefferson; joint; Juana; Juanita; Kris Kras; la verde; leña; lucas; macoña; mafufa; mani; Margarita; María; María Juanita; Mariana; mariguana; marijuana; marinola; mariola; Mary Poppins; meserole; monstuo verde; monte; mora; mostaza; mota; orégano; oro verde; panatela; pasto; pastura; pepita verde; petate; petate del soldado; pitillo; pito; pochola; podo; polillo; pot; queta; rollo; té; toque; tronadora; yedo; yerba; yerba de diablo; yerba de oro; yerba santa; yerba verde; yesca; zacate

marijuana cigarette frajo de seda; leñito

marijuana smoker yesco

marijuana user grifo; mariguano; marihuano; moto

marrow médula; tuétano

mask máscara

massage masaje *m*

massage, to dar masaje; masajar; masajear; masar; sobar

masturbate, to hacerse la casqueta *Chicano*; masturbarse; puñetear *vulgar*

masturbation casqueta *Chicano*; masturbación *f*

maternity de maternidad *adj*; maternidad *f*

maternity clothes ropa de maternidad

maternity floor piso de maternidad

maternity hospital casa de maternidad

matter, it doesn't no importa

mattress colchón *m*

maturity madurez *f*

maxilla maxilar *m*

maxillar maxilar *adj*

measles sarampión *m*; granuja *slang*; morbilia, tapetillo de los niños *fam*

German measles fiebre de tres días *f*; sarampión alemán

live measles virus vaccine vacuna antisarampión de virus vivo

measure medida

measure, to medir (i)

measuring cup taza de medir

medical médico *adj*

medical purposes fines médicos *m*

medical records archivo clínico

medication medicación *f*

medicine droga; medicamento; medicina; medicación

medicine, patent medicina de la botica; medicina de la farmacia; medicina patentada; medicina registrada

medicine cabinet (medicine chest) botiquín *m*; despensa *Chicano*

melancholia melancolía

member of police narcotics squad narco

membrane membrana; tela
  mucous membrane mucosa
menarche primera regla; menarquia
Ménière's disease enfermedad de
  Ménière *f*
meningitis meningitis *f*
menopause cambio de vida;
  menopausia; período climatérico
menstruate, to estar indispuesta; estar
  mala; estar mala de la garra; estar mala
  de la luna; menstruar; perder (ie)
  sangre; tener el mes; tener/traer la garra
menstruation administración *f, Mex.;*
  costumbre *f;* enferma *euph;* luna
  Chicano; menstruación *f, general;* mes
  m; período *fam;* regla *Mex., P.R.;*
  tiempo del mes *fam*
mentally retarded inocente *adj, euph;*
  retardado *adj;* simple *adj, euph*
mental retardation retardo mental;
  retraso mental
menthol mentol *m*
mentholatum mentolato *Chicano*
Mercurochrome mercurocromo; sangre
  de chango *f, Chicano*
Merthiolate mertiolato
mescaline mescalina
metabolize, to metabolizar
metastasis metástasis *f*
methadone metadona
midwife *(quack)* rinconera
  midwife *(trained)* partera
  midwife *(untrained)* comadrona
migraine jaqueca; migraña
mild leve *adj*
mile leche *f;* milque *f, Chicano;*
  milk of magnesia leche de
  magnesia *f*
milligram miligramo
milliliter mililitro
mineral mineral *m, adj*
  mineral water agua mineral
mint leaves hojas de hierbabuena
  yerbabuena
mirror writing escritura en espejo
miscarriage malparto; parto malogrado
mix, to mezclar
mixture mezcla
moderate moderado *adj*
moist húmedo *adj*
mold moho
mole *(birthmark)* lunar *m*
mononucleosis mononucleosis
  infecciosa *f*
morning sickness ansias matutinas *f;*
  enfermedad matutina *f;* mal de madre
  m; vómitos del embarazo *m*
morphine morfi *f;* morfina
moustache bigote *m;* mostacho
mouth boca; bucal *adj*
  mouth breathing respiración bucal *f*
  mouth mirror odontascopio
  mouthpiece bocal *m;* boquilla
  mouth-to-mouth resuscitation
  resucitación boca a boca *f*
mouthwash enjuagatorio; lavado bucal;
  listerina *fam*
move, to mover (ue)
MRI/Magnetic Resonance Images
  IRM/Imágenes por Resonancia
  Magnética *f*
mucos frío *slang, Mex.;* moco
multiple sclerosis esclerosis en placa *f;*
  esclerosis múltiple *f*

mumps paperas; parótidas *f, pl;* bolas
  Chicano; buche *m, Mex.;* coquetas *Mex.;*
  farfallota *P.R.;* mompes *m, pl, Chicano*
muscle músculo
  muscle, involuntary músculo
  involuntario
  muscle, smooth músculo liso
  muscle, striated músculo estriado
  muscle, voluntary músculo
  voluntario
muscular dystrophy distrofia muscular
  progresiva
mushroom hongo
mustard mostaza
  mustard bath baño de mostaza
  mustard plaster cataplasma de
  mostaza; sinapismo
  mustard water agua con mostaza
mute mudo *adj*
myocardial infarct infarto miocardíaco;
  infarto miocardiaco
myocardium miocardio
myometrium miometrio
myopia miopía
myopic miope *adj*
nail uña
nape of neck cogote *m;* nuca
narcotic droga estupefaciente; droga
  somnífera; narcótico *m, adj*
  narcotic pills pinguas *f, pl*
  narcotic substitute, any la otra cosa
nasal drip goteo nasal; moqueadera
  Chicano
nausea basca; náusea
  nausea, morning asqueo;
  enfermedad matutina *f;* malestares
  de la mañana *m*
navel ombligo
nearsighted corto de vista *adj;* miope *adj*
nearsightedness miopía
neck cuello
needle aguja
  needle, hypodermic aguja
  hipodérmica; jeringa
neglect, to descuidar
negroid negro *adj*
nephritis nefritis *f*
nerve nervio
  nerve, cranial nervio craneal
  nerve, motor nervio motor
  nerve, parasympathetic nervio
  parasimpático
  nerve, sensory nervio sensorial
  nerve, sympathetic nervio simpático
nervous nervioso *adj*
  nervous breakdown colapso;
  desarreglo nervioso; neurastenia
  nervous disorder desorden nervioso
  m
  nervous system, autonomic sistema
  nervioso autónomo *m*
  nervous system, central sistema
  nervioso central *m*
neuralgia neuralgia
neurasthenia neurastenia
neurasthenic neurasténico *adj*
neuritis neuritis *f*
neurosis neurosis *f*
neurotic neurótico *adj*
nightmare pesadilla
nipple *(breast)* pezón *m;* chichi *f, Arg.,*
  Mex.
  nipple *(female)* chichi *f, slang;* pezón
  m

nipple *(male)* tetilla
nipple *(of a baby nursing bottle)*
  chupón *m;* mamadera; tetera *Mex.,*
  Cuba, P.R.; tetilla; tetina
nipple, cracked grieta del pezón
nipple, engorged *(caked)* pezón
  enlechado
nipple shield escudo para el pezón;
  pezonera
nitric acid ácido nítrico
nitro(glycerin) nitro(glicerina)
noninfectious no infeccioso *adj*
no one nadie
nose nariz *f;* nayotas *f, pl, slang, Chicano*
nosebleed hemorragia nasal;
  nosebleed, to have a salirle sangre
  de la nariz
nose bleeding epistaxis *f*
nostril fosa nasal; ventana de la nariz;
  ventanilla de la nariz
Novocaine novocaína
nucleated leukocytes leucocitos
  nucleados
  acidophiles acidófilos
  basophiles basófilos
  blood platelets plaquetas
  sanguíneas
  eosinphiles eosinófilos
  lymphocytes linfocitos
  monocytes monocitos
  polymorphonuclear neutrophiles
  neutrófilos polimorfonucleares
  "polymorphs" «polimorfos»
  reticulocytes reticulocitos
  thrombocytes trombocitos
numb adormecido *adj;* entumecido *adj;*
  entumido *adj*
numbness adormecimiento
nurse *(for the sick)* enfermera;
  (nursemaid) niñera
  nurse, baby ama de cría; niñera;
  nodriza
  nurse, wet chichi *f, fam, Guat.,Mex.;*
  chichigua *vulgar, Sp.Am.;* nodriza
nurse, to amamantar; criar a los
  pechos; dar de mamar; dar el pecho al
  niño
nursery cuarto de los niños
  nursery, newborn sala de los recién
  nacidos
nursing amamantamiento; crianza; de
  crianza *adj;* lactancia; lactante *adj*
  nursing *(for the sick)* asistencia a los
  enfermos
  nursing bottle biberón *m;*
  mamadera; tetera
  nursing bra sostén de maternidad *m*
  nursing care cuidados auxiliares
  nursing home clínica de reposo;
  hospicio para ancianos
  nursing pad almohadita
obese gordo *adj;* obeso *adj*
obesity gordura; obesidad *f*
obstetric(al) obstétrico *adj*
obstetrician obstétrico; médico partero;
  tocólogo
obstetrics obstetricia; tocología
obstruction impedimento;
  obstrucción *f*
  obstruction, nasal mormación *f,*
  Chicano
  obstruction, stomach entablazón *f,*
  Chicano
obtain, to *(get, to)* conseguir (i)

occipital   occipital *adj*
occlusion   oclusión *f*
oil   aceite *m*
   oil, baby   aceite para niños
   oil, castor   aceite de ricino
   oil, cod liver   aceite de hígado de bacalao
   oil, mineral   aceite mineral
   oil of wintergreen   aceite de gaulteria
   oil, pine   aceite de pino *m*
ointment   crema; pomada; ungüento; unto
O.K.   O.K. *Sp.Am.*; está bien; vale *Spain*
old age   senectud *f*; vejez *f*
ol factory   olfatorio *adj*
one-eyed   tuerto *adj*; monocular *adj*; virulo *adj, Chicano*
onset   ataque *m*; comienzo; principio
operating room   quirófano; sala de operaciones
operation   operación *f*
ophthalmia (inflammation of the eye)   inflamación de los ojos *f*; oftalmía
ophthalmic   oftálmico *adj*
ophthalmoscope   oftalmoscopio
opium   chinaloa *slang*; opio
optic nerve   nervio óptico
organ   órgano
orgasm   orgasmo
oriental   oriental *adj*
osteomyelitis   inflamación de la médula del hueso *f*; osteomielitis *f*
otitis   otitis *f*
ounce   onza
outpatient   paciente ambulatorio/ambulatoria *m/f*; paciente externo/externa *m/f*
outside of   fuera de *prep*
ovary   ovario
overdose   dosis excesiva *f, inv*; sobredosis *f, inv*
overdose, to   dar una dosis excesiva
overdue   atrasado *adj*
overweight   exceso de peso; sobrepeso; *adj* excesivamente gordo *adj*; excesivamente grueso *adj*
ovulate, to   ovular
ovulation   ovulación *f*
ovum   huevo; óvulo
oxalic acid   ácido oxálico
oxygen   oxígeno
oxytocic   oxitócico *adj*
oxytocin   oxitocina
pacemaker   aparato cardiocinético; marcador de paso *m*; marcador de ritmo *m*; marcapaso; monitor cardíaco *m*; seno auricular
pacifier   chupete *m*; mamón *m, Chicano*
packet of heroin   gramo
pad   cojín *m*; cojincillo
paid   dolor *m*
   pain, ache   dolor
   pain, bearing-down   sensación de pesantez en el perineo *f*
   pain, boring   dolor penetrante
   pain, burning   dolor ardiente; dolor quemante; escozor *m*
   pain, colicky   dolor cólico
   pain, constant   dolor constante
   pain, dule   dolor sordo
   pains, expulsive   dolores expulsivos
   pain, false   dolor falso
   pain, growing   dolor de crecimiento
   pains, hunger   dolores de hambre

pains, intermenstrual   dolores intermenstruales
pain killer   calmante *m*
pain, labor   dolor de parto; dolores de parto
pain, mild   dolor leve
pain, moderate   dolor moderado
pain, phantom limb   dolor de miembro fantasma
pains, premonitory   dolores premonitorios
pain, pressure-like   dolor opresivo; dolor de presión
pain, prickling   hormigueo
pain, radiating   dolor que le corre
pain, referred   dolor referido
pain, root   dolor radicular
pain, severe   dolor severo
pain, sharp   dolor agudo; dolor clavado; punzada
pain, sharp internal   torzón *m*
pain, shooting   dolor fulgurante; punzada
pain, smarting   escozor *m*
pain, stabbing   dolor punzante
pain, steady   dolor continuo
pain, tearing   dolor desgarrante
pain, thoracic   dolor torácico
pain, twinge   latido
pain, wandering   dolor errante
painful   doloroso *adj*
painless   sin dolor
palate   paladar *m*; cielo de la boca
   palate, hard   bóveda ósea del paladar; paladar duro
   palate, soft   velo del paladar
pale   pálido *adj*
palliative   paliativo *m, adj*
palpitation   latido *Chicano*; palpitación *f*
palsy   parálisis *f*; paralización *f*
   palsy, Bell's   parálisis facial
   palsy, cerebral   parálisis cerebral
   palsy, shaking (Parkinson's disease)   enefermedad de Parkinson *f*; parálisis agitante
pancreas   páncreas *m*
pancreatic   pancreático *adj*
pancreatitis   pancreatitis *f*
pant, to   jadear; resollar (ue)
panting   jadeante *adj*
paralyzed, to be   estar paralizado (paralizada)
Pap smear   frotis de Papanicolaou *m*; untos de Papanicolaou *m*
paralysis   parálisis *f*; paralización *f*
paranoia   paranoia
paraplegia   parálisis de la mitad inferior de cuerpo *f*; paraplejía
parasite   parásito
   amoeba   ameba; amiba
   ascaris (roundworm)   ascáride *f*; ascaris *f*; lombriz grande redonda *f*
   chigger flea   garrapata; güina *Mex.*; nigua
   common name   nombre común *m*
   cysticercus (bladderworm)   cisticerco
   distribution   distribución *f*
   feces, form of parasite in   forma de los parásitos en heces
   flea   pulga
   focus of infection   foco de infección
   giardia   giardia
   gnat   bobito *Chicano*; jején *m, C.A.*

   louse   piojo
   louse, crab   ladilla
   nit   liendre *f*
   metazoon   metazoo
   mite   ácaro
   parasitic cyst   ladilla; quiste *m*
   pediculosis (infestation)   pediculosis *f*; piojería
   protozoa   protozoarios
   protozoa, flagellates   flagelados
   route of entry   vía de entrada
   schistosoma   bilharzia; esquistosoma *m*
   solium (tapeworm)   gusano tableado; solitaria
   sporozoa   esporozoarios
   tapeworm   lombriz solitaria *f*; solitaria; tenia
   threadworms   lombriz chiquita afilada *f*; oxiuro
   trichinosis   triquinosis *f*
   trichocephalus   lombriz de látigo *f*; tricocéfalo
   uncinaria (hookworm)   lombriz de gancho *f*; uncinaria
   worm   gusano; lombriz *f*
   worm, intestinal   verme *m*
paregoric   paregórico
parotid gland   glándula parótida
pass on (a disease), to   pegar
pass over, to   atravesar (ie); pasar por
patch   parche *m*
PCP   amiba; polvo (de ángel)
pear-shaped   piriforme *adj*
pediatric   pediátrico *adj*
pediatrician   pediatra *m/f*; pedíatra *m/f*
pediatrics   pediatría
pellagra   pelagra
pelvic   pelviano *adj*; pélvico *adj*
pelvimeter   pelvímetro
pelvis   pelvis *f*
penicillin   penicilina
penis   pene *m*; balone *m, Chicano*; chale *m, vulgar, Chicano*; chalito *vulgar, Chicano*; chicote *m, slang*; chile *m, slang*; chorizo *vulgar*; güine *m, vulgar*; miembro; palo *slang*; picha *vulgar* pichón *m, vulgar*; pija *slang, Arg.*; pilinga *vulgar*; pito *slang*; reata/riata *vulgar*; verga *slang*
pennyroyal leaves   hojas de poleo
perforated eardrum   tímpano perforado
perforation   perforación *f*
pericarditis   pericarditis *f*
perimetrium   perimetrio
perineal   perineal *adj*
perineum   perineo
periosteum   periostio
peritonitis   abdomen agudo *m, slang*; panza peligrosa *slang*; peritonitis *f*
permit   permiso
peroxide   peróxido
   peroxide, hydrogen   agua oxigenada; peróxido de hidrógeno
persist, to   persistir (en)
person   persona
   person getting on in years   persona entrada en años
   person high on drugs   cócono
perspiration   transpiración *f*
perspire, to   transpirar
pertussis   coqueluche *f*; tos convulsiva *f*; tos ferina *f*; tosferina

pesticide pesticida *m;* plaguicida *m*
phalanx falange *f*
phallus falo
pharmacist farmacéutico; boticario
pharmacy botica; farmacia
pharyngitis faringitis *f*
pharynx faringe *f*
phenobarbital fenobarbital *m*
phlebitis flebitis *f;* tromboflebitis *f*
phlegm flema; mocosidad *f;* moquera *fam*
phosphoric acid ácido fosfórico
phosphorus fósforo
photography fotografía
phthisis consunción *f;* tisis *f*
physical físico *adj*
physically físicamente *adv*
physician doctor *m;* doctora; médica; médico
  physician, attending médico/médica a cargo *m/f;* médico/médica de cabecera *m/f*
  physician, consulting médico consultor; médica consultora *m/f;* médico/médica de apelación *m/f*
  physician, resident (house) médico/médica residente *m/f*
pigeon toe dedo de pichón
pigeon-toed patizambo *adj*
pile almorrana; hemorroides *f, pl*
pill pastilla; píldora
  pill, birth control pastillas para no tener niños; píldora anticonceptiva; píldoras para control de embarazo
  pill, sleeping píldora para dormir; píldora somnífera; píldora soporífica sedativo; somnífero; soporífera; soporífero
  pill, thyroid medicación tiroides *f*
pillow almohada
  pillow *(inflatable rubber "doughnut")* almohadilla neumática en forma de anillo
pimple barrillo; buba; bubón *m;* grano de la cara; pústula
  pimple, blackhead barro; espinilla
pinched nerve nervio aplastado
pinkeye conjuntivitis catarral aguda *f;* mal de ojo *m;* oftalmía contagiosa
piperazine piperacina; piperazina
pitocin pitocín *m;* pitocina
pituitary gland glándula pituitaria
PKU/phenylketonuria fenilcetonuria; fenilquetonuria; prueba del pañal
place, to colocar; poner
placenta placenta; secundinas
  placenta previa placenta previa
placental placentario *adj*
plague peste *f;* plaga
  plague, bubonic peste bubónica; tifo de oriente
plannted parenthood natalidad dirigida *f;* procreación planeada *f*
plaque placa
plasma plasma *m*
plaster of Paris yeso mate
plate placa
platelet plaqueta
pleural tap toracentesis *f*
pleurisy pleuresía; inflamación de los bofes *f, Chicano*
pneumonia neumonía; pulmonía
pock cacaraña *Mex., Guat.;* postilla; viruela

point to, to indicar; señalar
poison intoxicante *m;* ponzoña; veneno
poisoning envenenamiento; intoxicación *f*
  poisoning, botulism intoxicación botulínica
  poisoning, carbon monoxide intoxicación por monóxido de carbono
  poisoning, food envenenamiento por comestibles; intoxicación con alimentos
  poisoning, lead envenenamiento plúmbico; envenanamiento del plomo; saturnismo
  poisoning, salmonella intoxicación por salmonelas
  poisoning, staphylococcal intoxicación por estafilococos
  poison ivy chechén *m;* hiedra venenosa; yedra venenosa; zumaque venonosa *m*
poison, to envenenar; emponzoñar; intoxicar
  poison oneself, to envenenarse
poisonous ponzoñoso *adj;* venenosa *adj*
polio(myelitis) parálisis infantil *f;* polio(mielitis) *f*
polish, to pulir
polyp pólipo
pomade pomada
poor health, in en mala salud
poreclain porcelana
pore poro
postnatal care cuidado postnatal
potassium potasio
  potassium iodide yoduro de potasio
  potassium permanganate permanganato de potasio
potbellied panzón *adj*
potion dosis *f, inv,* poción *f*
poultice cataplasma; emplasto
pound libra
powder polvo
powered en polvo *adj*
powdery empolvado *adj;* polvoriento *adj;* polvoroso *adj*
precipitate, to precipitar
predisposition predisposición *f*
pregnancy embarazo; estado interesante *euph;* gravidez *f;* preñez *f*
  pregnancy, ectopic embarazo ectópico; embarazo fuera de la matriz
  pregnancy, false embarazo falso
  pregnancy, hysteria embarazo histérico
  pregnancy, incomplete embarazo incompleto
  pregnancy, tubal embarazo en los tubos; embarazo tubárico
pregnant embarazada *adj;* encinta *adj;* grávida *adj;* gruesa *adj, fam;* panzona *vulgar;* preñada *adj*
premature prematuro *adj;* sietemesino *(literally "seven months") adj*
prenatal prenatal *adj*
  prenatal care cuidado prenatal
presbyopia hipermetropía; presbicia; presbiopía
prescribe, to prescribir; prescribir un remedio; recetar
  prescribe for oneself, to autorecetarse

prescription prescripción *f;* receta; receta médica
presentation presentación *f*
pressure presión *f*
  exert pressure on, to ejercer presión sobre
pressure sensations sensaciones de ser apretado/apretada
prevent, to impedir (i)
prick pinchazo; punzada; afilerazo
prick, to pinchar; punzar
prickly heat erupción debida al calor *f;* picazón *f;* sarpullido
probe estilete *m;* sonda; tienta
problem problema *m;* trastorno
procedure procedimiento
procreate, to procrear
proctitis proctitis *f*
produce, to producir
progeny progenie *f;* prole *f*
progesterone progesterona
prolapse caída de la matriz; prolapso
prophylactic profiláctico *m, adj*
prostatitis prostatitis *f;* tapado de orín *m*
prosthesis miembro artificial; prótesis *f*
prostration prostración *f*
  prostration, heat prostración del calor
prothrombin time tiempo de protrombina
prove, to (test, to; try out, to) probar (ue)
provide an addict with a fix, to curar
psilocybin hongos; mujercitas; niños
psoriasis mal de pintas *m;* soríasis *f*
psychedelic droga (p)sicodélica; sicodélico *adj*
psychosis sicosis *f*
psychosomatic sicosomático *adj*
psychotic sicótico *adj*
pterygium carnosidad *f, fam;* pterigión *m*
pubic púbico *adj;* pubiano *adj;* pelo púbico;
  pubic hair pelitos *m, pl, Chicano*
  pubic region partes ocultas *f;* verijas *pl*
puerile pueril *adj*
puerperal puerperal *adj*
puerperium puerperio; riesgo
pull, to jalar, tirar
  pull back foreskin of penis, to pelársela
  pull out, to extraer
  pull up (one's) knees, to encoger las rodillas
pulp pulpa
pulpotomy pulpotomía
pulse pulso
pump, to sacar (leche) por medio de una bomba
purgation purgación *f*
purgative catártico *adj;* purgante *m*
purge lavado; lavativo; purga; purgante *m*
pursue, to perseguir (i)
pus pus *m*
push, to *(shove, press)* empujar; *(strain)* pujar
pustule bubón *m;* grano; pústula
put, to colocar; poner
  put heroin in capsules, to capear; capiar
  put in a plaster cast, to enyesar
  put on *(clothing)*, **to** ponerse + *noun*

put to sleep, to adormecer por anestesia

pyorrhea mal de las encías *m*; piorrea

quadruplet cuadrúpleto; cuatrillizo

quarrel, to reñir (i)

quart cuarto

quinine quinina

quinsy *(sore throat)* amigdalitis supurativa *f*; esquinancia

quintuplet quintillizo; quíntuplo

quit cold turkey, to *(suddenly)* kickear

rabbit test examen de conejo *m*

rabies hidrofobia; rabia

radiation radiación *f*

  radiation shield blindaje contra la radiación *m*

  radiation therapy radioterapia

  radiation treatment radiaciones *f*

radius radio

rale estertor *m*

rape rapto *Chicano*; violación *f*

rash alfombra *P.R., Cuba*; erupción *f*; salpullido; sarpullido

  rash, diaper pañalitis *f*

  wheals *(hives)* ronchas

rat bite ordedura de rata *m*

RBC *(red blood count)* NGR (numeración de glóbulos rojos) *f*

realize, to darse cuenta de *algo*

recessive recesivo *adj*

  recessive character carácter recesivo *m*

recover, to curarse; sanar

rectal rectal *adj*

rectocele rectocele *m*

rectum recto

recur, to repetirse (i); volver (ue) a ocurrir

red blood cells hematíes *m*

reddish bermejizo *adj, hair*; rojizo *adj*

red-haired pelirrojo *adj*

redness rubor *m*

reduce, to reducir(se)

  reduce a fracture, to enderezar

reducing exercises ejercicios físicos para adelgazar; ejercicios físicos para reducir peso

refer, to referir (ie)

refined refinado *adj*

reflex reflejo

regenerate, to regenerar

regulate, to regular

regurgitation regurgitación *f*

reimplantation reimplantación *f*; reinjertación *f*

relapse atrasado *adj*; recaída; recidiva

  relapse, to cause to suffer atrasar

  relapse, to have a atrasarse

relation parentesco; pariente *f*; relación *f*

relations, to have sexual tener relaciones sexuales; coger / cojer *vulgar, Arg., P.R., Mex.*; conocer; chingar *vulgar*; chopetear *slang*; dar una atascada *vulgar*; dar pá dentro *vulgar*; dormir (ue) con *alguien*; echar un palito *Chicano*; estar con *alguien*; hacer cositas *euph, Chicano*; tumbar

relationship parentesco; relación *f*

relax, to aflojarse; calmarse; relajar el cuerpo; relajarse

relaxation descanso; relajación *f*

  relaxation of tension disminución de la tirantez *f*

release descargo

release, to soltar (ue)

remedy medicamento; remedio

remember, to acordarse (ue) (de); recordar (ue)

remove, to quitar

remove the nerve, to matarle el nervio a *alguien*; sacarle el nervio a *alguien*

renal renal *adj*

repeat, to repetir (i)

repent, to arrepentir(se) (ie)

reproduction reproducción *f*

reproductive reproductivo *adj*

request pedido; petición *f*

require, to requerir (ie)

respiratory system aparato respiratorio; sistema respiratorio *m*

rest *(repose)* descanso; reposo; *(support)* apoyo; soporte *m*

rest, to descansar; reposar

rest on, to apoyarse en

restraining device coercitivo; medio de restricción

restroom baño; comodidades *f, pl*; cuarto de baño; excusado; servicios *m*; WC *m*

resusitation, cardiopulmonary (CRP) resucitación cardiopulmonar (RCP) *f*

return, to *(give back, to)* devolver (ue)

RH factor factor RH *m*; factor Rhesus *m*

  RH negative RH-negativo *adj*

  RH positive RH-positivo *adj*

rheum reuma *m*

rheumatism reuma *m*; reumatismo

rheumatoid arthritis artritis reumatoidea *f*

rhinitis escurrimiento de la nariz; rinitis *f*

rhogam rogam *m*

rhythm method método del ritmo; ritmo

rib costilla

  rib, false (floating) costilla falsa (flotante)

  rib, true costilla verdadera

rickets raquitis *m*; raquitismo

ridge elevación *f*; reborde *m*

ring *(IUD)* anillo

rinse (out), to enjuagar(se)

rise, to subir

risk riesgo

roll up one's sleeve, to arremangarse; subirse la manga

roof of the mouth cielo de la boca; paladar *m*

root raíz *f*

  root canal canal radicular *m*

    root canal work curación del nervio *f*; extracción del nervio *f*

roseola roséola; rubéola

rough áspero *adj*; raposo *adj* calloso *adj*

rub fricción *f*; frotación *f*

rub, to frotar; frotarse; pasar la mano sobre la superficie de; restregar

rubella alfombría *Chicano*; fiebre de tres días *f*; peluza *Mex.*; roséola epidémica; rubéola; sarampión alemán *m*

rubber *(material)* caucho; goma; *(condom)* condón *m*; goma; hule *m*; preservativo

  rubber bulb, syringe pera de goma

  rubber gloves guantes de goma *m, pl*

rubbing alcohol alcohol para fricciones *m*

rupture *(hernia)* hernia; quebradura; relajación *f*; reventón *m*; rotadura *Chicano*; rotura; ruptura

rupture, to *(burst, to)* romper

ruptured roto *adj*

sac saco

saccharine sacarina

sacro-iliac sacroilíaco *adj*

sacrum sacro

saline solution agua con sal; agua salina

saliva esputo; expectoración *f*; saliva

salivary gland glándula salival

salt sal *f*

  salt, iodized sal yodada

  salt, noniodized sal corriente

  salts, smelling sales aromáticas; sales perfumadas

  salt water agua salada

salve pomada; ungüento

sample muestra

sanitary higiénico *adj*; sanitario *adj*

  sanitary napkin absorbente higiénico *m*; almohadilla higiénica; kotex *m*; servilleta sanitaria paño higiénico

  sanitary pad kotex *m*; servilleta sanitaria

sarcoma sarcoma *m*

  sarcoma, Kaposi's sarcoma de Kaposi

say goodbye to, to despedirse (i) (de)

scab costra; cuerín *m, Chicano*; cuerito *Chicano*; postilla

scabies guaguana *slang*; gusto *slang*; sarna

scale escama

scalp casco; cuero cabelludo; piel de la cabeza *f*

scalpel bisturí *m*; escalpelo

scar cicatriz *f*

scarred cicatrizado *adj*

schizophrenia esquizofrenia

schizophrenic esquizofrénico *adj*

sciatic ciático *adj*

sciatica ciática

scorpion bite mordedura de escorpión

scotoma *(spots before the eyes)* escotoma *m*; manchas frente a los ojos

scratch rascado; rasguño; raspón *m, Sp.Am.*

scratch to *(to relieve itch)* rascar(se); *(to hurt)* rasguñar

scrotum bolsa de los testículos; escroto

scrub, to *(surgically)*, fregar; lavar; refregar

scurvy escorbuto

seasickness mal de mar *m*; mareo

seat belt cinturón de seguridad *m*

  buckle the seat belt, to abrocharse el cinturón

seborrhea seborrea

seconal capsule colorada

secrete, to secretar

sedative calmante *m*; sedante *m*; sedativo

sedimentation sedimentación *f*

  erythrosedimentation eritrosedimentación *f*

seizure ataque *m*; convulsión *f*

semen esperma; leche *f, vulgar*; mecos *m, pl, vulgar*; semen *m*

seminal vesicle vesículo seminal

senile senil *adj*

  senile, to be estar chocho

senility caduquez *f*; senectud *f*;
senilidad *f*
sense sentido
  sense, of feel *(tactile)* sentido del tacto
  sense, of hearing *(auditory)* sentido
del oído
  sense, of sight *(visual)* sentido de la
vista
  sense, of smell *(olfactory)* sentido
del olfato
  sense, of taste *(gustatory)* sentido
del gusto
sensorial sensorial *adj*
septicemia infección en la sangre *f*,
fam; piemia; septicemia; toxemia
septum tabique *m*
serious grave *adj*; serio *adj*
serum suero
  serum, antivenin suero antiviperino
  serum, black widow spider antivenin
suero antialacrán
serve, to servir (i)
set a fracture, to componer una
fractura; reducir una fractura
severe agudo *adj*; fuerte *adj*; severo *adj*
shape forma
be in shape, to estar en forma
be out of shape, to estar en baja forma
get in shape, to ponerse en forma
keep in shape, to mantenerse en forma
shave *(oneself)*, **to** afeitar (se);
rasurar(se)
shield *(IUD)* escudo
shin canilla; espinilla
shinbone tibia
shingles herpes *m/f*; zona; zoster *f*;
jiotes *f, Mex., C.A.*
shiver, to temblar; tiritar
shock choque *m*; conmoción nerviosa
f; sobresalto; susto
  shock, anaphylactic choque alérgico
fam; choque anafiláctico
shoot up heroin, to filerearse;
inyectarse; picarse
shortness of breath ahoguijo; ahoguío
fam
shortsighted cegato *adj, fam*; miope *adj*
short-winded *adj* corto de resuello
shot chot *m, Chicano*; inyección *f*
shoulder hombro
shoulder blade *(scapula)* escápula;
espaldilla; omóplato; paletilla
show, to mostrar (ue)
shower, to *(take a shower, to)* ducharse
show one's teeth, to enseñar los
dientes; mostrar (ue) los dientes
sick enfermo *adj*; malo *adj*
sickliness achaque *m*
sickly cholenco *adj, Chicano*;
demacrado *adj*; enfermizo *adj*; farruto
adj. Arg., Bol., Chile; pálido *adj*
sickness dolencia; enfermedad *f*; mal
m; padecimiento
side costado; lado
  side, left lower lado izquierdo
inferior
  side, left upper lado izquierdo
superior
  side, right lower lado derecho
inferior
  side, right upper lado derecho
superior
silver nitrate nitrato de plata
simulation fingimiento

single out, to separar
sinus seno
  sinus congestion congestión nasal *f*;
sinusitis *f*
sit down, to sentarse (ie)
sitz bath baño de asiento; semicupio
size tamaño
  size, assorted tamaño surtido
  size, large tamaño grande
  size, small tamaño pequeño
skeleton armazón *m*; esqueleto
skin piel *f*
  skin, flap of the colgajo
  skin, of the face cutis *m/f, inv*
skinned *(complexioned)*, **dark** moreno
adj
skinned *(complexioned)*, **light** de piel
blanca; de tez blanca
skinned *(complexioned)*, **olive** trigueño
adj
**skinned, very dark, lacking negroid
features** pinto *adj*; retinto *adj*
skull calavera; cráneo
  skull, top of tapa de los sesos *fam*
  sleep, to dormir (ue)
  fall asleep, to dormirse (ue)
sleeping sickness enfermedad del
sueño *f*
sling cabestrillo; hondo
slipped disc disco desplazado; disco
intervertebral luxado
smallpox viruela
smear cultivo frote *m*; frotis *m*
smegma esmegma *m*; queso *slang*
smell, to oler (ue)
smile, to sonreír (i)
smoke humo
smoke, marijuana, to motear; motiar;
tronar
smooth, to limar
snake bite mordedura de culebra
sneeze, to estornudar
sniff, to aspirar por la nariz; sorber por
la nariz
  sniff glue, to hacer(se) a la glu(fa);
sesonar
  **sniff residue of powdered narcotics,
to** estufear; estufiar
sniffle, to sorberse los mocos *(because
of a cold)*; sorberse las lágrimas *(when
crying)*
soak, to remojar
soap jabón *m*
soapy water agua jabonosa
sodium sodio; sódico *adj*
  sodium carbonate carbonato de
sodio
  sodium hydroxide hidróxido de
sodio
  sodium hypochlorite *(bleach)*
blanqueador de ropa *m*; hipoclorito
de sodio
  sodium pentothal pentotal sódico
m; pentotal de sodio *m*
  sodium peroxide peróxido de sodio
  sodium sulfate *(in toilet cleaners)*
sulfato de sodio (en limpiadores de
inodoros)
soft blando *adj*; suave *adj*; *(pliant)*
blando *adj*
solution solución *f*
soporific narcótico; soporífico
sore aflicción *f*; dolor *m*; pena;
doloroso *adj*;

(wound) grano; llaga; úlcera
  sore ears mal (dolor) de oídos *m*
  sore eyes dolor de ojos *m*
  sore throat garganta inflamada; mal
(dolor) de garganta *m*
souffle pilido *Mex.*; silbido
sound *(harsh, raucous)* ronquido
spasm contracción muscular *f*;
espasmo; latido *Chicano*
spasmodic espasmódico *adj*;
intermitente *adj*; irregular *adj*
spastic espasmódico *adj*; espástico *adj*
specimen espécimen *m*; muestra
  specimen, urine muestra de orina
spectacles anteojos *(general term)*;
espejuelos *Cuba*; gafas; lentes *m, pl,
Mex.*; quevedos *m, wire-rimmed*
speculum espéculo; espejo vaginal
spell, to deletrear
sperm espermatozoide *m*; mecos;
semen *m*; semilla *slang, Mex.*
spermaticide, vaginal espermaticida
vaginal *m*
sphincter esfínter *m*
spinal column columna vertebral;
espina dorsal
spinal cord médula espinal
spiral *(IUD)* espiral *m*
spit, to escupir; *(phlegm)* gargajear
  spit in the bowl, to escupir en la
taza
spitting gargajeo
spleen bazo; esplín *m, Chicano*
splint férula; tablilla
  splint, in a entablillado *adj*
splinter *(in the eye)* astilla (en el ojo);
esquirla
spoonful cucharada
spot mancha
spotted/spotty manchado *adj*
spotted sickness mal de pinto *m*; pinta
spotting manchas de sangre
sprain dislocación *f*; esguince *f*; falseo
Chicano; torcedura
sprain, to desconcertar (ie); falsear;
torcer (ue)
spray pulverización *f*; pulverizador *m*;
rociador *m*
spread (out), to tender (ie) (con)
spread limbs, to extender (ie)
sputum esputo; desgarro *Sp.Am.*;
gargajo; pollo *Chicano*; saliva
squat, to acuclillarse; ponerse de
cuclillas
squeeze, to apretar (ie)
squint-eyed bisojo *adj*; bizco *adj*;
ojituerto *adj*
stain/staining coloración *f*; colorante
m; tinción *f*
  stain, acid-fast coloración
acidorresistente
stand up, to levantarse; parar(se);
ponerse de pie
starch almidón *m*
starchy almidonado *adj*; amiláceo *adj*
stay, to quedarse
  stay awake, to desvelarse
sterile estéril *adj*; infecundo *adj*
sterility esterilidad *f*; infecundidad *f*
  sterility, female frío de la matriz
  sterility, permanent esterilidad
permanente
sterilization esterilización *f*
sterilize, to esterilizar

sterilize the bottles, to esterilizar las botellas
sterilized esterilizado *adj*
sterilizer esterilizador *m*
stethoscope estetoscopio
stick to clavar; picar
   stick out, to sacar
stiff tieso *adj*
   stiff neck nuca tiesa *fam*; torticolis *m*; tortícolis *m*
   stiff ("frozen") joint articulación envarada *f*; articulación trabada *f*
stillbirth nati-muerto; parto muerto
stillborn mortinato *adj*; nacido muerto *adj*
stimulant estimulante *m*
sting (*of an insect*) picadura; piquete *m*; punzada
   sting, ant picadura de hormiga
   sting, bee picadura de abeja
   sting, black widow spider picadura de ubar *fam*; picadura de viuda negra
   sting, botfly picadura de moscardón
   sting, chigoe/jigger/sandflea picadura de nigua
   sting, flea picadura de pulga
   sting, hornet picadura de avispón
   sting, mosquito picadura de mosquito
   sting, scorpion picadura de alacrán
   sting, spider picadura de araña
   sting, tick picadura de garrapata
   sting, wasp picadura de avispa
sting, to picar
stir, to revolver (ue)
stitch puntada *Sp.Am.*; punto; sutura
stocking, elastic calceta elástica
stomach estómago; panza *Chicano*; vientre *m*
   stomach, on an empty en ayunas
   stomach, pit of boca de estómago; epigastrio
   stomach ache dolor de estómago *m*
   stomach pump bomba estomacal
   stomach ulcer úlcera del estómago
stool deposición *f*; evacuación intestinal *f*; excremento; heces fecales *f, pl*
   stool softener cápsula para ablandar evacuaciones; copro-emoliente *m*
   stool specimen muestra de excremento; muestra de heces fecales
stop, to pararse
strabismus bizco *C.A.*; estrabismo
straighten the teeth, to enderezar los dientes
strain tensión *f*; torcedura
straining, tenesmus pujos
strength fuerza
strep throat estreptococia; mal (dolor) de garganta por estreptococo
streptomycin estreptomicina
stretch, to (*unfold, to*) tender (ie)
stretch marks (*strias*) estrías
stricture constricción *f*; estenosis *f*; estrechez *f*; estrictura
stroke accidente cerebral *m*; apoplejía, ataque fulminante *m*; derrame cerebral *m*; embolia cerebral; embolio *Chicano*; estroc *m*, *Chicano*; hemorragia vascular; parálisis *f*
strong tea té cargado *m*; té fuerte *m*
strychnine estricnina
stuttering balbucencia; tartamudez *f*

sty orzuelo; perrilla *fam*
stylet estilete *m*
sublingual gland glándula sublingual
submaxillary gland glándula submaxilar
subside, to calmarse
substitute substituto
subtract, to deducir; sustraer
suck, to chupar; mamar
sudden súbito *adj*
suffer, to padecer (de); sufrir (de)
suffocation asfixia; sofocación *f*
sugar azúcar *m/f*
sugary azucarado *adj*
suggest, to sugerir (ie)
suicide suicidio
sulfathiazole sulfatiazol *m*
sulfonyluria sulfoniluria
sulphur (sulfur) azufre *m*
   sulphur/sulfur powder polvo de azufre
sulphuric/sulfuric acid ácido sulfúrico
sunglasses anteojos oscuros; gafas de sol
sunstroke insolación *f*; asoleada *Sp.Am.*
suntan lotion loción bronceadora *f*; loción para el sol *f*
suntanned bronceado *adj*; tostado *adj*
supplementary feedings alimentación suplementaria *f*
support apoyo; soporte *m*; sostén *m*
supporter faja médica
   supporter, athletic suspensorio
suppository cala; calilla; supositorio
suppository, vaginal óvulos
suppuration supuración *f*
surface superficie *f*
surgical quirúrgico *adj*
suture comisura; sutura
   suture, dental sutura
   suture dissolving sutura absorbible
suture, to suturar
swallow trago
swallow, to tragar
sweat sudor *m*
sweat, to sudar
sweetener dulcificante *m*
sweets dulces *m, pl*; golosinas *f; pl*
swell, to hinchar
swelling hinchazón *f*; tumefacción *f*; tumor *m*
   swelling on the head chichón *m*
swollen hinchado *adj*
symptom síntoma *m*
syndrome síndrome *m*
syphilis avariosis *f, Sp.Am.*; infección de la sangre *f, euph*; lúes *f*; mal de bubas *m, slang*; mal francés *m, slang*; sangre mala *f, slang*; sífilis *f*
syringe jeringa; jeringuilla
   syringe, disposable jeringa desechable; jeringuilla descartable
   syringe, glass cylinder jeringa con cilindro de cristal
   syringe, hollow needle jeringa con aguja hueca
   syringe, hypodermic jeringuilla hipodérmica
   syringe-piston, plunger émbolo
syrup of ipecac jarabe de ipeca *m*
systole sístole *f*
tablespoonful cucharada
tablet comprimido; pastilla; tableta
tachycardia taquicardia

tactile táctil *adj*
take, to tomar
   take advantage of, to aprovecharse de
   take (drugs), to administrarse; ingerir/injerir (ie); tomar
   take a risk, to arriesgarse
   take care of, to cuidar
   take hold, to agarrar
   take marijuana, to amarihuanarse; engrifarse; enmarihuanarse
   take off, to (*undress, to*) quitarse
   take place, to tener lugar
Tampax tampax *m*
tampon ta(m)pón *m*
tantrum berrinche *m, fam*
   tantrum, temper pataletas
tartar sarro
   tartar, dental saburra; sarro; tártaro
taste sabor *m*
taste, to (*try, to*) probar (ue); (*to savour*) saborear; saber
   taste like, to saber a
   taste good (bad), to tener buen (mal) sabor
tasteless desabrido *adj*
tattoo(ing) tatuaje *m*
tea té *m*
   tea, chamomile agua de manzanilla; té de manzanilla
tear (*split*) desgarramiento; desgarrón *m*; (*drop of liquid*) lágrima
   tear gland glándula lagrimal
tear, to romper; derramar lágrimas
teaspoonful cucharadita
   teaspoonful, level cucharadita llena al ras
teeth dientes *m*; mazorca *sg, slang*
   teeth, artificial (false) dientes postizos
   teeth, bicuspids bicúspides *m*; premolares *m*
   teeth, canine (eyeteeth) canino; colmillo
   teeth, deciduous dientes de leche
   teeth, even dientes parejos
   teeth, front (incisors) incisivos
   incisor, central incisivo central
   incisor, lateral incisivo lateral
   teeth, lacking chimuelo *adj, Chicano*
   teeth——molars molares *m*
   teeth, stained dientes manchados
   teeth——third molar tercer molar
   teeth, white dientes blancos
   teeth, wisdom muelas cordales *f*; muelas del juicio *f*
teethe, to dentar (ie); echar dientes; endentecer
teething dentición *f*; salida de los dientes
tell, to (*say, to*) decir
temperature calentura; temperatura
temple sien *f*
tendon tendón *m*
tepid tibio *adj*
Terramycin terramicina
test examen *m*; prueba
   test of análisis de *m, inv*
   test, angiography angiografía; radiografía de los vasos sanguíneos
   test, cardiac function prueba de función cardíaca
   test, serology prueba serológica
   test, sputum análisis de esputos
   test, tuberculin tuberculina

test, urinalysis   análisis de la orina; urinálisis *m, inv*
test, to   examinar; poner a prueba
testicle   testículo; blanquillo *slang, Chicano*; bolas *f, pl, slang, Chicano*; compañones *m, pl, slang*; cuates *m, pl, slang, Chicano*; huevos *m, pl, slang*
testis   testis *m*; testículo
tetanus   tétano(s); mal de arco *m, slang*; pasmo seco; trimo
   tetanus, infantum   moto *slang; Mex.*; mozusuelo *Mex.*; siete días (7 días) *m*
tetracycline   tetraciclina
therapeutic   terapéutico *adj*
therapist   terapeuta *m/f*
therapy   terapia; tratamiento
   therapy, x-ray   radioterapia
thermometer   termómetro
   thermometer, axillary   termómetro axilar
   thermometer, oral   termómetro oral
   thermometer, rectal   termómetro rectal
thicken, to   espesar
thigh   muslo
think, to   pensar (ie)
thoracic cavity   caja torácica
thorax   tórax *m*
throat   garganta
thrombophlebitis   flebitis *f*; tromboflebitis *f*
thrombosis   trombosis *f*
   thrombosis, coronary   trombosis coronaria
thrombus   coágulo; cuajo; cuajarón *m*
thrush   afta; algodoncillo *fam*
thymus   timo
thyroid   tiroides *m*; tiroideo *adj*
tic   tic *m*; tirón *m*; sacudida
   tic douloureux   tic doloroso de la cara
tie the tubes, to   ligar los tubos de Falopio; ligar los tubos uterinos; ligar trompas
tingling   hormigueo
tinnitus   zumbido del oído
tire, to   cansar(se)
tissue   tejido
toe   dedo (del pie)
   toe, big   dedo grueso
   toe, hammer   dedo en martillo
   toe, pigeon   dedo de pichón
toilet   baño; común *m*; excusado; inodoro; privado; retrete *m, Spain*; servicios
toiletries   artículos de tocador
tolerance   tolerancia
tongue   lengua
   tongue depressor   abatelengua *m, inv*; bajalengua *m*; depresor de la lengua *m*; pisa-lengua *m*
tonic   tónico
tonsilitis   amigdalitis *f*; tonsilitis *f*
tonsils   amígdalas; anginas *Mex., Ven.*; tonsils *m, Chicano*
tooth   diente *m*
   tooth, baby   diente de leche; diente mamón; diente temporal
   tooth, back   muela; molar *m*
   tooth decay   caries *f, inv*; dientes podridos; guijón *m*; neguijón *m*
   tooth, impacted   diente impactado
   tooth, large, misshapened   diente de ajo *fam*

tooth, lower   diente inferior
tooth, neck of   cuello del diente
tooth, socket   alvéolo
tooth, upper   diente superior
toothache   dolor de dientes *m*; dolor de muelas *m*; odontalgia
toothbrush   cepillo de dientes
toothpaste   pasta de dientes; pasta dentífrica
toothpick   mondadientes *m, inv*; palillo de dientes
touch, to   tocar
tourniquet   liga; torniquete *m*
toxemia   toxemia
   toxemia of pregnancy   intoxicación del embarazo *f*; toxemia del embarazo
trachea   gaznate *m*; tráquea
tracheostomy   traqueostomía
tracks   trakes *m*; traques *m*
traction   tracción *f*
trade, to   cambiar
traffic in drugs, to   dilear; diliar; traficar
tranquilizer   apaciguador *m*; calmante *m*; tranquilizante *m*
transfer, to   transferir (ie)
transfusion   transfusión *f*
transmission   transmisión *f*
   transmission by contact   transmisión mediante contacto
   transmission, droplet   transmisión por gotillas
   transmission, vector   transmisión mediante vector
   transmission vehicle   vehículo
trauma   trauma *m*; traumatismo
treatment   tratamiento
tremor   tremblor *m*; tremor *m*
triplet   trillizo
truss   braguero; faja
tub   bañera; tina de baño
tube   tubo
   tube, fallopian   trompa de Falopio; tubo de Falopio
   tube (for feeding)   sonda
tubercular   afectado *adj, Chicano*; tuberculoso *adj*
tuberculosis   tisis *f*; tuberculosis *f*; afectado del pulmón *Chicano, Mex.*; manchado del pulmón *Mex.*; peste blanca *f*
tumefaction   edema *m*; hinchazón *f*; tumefacción *f*
tumor   tumor *m*; neoformación *f*; neoplasma *m*; tacotillo *Chicano*
   tumor on the head   chiporra *Guat., Hond.*
tuning fork   diapasón *m*
turn (over), to   darse vuelta; volverse (ue)
turn into, to   convertir(se) (ie)
turpentine   esencia de trementina; trementina
twin   cuate *m/f, Mex.*; gemelo; mellizo
twist, to (bend, to)   bornear
twist, to (turn, to)   torcer (ue)
twisted   torcido *adj*; zambo *adj*
ulcer   úlcera
   ulcer, gastric   úlcera gástrica
   ulcer, peptic   úlcera péptica
ulna   cúbito
ultrasound   ultrasonda
ultraviolet lamp   lámpara de rayos ultravioletas
umbilical cord   cordón umbilical *m*

umbilical hernia, (to have an)   (estar) desombligado/desombligada
umbilicus   ombligo
unconscious   inconsciente *adj*
unconsciousness   inconsciencia; insensibilidad *f*
undernourished   desnutrido *adj*
underside   superficie inferior *f*
undersigned   abajo firmado *adj*
understand, to   comprender; entender (ie)
underweight   falta de peso; peso escaso
undress, to   desnudarse; desvestirse (i); encuerarse *Chicano*
unguent   pomada; ungüento
unplug, to   destapar
untreated   no tratado *adj*
uremia   intoxicación de orín *f*; uremia
ureter   uréter *m*
urethra   canal urinario *m*; caño urinario; uretra
urinalysis   análisis de la orina *m, inv*
urinary bladder   vejiga de la orina
urinary problem   mal de orín *m*
urinary tract   vías urinarias
urinate, to   orinar; hacer agua *Chicano*; hacer (la) chi(s) *vulgar, Chicano*; hacer (la) pipi/pipí; mear; tirar (el) agua *slang*
urine   orina; orines *m, pl*; "aguas menores" *f*; chi *f, vulgar*
   collection of the urine specimen   acumulación de la muestra *f*
   color: straw   de paja *adj*
   color: yellow   amarillo *adj*
   frequent urinating   meadera *Chicano*; orinar muy de seguido
   urine constituents   componentes *m*
      acetone   acetona
      albumin   albúmina
      ammonia   amoníaco
      bile   bilis *f*
      bilirubin   bilirrubina
      blood   sangre *f*
      calcium   calcio
      chlorides   cloruro
      creatine   creatina
      crystal(s)   cristal(es) *m*
      glucose   glucosa
      phosphate   fosfato
      solids   sólidos *m*
      total nitrogen   nitrógeno total
      total sulfur   azufre total *m*
      urea   urea
      urobilin   urobilina
      urobilirubin   urobilirrubina
urticaria   urticaria
user of pills   pildoriento
user of marijuana, cocaine, morphine   maricocaimorfi
user of morphine   morfiniento
uterus   matriz *f*; útero
   uterus prolapse   caída de la matriz; prolapso de la matriz; prolapso del útero
uvula   campanilla *fam*; galillo *fam*; úvula
vaccinate, to   vacunar
vaccination   inoculación *f*; vacunación *f*
   vaccination, booster   refuerzo
   vaccination, DPT   triple *f*
vaccine, immunization   immunización *f*; vacuna
   vaccine, oral polio   gotas para polio; vacuna oral contra la polio

vagina   vagina; agujero *vulgar, Chicano;*
concha *vulgar, Arg., Chile, Urug.;* cueva
slang, vulgar, Chicano; linda *slang;* pan
m, slang, vulgar; panocho *slang;* partida
vulgar

vaginal   vaginal *adj*

vaginitis   vaginitis *f*

valve   válvula

vapor   vapor *m*

varicose   varicoso *adj*

   varicose vein   várice *f;* variz *m;* vena
varicosa

variocosity   varicosidad *f*

vas deferens   conducto deferente

vaseline   vaselina

vein   vena

velum   velo

veneral disease   enfermedad venérea *f;*
secreta *slang*

   **AIDS/Acquired Immune Deficiency
Syndrome**   SIDA Síndrome de
Inmuno[logía] Deficiencia
Adquirida *m*

   canker sore   postemilla; úlcera
gangrenosa

   chancre   chancro; grano

   chancre, hard   chancro duro; chancro
sifilítico

   chancre, noninfecting   chancro
blando; chancro simple

   chlamidia   clamidia

   cold sore   fuegos en la boca (en los
labios); herpes labial *m*

   conduloma   condiloma *m*

   genital wart   verruga genital; verruga
venérea

   gonorrhea   gonorrea; blenorragia;
chorro *euph, Chicano;* gota *slang;*
mal de orín *m, slang;* purgaciones *f,
pl, slang*

   herpes   herpe(s) *m/f*

   herpes genitalis   herpes genital

   herpes menstrualis   herpes menstrual

   herpes zoster   herpes zoster

   HIV/Human Immunodeficiency Virus
VIH *m;* Virus de (la)
Inmunodeficiencia Humana *m*

   human papilloma virus   virus de(l)
papiloma humano *m*

   lymphogranuloma venereum
bubones *m;* linfogranuloma venéreo
m

   moniliasis   algodoncillo; boquera;
candidiasis *f;* moniliasis *f;* muguet
m

   nongonococcal urethritis   uretritis
no gonococal *f*

   nonspecific urethritis   uretritis
inespecífica *f;* uretritis no específica *f*

sexually transmitted diseases
enfermedades pasadas sexualmente *f*

syphilis   infección de la sangre *f,
euph;* sangre mala *f, slang;* sífilis *f*

trichomonas   tricomonas

venereal lesion   chancro; grano;
úlcera

vesicular eruption   erupción
vesicular *f*

vermifuge   antihelmíntico *m, adj;*
vermífugo *m, adj*

vertebra   vértebra

vial   ampolla; botella; frasco; vial *m*

victim   víctima

vinegar   vinagre *m*

virus   virus *m*

vision   visión *f;* vista

   vision, blurred   vista borrosa

   vision, double   vista doble

vitamin   vitamina

   vitamin B$_1$ tiamina

   vitamin B$_2$ riboflavina

   vitamin B$_6$ piridoxina

   vitamin C   ácido ascórbico

   vitamin: calcium   calcio

   vitamin: iron   hierro; sulfato ferroso

   vitamin: niacin   ácido nicotínico;
niacina

vitiligo   ciricua *fam;* jiricua *slang;* vitíligo

vitreous humor   humor vitreo *m*

vocal cord   cuerda vocal

vomit (vomiting)   vómito; arrojadera
vulgar; basca

vomit, to   vomitar; arrojar *fam;* devolver
(ue); dompear *Chicano;* tirar las tripas

vomitive   emético *m, adj;* vomitivo *m,
adj*

vulva   vulva; panocha *slang;* rajada
vulgar

waist   cintura

wait (for), to   esperar

waiver   renuncia voluntaria

wake up, to   despertar(se) (ie)

walk, to   andar; caminar

walker   andador *m*

walking cane   bastón de paseo *m*

want, to/ love, to   querer (ie)

warm   templado *adj;* tibio *adj*

warmer   calentador *m;* más caliente *adj*

warn, to   advertir (ie)

warning   aviso

warning sign   signo de advertencia

warrant, to   hacer certificación

wart   mezquino *Mex.; C.A., Col.* verruga

   wart, plantar   ojo de pescado *fam*

wash, to   lavar

   wash oneself, to   lavarse

waste   desecho

watch, to (care for, to)   cuidar

water   agua

   water pick   limpiador de agua a
presión *m*

watery   acuoso *adj;* blandito *adj*

WBC (white blood count)   NGB
(numeración de glóbulos blancos) *f*

weak   débil *adj*

weakness   debilidad *f*

weal (large welt)   cardenal *m;* verdugón
m

wean, to   destetar

weigh, to   pesar

weight   peso

well-being   bienestar *m*

wen   lobanillo; lupia

wet   mojado *adj*

wet the bed, to   mojar la cama

wheal   pápula; roncha

wheelchair   silla de ruedas

wheeze, to   respirar asmáticamente;
respirar con dificultad

whooping cough (pertussis)
coqueluche *f;* tos ahogona *f, Mex.;* tos
convulsiva *f;* tos ferina *f;* tosferina

wire, to   atar con alambre

witness   testigo

womb   matriz *f;* útero

worry   pena; preocupación *f*

worry, to   apenarse *Chicano;*
preocuparse

wound   herida; llaga; coco

   abrasion   abrasión *f*

   chafe   rozadura

   cut   cortadura

   incised   herida incisa

   incision   cisura; incisión *f*

   knife wound   filorazo *Chicano*

   laceration   laceración *f*

   puncture wound   herida penetrante;
herida punzante

   scrape   raspadura

   tear (torn wound)   desgarro;
desgarrón *m*

wound, to (hurt, to)   herir (ie)

wrapping in a cold (wet) sheet
empacamiento en sábana fría
(mojada)

wrinkle   arruga

wrist   muñeca

xerosis   resequedad de los ojos *f;* xerosis
f

x-ray   radiografía; rayos equis; retrato
del x-ray *Chicano*

   x-ray, chest   radiografía del tórax;—
del pecho

x-ray, to   radiografiar

zinc oxide   radióxido de zinc

Spanish-English Vocabulary

Vocabulario español-inglés

ABBREVIATIONS

ABBREVIATURAS

adj	adjective	**adjetivo**
adv	adverb	**adverbio**
euph	euphemism	**eufemismo**
fam	familiar	**familiar**
f	feminine noun	**sustantivo feminino**
inv	invariable	**invariable**
m	masculine noun	**sustantivo masculino**
m/f	masculine or feminine noun	**sustantivo masculino** o **feminino**
med	medicine	**medicina**
pl	plural	**plural**
sg	singular	**singular**

Unless specified, words ending with **a** are feminine, words ending with **o** are masculine.

SPECIAL WORDS USED TO INDICATE REGIONAL OCCURRENCES
PALABRAS ESPECIALES USADAS PARA INDICACION REGIONAL

Arg.	Argentina	**la Argentina**
Bol.	Bolivia	**Bolivia**
C.A.	Central America (Guatemala, El Salvador, Honduras, Costa Rica, Nicaragua)	**Centroamérica (Guatemala, el Salvador, Honduras, Costa Rica, Nicaragua)**
Carrib.	(Cuba, Puerto Rico, Dominican Republic)	**(Cuba, Puerto Rico, la República Dominicana)**
Chicano	Chicano (southwestern U.S.)	**Chicano**
Chile	Chile	**Chile**
Col.	Colombia	**Colombia**
C.R.	Costa Rica	**Costa Rica**
Cuba	Cuba	**Cuba**
Ec.	Ecuador	**el Ecuador**
Guat.	Guatemala	**Guatemala**
Hond.	Honduras	**Honduras**
Mex.	Mexico	**México**
Nic.	Nicaragua	**Nicaragua**
Pan.	Panama	**Panamá**
Para.	Paraguay	**Paraguay**
Peru	Peru	**Perú**
P.R.	Puerto Rico	**Puerto Rico**
Riopl.	Rio de la Plata region (Eastern Argentina, Uruguay)	**Río de la Plata (la Argentina Oriental, el Uruguay)**
Sal.	El Salvador	**el Salvador**
SpAm	Spanish America	**América del Sur**
Spain	Spain	**España**
Ur.	Uruguay	**el Uruguay**
Ven.	Venezuela	**Venezuela**

VOCABULARY

VOCABULARIO

a *f* amphetamines
a término at term (birth)
a tierra electrical grounding
abajo firmado *adj* undersigned
abatelengua *m, inv* tongue depressor
abatimiento depression
abdomen *m* abdomen
   abdomen agudo *slang* acute abdomen; bowel obstruction; peritonitis; appendicitis

aborto abortion
   aborto espontáneo spontaneous abortion
   aborto inducido induced abortion
   aborto provocado induced abortion
   aborto terapéutico therapeutic abortion
abotagar to become bloated
   abotagarse to bloat; to swell
abrasión *f* abrasion

abrelatas *m, inv* can opener
absceso abscess
absorbente higiénico *m* sanitary napkin
abstenerse de las relaciones sexuales to abstain from sexual relations
abuja fix; injection (of a narcotic substance); joint (of a narcotic substance)
abujazo fix; injection (of a narcotic substance)

abuso de (las) drogas drug abuse

acabarse *C.A., Mex., Ríopl.* to decline in health

ácaro parasite; mite

accidente *m* accident; complication

    accidente cerebral stroke

acedía heartburn

aceite *m* oil

    aceite de gaulteria oil of wintergreen

    aceite de hígado de bacalao cod liver oil

    aceite de pino pine oil

    aceite de ricino castor oil

    aceite mineral mineral oil

    aceite para niños baby oil

acercarse to get close

acetaminofén *m* acetaminophen

acetona acetone

acidez *f* acidity; heartburn

ácido acid

    ácido *slang* amphetamines

    ácido acético (puro) acetic acid

    ácido acetilsalicílico acetylsalicylic acid

    ácido arsénico arsenic acid

    ácido ascórbico ascorbic acid; vitamin C

    ácido bórico boric acid

    ácido carbólico carbolic acid

    ácido clorhídrico hydrochloric acid

    ácido fluorhídrico hydrofluoric acid

    ácido fólico folic acid

    ácido fosfórico phosphoric acid

    ácido lisérgico LSD

    ácido nicotínico niacin

    ácido nítrico nitric acid

    ácido oxálico oxalic acid

    ácido paramino salicílico p-aminosalicylic acid (PAS)

    ácido sulfúrico sulphuric acid

    ácido tánico tannic acid

    ácido úrico uric acid

acidófilos acidophiles

acné *f* acne

acordarse (ue) de to remember

acostarse (ue) to go to bed; to lie down

acrílico *adj* acrylic

acromatopsia color blindness

acuclillarse to squat

acumulación de la muestra *f* collection of the specimen

acumular to accumulate; to collect

acupuntura acupuncture

achaque *m, C.R.* sickliness; fainting spell during pregnancy

adelgazar to lose weight

adicto (drug) addict; *adj* addicted

    adicto a droga(s) drug addict

    adicto a las drogas narcóticas (drug) addict

administración *f, Mex.* menstruation

administrarse to take (drugs)

adolorado *adj, Chicano* hypochondriac

adormecer to make sleepy

    adormecer el nervio to deaden the nerve

    adormecer por anestesia to put to sleep

adormecido *adj* numb

adormecimiento numb, numbness

adquirir (ie) to acquire

adrenalina adrenalin

advertir (ie) to warn

afasia aphasia

afectado *adj, Chicano* tubercular; *Arg.* **estar afectado** to be hurt

afectado del pulmón *Chicano, Mex.* tuberculosis

afeitar(se) to shave

aflicción *f* sore

aflojarse to relax

afonia aphonia; hoarseness

afónico *adj* hoarse

afta oral lesion; thrush

agacharparse to bend over; to crouch

agacharse to bend over

agarraderas *Chicano* breast

agotamiento exhaustion

    agotamiento por calor heat exhaustion

agrandamiento enlargement

agravamiento change for the worse

agregar to add

agriera *Sp.Am.* heartburn

agrietar to crack

    agrietarse to chap

agruras heartburn

agua water

    agua con azúcar glucose water

    agua con mostaza mustard water

    agua con sal saline solution

    agua de amnios amniotic fluid

    agua de manzanilla chamomile tea

    agua jabonosa soapy water

    agua mineral mineral water

    agua oxigenada peroxide; hydrogen peroxide

    agua salada salt water

    agua salina saline solution

    "aguas mayores" *euph* feces; stool

    "aguas menores" *euph* urine

agudo *adj* severe

aguja needle

    aguja hipodérmica hypodermic needle

agujero foramen; hole; *vulgar, Chicano* anus; vagina

aguoso *adj* watery

ahogamiento dropsy

ahogarse to choke

ahoguijo congestion of the chest; shortness of breath

ahogío *fam* congestion of the chest; shortness of breath; asthma *fam, Mex.*

aislamiento por cuarentena isolation

aislar to isolate

al ras level

alambre de contacto *m* (electrical) lead wire

alambrito loop

albúmina albumin

alcanfor *m* camphor

alcohol *m* alcohol

    alcohol para fricciones rubbing alcohol

alcoholismo alcoholism

alergia allergy; hay fever

alfombra *P.R., Cuba* rash

alfombría *Chicano* German measles; rubella

alfombrilla *Chicano* German measles

algodón *m* cotton

    algodón absorbente absorbent cotton

algodón estéril sterile cotton

algodoncillo *fam* thrush; moniliasis

aliento breath

alimentación *f* feeding

    alimentación suplementaria supplementary feeding

alimentar to feed

aliviando *adj* "high" on narcotics; "turned on"

aliviar to cure; to make better; to relieve

    aliviarse to get well; *Chicano* to deliver a child

alivio relief

almacenar to store

almidón *m* starch

    almidón animal glycogen

almidonado *adj* starchy

almohada pillow

    almohadilla caliente eléctrica electric heating pad

    almohadilla higiénica sanitary napkin

    almohadilla neumática en forma de anillo inflatable rubber "doughnut"

almohadita nursing pad

almorrana pile; hemorrhoid

almorzar (ue) to have lunch

alucinación *f* hallucination

alucinógeno hallucinogenic drug; hallucinogen

alumbrado *adj, slang, Chicano* drunk

alumbramiento childbirth; confinement

alumbrar to give birth

alvéolo tooth socket; alveolus

ama de cría baby nurse

amalgama amalgam

amamantamiento nursing

amamantar to nurse (breastfeed)

amarihuanarse to take marijuana

amarillo *adj* yellow

amarrar to bind

ambliopia amblyopia

ameba amoeba

amenaza de aborto threatened abortion

amenorrea amenorrhea

amiba *slang* amoeba; PCP

amígdalas tonsils

amigdalitis *f* tonsilitis

    amigdalitis supurativa quinsy (sore throat)

amiláceo *adj* starchy

aminoácidos amino acids

amoníaco ammonia

amoratado *adj* black and blue

ampicilina ampicillin

ampliación *f* enlargement

ampolla blister; vial; ampoule

ampolleta ampoule

analgésico *m, adj* analgesic

análisis *m, inv* test

    análisis de esputos sputum test

    análisis de laboratorio laboratory test

    análisis de orina urinalysis

    análisis de sangre blood chemistry (analysis of blood); blood test

analizador del oxígeno de la sangre *m* blood oxygen analyzer

anca haunch

andador *m* walker

andar to walk
  andar + *adj* to be high *See high Appendix A.*
  andar andando to be up and about after an illness
  andar bombo (bomba) to be drunk; to get drunk
  andar carga to be carrying narcotic drugs
  andar cargado (cargada) to be carrying narcotic drugs
  andar crudo (cruda) to have a hangover
  andar el cuerpo to defecate
  andar eléctrico (eléctrica) to be drunk; to get drunk
  andar en la línea to be drunk; to get drunk
  andar loco (loca) to be drunk; to get drunk
anemia anemia
  anemia aplástica aplastic anemia
  anemia drepanocítica sickle cell anemia
  anemia perniciosa pernicious anemia
anestesia anesthesia
  anestesia caudal caudal anesthesia
  anestesia de bloque block anesthesia
  anestesia en silla de montar saddle block anesthesia
  anestesia epidural epidural anesthesia
  anestesia espinal spinal anesthesia
  anestesia local local anesthesia
  anestesia por inhalación inhalation anesthesia
  anestesia raquídea spinal anesthesia
  anestesia regional regional anesthesia
  anestesia total general anesthesia
anestésico *m, adj* anesthetic
anestético *m, adj* anesthetic
aneurisma *m* aneurysm
anfetamina amphetamine
angina angina; *Mex., Ven.* tonsil
  angina de pecho angina pectoris
angustia anguish
anillo IUD ring
ano anus
anomalía congénita congenital anomaly
ansias matutinas morning sickness
ansiedad *f* anxiety
antebrazo forearm
anteojos *m, pl, general term* eyeglasses; spectacles
  anteojos oscuros sunglasses
antiácido *m, adj* antacid
antibiótico *m, adj* antibiotic
  antibiótico de alcance amplio broad-spectrum antibiotic
  antibiótico de espectro amplio broad-spectrum antibiotic
anticoagulante *m, adj* anticoagulant
anticolinérgico *m, adj* anticholinergic
anticonceptivo *m, adj* contraceptive
anticuerpo antibody
antidoto antidote
  antidoto universal universal antidote
antiemético *m, adj* antiemetic
antiespasmódico *m, adj* antispasmodic
antígeno antigen

antihelmíntico *m, adj* vermifuge
antihemorrágico *adj* antihemorrhagic
antihistamínico *m, adj* antihistamine
antipalúdico *m, adj;* antimalarial
antipirético *m, adj* antipyretic
antiséptico *m, adj* antiseptic
antitetánico *adj* antitetanic; anti-tetanus
antitoxina antitoxin
añadir to add
apaciguador *m* tranquilizer
aparatito *Chicano* IUD
aparato apparatus; system; *Chicano* buttock
  aparato auditivo hearing aid
  aparato cardiovascular cardiovascular system
  aparato circulatorio circulatory system
  aparato digestivo digestive system
  aparato endócrino endocrine system
  aparato gastrointestinal gastrointestinal system
  aparato genitourinario genitourinary system
  aparato intrauterino intrauterine device
  aparato para la sordera hearing aid
  aparato reproductivo reproductive system
  aparato respiratorio respiratory system
apartar to isolate
apenarse *Chicano* to worry
apéndice *m* appendix
apendicitis *f* appendicitis
apendix *f* appendix
apestoso *adj* foul-smelling
apetito appetite
aplicación *f* application
  aplicación de hielo empaquetado ice pack
apoplejía apoplexy; stroke
apósito dressing
apostemado *adj* abscessed
apoyo support
  apoyo para la cabeza headrest
apretar (ie) to squeeze
arca *Mex.* armpit
ardor de estómago *m* heartburn
armazón *m/f* skeleton
  armazón de calentamiento *f* warming crib
arrebato fit
arremangarse to roll up one's sleeve
arrepentirse (ie) to repent
arritmia irregular heartbeat; arrhythmia
  arritmia cardíaca cardiac arrhythmia
arrojar *fam* to vomit
arruga wrinkle
arsénico arsenic
arteria dental dental artery
arteriosclerosis *f* arteriosclerosis
articulación *f* articulation; joint
  articulación envarada stiff or "frozen" joint
  articulación trabada stiff or "frozen" joint
artificial *adj* artificial
artritis *f* arthritis
  artritis reumatoidea rheumatic arthritis
asa loop
ascáride *f* ascaris; roundworm
ascaris *f* ascaris; roundworm
aseo cleanliness

asfixia suffocation, choking
asientos *slang* diarrhea
asintomático *adj* asymptomatic
asma asthma
  asma bronquial bronchial asthma
asoleada *Sp.Am.* sunstroke
áspero *adj* rough
aspirar por la nariz to sniff
aspirina aspirin
  aspirina para niños children's aspirin
asqueo morning nausea
astigmatismo astigmatism
astilla (en el ojo) splinter (in the eye)
astringente *m, adj* astringent
asumir to assume
asustarse to get frightened
ataque *m* attack; convulsion; onset; seizure
  ataque (de epilepsia) epilepsy
  ataque al corazón heart attack
  ataque asmático asthmatic attack; seizure
  ataque cardíaco heart attack
  ataque del corazón heart attack
  ataque epiléptico epileptic attack
  ataque fulminante stroke
  ataque vesicular gallbladder attack
atar to bind
  atar con alambre to wire
atarantado *adj* dizzy
atorarse to choke
atragantarse to choke
atrasado *adj* overdue; relapse
atrasar to cause to suffer a relapse
  atrasarse to have a relapse
atravesar (ie) to pass over
atrofia atrophy
atropina atropine
audífono hearing aid
auditivo *adj* auditory
aumentar to increase
aumento increase
aurícola external ear
autorización *f* authorization
autorizar to authorize
avariosis *f, Sp.Am.* syphilis
axila armpit
ayuda enema
ayunas, en fasting
ayuno fasting
azúcar *m/f* sugar
  azúcar de uva dextrose
  azúcar sanguíneo blood sugar
azucarado *adj* sugary
azufre *m* sulphur; *slang* heroin
  azufre total total sulphur
bachica cigarette butt (especially marijuana)
bacteria bacterium
bacteriemia bacteremia
báculo cane
bajar el nivel del colesterol to lower the cholesteral count
bala bullet
bálano glans (penis)
balazo bullet wound
balbucencia stuttering
balone *m, Chicano* penis
bálsamo balsam
banco de sangre blood bank
bañar to bathe
  bañar(se) to bathe; to take a bath
bañera tub

baño bath; restroom; toilet
  baño de almidón starch bath
  baño de asiento sitz bath
  baño de azufre sulphur bath
  baño de brea tar bath
  baño de esponja sponge bath
  baño de harina de avena oatmeal bath
  baño de mostaza mustard bath
  baño de permanganato de potasio potassium permanganate bath
  baño de regadera *Chicano* shower bath
  baño de salvado bran bath
  baño de sodio sodium bath
  baño de toalla *Chicano* sponge bath
  baño emoliente emollient bath
  baño salino saline bath
barba beard; chin
barbilla chin
barbiturato barbiturate; barbiturate pill
barbitúrico barbiturate pill
barriga belly
barrillo pimple
barro pimple; blackhead
basca nausea
base del cráneo *f* base of the cranium
basófilos basophiles
bastón *m* cane
  bastón de paseo walking cane
bastoncillo rod (of the retina)
bata gown, robe
bazo spleen
bebé *m* baby; infant
beber mucho . . . to drink plenty of . . .
belladona belladonna
bencedrina benzedrine
benjuí *m* benzoin
benzoína benzoin
béquico cough suppressant
bermejizo *adj* reddish (hair)
berrinche *m, fam* tantrum
biberón *m* baby bottle; nursing bottle
bicarbonato de soda bicarbonate of soda
bíceps *m* biceps
bicúspide *m, adj* bicuspid
bienestar *m* well-being
bigote *m* moustache
bilharzia schistosoma
bilirrubina bilirubin
bilis *f* bile; irritability *(not related to bile)*
biometría hemática blood count
bisojo *adj* cross-eyed; squint-eyed
bisturí *m* scalpel
bizco *m, adj, C.A.* cross-eyed; squint-eyed; strabismus
bizquera cross-eyes; strabismus
blandito *adj* watery
blando *adj* soft *(pliant)*
blanqueador de ropa *m* sodium hypochlorite *(bleach)*
blanqueo bleach
blanquillo *slang, Chicano* testicle
blefaritis *f* blepharitis
blenorragia gonorrhea
blindaje contra la radiación *m* radiation shield
bloquear to block
bobas chicken pox
bobita *Chicano* gnat
boca mouth
  boca del estómago pit of stomach
bocado de Adán Adam's apple

bocal *m* mouthpiece
bocio goiter
bofe *m, Chicano, Sp.Am.* lung
bola lump; **bolas** *Chicano* mumps; knot (type of tissue swelling); *slang, Chicano* testicle
bolo *adj, C.A.* drunk
bolsa bag
  bolsa de agua caliente hot water bag
  bolsa de caucho para hielo ice bag; ice pack
  bolsa de hielo ice bag; ice pack
  bolsa de lágrimas tear sac
  bolsa de las aguas bag of waters
  bolsa de los testículos scrotum
  bolsa membranosa bag of waters
  bolsa para enema enema bag
bomba pump
  bomba de ordeñar breast pump
  bomba estomacal stomach pump
bombido *slang* amphetamines
bombita *slang* amphetamine + heroin + barbiturate IV amphetamine
bombo *Ur.* buttock
boquera fungus; moniliasis
boquilla cheilosis *(sore at corner of mouth)*; mouthpiece
boquineta *m, Chicano* cleft palate; hairlip
bornear to twist; to bend
borrachera drunkenness
borracho *adj* drunk
borujo lump
borujón *m* large lump
bote *m, slang, Chicano* baby bottle
botella bottle; vial
botica drug store; pharmacy
botiquín *m* kit; medicine cabinet; medicine chest
  botiquín de emergencia emergency kit
  botiquín de primeros auxilios first aid kit
bóveda ósea del paladar hard palate
braga diaper
braguero brace; truss
brazo arm
brea de hulla coal tar
bromuro bromide
bronceado *adj* suntanned
bronquios bronchia
bronquitis *f* bronchitis
brucelosis *f* Malta fever
búa bubo
buba pimple
bubón *m* pustule; **bubones** lymphogranuloma venereum
buche *m, Mex.* mumps; *slang* goiter
buena salud *f* fitness (good health)
bulla blister
bulto lump
bursitis *f* bursitis
buscatoques *m/f, inv, slang* addict in search of a fix
búster *m* booster shot
busto breast
butón *m* pimple
caballete *m* bridge (of the nose)
caballo heroin
caballón *adj* "high" on narcotics; "turned on"
cabecita de vena *Chicano* angiomata
cabello hair
cabestrillo sling

cabeza head; *slang* glans (penis)
cabezal *m* compress
caca *slang* feces; stool
ca-ca *slang* heroin
cacahuate *m* barbiturate pill
cácara *Chicano* acne
cacaraña *Mex. Guat.* pock
cachete *m* cheek
cachucha drug supply; heroin capsule
cada every
cadáver *m* corpse
cadera hip
caduquez *f* senility
caer to fall
  caer con algo to catch; to come down with a disease
  caerse to fall down
café *m* coffee; *slang* LSD
  café caliente hot coffee
cafeína caffeine
cagada *vulgar* feces; stool; *slang* heroin
cagadera *vulgar, Chicano* diarrhea
caída fall
  caída de la matriz prolapse; uterus prolapse
  caída de la mollera fallen fontanel
  caída de los dientes loss of one's teeth
caja torácica thoracic cavity
cajetuda *Chicano* headache
cala suppository
calambres *m* cramps; menstrual cramps; muscular cramps
  calambres de los cortadores de caña cane-cutter's cramps
  calambres térmicos heat cramps
calamina calamine
calavera skull
calcañar *m* heel
calceta elástica elastic stocking
calcio calcium
cálculo stone
  cálculo biliar gallstone
  cálculo en el riñon kidney stone
  cálculo en la vejiga gallstone
  cálculo renal kidney stone
calentador *m* warmer
calentura fever; temperature
callarse to be quiet
callo callus; corn
calloso *adj* calloused; rough
calmante *m* pain killer; sedative; tranquilizer
  calmante para la tos cough suppressant
calmar(se) to calm down
  calmarse to relax
calofrío *Chicano* hot flashes
calor *m* heat
  calores hot flashes
calostro colostrum
calote *m* cast
calvicie *f* baldness
calvo *adj* bald
calzar to put on (footwear, gloves) to wear
cama bed
cámara chamber; *slang* diarrhea, feces; stool
  cámara anterior del cerebro anterior chamber of cerebrum
  cámara posterior del cerebro posterior chamber of cerebrum
cambiar to trade

cambiar el pañal to diaper
cambiar(se) to change (oneself)
cambio de vida change of life; menopause
camilla calentadora de niño warming crib
camilla de niño crib
caminar to walk
camisón *m* gown
campanilla *fam* uvula
canal *m* canal; duct
   canal de la oreja *fam* external ear canal
   canal del parto birth canal
   canal radicular root canal
   canal urinario urethra
canas (verdes) (premature) gray hair
cáncer *m* cancer
   cáncer en la sangre leukemia
canceroso *adj* cancerous
candidiasis *f* fungus, moniliasis
cangrena gangrene
canilla shin
canino canine tooth; eyetooth
cano urinario urethra
cansado *adj* tired
cansar to tire
   cansarse to get tired
capa *slang* heroin capsule
capear to put heroin in capsules
capiar to put heroin in capsules
capilar *m* capillary
capón *adj, Chicano* infertile
cápsula capsule
   cápsula para ablandar evacuaciones stool softener
cara face
caracol *m, fam* cochlea
carácter recesivo *m* recessive character
carátula *slang, Chicano* face
carbohidrato carbohydrate
carbón activado *m* activated charcoal
carbonato de sodio sodium carbonate
carcinoma *m* carcinoma
cardenal *m* weal (large welt)
cardialgia heartburn
cardiopatías heart disease
cardioscopio cardioscope
carencia deficiency
carga *slang* load of narcotics
cargar la calentura *Chicano* to increase; to persist (fever)
caries f, *inv* cavity; caries; tooth decay
carne *f* flesh
carnosidad f, *fam* pterytium
carraspera *fam* hoarseness
carrasposo *adj* chronically hoarse
carrillo cheek
cartílago cartilage
casa de maternidad maternity hospital
casarse (con) to get married; to marry
casco scalp
caso case
   caso límite borderline case
   caso urgente emergency
caspa dandruff
casqueta *Chicano* masturbation
cataplasma cataplasm; poultice
   cataplasma de mostaza mustard plaster
catarata cataract
catarro cold
   catarro constipado *Chicano* hay fever
catártico *m, adj* purgative
catéter *m* catheter

cateterizar to catheterize
caucásico *m, adj* caucasian
cauterización *f* cauterization
cavidad *f* cavity
   cavidad dental caries
ceceo lisp; stutter
ceder to give up (a claim)
cegato *adj, fam* shortsighted
ceguedad *f* blindness
ceguera blindness
   ceguera del río river blindness
   ceguera para los colores color blindness
ceja brow; eyebrow
celíaca celiac disease
célula cell
   célula ciliada ciliated cell
   células falciformes sickle cells
cemento cementum
cepillarse los dientes to brush one's teeth
cepillo de dientes toothbrush
cera de los oídos earwax
cerebro cerebrum
cerilla earwax
cerrar (ie) to close
certificado de nacimiento birth certificate
certificar to certify
cerumen *m* earwax
cerviz *f* cervix
chale *m, vulgar, Chicano* penis
chalito *m, vulgar, Chicano* penis
chamorro *Chicano* calf of leg
chancro chancre; veneral lesion
   chancro blando soft chancre
   chancro duro hard chancre
   chancro sifilítico hard chancre
   chancro simple non-infecting chancre
chechén *m* poison ivy
cheuto *adj, Chile* hairlip
chi *f, vulgar* urine
chichas *f, pl, C.R.* breast
chiche *m, Mex., Guat.* breast of a wet nurse
chichi *f, fam, Arg.* nipple (of female breast); *Guat., Mex.* wet nurse; *Mex.* breast
chichigua *vulgar, Sp.Am.* wet nurse
chichón *m* lump; bump on head; swelling on the head
chicloso *vulgar, Chicano* anus
chicote *m, slang* penis
chile *m, slang* penis
chimpa *Chicano* hair
chimuelo *adj, Chicano* lacking teeth
chinaloa *slang* opium
chiche *f* bedbug
chingar *vulgar* to have sexual relations
chino *Mex.* fine-toothed comb
chiporra *Guat., Hond.* tumor on the head
chiquito *vulgar, Chicano* anus
chiva *slang* heroin
cholenco *adj* sickly
chopetear *slang* to have sexual relations
choque *m* shock
   choque alérgico *fam* anaphylactic shock
   choque anafiláctico anaphylactic shock
choquezuela knee cap
chorizo *vulgar* penis

chorrillo *slang* diarrhea
chorro *euph, Chicano* gonorrhea; *slang* diarrhea
chot *m, Chicano* shot, injection
chucho *Chile, Arg.* malarial fever
chueco, andar to deal in illegal transactions
chupar to suck
chupete *m* pacifier
chupón *m* nipple (of a baby/nursing bottle)
chutear to mainline drugs
ciática sciatica
ciático *adj* sciatic
cicatriz *f* scar
cicatrizado *adj* scarred
ciego *adj* blind
cielo de la boca roof of the mouth
cinta band; tape
   cinta adhesiva adhesive tape
cintura binder; waist
circulación *f* circulation
   circulación sanguínea blood circulation
circuncidar to circumcise
circuncisión *f* circumcision
ciricua *fam* vitiligo
cirrosis del hígado *f* cirrhosis of the liver
   cirrosis hepática cirrhosis of the liver
cirugía surgery
cisticerco cysticercus; bladderworm
cistitis *f* cystitis
cistoscopía/cistoscopia cystoscopy
cistoscopio cystoscope
cisura fissure; incision
cita appointment
clamidia chlamidia
clara de huevo egg white
clavar to stick
clavícula collar bone; clavicle
clavija de contacto electrical plug
clínica clinic; private hospital; doctor's office
   clínica dental dental office
   clínica de reposo nursing home
clítoris *m* clitoris
cloasma *m* chloasma (*facial discoloration*); mask of pregnancy
cloranfenicol *m* chloramphenicol
cloro bleach; chlorine
clorofila chlorophyll
cloromicetín *m* chloromycetin
cloromicetina chloromycetin
cloroquina chloroquinine
cloruro chlorine
   cloruro mercúrico bichloride of mercury
coagulante *m, adj* coagulant
coágulo sanguíneo blood clot
cocaína cocaine
cóccix *m, Chicano* coccyx
cóclea cochlea
cócono person high on drugs
codeína codeine
codo elbow
coercitivo restraining device
coger (cojer) *vulgar, Arg., P.R., Mex.* to have sexual relations
coil *m, Chicano* coil
coito coitus
cojear to limp; to hobble
cojera lameness

cojincillo pad
cojo *adj* crippled; lame
cola glue
colgajo flap of skin
colapso collapse; nervous breakdown
  colapso físico physical collapse
colchón *m* mattress
colecistograma *m* cholecystogram
cólera *f* anger; *m* cholera
colesterol *m* cholesterol
  colesterol elevado high cholesterol
colgar (ue) to hang
  colgar (ue) las piernas to dangle
  one's legs
cólico *m adj* colic
colita *slang* coccyx
colitis *f* colitis
  colitis ulcerosa diverticulitis
colmillo canine tooth; eyetooth
colocar to place
colon *m* colon
  colon sigmoide sigmoid colon
color *m* color
coloración *f* stain; staining
colorada barbiturate pill; seconal
  capsule; *slang, Chicano* blood
colorante *m* stain, staining
colostomía colostomy
columna vertebral backbone; spinal
  column
coma *m* coma
comadrona midwife (untrained)
combustible *m* fuel
comenzar (ie) to begin
comezón *f* itch
comienzo onset
comisura suture
cómodo *adj* comfortable
compañones *m, slang* testicle
competir (i) to compete
complicación *f* complication
componente *m* constituent;
  component
  componente de sangre blood
  component
  componente sanguíneo blood
  component
componer una fractura to set a
  fracture
comprender to understand
compresa compress
  compresa fría cold pack
comprimido tablet
común *m* toilet; *Mex.* buttock
concebir (i) to conceive
concepción *f* conception
concha *vulgar, Arg., Chile, Urg.* vagina;
  fam external ear
concusión *f* concussion
condiloma *m* condyloma
condón *m* rubber; condom
conducto duct; canal
  conducto auditivo external ear canal
  conducto deferente vas deferens
  conducto lacrimal tear duct
  conducto lagrimal tear duct
  conducto semicircular semicircular
  canal
conejo *slang, Chicano* biceps
conexionar to connect
confesar (ie) to confess
confusión *f* confusion
congelación *f* frostbite
congénito *adj* congenital

congestión *f* congestion
  congestión nasal sinus congestion
congoja anguish
conjuntiva conjunctiva
conjuntivitis *f* conjuctivitis
  conjuntivitis catarral aguda pink eye
conmoción nerviosa *f* shock
cono cone
conocer to know; to be acquainted
  with; to have sexual relations
conocimiento consciousness;
  knowledge
conseguir (i) to obtain; to get
consentir (ie) to consent
constipación *f* constipation
constipado *m, adj* "stopped-up"; head
  cold
constricción *f* stricture
consunción *f* phthisis
contacto contact
contagiar to communicate a disease; to
  infect
contagioso *adj* contagious
contaminación *f* contamination
contar (ue) to count
continuar to continue
contracción *f* contraction
  contracción muscular spasm
  contracciones de la matriz
  contractions
contraceptivo *m, adj* contraceptive
contraer una enfermedad to catch a
  disease
contraveneno antitoxin
control de la natalidad *m* birth control
controlar to control
contusión *f* bruise, contusion
convalecencia convalescence;
  convalescent hospital
convaleciente *adj* convalescent
convertir (ie) to convert
  convertir(se) (ie) to turn into
convulsión *f* convulsion; epileptic
  attack; fit; seizure
copa ocular eyecup
coqueluche *f* whooping cough; pertussis
coquetas *Mex.* mumps
coraje *m* anger
coramina coramine
corazón *m* heart
cordón *m* cord
  cordón del ombligo umbilical cord
  cordón dental dental floss
  cordón umbilical umbilical cord
corea chorea
corioide *f* chorioid
coriodes *f, inv* chorioid
córnea cornea
  córnea opaca sclera
corona crown; crown of tooth
  corona acrílica acrylic jacket crown
  corona de porcelana porcelain
  jacket crown
coronamiento crowning
coronar to crown
coronario *adj* coronary
corredera *Chicano* diarrhea
correr el cuerpo to defecate
corriente *f, adj* electrical current; stream
  corriente de aire caliente flow of
  warm air
  corriente sanguínea bloodstream
cortada incision; laceration; *Sp.Am.* cut
cortadura cut

cortarse to cut (oneself)
corte *m* cut
  corte de las partes episiotomy
  corte por congelación frozen section
corteza cerebral cerebral cortex
corticoesteroide *m* corticosteroid
cortisona cortisone
corto *adj* defective
  corto de oído hard of hearing
  corto de vista nearsighted
corva back of knees
costado flank; side
costar (ue) to cost
costilla rib
  costilla flotante false (floating) rib
  costilla verdadera true rib
costra scab
costumbre *f* menstruation
cotidiano *adj* daily
coxis *m* coccyx
coyuntura articulation; joint
cráneo skull; cranium
creatina creatine
crema ointment
  crema vaginal vaginal cream
creta pulverizada en agua ground
  chalk in water
cretinismo cretinism
crianza nursing; lactation period
criar to feed; to bring up
  criar a los pechos to nurse (a baby)
  criar con pecho *Chicano* to
  breastfeed
criatura baby; infant
cristal(es) *m* crystal(s)
cristalino crystaline; lens of eye
crónico *adj* chronic
cruento *adj* bloody
crup *f* croup
cuadril *m, Mex., Chicano* hip
cuadrúpleto quadruplet
cuajar to clot
cuajarón *m* blood clot
  cuajarón de sangre blood clot
cuarentena forty days following
  parturition; confinement
cuarteado *adj* chapped
cuarto quart; room
  cuarto de baño restroom
  cuarto de los niños nursery
cuate *Mex.* twin
  cuates *m, pl, slang, Chicano* testicles
cuatrillizo quadruplet
cúbito ulna
cucharada spoonful; tablespoon
cucharadita teaspoon
  cucharadita llena al ras level
  teaspoonful
cuchillada gash
cuchillo knife
cuello neck; neck of tooth
  cuello de la matriz cervix
  cuello del útero cervix
cuenca *Chicano* collarbone; clavicle
  cuenca de los ojos eye socket
cuentagotas *m, inv* eye dropper;
  medicine dropper
cuerda vocal vocal chord
cuerín *m, Chicano* scab
cuero skin
  cuero cabelludo scalp
cuerpo body
cuertito *Chicano* scab
cueva *slang, vulgar, Chicano* vagina

cuidado   care
   cuidado cardíaco   cardiac care
   cuidado intensivo   intensive care
   cuidado posnatal-postnatal
     postnatal care
   cuidado prenatal   prenatal care
cuidar   to take care of; to watch; to care
   for
culebrilla   fungus; ringworm; tinea
culo   *fam, Arg.* buttock
cuna   crib
cura   *f* cure; dressing; fix; *m* priest
curación   *f* dressing; healing
   curación del nervio   root canal work
curar   to heal; *slang* to provide an addict
   with a fix
   curarse   to recover
curetaje   *m* curettage
curita   Band-Aid
cursera   *slang* diarrhea
cúspide   *m* cuspid
cutícula   cuticle
   cutícula desgarrada   hang nail
cutis   *m/f, inv* skin (of the face)
daltonismo   color blindness
daño   damage
   daño sufrido por causa de helada
     frostbite
dar   to give
   dar a luz   to give birth; to deliver
   dar de alta   to discharge (from the
     hospital)
   dar de mamar   to brestfeed; to nurse
   dar el pecho   to breastfeed
   dar el pecho al niño   to nurse
   dar una dosis excesiva   to overdose
   darse un piquete   to inject onself
     with drugs
   darse vuelta   to turn (over)
de   *prep* of; from
   de crianza   *adj* nursing
   de maternidad   *adj* maternity
   de paja   *adj* straw
débil   *adj* weak
debilidad   *f* weakness
decir   to tell; to say
dedo   finger
   dedo anular   ring finger
   dedo del corazón   middle finger
   dedo del medio   middle finger
   dedo (del pie)   toe
   dedo gordo   thumb
   dedo gordo en matrillo   hammer toe
   dedo grueso   big toe
deducir   to subtract
defecto   defect
defibrilador   *m* defibrillator
deficiencia   deficiency
   deficiencia de hierro   anemia; iron
     deficiency
deforme   *adj* deformed
deformidad   *f* deformity
delantal   *m* apron
deletrear   to spell
delirio   delirium
demacración   *f* emaciation
demacrado   *adj* sickly
demencia   dementia; insanity
demostrar (ue)   to demonstrate; to show
dengue   *m* dengue
dentadura   denture; set of teeth
   dentadura (postiza)   denture
   dentadura completa   full denture
   dentadura parcial   partial denture

dentellada   bite *(toothmark)*
dentición   *f* dentition; teething
dentífrico   *m, adj* dentifrice
dentina   dentine
dependencia farmacológica   drug
   addiction
depilatorio   *m, adj* depilatory
deposiciones   *f* feces; stool
depósito de sangre   blood stock
depresión   *f* depression
depresor de la lengua   *m* tongue
   depressor
deprimido   *adj* depressed
dermatitis   *f* dermatitis
derramar   to spill; to shed
derrame   *m* discharge (bloody)
   derrame biliar   jaundice
   derrame cerebral   stroke
desabrido   *adj* tasteless
desagüe   *m* drainage
desaldillado   *Mex.* hernia
desangramiento   bleeding to excess;
   hemorrhage
desangrar   to bleed excessively; to bleed
   in excess
desojar   to cure from the evil eye
desarreglo nervioso   nervous
   breakdown
desayunarse   to eat breakfast
descansar   to rest
descanso   relaxation; *Chile* toilet
descargo   release
desconcertar (ie)   to sprain
descongestionante   *m, adj* decongestant
descubrimiento   discovery
descubrir   to detect
descuidado   *adj* careless; neglected
descuidar   to neglect
desecación   *f* dehydration
desecho   waste; secretion
desequilibrio   imbalance
desfallecimiento   fainting spell
desgarradura   laceration
desgarramiento   tear
desgarrar   *Chicano* to cough up phlegm
desgarro   tear, laceration; *Sp.Am.*
   sputum
deshidratación   *f* dehydration
deshidratar   to dehydrate
desinfectante   *m, adj* disinfectant
desmayarse   to faint
desmayo   fainting spell
desnudarse   to undress
desnutrición   *f* malnutrition
desnutrido   *adj* malnourished; *fam*
   undernourished; emaciated
desodorante   *m, adj* deodorant
desorden   *m* disorder
   desorden nervioso   nervous disorder
despedirse (i) (de)   to say goodbye (to)
despensa   *Chicano* medicine cabinet;
   medicine chest
despertar(se) (ie)   to wake up
desprender   to release
destetar   to wean
destruido   *adj* destroyed
desvanecimiento   fainting spell
desvelarse   to stay awake
desvestirse (i)   to get undressed
detectar   to detect
detergente   *m, adj* detergent
determinación   *f* determination
   determinación del grupo sanguíneo
     blood type

determinación del tiempo de
   circulación   determination of
   circulating time
dextrosa   dextrose
diabetes   *f* diabetes
diabetes adquirida durante la
   madurez   adult-onset diabetes
diabetes insípida   diabetes insipidus
diabetes mellitus   diabetes mellitus
diabetes (del principio) precoz
   juvenile-onset diabetes
diabetes sacarina   diabetes mellitus
   diabetes sacarina dependiente de
    la insulina   insulin dependent
    diabetes
   diabetes sacarina no dependiente
    de la insulina   non-insulin
    dependent diabetes
diabético   *m, adj* diabetic
diafragma   *m* diaphragm
diafragma anticonceptivo
   diaphragm (birth control device)
diagnosis   *f, inv* diagnosis
diagnosticar   to diagnose
diagnóstico   *m, adj* diagnosis
diagrama   *m* chart
diapasón   *m* turning fork
diario   *adj* daily
diarrea   diarrhea
diástole   *f* diastole
dicipela   *Chicano* erysipelas
diente   *m* tooth
   diente cariado   cavity
   diente de ajo   *fam* large,
    misshapened tooth
   diente de leche   baby tooth
   diente impactado   impacted tooth
   diente inferior   lower tooth
   diente mamón   baby tooth
   diente picado   cavity
   diente podrido   caries
   diente superior   upper tooth
   dientes blancos   white teeth
   dientes de leche   *pl* baby teeth;
    deciduous teeth
   dientes manchados   stained teeth
   dientes parejos   even teeth
   dientes podridos   tooth decay
   dientes postizos   artificial (false)
    teeth
dieta   diet
   dieta de líquidos   liquid diet
difenhidramina   diphenydramine
dificultad al respirar   *f* dyspnea
dificultoso   *adj* labored
difteria   diphtheria
digerir (ie)   to digest
digestión   *f* digestion
digitalina   digitalin
dilatación del cuello de la matriz   *f*
   dilation (of cervix)
dilear   to deal in drugs; to traffic in
   drugs
diliar   to deal in drugs; to traffic in
   drugs
discernir (ie)   to discern
disco   disc
   disco calcificado   calcified disc
   disco desplazado   slipped disc
   disco intervertebral luxado   slipped
    disc
disentería   dysentery
   disentería amebiana   amoebic
    dysentery

disentería amibiana amoebic dysentery
disentería bacilar bacillary dysentery
dislocación *f* sprain
dismenorrea dysmennorrhea
disminución de la tirantez *f* relaxation of tension
disolver (ue) to dissolve
dispepsia indigestion
dispositivo intrauterino intrauterine device (IUD)
distribución *f* distribution
distrofia muscular progresiva muscular dystrophy
DIU *m* IUD
diurético *m, adj* diuretic
diverticulitis *f* diverticulitis
divertirse (ie) to amuse oneself; to have a good time
doblarse to bend over
doctor *m* physician
doctora physician
dolencia ailment; disease; sickness
doler (ue) to hurt; to ache
dolor *m* pain; ache; sore
  dolor agudo sharp pain
  dolor al orinar dysuria
  dolor ardiente burning pain
  dolor cólico colicky pain
  dolor constante constant pain
  dolor continuo steady pain
  dolor de cabeza headache
  dolor de crecimiento growing pain
  dolor de dientes toothache
  dolor de estómago stomachache
  dolor de hambre hunger pain
  dolor de la vesícula gallbladder attack
  dolor de miembro fantasma phantom limb pain
  dolor de muelas toothache
  dolor de oído earache
  dolor de ojos sore eyes
  dolor de parto labor pain
  dolor errante wandering pain
  dolor falso false pain
  dolor fulgurante shooting pain
  dolor leve mild pain
  dolor moderado moderate pain
  dolor opresivo pressure-like pain
  dolor penetrante boring pain
  dolor radicular root pain
  dolor referido referred pain
  dolor severo severe pain
  dolor sordo dull pain
  dolor torácico thoracic pain
  dolores de parto contractions; labor pains
  dolores del período menstrual pains
  dolores expulsivos expulsive pains
  dolores intermenstruales intermenstrual pain
  dolores premonitorios premonitory pains
doloroso *adj* painful
donador de sangre *m* blood donor
donante de sangre *m/f* blood donor
  donante universal universal donor
doña juanita *slang* marijuana
dormir (ue) to sleep
  dormir (ue) con *alguien* to have sexual relations
  dormirse (ue) to fall asleep; to doze off

dorso back
  dorso de la mano back of the hand
dosificación *f* dosage
dosis *f, inv* dosage; dose; potion
  dosis de refuerzo booster dose
  dosis excesiva excessive dose
dracma *m* dram
drenaje *m, surgical* drainage; *Chicano* catheter
droga drug; medicine
  droga alucinadora hallucinogen; hallucinogenic drug
  droga antihistamínica antihistamine
  droga estupefaciente narcotic
  droga LSD LSD
  droga psicodélica psychedelic
  drogma somnífera narcotic
drogadicto addict; drug addict
droguería *Sp.Am.* drugstore
ducha shower; bath; douche
  ducha interna douche
  ducha vaginal douche
ducharse to shower; to take a shower
dulces *m, pl* sweets
dulcificante *m* sweetener
duodeno duodenum
duración del embarazo *f* length of pregnancy (LOP)
duradero *adj* chronic
dureza lump
duro de oído hard of hearing
eccema *m/f* eczema
eclampsia eclampsia
eclipsado *adj* deformed
edema *m* edema; tumefaction
efedrina ephedrine
ejercer to exercise
  ejercer presión sobre to exert pressure on
ejercicio exercise
  ejercicios físicos para adelgazar reducing exercises
  ejercicos físios para reducir peso reducing exercises
electricidad *f* electricity
electrocardiograma *m* electrocardiogram
electroencefalograma *m* electroencefalogram
elegir (i) to choose
elevación *f* ridge
embarazada *adj* pregnant
embarazo pregnancy
  embarazo ectópico ectopic pregnancy
  embarazo en los tubos tubal pregnancy
  embarazo falso false pregnancy
  embarazo fuera de la matriz ectopic pregnancy
  embarazo histérico hysteria pregnancy
  embarazo incompleto incomplete pregnancy
  embarazo tubárico tubal pregnancy
embolia embolism
  embolia cerebral stroke
embolio *Chicano* stroke
embolismo embolism
émbolo piston; plunger of syringe
embriaguez *f* intoxication
embrión *m* embryo
embudo funnel
emergencia emergency

emético *m, adj* emetic; vomitive
emoliente *m, adj* emollient
empacamiento en sábana fría/mojada wrapping in a cold/wet sheet
empaque *m, Chicano* temporary filling
empastadura filling
empastar to fill
empaste *m* filling
  empaste provisional temporary filling
empeine *m* instep; groin; ringworm; tinea
empeorar to make worse
empezar (ie) to begin
emplaste *m, Med* plaster, poultice
emplasto poultice
  emplasto adhesivo adhesive plaster
  emplasto frío cold pack
  emplasto para callos corn plaster
emplomadura *Arg.* to fill (teeth)
empolvado *adj* powdery
empujar *(to shove/press)* to push
emulsión *f* emulsion
en *prep* in; at; on; upon
en ayunas fasting
  en casa at home
  en diálisis dialysis
  en la mesa on the table
  en polvo powdered
enano dwarf
encachucha homemade drug capsule
encajarse to go down in birth canal
encefalitis *f* encephalitis
encender (ie) to light; to turn on
enchufe *m* electrical plug; electrical socket
encía gum
encinta *adj* pregnant
encoger las rodillas to pull up (one's) knees
enconarse to fester
encono *Chile* inflammation
encontrar (ue) to find
encuerarse *Chicano* to undress
enderezar los dientes to straighten the teeth
endometrio endometrium
endoscopio endoscope
enema *f/m* enema
  enema de bario barium enema
  enema de limpieza cleansing enema
  enema de retención retention enema
  enema jabonosa soapsuds enema
  enema nutritiva nutritive enema
  enema opaca barium enema
energía energy
enfadarse to get angry
enferma *euph.* menstruation
enfermarse to get sick; *Chicano* to be in labor
enfermedad *f* disease; illness; sickness
  enfermedad aguda acute illness
  enfermedad cardíaca heart disease
  enfermedad contagiosa contagious illness (disease)
  enfermedad crónica chronic illness
  enfermedad de Altzheimer Altzheimer's disease
  enfermedad de andancia *Chicano* disease that is "going around"
  enfermedad de Chagas Chagas's disease
  enfermedad de Ménière Ménière's disease

enfermedad de notificación notifiable disease

enfermedad de Parkinson Parkinson's disease

enfermedad del corazón heart disease

enfermedad del sueño sleeping sickness

enfermedad endañada *Chicano* disease due to act of witchcraft

enfermedad grave serious illness

enfermedad leve minor illness

enfermedad matutina morning sickness; morning nausea

enfermedad mental mental illness

enfermedad pasada sexualmente sexually transmitted disease

enfermedad obligatoria reportable disease

enfermedad orgánica organic illness (disease)

enfermedad tra(n)smisible contagious illness (disease)

enfermedad tropical tropical illness (disease)

enfermedad venérea veneral disease

enfermera nurse

enfermería infirmary; patients of a hospital

enfermizo *adj* feeble; sickly

enfermo *adj* ill; sick; *m* sick person

enfisema *m* emphysema

enflaquecimiento emaciation

engordar to gain weight

engrifar to administer marijuana to someone

engrifarse to take marijuana

enjuagar to rinse

enjuagar(se) to rinse (out)

enjuagatorio mouthwash

enmarihuanar to administer marijuana to someone

enmarihuanarse to take marijuana

enojarse to get angry

enrojecido *adj* flushed

ensanchamiento enlargement

enseñar los dientes *fam* to show one's teeth

ensordecimiento deafness

entablazón *f, Chicano* constipation; stomach obstruction

entablillado *adj* in a splint

entender (ie) to understand

entierro funeral

entrañas bowels

entrepiernas *pl* crotch

entuertos postpartum pains; cramps

entumecido *adj* numb

envenenamiento poisoning

envenenamiento de la sangre blood poisoning

envenenamiento del plomo lead poisoning

envenenamiento plúmbico lead poisoning

envenenamiento por comestibles food poisoning

envenenar(se) to poison (oneself)

enyesar to put in a plaster cast

enzima enzyme

eosinófilo eosinophile

epidemia epidemic

epidémico *adj* epidemic

epidermis *f* epidermis

epidídimo epididymis

epilepsia epilepsy

episiotomía episiotomy

epistaxis *f* nosebleeding

equipo de urgencia first-aid kit

erisipela erysipelas

eritema solar *m* sunburn

eritrocito erythrocyte (red blood cell)

eritromicina erythromycin

eritrosedimentación *f* sedimentation; erythrosedimentation

eructar to belch; to burp

eructo burp

erupción *f* rash

erupción cutánea impetigo

erupción debida al calor prickly heat

erupción vesicular vesicular eruption

escaldadura scald

escaldadura (en los bebés) diaper rash

escalofrío chill

escalpelo scalpel

escama scale

escápula shoulder blade; scapula

escarrar to cough up phlegm

escayola calcium sulfate

esclerosis *f* sclerosis

esclerosis en placa multiple sclerosis

esclerosis múltiple multiple sclerosis

esclerótica sclera

esconderse to hide

escorbuto scurvy

escotoma *m* scotoma; spots before the eyes

escozor *m* itching; burning pain; smarting pain; sting

escritura en espejo mirror writing

escroto scrotum

escuchar to listen (to)

escudo shield (IUD)

escudo ocular eye shield

escudo para el pezón nipple shield

escupir en la taza to spit in the bowl

escurrimiento draining; dripping

escurrimiento de la nariz rhinitis; runny nose

esencia de trementina turpentine

esfínter *m* sphincter

esguince *f* sprain

esmalte *m* enamel

esmegma *m* smegma

esófago esophagus

espalda back

espaldilla shoulder blade; scapula

esparadrapo adhesive tape

espasmo spasm

espasmódico *adj* spasmodic; spastic

espástico *adj* spastic

espécimen *m* specimen

espéculo speculum

espejo vaginal speculum

espejuelos *pl* eyeglasses; *Cuba* spectacles

esperar to hope (for); to wait (for)

esperma semen

espermaticida vaginal *m* vaginal spermaticide

espermatozoide *m* sperm

espesar to thicken

espina dorsal spinal column

espinilla blackhead; shin bone

espinillas acne

espiral *m* spiral (IUD)

espiral intrauterino intrauterine loop

espirar to exhale

esporozoarios sporozoa

espulgar to delouse

espuma foam

espuma vaginal vaginal foam

esputo saliva; sputum

esqueleto skeleton

esquinancia quinsy (sore throat)

esquirla splinter (bone)

esquistosoma *m* schistosoma

esquizofrenia schizophrenia

esquizofrénico *adj* schizophrenic

estado interesante *euph.* pregnancy

estancamiento engorgement

estar to be

estar a dieta to be on a diet

estar con *alguien* to have sexual relations

estar coronando to crown

estar de parto to be in labor

estar indispuesta to menstruate

estar mala to menstruate

estar mala de la garra to menstruate

estar mala de la luna to menstruate

estar mediagua to be (to get) drunk

estenosis *f* stricture

estéril *adj* infertile; sterile

esterilidad *f* sterility

esterilidad permanente permanent sterility

esterilización *f* sterilization

esterilizado *adj* sterilized

esterilizador *m* sterilizer

esterilizar to sterilize

esterilizar las botellas to sterilize the bottles

esternón *m* breastbone

estertor *m* rale

estertor agónico death rattle

estetoscopio stethoscope

estetoscopio fetal fetoscope

estilete *m* probe; stylet

estimulante *m* stimulant

estómago stomach

estómago sucio *Chicano* indigestion

estornudar to sneeze

estrabismo strabismus

estrechez *f* stricture; narrowness

estreñido *adj* constipated

estreñimiento constipation

entreptococia strep throat

estreptomicina streptomycin

estrías stretch marks (strias)

estribo stirrup; stapes

estricnina strychnine

estrictura stricture

estroc *m, Chicano* stroke

estrógeno estrogen

estuche *m* kit

estufa warming crib; incubator

estufear to sniff residue of powdered narcotics

estufiar to sniff residue of powdered narcotics

etiqueta label

evacuación del vientre *f* feces; stool

evacuar to defecate

examen *m* test

examen de conejo rabbit test

examinación *f* examination

examinar to examine; to test
excesivamente *adv* excessively
  excesivamente gordo *adj* overweight
  excesivamente grueso *adj* overweight
excesivo *adj* excessive
exceso de peso overweight
excreción *f* excretion
excremento excretion; feces; stool
excusado toilet
exhalar to exhale
exhalarse to breathe hard
eximir to exempt; to release
expectoración *f* saliva
expectorante *m, adj* expectorant
expulsión *f* expulsion
extender (ie) to spread limbs
externo *adj* external
extracción *f* extraction; removal
  extracción con fórceps forceps
    delivery
  extracción de nalgas breech delivery
  extracción del nervio root canal
    work
extracto extract
  extracto de hígado liver extract
extraer to pull out
extremidad *f* limb
eyacular to ejaculate
facciones *f* features
factor RH *m* RH factor
  factor rhesus RH factor
faja band; binder; truss
  faja abdominal swathing bandage
  faja médica supporter
fajero "belly" binder
falange *f* phalanx
fallecimiento death
fallo *Med* failure
  fallo cardíaco cardiac arrest
  fallo del corazón *m* heart failure
falo penis; phallus
falseo *Chicano* sprain
falta de peso underweight
familia family
farfallota *P.R.* mumps
faringe *f* pharynx
faringitis *f* pharingitis
farmacia pharmacy; *Spain* drugstore
fatiga exhaustion; fatigue; *slang* asthma
fatigarse to get tired
fauces *f, pl* fauces
febrífugo *m, adj* antipyretic
fecha de caducidad expiration date
fecundación del huevo *f* conception
fémur *m* femur
fenilcetonuria phenylketonuria; PKU
fenilquetonuria phenylketonuria; PKU
fenobarbital *m* phenobarbital
férula splint
feto fetus
fetoscopio fetoscope
fibrilación auricular *f* atrial fibrillation
fibrina fibrin
fibroideo *adj* fibroid
fibroma *m* fibroma
fibrosis quística *f* cystic fibrosis
fiebre *f* fever; *fam, Mex.* hepatitis
  fiebre amarilla yellow fever
  fiebre de Colorado Colorado tick
    fever
  fiebre de conejo rabbit fever
  fiebre de las cotorras parrot fever
  fiebre de las Montañas Rocosas
    Rocky Mountain spotted fever

fiebre de Malta Malta fever
fiebre de tres días German Measles;
  rubella
fiebre de(l) heno hay fever
fiebre de valle valley fever;
  coccidioidomycosis
fiebre entérica enteric fever
fiebre escarlatina scarlet fever
fiebre ganglionar acute infectious
  adenitis fever
fiebre glandular glandular fever
fiebre intermitente intermittent
  fever
fiebre manchada spotted fever
fiebre ondulante Malta fever;
  undulant fever
fiebre palúdica malarial fever
fiebre paratífica paratyphoid fever
fiebre paratifoidea paratyphoid
  fever
fiebre por mordedura de rata rat-
  bite fever
fiebre purpúrea (de las montañas)
  spotted fever
fiebre reumática rheumatic fever
fiebre rompehuesos dengue;
  breakbone fever
fiebre térmica thermic fever
fiebre tifoidea typhoid fever
fiebre tra(n)smitida por garrapatas
  Colorado tick fever
fiebre tropical yellow fever
filerazo fix
filerearse to shoot up heroin
filete *m* crown of tooth
filorazo *Chicano* knife wound
filtrar to filter
fines médicos *m* medical purposes
fingimiento simulation
físicamente *adj* physically
fístula fistula
fisura fissure
flác(c)ido *ajd* limp
flagelados flagellates
flato flatus
flatulencia flatulence
flebitis *f* phlebitis
flema phlegm
flexura bend
  flexura de la pierna back of the knee
  flexura del brazo bend of the arm
flores blancas *f* white discharge
fluido *adj* fluent, free-flowing
flúido *adj* fluid; fluent; *m* fluid; *(Elec)*
  current
fluir to flow
flujo discharge
  flujo blanco white discharge
  flujo de sangre bleeding
  flujo inesperado de sangre por la
    vagina breakthrough bleeding
  flujo vaginal vaginal discharge
flúor *m* fluoride
fluoruro fluoride
foco de infección focus of infection
folículo follicule
fondillo *Cuba* buttock
fondo del útero fundus
fontanela fontanel
foramen *m* foramen
fórceps *m, inv* (obstetrical) forceps
fórmula formula
fosa fossa
  fosa nasal nostril

fosfato phosphate
fósforo phosphorus
fotografía photography
fóvea central fovea centralis
fractura fracture
  fractura abierta open fracture
  fractura cerrada closed fracture
  fractura complicada complicated
    fracture; open fracture
  fractura compuesta compound
    fracture
  fractura conminuta comminuted
    fracture
  fractura del cráneo skull fracture
  fractura en tallo verde green-stick
    fracture
  fractura espiral spiral fracture
  fractura espontánea spontaneous
    fracture
  fractura grave serious fracture
  fractura impactada impacted fracture
  fractura mayor serious fracture
  fractura múltiple multiple fracture
  fractura oblicua oblique fracture
  fractura por arrancamiento avulsion
    fracture
  fractura simple closed fracture;
    simple fracture
  fractura transversa transverse fracture
fracturar to fracture
frajo de seda marijuana cigarette
frasco flask; jar; vial
frazada blanket
fregar to scrub (surgically)
frenillo frenum of the tongue
frente *f* forehead
fresa burr
fricción *f* rub
frigidez *f* frigidity
frío cold; *slang, Mex.* mucus
  frío de la matriz female sterility
  fríos *Sp.Am.* malaria
frontal *adj* frontal
frotación *f* rub
frotar to rub
frote/frotis *m* smear
  frotis de Papanicolaou Pap smear
  frotis sanguíneo blood smear, film
fuegos en la boca (en los labios) cold
  sores
fuente *f* source; *fam* bag of waters
fuera de *prep* outside of
fuerte *adj* severe; strong
fuerza strength
fumigación *f* fumigation
fundillo *Mex.* buttock
funeraria funeral home
fungicida *m, adj* fungicide
furúnculo boil
gafas *pl* eyeglasses; spectacles
  gafas del sol sunglasses
galillo *fam* uvula
gallazo fix
gancho clasp
ganglio bubo; ganglion
gangrena gangrene
gargajear to spit phlegm
gargajeo spitting
gargajo sputum
garganta throat
  garganta inflamada sore throat
gargantada liquid or blood ejected
  from the throat
gárgara gargle; gargling

gargarismo   gargle (liquid); gargling solution
garrapata   chigger flea; tick
garrotillo   diphtheria; inflammation of the throat
gas   *m* gas
gasa   gauze
gastritis   *f* gastritis
gaznate   *m* trachea
gemelo   twin
germen   *m* germ; *slang* sperm
germicida   *m, adj* germicide
gestación   *f* gestation
ginecólogo   gynecologist
glande   *m* glans (penis)
glándula   gland
  glándula carotídea/carótida   carotid gland
  glándula de Cowper   Cowper's gland
  glándula de la próstata   prostate gland
  glándula lacrimal/lagrimal   tear gland
  glándula linfática   lymph gland
  glándula mamaria   mammary gland
  glándula paratiroides   parathyroid gland
  glándula parótida   parotid gland
  glándula pineal   pineal gland
  glándula pituitaria   pituitary gland
  glándula prostática   prostate gland
  glándula salival   salivary gland
  glándula sebácea   sebaceous gland
  glándula sublingual   sublingual gland
  glándula submaxilar   submaxillary gland
  glándula sudorípara   sweat gland
  glándula suprarrenal   adrenal gland
  glándula tiroides   thyroid gland
glaucoma   *m* glaucoma
glicerina   glycerine
glicógeno   glycogen
globo   sphere; balloon (of heroin); barbiturate pill
  globo del ojo   eyeball
  globo ocular   eyeball
glóbulo   corpuscle
  glóbulos blancos   leukocytes (white blood cells)
  glóbulos rojos   erythrocytes (red blood cells)
glucagón   *m* glucagon
glucemia   blood sugar
  glucemia en ayunas   fasting blood sugar
glucógeno   glycogen
glucosa   glucose
glufo   *m, adj* glue sniffer; "high" from glue sniffing
gluteo   gluteal region
golosinas   *pl* sweets
golpe   *m* concussion
  golpe de calor   heat stroke
golpearse   to hit oneself
goma   condom; rubber; glue
gonorrea   gonorrhea
gordo   *m, adj* fat; obese
gordura   obesity
gorra   *slang* heroin capsule
gorro cervical   cervical cap
gota   drop; gout; *slang* gonorrhea
  gotas para la tos   cough drops
  gotas para polio   oral polio vaccine

goteador   *m* eye dropper; medicine dropper
goteo nasal   nasal drip
gotera (para los ojos)   *Sp.Am.* eye dropper; medicine dropper
gramo   *slang* packet of heroin
granizo   cataract
grano   pustule; open skin wound; chancre; veneral lesion
  grano de la cara   pimple
grasa   fat
  grasa en las venas   cholesterol
gratis   *adj* free
grave   *adj* serious
grávida   *adj* pregnant
gravidez   *f* gestation; pregnancy
griefo   marijuana
grieta   fissure
  grieta del pezón   cracked nipple
  grietas en el paladar   cleft palate
grifa   marijuana
grifo   marijuana user
gripa   influenza; flu
gripe   *f* flu, influenza
gruesa   *adj. fam* pregnant
grueso   *adj* coarse; stout
grupo sanguíneo   blood group
guagua   *m/f, Chile, Ec., Perú, Bol.* infant; baby
guaguana   *slang* scabies
guantes de goma   *m, pl* rubber gloves
guayacol   *m* guaiacol
güegüecho   goiter
güina   *Mex.* chigger flea
gusano   worm
  gusano tableado   solium; tapeworm
gusto   taste; *slang* scabies
hacer   to do; to make
  hacer agua   *Chicano* to urinate
  hacer bajar por fuerza   to bear down
  hacer buches   *fam* to gargle
    hacer buches de sal   to gargle
  hacer caca   *Chicano* to defecate
  hacer caquis maquis   to defecate
  hacer certificación   to warrant
  hacer daño   to injure
  hacer ejercicios moderadamente   to exercise moderately
  hacer el cuerpo   to defecate
  hacer garantías   to guarantee
  hacer gárgaras   to gargle
  hacer (la) pipi/pipí   to urinate
  hacer(se) a la glu(fa)   to sniff glue
  hacerse + *noun of profession* to become (*something*)
hachís   *m* hash; hashish
hallazgos de laboratorio   laboratory findings
harina   flour
haschich   *m* hash, hashish
heces fecales   *f, pl* feces; stool
hematíe   *m* erythrocyte (red blood cell)
hematimetría   blood count
hemisferio cerebral   cerebral hemisphere
hemocultivo   blood culture
hemofilia   hemophilia
hemoglobina   hemoglobin
hemorragia   bleeding; hemorrhage
  hemorragia detrás de la córnea   hyphemia
  hemorragia inesperada   breakthrough bleeding
  hemorragia interna   internal bleeding

hemorragia nasal   nosebleed
hemorragia vascular   stroke
hemorroides   *f, pl* hemorrhoids; piles
hemostato   hemostat
hepatitis   *f* hepatitis
  hepatitis infecciosa   infectious hepatitis
  hepatitis viral   viral hepatitis
herbicida   *m* herbicide
herida   injury, wound
  herida incisa   incised wound
  herida penetrante   puncture wound
  herida punzante   punture wound
herido   *adj* injured
herir (ie)   to wound; to hurt
hernia   hernia; rupture
  hernia del ombligo   umbilical hernia
  hernia femoral   femoral hernia
  hernia inguinal   inguinal hernia
heroína   heroin
herpe(s)   *m/f* herpes; shingles
  herpe febril   fever blister
  herpes genital   herpes genitalis
  herpes labial   cold sore
  herpes menstrual   herpes menstrualis
  herpes zoster   herpes zoster
hervir (ie) las botellas   to boil the bottles
hidrofobia   rabies
hidropesía   dropsy
hidróxido de sodio   sodium hydroxide
hiedra venenosa   poison ivy
hiel   *f* bile
hielo   ice
hierba   *slang* marijuana
hierro   iron
hígado   liver
higienista dental   *m/f* dental hygienist
hilo dental   dental floss
himen   *m* hymen
hinchado   *adj* bloated; swollen
hinchar   to swell
hinchazón   *m/f* abscess; swelling; edema; lump
hiperópico   *adj* farsighted
hipermetropía   farsightedness; presbyopia
hipertensión   *f* hypertension
  hipertensión arterial   high blood pressure
hipo   hiccough; hiccup
hipoclorito de sodio   sodium hypochlorite (bleach)
hipocondría/hipocondria   hypochondria
hipocóndrico   *m, adj* hypochondriac
hipotensión   *f* hypotension
  hipotensión arterial   low blood pressure
hipsus   *m* hiccough; hiccup
hisopillo   cotton swab
hisopo de algodón   cotton swab
hoja   leaf
  hojas de eucalipto   eucalyptus leaves
  hojas de poleo   pennyroyal leaves
  hojas de hierbabuena/yerbabuena   mint leaves
hombro   shoulder
hongo   fungus
  hongos   *slang* mushrooms; magic mushrooms; psilocybin
hormigueo   tingling
hormón   *m* hormone

hormona hormone
hueso bone
huevo ovum
  huevos *pl, slang* testicle
hule *m, slang* condom; "rubber" (birth control)
húmedo *adj* moist
húmero humerus
humo smoke
humor *m* humor
  humor acuoso aqueous humor
  buen humor good humor
  humor vítreo vitreous humor
ictericia jaundice
ictiol *m* ichthyol
íleom *m* ileum
ilion *m* ilium
Imagenes por Resonancia Magnética/IRM *f* Magnetic Resonance Images/MRI
impacción *f* impaction
impedimento handicap; obstruction
impedir (i) to prevent
impericia malpractice
impétigo impetigo
impotencia impotence
impresión *f* impression
incapacidad *f* disability
incisión *f* incision
incisivos front teeth; incisors
incomodidad *f* discomfort
incómodo *adj* bothersome; inconvenient
incompatible *adj* incompatible
inconsciencia unconsciousness
inconsciente *adj* unconscious
incordio bubo
incrustación *f* inlay
incubadora warming crib
indección *f, Chicano* injection
índice *m* index finger
indigestión *f* indigestion
indolente *adj* lazy (*indolent*)
infarto heart attack; infarct
  infarto miocardíaco/miocardiaco myocardial infarct
infección *f* infection
  infección de la bolsa de lágrimas dacrycystitis
  infección de la sangre *euph.* syphillis
  infección de la vejiga cystitis
  infección de serpigo athlete's foot
  infección en la sangre *fam* septicemia
infeccioso *adj* infectious
infectar to infect
infecundidad *f* sterility
infecundo *adj* sterile
infértil *adj* infertile
inflamación *f* inflammation
  inflamación de la médula del hueso osteomyelitis
  inflamación de los ojos ophthalmia (*inflammation of the eye*)
  inflamación del hígado hepatitis
inflamar to inflame
influenza flu; influenza
  influenza asiática Asiatic flu
ingerir (ie) *slang* to take (drugs)
ingle *f* groin
ingrediente *m* ingredient
inhabilidad *f* disability
injerir (ie) *slang* to take (drugs)
injerto graft

inmovilización *f* immobilization
inmune *adj* immune
inmunización *f* vaccine; immunization
inocente *adj, euph.* mentally retarded; *Mex.* deformed
inoculación *f* inoculation; vaccination
inodoro restroom; toilet
insecticida *m* insecticide
insensibilidad *f* unconsciousness
insidioso *adj* insidious
insolación *f* heat stroke; sunstroke
insomnio insomnia
instrumento afilado sharp-edged instrument
insuficiencia lack; shortage
  insuficiencia aórtica aortic failure
  insuficiencia cardíaca heart failure
insulina insulin
insulínico *adj* insulin
insulto *Chicano* indigestion
intermitente *adj* spasmodic
internamente *adv* internally
interrupción de coito *f* coitus interruptus
intervalo interval
intestino intestine
  intestino ciego caecum
  intestino delgado small intestine
  intestino grueso large intestine
  intestino inferior bowel
intolerancia intolerance
intoxicación *f* poisoning
  intoxicación alimenticia food poisoning
  intoxicación botulínica botulism poisoning
  intoxicación con alimentos food poisoning
  intoxicación de la sangre blood poisoning
  intoxicación de orín uremia
  intoxicación del embarazo toxemia of pregnancy
  intoxicación por estafilococos staphylococcal poisoning
  intoxicación por monóxido de carbono carbon monoxide poisoning
  intoxicación por salmonela salmonella poisoning
intoxicado *adj* drunk
intususcepción *f* intussusception
invalidez *f* disability
inválido *adj* cripple
inyección *f* shot; injection
  inyección de refuerzo booster shot
  inyección endovenosa intravenous injection
  inyección hipodérmica hypodermic injection
  inyección intracutánea intracutaneous injection
  inyección intramuscular intramuscular injection
  inyección intravenosa intravenous injection
  inyección secundaria booster shot
  inyección subcutánea subcutaneous injection
inyectar(se) to inject (oneself)
  inyectarse *slang* to inject oneself with drugs
ir al inodoro *fam* to defecate

iris *m* iris
IRM/Imágenes por Resonancia Magnética *f* MRI/Magnetic Resonance Images
irregular *adj* irregular; spasmodic
irrigación *f* douche; irrigation
irrigar *Med* to irrigate
irritación *f* irritation
irritar to irritate
irse to go away
isolote *m* islet
jabón *m* soap
jadeante *adj* panting
jadear to pant
jaipo *slang* "mainliner"; hypodermic needle used to inject drug
jalar to pull
  jalarse *Sp.Am.* to get drunk; *P.R.* to leave; to go away
jalea jelly
  jalea vaginal vaginal jelly
jane *adj, Hond.* harelip
jaqueca severe headache; migraine
jarabe *m* syrup
  jarabe de ipeca syrup of ipecac
  jarabe para la tos cough syrup
jején *m, Sp.Am.* gnat
jeringa hypodermic needle; syringe
  jeringa con aguja hueca hollow needle syringe
  jeringa con cilindro de cristal glass cylinder syringe
  jeringa desechable disposable syringe
jeringuilla syringe
  jeringuilla descartable disposable syringe
  jeringuilla hipodérmica hypodermic syringe
jey fíver *m, Chicano* hay fever
jimagua twin
jiotes *f, fam* tinea corporis; *m, C.A., Mex.* shingles
jiricua *slang* vitiligo
jorobado *m, adj* hunchback
juanete *m* bunion
juanita *slang* marijuana
jugo juice
  jugo digestivo enzyme
  jugo gástrico gastric juice
keroseno kerosene
kickear *slang* to quit cold turkey
kilogramo kilogram
la otra cosa any narcotic substitute
labio lip
  labio cucho *Chicano* hairlip
  labio leporino harelip
laboratorio laboratory
laceración *f* laceration
lacrimal *adj* lachrymal
lactancia lactation
  lactancia maternal breastfeeding
lactante *adj* nursing
ladilla crab louse; parasitic cyst
lado side
  lado derecho inferior lower right side
  lado derecho superior upper right side
  lado izquierdo inferior lower left side
  lado izquierdo superior upper left side
lagrimal *adj* lachrymal

lágrimas tears
lámpara de rayos ultravioletas ultraviolet lamp
laringe *f* larynx
laringitis *f* laryngitis
laringoscopio laryngoscope
lastimadura bruise; injury; wound
lastimar to injure
latido *(of heart)* beat; beating twinge of pain; throb; throbbing *Chicano* palpitation; spasm
  latido cardíaco heartbeat
  latido del corazón fetal fetal heart tone
  latido irregular irregular heartbeat; arrhythmia
lavado enema; lavage; purge
  lavado bucal mouth wash
  lavado interno douche
  lavado vaginal douche
lavamanos *m, inv, slang* lavatory
lavaojos *m, inv* eye cup
lavar to scrub (surgically); to wash
  lavarse to wash onself
lavativa enema
lavativo purge
laxante *m* laxative
laxativo laxative
lazarín *m* leprosy
lazarino *m* leper; *adj* leprous
lazo loop (IUD)
leche *f* milk
  leche de magnesia milk of magnesia
lecho bed
legrado *fam* D&C
lejía lye
lengua tongue
  lengua saburrosa coated tongue
  lengua sucia coated tongue
lente *m* lens
  lente de contacto contact lens
  lentes *pl* eye glasses; *Mex.* spectacles
  lentilla contact lens
leña marijuana
leñito marijuana cigarette
lepra leprosy
leproso *adj* leprous
lesión *f* injury; lesion
leucemia leukemia
leucocitos leukocytes (white blood cells)
levadura de cerveza Brewer's yeast
levantar to lift
  levantarse to get up; to stand up
leve *adj* mild
líquido liquid
libra pound
libre *adj* free
  libre albedrío free will
liendre *f* louse, nit
liga tourniquet
ligadura de trompas tubal ligation
ligamento ligament
ligar to bind; to tie
  ligar los tubos de falopio to tie the tubes
  ligar trompas to tie the tubes
limar to file down; to polish; to smooth
limpiador de agua a presión *m* waterpick
limpiarse to clean oneself
limpieza cleanliness; cleaning
lindano lindane

linfocito lymphocyte
linfogranuloma venéreo *m* lymphogranuloma venereum
lingual *adj* lingual
linimento liniment
lisiado *adj* crippled; injured; lame
lista de intercambios exchange list
listerina *fam* mouthwash
litro liter
llaga sore; wound
  llaga de cama bedsore
  llaga de fiebre fever blister
  llaga ulcerosa canker sore
llamaradas hot flashes
llamar to call
  llamarse to be called; to be named
llenar to fill
llorar to cry
lo demás *fam* placenta
lobanillo wen
lóbulo earlobe
loción *f* lotion
  loción bronceadora suntan lotion
  loción para el sol suntan lotion
loco *adj* crazy; *slang* "high" on narcotics; "turned on"
locote *adj, slang* "high" on narcotics; "turned on"
locura insanity; madness
  locura de doble forma manic-depressive insanity
lombriz *f* worm
  lombriz chiquita afilada threadworm
  lombriz de gancho uncinaria; hookworm
  lombriz de látigo trichocephalus
  lombriz grande redonda ascaris; roundworm
  lombriz solitaria tapeworm
lomo loin
lubricante *m* lubricant
lubricativo *adj* lubricant
lúes *f* syphilis
luna *Chicano* menstruation
lunar *m* birthmark; blemish; mole
lupa magnifying glass
lupia wen
lupo loop
machar to crush; to mash; to pound
machucar to crush; to bruise
maculosa de las Montañas Rocosas Rocky Mountain spotted fever
madurez *f* maturity
magnesia nagnesia
magulladura bruise
mal *m* disease; illness; sickness
  mal de arco *slang* tetanus
  mal de bubas *slang* syphilis
  mal de Down Down's Syndrome
  mal (dolor) de garganta sore throat
    mal (dolor) de garganta por estreptococo strep throat
  mal de Hansen leprosy
  mal de las encías pyorrhea
  mal de madre morning sickness
  mal de mar seasickness
  mal (dolor) de oídos *m* sore ears; earache
  mal de ojo evil eye; *fam* conjunctivitis
  mal de orín urinary problem; *slang* gonorrhea
  mal de pintas psoriasis

mal de riñón kidney disease
mal (baile) de San Guido (de San Vito) chorea
mal de San Lázaro leprosy
mal francés *slang* syphilis
mal *adv* badly; poorly
  mal nutrido *adj* malnourished
mal/malo/mala *adj* bad
  mala alimentación *f* malnutrition
    mala alimentación mojada kwashiokor (malnutrition)
    mala alimentación seca marasmus (malnutrition)
  mala digestión *f* indigestion
malaria malaria
malestar *m* discomfort; malaise
  malestar de la mañana morning nausea
  malestar general general malaise
  malestar post-alcohólico/posalcohólico hangover
malformación congénita *f* congenital malformation
malignidad *f* malignancy
maligno *adj* malignant
malnutrición *f* malnutrition
malo *adj* ill; sick *See «mal» above.*
malparto miscarriage
malpraxis *f* malpractice
mamadera breast pump; nipple (of a baby nursing bottle); nursing bottle; *Sp.Am.* baby bottle
mamar to suck
mamón *m* baby still at the breast; *Chicano* pacifier
mancha blemish; spot
  mancha de la preñez chloasma *(facial discoloration)*
  mancha de la sangre blood stain
  mancha del embarazo chloasma *(facial discoloration)*
  mancha volante floater
  manchas de sangre spotting
  manchas frente a los ojos scotoma; spots before the eyes
  manchas oscuras en la piel skin blotches
manchado *adj* spotted; stained
  manchado de sangre bloodstained
  manchado del pulmón *Mex.* tuberculosis
manco *adj* crippled hand
mandíbula jawbone; jaw
manía madness, mania
maníaco *adj* maniac
maniamelancolía manic depressive insanity
mano *f* hand
manteca de cacao cocoa butter
manzana apple; block; *Mex.* Adam's apple
maquillarse to put on makeup
marasmo marasmus
marcador *m* marker
  marcador de paso pacemaker
  marcador de ritmo pacemaker
marcapaso pacemaker
marcha gait
marcharse to go away
mareo seasickness; fainting spell
María Juanita *slang* marijuana
maricocaimorfi *m/f* user of marijuana, cocaine, morphine

mariguana marijuana
mariguano marijuana user
marihuanar to administer marijuana to someone
marihuano marijuana user
marijuana marijuana
mariola *slang* marijuana
martillo hammer (malleus)
más caliente *adj* warmer
masaje *m* massage
mascar to chew
máscara mask
masticar to chew
mastitis por estasis *f* caked breast
masturbación *f* masturbation
masturbar(se) to masturbate
matarle el nervio a *alguien* to remove the nerve
matayerbas *m, inv* herbicide
materia matter
    materia fecal feces; stool
    materia gris *fam* cerebral cortex
maternidad *f* maternity
matriz *f* uterus; womb
maxilar *adj* maxillary
mazorca *slang* teeth
meadera *Chicano* frequent urination
médica; médico physician
    médico, médica a cargo attending physician
    médico, médica asistente attending physician
    médico, médica consultor(a) consulting physician
    médico, médica de apelación consulting physician
    médico, médica de cabecera attending physician
    médico, médica forense coroner
    médico, médica partero, partera obstetrician
    médico, médica residente resident (house) physician
medicación *f* medication
    medicación tiroides thyroid pill
medicamento medicine; remedy
medicina drug; medicine
    medicina de la botica patent medicine
    medicina de la farmacia patent medicine
    medicina deportiva sports medicine
    medicina interna internal medicine
    medicina patentada patent medicine
    medicina profiláctica preventive medicine
    medicina registrada patent medicine
    medicina socializada socialized medicine
medida dose
medio de restricción restraining device
medir (i) to measure
médula marrow
    médula espinal spinal cord
mejilla cheek
mejorarse to improve; to get better
melancolía melancholia
mellizo twin
membrana membrane
meningitis cerebroespinal *f* cerebrospinal meningitis
menopausia menopause
menstruación *f* menstruation

menstruación dolorosa dysmenorrhea
menstruar to menstruate
mentir (ie) to lie
mentol *m* menthol
mentolato *Chicano* mentholatum
mentón *m* chin
meñique *m* little finger
mercurocromo mercurochrome
mertiolato merthiolate
mes *m* menstruation
mesa del parto delivery table
mescalina mescaline
meta goal
metabolizar to metabolize
metadona methadone
metástasis *f* metastasis
método method
    método curativo cure
    método de Billing Billing's method of birth control
    método del ritmo rhythm method
mezcla mixture
mezclar to mix
mezquino *Mex., C.A., Col.* wart
microbio germ
miedo fear
miembro penis; limb
    miembro artificial artificial limb; prosthesis
mierda *vulgar* feces; stool
migraña migraine
miligramo milligram
mililitro milliliter
milque *f, Chicano* milk
miometrio myometrium
mineral *m* mineral
miocardio *adj* myocardium
miope *adj* myopic; nearsighted; shortsighted
miopía myopia; nearsightedness
moco mucus
moderado *adj* moderate
modorra drowsiness
moho mold
mojado *adj* wet; damp; soaked
mojar to wet; to soak; to damp(en)
molar *m* molar
mollera fontanel; crown of the head
mompes *m, pl, Chicano* mumps
mondadientes *m, inv* toothpick
mongolismo Down's syndrome
moniliasis *f* moniliasis
monitor *m* monitor
    monitor cardíaco pacemaker
monocitos monocytes
mononucleosis infecciosa *f* mononucleosis
morbilia measles
mordedura (animal) bite
    mordedura de culebra snake bite
    mordedura de escorpión scorpion bite
    mordedura de gato cat bite
    mordedura de perro dog bite
    mordedura de rata rat bite
    mordedura de serpiente snake bite
    mordedura humana human bite
morder (ue) to bite
mordida *Sp.Am.* (animal) bite
mordisco dental impression
morete *m, Mex., Hond.* bruise
moreteado *adj, Chicano* bruised
moretón *m* bruise

morfi *f, slang* morphine
morfina morphine
morfiniento user of morphine
morfinomanía drug habit
morfinómano (drug) addict
moribundo *adj* dying
morir (ue) to die
mormación *f, Chicano* nasal obstruction
morragia *Chicano* hemorrhage
mortinato *adj* stillborn
mosco volante floater
mostacho moustache
mostaza mustard
mostrar (ue) to show
    mostrar (ue) los dientes to show one's teeth
mota *slang* marijuana
mote *m* nickname
motear to smoke marijuana
motiado *adj* "high"; "turned on" marijuana
motiar to smoke marijuana
moto marijuana user; *slang, Mex.* infantum tetanus
mover (ue) to move
mozusuelo *Mex.* infantum tetanus
mudo *adj* mute
muela back tooth; molar
    muelas cordales wisdom teeth
    muelas de juicio wisdom teeth
muerte *f* death
muerto *adj* dead
muestra sample; specimen
    muestra de excremento stool specimen
    muestra de heces fecales stool specimen
    muestra de la orina urine specimen
    muestra de la sangre bloody show
muguet *m* moniliasis
mujercitas *slang* psilocybin
muleta crutch
muñeca wrist
murmullo heart murmur
músculo muscle
    músculo estriado striated muscle
    músculo involuntario involuntary muscle
    músculo liso smooth muscle
    músculo voluntario voluntary muscle
muslo thigh
nacido *m (inflamed)* boil; *adj* born
    nacido muerto *adj* stillborn
nacimiento birth
    nacimiento múltiple multiple birth
    nacimiento prematuro premature birth
    nacimiento tardío post-term birth
nadie no one
nalga buttock
naqueado *adj. Chicano* unconscious
naranjas *slang* amphetamines
narco member of police narcotics squad
narcomanía drug addiction
narcótico *m, adj* narcotic; soporific
narcotraficante *m/f* dope pusher
nariz *f* nose
natalidad *f* birth rate
    natalidad dirigida planned parenthood
nati-muerto stillbirth

náusea nausea
nayotas *pl, slang, Chicano* nose
nefritis *f* nephritis
negar (ie) to deny
negro *adj* negroid
nena infant
nene *m* infant
neoformación *f* tumor
neoplasma *m* tumor
nervio nerve
  nervio aplastado pinched nerve
  nervio craneal cranial nerve
  nervio dental dental nerve
  nervio motor motor nerve
  nervio óptico optic nerve
  nervio parasimpático
    parasympathetic nerve
  nervio sensorial sensory nerve
  nervio simpático sympathetic nerve
neumonía pneumonia
neuralgia neuralgia
neurastenia nervous breakdown;
  neurasthenia
neurasténico *adj* neurasthenic
neuritis *f* neuritis
neurosis *f* neurosis
neurótico *m, adj* neurotic
neutrófilos polimorfonucleares
  polymorphonuclear neutrophiles
NGB *f* WBC (white blood count)
NGR *f* RBC (red blood count)
niacina niacin
nictalopia night blindness; nyctalopia
nieve *f, slang* heroin; cocaine
nigua chigger flea
niña del ojo pupil of eye
niñera nursemaid; baby nurse
niños *slang* psilocybin
nitrato de plata silver nitrate
nitro(glicerina) *f* nitro(glycerin)
nitrógeno total total nitrogen
no infeccioso *adj* noninfectious
no sentir (ie) nada to feel nothing
no tener razón to be wrong
no tratado *adj* untreated; not treated
nodriza baby nurse; wet nurse
nódulo linfático lymph node
nombre común *m* common name
novocaína Novocaine
nuca nape of neck
  nuca tiesa *fam* stiff neck
nudillo knuckle
nudo knot; node; protuberance
  nudo linfático *fam* lymph node
nuez de Adán *f* Adam's apple
numeración *f* numeration
  numeración de glóbulos blancos
    white blood count (WBC)
  numeración de glóbulos rojos red
    blood count (RBC)
órgano organ
  órganos genitales genitals
óvulo ovum
  óvulos *pl. Sp. Am.* vaginal suppository
obesidad *f* obesity
obeso *adj* obese
objetivo goal
obrar *Mex.* to defecate
obstetricia obstetrics
obstétrico *adj* obstetric; obstetrical
  obstétrico *m* obstetrician
obstrucción *f* blockage; obstruction
  obstrucción de la tripa bowel
    obstruction

obstruir to block
  obstruir el nervio to block the nerve
occipital *adj* occipital
oclusión *f* occlusion
odontalgia toothache
odontología dentistry; odontology
odontólogo dentist, odontologist
oftalmía ophthalmia; inflammation of
  the eye
  oftalmía contagiosa pinkeye
oftálmico *adj* ophthalmic
oftalmoscopio ophthalmoscope
oído ear (organ of hearing)
  oído externo external ear
  oído interno internal ear
  oído medio middle ear
ojera eye cup
ojituerto *adj* squint-eyed
ojo eye
  ojo de pescado *fam* plantar wart
  ojo de vidrio glass eye
  ojo de morado blackeye
  ojos capotudos *Chicano* bulging
    eyes
  ojos saltones bulging eyes
oler (ue) to smell
olfatorio *adj* olfactory
ombligo navel; umbilicus
  ombligo salido *slang* umbilical
    hernia
  ombligón *m, slang* umbilical hernia
  ombliguero "belly" binder
omóplato shoulder blade; scapula
oncocerciasis *f* onchocerciasis; river
  blindness
oncocercosis *f* river blindness;
  onchocerciasis; onchocerocosis
onza ounce
operación *f* operation
  operación cesárea cesarean section
opio opium
oreja ear; outer ear
orgasmo orgasm
orificación *f* inlay
orificar to fill with gold
orín *m* urine; rust (*caused by dampness*);
  orines *m, pl* urine
orina urine
orinal *m* urinal
orinar to urinate
  orinarse to urinate (involuntarily);
    to wet oneself
oro gold
orzuelo sty
osteomielitis *f* osteomyelitis
otitis *f* otitis
ovar to ovulate
ovario ovary
ovulación *f* ovulation
oxígeno oxygen
oxitócico *adj* oxytocic
oxitocina oxytocin
oxiuro threadworm; oxyurid
pabellón externo de la oreja *m*
  external ear
pacha *Chicano* baby bottle
paciente *m/f, adj* patient
  paciente ambulatorio outpatient
  paciente externo outpatient
padecimiento illness; sickness
padrastro stepfather; *fam* hangnail
paladar *m* palate; roof of the mouth
  paladar hendido cleft palate
  paladar partido cleft palate

paletilla shoulder blade; scapula
paliativo *m, adj* palliative
pálido *adj* pale; sickly
palillo de dientes toothpick
palma de la mano palm of the hand
palpitación *f* heartbeat; palpitation
  palpitación irregular irregular
    heartbeat; arrhythmia
  palpitación lenta slow heartbeat
  palpitación rápida rapid heartbeat;
    tachycardia
  palpitación rítmica rhythmical
    heartbeat
paludismo malaria
páncreas *m* pancreas
pantorrilla calf of the leg
panza *Chicano* stomach; *fam*
  abdomen; belly
  panza peligrosa *slang* bowel
    obstruction; peritonitis;
    appendicitis
panzón *adj* potbellied
pañal *m* diaper
paño cloth; pad; *Med* chloasma *(facial
  discoloration)*; mask of pregnancy
  paños en los ojos eyepads
  paño higiénico sanitary napkin
pañalitis *f* diaper rash
paperas mumps
pápula wheal
parálisis *f* palsy; paralysis; stroke
  parálisis agitante shaking palsy;
    Parkinson's disease
  parálisis cerebral cerebral paralysis
  **parálisis de la mitad inferior del
    cuerpo** paraplegia
  parálisis facial Bell's palsy
  parálisis infantil infantile paralysis;
    polio(myelitis)
paralización *f* palsy; paralysis
paranoia paranoia
paraplejía paraplegia
parar(se) to stand up; to stop
parásito parasite
parche *m* dressing; patch
  parchecito Band-Aid
  parche para callos corn plaster
paregórico paregoric
parentesco relation; relationship
parienta *f* relation; relative
pariente *m* relation; relative
parir to give birth; to deliver
paro stoppage
  paro cardíaco cardiac arrest
  paro del corazón heart failure
parótidas *f, pl* mumps
paroxismo fit
parpadear to blink
párpado eyelid
partes *f, slang* genitals
  partes ocultas *slang* genitals
partida certificate
  partida de nacimiento birth
    certificate
partidura fissure
parto childbirth; delivery; labor
  parto abdominal abdominal labor
  parto artificial artificial labor
  parto cesáreo cesarean delivery
  parto complicado complicated labor
  parto espontáneo spontaneous
    labor
  parto inducido induced labor
  parto inmaturo immature labor

parto instrumental instrumental labor
parto malogrado miscarriage
parto muerto stillbirth
parto múltiple multiple labor
parto por operación cesarean delivery
parto prematuro premature labor; premature delivery
parto prolongado prolonged labor
parto seco dry labor
pasar to pass; to transfer
pasar la mano sobre la superficie de to rub
pasar por to pass over
pase del cuerpo *m* feces; stool
pasta de dientes toothpaste
pasta dentífrica toothpaste
pastilla (birth control) pill; lozenge; tablet
pastilla de chupar lozenge
pastillas anticonceptivas contraceptive pills
pastillas para la tos cough drops; cough lozenges
pastillas para no tener niños birth control pills
patada kick
pataletas temper tantrum; *fam* fit of kicking or stamping
patas de gallo crow's feet
patizambo *adj* pigeon-toed
pavico *Chicano* diaper
peca freckle
pecho breast; chest
pedíatra/pediatra *m/f* pediatrician
pediatría pediatrics
pediátrico *adj* pediatric
pediculosis *f* pediculosis; infestation
pedir (i) to ask (for); to request
pedo *slang* flatus
pegadizo *adj* contagious
pegar to pass on (a disease)
peinarse to comb one's hair
pelagra pellagra
pelársela *Chicano* to pull back foreskin of penis
peligroso *adj* dangerous
pelirrojo *adj* red-haired
pellejo flap of skin
pellín *m, Chicano* buttock
pelo hair
pelitos *pl, Chicano* pubic hair
pelo crespo curly hair
pelo chino *Mex.* curly; *Col.* straight hair
pelo grifo *Chicano* kinky hair
pelo liso straight hair
pelo púbico pubic hair
pelo quebrado wavy hair
pelotita *slang* clitoris
peludo *adj* hairy
peluza *Mex.* German measles; rubella
pelviano adj pelvic
pélvico *adj* pelvic
pelvímetro pelvimeter
pelvis *f* pelvis
pena sore; worry
pene *m* penis
penicilina penicillin
pensar (ie) to think
pentotal *m* pentothal
pentotal de sodio sodium pentothal
pentotal sódico sodium pentothal

pepa *slang* clitoris
pera de goma rubber bulb; syringe
perder (ie) to lose
perder (ie) flúidos del cuerpo to dehydrate
perder (ie) peso to lost weight
perder (ie) sangre to menstruate
pérdida del sueño insomnia
perforación *f* perforation
perforar to drill
pericarditis *f* pericarditis
perimetrio perimetrio
perineal *adj* perineal
perineo perineum
período *fam* menstruation
período climatérico menopause
periostio periosteum
peritonitis *f* peritonitis
perleche *m* oral lesion
permanganato de potasio potassium permanganate
permiso permission; permit
peroné *m* fibula
peróxido peroxide
peróxido de hidrógeno hydrogen peroxide
peróxido de sodio sodium peroxide
perrilla *fam* sty
perseguir (i) to pursue
persistir (en) to persist
pesadilla nightmare
pesar to weight
peso weight
peso del nacimiento birthweight
peso escaso underweight
pestaña eyelash
peste *f* plague
peste blanca tuberculosis
peste bubónica bubonic plague
pesticida *m* pesticide
petición *f* request
pezón *m* nipple of female (breast)
pezón enlechado engorged (caked) nipple
pezonera nipple shield
picadura cavity; bite (of insect); sting (of insect)
picadura de abeja bee sting
picadura de alacrán scorpion sting
picadura de araña spider bite; spider sting
picadura de avispa wasp sting
picadura de avispón hornet sting
picadura de garrapata tick sting
picadura de hormiga ant sting
picadura de moscardón botfly sting
picadura de mosquito mosquito sting
picadura de nigua chigoe/jigger/sandflea sting
picadura de pulga flea sting
picadura de ubar *fam* black-widow spider sting
picadura de viuda negra black-widow spider sting
picadura de zancudo *Mex.* mosquito sting
picar to stick; to bite
picarse *slang* to inject oneself with drugs
picazón *f* itch
picor *m* itching
pie *m* foot
pie de atleta athlete's foot

pie hueco high arched foot
pie plano flatfoot
piedra stone
piedra en la vejiga gallstone
piedra en los riñones kidney stone
piel *f* skin
piel amarilla *fam* jaundice
piel de la cabeza scalp
pielograma *m* pyelogram
pielograma intravenoso intravenous pyelogram
piemia septicemia
pierna leg
píldora (birth control) pill
píldora anticonceptiva birth control pill
píldora diurética diuretic
píldora para control de embarazo birth control pill
píldora para dormir sleeping pill
píldora somnífera sleeping pill
píldora soporífica sleeping pill
pildorear(se) to ingest narcotic pills
pildoriar(se) to ingest narcotic pills
pildoriento user of pills
píldoro *adj, slang* "high" on pills
pillido *Mex.* souffle
pinchar to prick
pinchazo prick
pinguas *pl* narcotic pills
pinta spotted sickness
pinto *adj* very dark-skinned; lacking negroid features
pinzas *pl* dental forceps
piocha chin
piojería pediculosis; infestation
piojo louse
piorrea pyorrhea
piperacina/piperazina piperazine
piquete *m (insect)* bite; sting (from an insect); *slang* injection *(of a narcotic substance)*
piridoxina vitamin B-6
piriforme *adj* pear-shaped
pirosis *f* heartburn
pisa-lengua *m* tongue depressor
piso floor
piso de maternidad maternity floor
piso ginecológico gynecological floor
pisporr(i)a *Chicano* lump; bump on head
pisto *adj* drunk
pitocín *m* pitocin
pitocina pitocin
PIV (pielograma intravenoso) *m* IVP (intravenous pyelogram)
placa plaque; plate
placenta afterbirth; placenta
placenta previa placenta previa
placentario *adj* placental
plaga plague
plaguicida *m* pesticide
planificación *f* planning
planificación de la familia family planning
planificación familiar family planning
planta del pie sole of the foot
plaqueta platelet
plaquetas sanguíneas blood platelets
plasma *m* plasma
plasma sanguíneo blood plasma

pleito lawsuit
pleuresía pleurisy
poción *f* potion
podo *slang* marijuana
poloridad *f* polarity
poliomielitis *f* polio(myelitis)
pólipo polyp
pollo *fam, Chicano, Arg.* sputum
polvo powder; *slang* PCP; cocaine
  polvo de azufre sulphur powder
polvoriento *adj* powdery
polvoroso *adj* powdery
pomada ointment; pomade; salve; unguent
pómulo cheekbone
poner to place
  poner a dieta to put on a diet
  poner a prueba to test
  ponerse + adj of emotion/mental state to become; turn + *adj*
  ponerse + noun to put on (*clothing*)
  ponerse alto *fam* to be drunk; to get drunk
  ponerse de pie to stand up
ponzoña poison
ponzoñoso *adj* poisonous
por día daily
porcelana porcelain
poro pore
portador, portadora de enfermedad
  m/f carrier (of an illness)
porte *m* bearing
postemilla canker sore
postilla pock; scab
postizo *adj* artificial
postración *f* prostration
  postración del calor heat prostration
potasio potassium
práctica impropia (inhábil) malpractice
precipitar to precipitate
predisposición *f* predisposition
prematuro *adj* premature
premolar *f* bicuspid
prenatal prenatal
prender *slang* to hook on narcotics
prendido *adj, slang* hooked on drugs
preñada *adj* pregnant
preñez pregnancy
preocupación *f* worry
preocuparse to worry
prepucio foreskin
presbicia farsightedness; presbyopia
presbiopía farsightedness; presbyopia
présbita *adj* farsighted
prescribir to prescribe
  prescribir un remedio to prescribe
prescripción *f* prescription
presentación *f* presentation
  presentación de nalgas breechbirth (frank breech)
  presentación trasera breechbirth (frank breech)
preservativo condom
presión *f* pressure
  presión arterial alta high blood pressure
  presión arterial baja low blood pressure
primer/primero/primera *adj* first
  primer período del parto first stage of labor
  primera ayuda first aid
  primera regla menarquia menarche
  primeros auxilios *pl* first aid

principio onset; beginning
privado toilet
privar to deprive
probar (ue) to prove; to test; to try out
procedimiento procedure
procreación planeada *f* planned parenthood
procrear to procreate
proctitis *f* proctitis
producir to produce
profiláctico *m, adj* prophylactic; condom
profundo *adj* deep
progenie *f* progeny
progesterona progesterone
prolapso prolapse
  prolapso de la matriz uterus prolapse
  prolapso de útero uterus prolapse
prole *f* progeny
próstata prostate gland
prótesis *f* prosthesis
  prótesis acústica hearing aid
  prótesis auditiva hearing aid
protozoarios protozoa
protuberancia lump
proveer con pañal to diaper
provocarse el vómito to cause vomiting
prueba test
  prueba del pañal PKU (phenylketonuria)
  prueba selecta de la sangre blood screening
  prueba serológica serology test
  pruebas cruzadas cross match
prurito itching
pterigión *m* pterygium
pubiano *adj* pubic
púbico *adj* pubic
puente *m* (dental) bridge
  puente fijo fixed dental bridge
  puente movible removable dental bridge
pueril *adj* puerile
puerperal *adj* puerperal
puerperio confinement; puerperium
pujar to bear down; to push
pujos straining; tenesmus
pulga flea
pulgada inch
pulgar *m* thumb
pulimento para muebles furniture polish
pulmón *m* lung
pulmonía pneumonia
pulpa pulp
pulpejo ball of thumb; earlobe; fleshy part
pulpotomía pulpotomy
pulso pulse
pulverización *f* spray
pulverizador *m* spray
puntada stitch; suture; *Sp.Am.* sharp, stabbing pain
punta del corazón apex of heart
punto stitch
punzada sharp pain; prick; sting (*of an insect*)
puñetear *vulgar* to masturbate
puño fist
pupa oral lesion
pupila pupil (eye)
purga purge
purgación *f* purgation; *slang* gonorrhea

purgante *m* cathartic; laxative; purgative; purge
pus *m* pus
  pus detrás de la córnea hypopyon
pústula pimple; pustule
quebradura hernia; rupture
  quebradura de huesos fracture
  quebradura en la ingle inguinal hernia
quebrarse to fracture
quedarse to stay
quejarse (de) to complain (about)
quemadura burn
  quemadura por ácido acid burn
  quemadura por álcali alkali burn
  quemadura por calor seco dry heat burn
  quemadura química chemical burn
  quemadura solar sunburn
quemarse to burn oneself
quemazón *f* sunburn; burn
querer (ie) to want; to love
queso *slang* smegma
quetosis *f* ketosis
quevedos *pl* (wire-rimmed) eyeglasses; spectacles
quijada jaw
  quijada (mandíbula) rota broken jaw
quinina quinine
quintillizo quintuplet
quíntuplo quintuplet
quirófano operating room
quirúrgico *adj* surgical
quiste *m* cyst; parasitic cyst
quitar to remove
  quitarse to take off; to undress
rabadilla coccyx
rabia anger; rabies
radiaciones *f* radiation treatment
radio radius; radium; *f* radio
radiografía x-ray
  radiografía del tórax chest x-ray
radiografiar to x-ray
radioterapia radiation therapy; x-ray therapy
radióxido de zinc zinc oxide
raíz *f* root
rajar to crack
rampa charleyhorse
raposo *adj* rough
rapto *Chicano* rape
raquitis *m* rickets
raquitismo *adj Ven.* drunk; *m* scratch
rascado *adj, Ven.* drunk; *m* scratch
rascar *Sp.Am.* to be drunk; to get drunk
  rascar(se) to scratch (*relieve itch*)
rasguñar to scratch (*hurt*)
rasguño scratch
raspa *fam* D&C
raspado curettage
raspadura scrape
raspón *m, Sp.Am.* scratch
rasurar(se) to shave
rayos equis x-ray
razpón *m* abrasion
reacción alérgica *f* allergic reaction
reactivación *f* booster shot
reborde *m* ridge
recaída relapse
receptor universal *m/f* universal recipient
recesivo *adj* recessive
receta prescription
  receta médica prescription
recetar to prescribe

recidiva relapse
reconocimiento examination
recordar (ue) to remember
rectal *adj* rectal
recto rectum
rectocele *m* rectocele
recuento sanguíneo blood count
reducir(se) to reduce
  reducir una fractura to set a fracture
referir (ie) to refer
refinado *adj* refined
reflejo reflex
  reflejo de convergencia convergence
  reflex
refregar to scrub (surgically)
refuerzo booster shot
regazo lap
regenerar to regenerate
régimen *m* diet
región glútea *f* gluteal region
regla *Mex., P.R.* menstruation
regoldar (ue) to belch
regüeldo burp
regular to control; to regulate
regurgitación *f* regurgitation
regurgitar to belch
reimplantación *f* reimplantation
reinjertación *f* reimplantation
reír (i) to laugh
relación *f* relation; relationship
  relación sexual intercourse
relajación *f* relaxation; rupture (hernia)
relajar el cuerpo to relax
  relajarse to relax
rellenar to fill
relleno filling
remedio remedy
  remedio casero home remedy
remojar to soak
renal *adj* renal
rengo *adj* lame
renguear *Sp.Am.* to limp
renovar (ue) el pañal de to diaper
renuncia voluntaria waiver
reñir (i) to quarrel
repelente de insectos *m* insect
  repellent
repetir (i) to repeat; *fam* to burp
  repetirse (i) to recur
reposo rest
requerir (ie) to require
resequedad de los ojos *f* xerosis
resfriado cold
  resfriado común common cold
resollar (ue) to breathe; to pant
respiración *f* breathing; respiration
  respiración artifical artificial
  respiration
respirar to breath
  respirar asmáticamente to wheeze
  respirar con dificultad to wheeze
restregar to rub
resucitación *f* rususcitation
  resucitación boca a boca mouth-to-
  mouth resuscitation
  resucitación cardiopulmonar (RCP)
  cardiopulmonary resuscitation
  (CPR)
resucitador cardiopulmonar *m*
  cardiopulmonary resuscitator
resuello breath; breathing
  corto de resuello short of breath;
  short-winded
  resuello asmático asthmatic wheeze

resultados adversos adverse results
retardado *adj* mentally retarded
retardo mental mental retardation
reticulocitos reticulocytes
retina retina
  retina desprendida detached retina
retinto *adj* very dark-skinned, lacking
  negroid features
retirarse *m* coitus interruptus
retortijón *m* abdominal cramps
  retortijón de tripas stomach cramps
retraso mental mental retardation
retrato del x-ray *Chicano* x-ray
retrete *m, Spain* restroom; toilet
retroceder to drop back into
reuma *m* rheum
reumas *m* rheumatism
reumatismo rheumatism
reventón *m* rupture; hernia
revolver (ue) to stir
rezumamiento eczema
rh-negativo *adj* rh negative
rh-positivo *adj* rh positive
riboflavina vitamin B_2
riesgo confinement; puerperium
rinconera midwife (quack)
rinitis *f* rhinitis
riñón *m* kidney
riñonera emesis basin
ritmo rhythm method
rociador *m* spray
rodilla knee
rogar (ue) to beg
rojizo *adj* reddish
romper to rupture; to burst; to tear
roncha wheal; hive
  roncha hulera leishmaniasis
  roncha mala leishmaniasis
ronco *adj* hoarse
ronquera aphonia; hoarseness; croup
ronquido harsh, raucous sound; snore
ropa de maternidad maternity clothes
roséola roseola
  roséola epidémica rubella
rostro face
rotadura *Chicano* rupture; hernia
roto *adj* ruptured
rótula kneecap
rotura rupture; hernia
rozadura abrasion; chafing; chafe
rozarse to chap skin
rubéola German measles; roseola;
  rubella
rubor *m* redness
ruptura rupture (hernia)
sabañón *m* chiliblain
saborear to taste
saburra dental tartar
sacar to take; to stick out
  sacar aire *Chicano* to burp
  sacarle el nervio a *alguien* to remove
  the nerve
  sacar (leche) por medio de una
  bomba to pump (milk)
sacarina saccharine
saco sac
  saco amniótico amniotic sac
sacro sacrum
sacrilíaco *adj* sacro-iliac
sacudida tic
sáculo saccule
sal *f* salt
  sal biliar bile salt
  sal corriente noniodized salt

sal de epsom epsom salt
sal de higuera epsom salt
sal yodada iodized salt
sales aromáticas smelling salts
sales perfumadas smelling salts
sala room
  sala de los recién nacidos newborn
  nursery
  sala de operaciones operating room
  sala de partos delivery room
  sala prenatal labor room
salida exit; electrical outlet
  salida de los dientes teething
salir to leave *(exit)*
  salir de su cuidado *Chicano* to give
  birth
  salirle sangre de la nariz to have a
  nosebleed
  salirse *m, slang* coitus interruptus
saliva saliva; sputum
salpullido diaper rash; prickly heat;
  rash
salvohonor *m, fam* buttock
sanar to heal; to recover; *euph.* to give
  birth
  sanarse *adj* to get well
sangrante *adj* bleeding
sangrar to bleed
sangre *f* blood
  sangre clara anemia
  sangre débil *fam* anemia
  sangre de chango *Chicano*
  mercurochrome
  sangre en la orina hematuria
  sangre entera whole blood
  sangre mala *slang* syphilis
  sangre oxalatada oxalated blood
  sangre pobre *fam* anemia
  sangre pura whole blood
  sangre umbilical cord blood
sarampión *m* measles
  sarampión alemán German measles;
  rubella
  sarampión bastardo German
  measles
sarcoma *m* sarcoma
  sarcoma de Kaposi Kaposi's sarcoma
sarna itch; scabies
sarpullido rash
sarro tartar; dental tartar
saturnismo lead poisoning
seborrea seborrhea
seca *fam* bubo
secar to dry
sección cesárea *f* cesarean section
secreción *f* discharge
secreta *slang* venereal disease; VD
secretar to secrete
secundinas placenta; *Mex.* afterbirth
seda encerada dental floss
sedante *m* sedative
sedativo sleeping pill; sedative
sedimentación *f* sedimentation
seguir (i) to follow
  seguir (i) trabajando to continue
  working
segundo *adj* second
  segundo parto *Chicano* afterbirth
  segundo período del parto second
  stage of labor
semen *m* semen
semicupio sitz bath
semilla *slang, Mex.* sperm
senectud *f* old age; senility

senil *adj* senile
senilidad *f* senility
seno breast; sinus
  seno auricular pacemaker
  seno doloroso painful breast
  senos *pl* bosom
sensación *f* sensation
  sensación de pesantez en el perineo bearing-down pain
  sensaciones de ser apretado, apretada pressure sensations
sensorial *adj* sensorial
sentadera buttock
sentarse (ie) to sit down
sentido sense
  sentido de la vista sense of sight *(visual)*
  sentido del gusto sense of taste *(gustatory)*
  sentido del oído sense of hearing *(auditory)*
  sentido del olfato sense of smell *(olfactory)*
  sentido del tacto sense of feel *(tactile)*
sentir (ie) to feel; to regret
  sentirse (ie) to feel *(emotion, pain)*
separar to single out
sepsis *f* blood poisoning
septicemia blood poisoning; septicemia
ser garantizado to be guaranteed
serio *adj* serious
serpigo ringworm; tinea
servicios restroom; toilet
servilleta sanitaria sanitary napkin; sanitary pad
servir (i) to serve
sesonar *slang* to sniff glue
sesos brains
severo *adj* severe
sicodélico *adj* psychodelic
sicosis *f* psychosis
  sicosis maníacodepresiva manic-depressive insanity
sicosomático *adj* psychosomatic
sicótico *adj* psychotic
SIDA *m* AIDS
sien *f* temple
siete (7) días *m* infantum tetanus
sietecueros *inv, slang* blister on sole of foot
sietemesino *adj* premature (literally "seven month")
sífilis *f* syphilis
signo de advertencia warning sign
silbido souffle
silla de ruedas wheelchair
simple *adj, euph* mentally retarded
sinapismo mustard plaster
síndrome *m* syndrome
síntoma *m* symptom
sinusitis *f* sinus congestion
sisote *m* boil; *Chicano* ringworm; tinea
sistema *m* system
  sistema nervioso autónomo autonomic nervous system
  sistema nervioso central central nervous system
sístole *f* systole
sobaco armpit
sobar to massage
sobredosis de drogas *f, inv* drug overdose

sobreparto lying-in after childbirth
sobrepeso overweight
sobresalto shock
sofocación *f* suffocation
solanera sunburn
soler (ue) to be in the habit of
solicitar admisión a to apply for admission
sólidos solids
solitaria solium; tapeworm
soltar (ue) to let go of
soltura *Chicano* diarrhea
solución *f* solution
  solución endovenosa IV (intravenous solution)
somnífero sleeping pill
somnolencia drowsiness
sonado *adj* "high" on narcotics; "turned on"
sonámbulo *adj, slang* "high" on narcotics; "turned on"
sonarse la nariz to blow one's nose
sonda catheter; probe; tube (for feeding)
sonreír (i) to smile
soñar (ue) (con) to dream (of)
soplarse la nariz to blow one's nose
soplo heart murmur
soporífera/soporífero sleeping pill
soporífico soporific
soporte *m* support
  soportes para el arco del pie arch supports
sorber *(with lips)* to sip; to suck up
  sorber por la nariz to sniff (in, up); *Med* to inhale
  sorberse los mocos to sniffle *(a causa de catarro)*
  sorberse las lágrimas to sniffle *(al llorar)*
sordera deafness
sordo *adj* deaf
sordomudo deaf mute
soríasis *f* psoriasis
sostén *m* support
  sostén de maternidad nursing bra
suave *adj* soft
subir to rise
  subirse to climb up
  subirse la manga to roll up one's sleeve
súbito *adj* sudden
su(b)stituto substitute
sudar to perspire; to sweat
sudor *m* sweat; perspiration
sueño crepuscular twilight sleep anesthesia
suero serum
  suero antialacrán black widow spider antivenom serum
  suero antiviperino antivenom serum
  suero por la vena IV (intravenous solution)
  suero sanguíneo blood serum
sugerir (ie) to suggest
suicidio suicide
sulfatiazol *m* sulfathiazole
sulfato sulfate
  sulfato de calcio calcium sulfate
  sulfato de sodio sodium sulfate (in toilet cleaners)
  sulfato ferroso iron
sulfoniluria sulfonyluria

superficie *f* surface
  superficie inferior underside
supositorio suppository
supuración *f* discharge; drainage; suppuration
suspensorio athletic supporter
susto shock
  susto con resuello duro *fam* hyperventilation
sustraer to subtract
sutura stitch; suture; (dental) suture
  sutura absorbible dissolving suture
tableta tablet
tablilla splint
tacotillo *Chicano* boil; tumor
táctil *adj* tactile
tacuache *adj* drunk
tajo *slang* episiotomy
talache *m* chin
taladrar to drill
taladro dental drill
talasemia anemia, thalassemia
talón *m* heel
tamaño size
  tamaño grande large size
  tamaño pequeño small size
  tamaño surtido assorted size
tampax *m* Tampax
tampón *m* tampon
tapa de los sesos *fam* top of skull
tapado de orín prostatitis
tapadura filling
tapar to fill
tapón *m* tampon
  tapón de cera impacted earwax
  tapón de moco *Mex.* bloody show
taquicardia rapid heartbeat; tachycardia
tarantas *Mex., Hond.* dizziness
  tarántula *Chicano* hairy
tartamudeo lisp; stutter
tartamudez *f* stuttering
tartamudo *m* stutterer; *adj* stuttering
tártaro dental tartar
tatuaje *m* tattoo(ing)
taza de medir measuring cup
té *m* tea; *slang* marijuana
  té cargado strong tea
  té de manzanilla chamomile tea
  té fuerte strong tea
tecato heroine user; junkie
tecla cigarette butt
tecolota cigarette butt
tecunda *Mex.* chicken pox
tejido tissue
tela tape; *Med* membrane
  tela adhesiva adhesive tape
tele *f, Chicano* baby bottle; breast
temblar to shiver
temblor *m* tremor
templado *adj* lukewarm
temporal *adj* deciduous
tenazas de extracción *pl* dental forceps
tendencias a sangrar bleeding tendencies
tender (ie) (con) to spread (out); to stretch; to unfold
tendón *m* tendon
tener to have
  tener . . . años to be . . . years
  tener buen (mal) sabor) to taste good (bad)
  tener buena cara to look (appear) well

tener calor *m* to be warm
tener cuidado to be careful
tener deseos (de) to desire (to)
tener el mes to menstruate
tener el niño to deliver (a baby)
tener éxito to be successful
tener frío to be cold
tener ganas (de) to feel like
tener (mucha) hambre *f* to be (very) hungry
tener la culpa to be guilty; to be at fault
tener (traer) la garra to menstruate
tener lugar to take place
tener miedo to be afraid
tener murria to be blue
tener prisa to be in a hurry
tener que + *infinitive* to have to (must)
no tener razón to be wrong
tener razón to be right
tener relaciones sexuales to have sexual relations
tener retraso to be late
tener (mucha) sed *f* to be (very) thirsty
tener sueño to be sleepy
tener vergüenza to be ashamed
tenia tapeworm
tensión *f* strain
terapeuta *m/f* therapist
terapéutico *adj* therapeutic
terapia therapy
tercer/tercera *adj* third
tercer molar *m* third molar
tercer período del parto third stage of labor
termómetro thermometer
termómetro oral oral thermometer
termómetro rectal rectal thermometer
termoterapia heat therapy
terramicina Terramycin
testículo testicle, testis
testigo witness
testis *m* testis
teta *slang* breast
tétanos tetanus; lockjaw
tetera nursing bottle; *Mex., Cuba, P.R.* nipple (of baby/nursing bottle)
tetilla male nipple; nipple (of a baby/nursing bottle)
tetina nipple (of a baby/nursing bottle)
tetraciclina tetracycline
tetracloruro de carbono carbon tetrachloride
tez *f* complexion
tromboflebitis *f* phlebitis
tiamina vitamin B_1
tibia shinbone
tibio *adj* lukewarm; tepid; warm
tic *m* tic
tic doloroso de la cara tic douloureux
tiempo time
tiempo de coagulación coagulation time
tiempo de hemorragia bleeding time
tiempo de protrombina prothrombin time
tiempo de retracción del coágulo clot reaction time
tiempo del mes *fam* menstruation
tienta probe
tieso *adj* stiff

tifo typhus fever
tifo abdominal typhoid fever
tifo de América yellow fever
tifo de oriente bubonic plague
tifus *m* typhus fever
tifus exantemático spotted fever; typhus fever
tifus icterodes yellow fever
timba *slang* heroin capsule
timo thymus
tímpano eardrum; tympanic membrane
tímpano perforado perforated eardrum
tina de baño tub
tinción *f* stain; staining
tiniado *adj, slang;* "high" from sniffing paint thinner
tinte *m* dye
tiña ringworm; tinea
tiraleches *f, inv* breast pump
tirar to shoot; to throw *(accidentally)* to drop
tirar (el) agua *slang* to urinate
tirar (la) basura *slang* to defecate
tirarse flato to expel anal gas
tirarse un pedo to expel anal gas
tiritar to shiver
tiroides *m* thyroid
tirón *m* tic
tisis *f* phthisis; tuberculosis
tlacuache *adj* drunk
toalla towel
toallas en los ojos eyepads
tobillera ankle support
tobillo ankle
tocar to feel; to touch
tocología obstetrics
tocólogo obstetrician
tolerancia tolerance
tomacorriente *m, Sp.Am.* electrical socket
tomada electrical socket
tomar to take; *slang* to take drugs
tomate *m, slang, Chicano* eyeball
tónico tonic
tonsilitis *f* tonsilitis
tonsils *m, Chicano* tonsils
toque *m* drag; puff of (marijuana) cigarette
toracentesis *f* pleural tap
tórax *m* chest, thorax
torcedura sprain; strain
torcer (ue) to sprain; to twist; to turn
torcido *adj* twisted
torcijón cólico *m, Mex.* stomach cramps
torniquete *m* tourniquet
torrente *m* stream
torrente circulatorio bloodstream
torrente de sangre bloodstream
torrente sanguíneo bloodstream
torsón *m* abdominal cramps
tortícolis *m* stiff neck
torzón *m* sharp intestinal cramps
tos *f* cough
tos ahogona *Mex.* whooping cough; pertussis
tos convulsiva whooping cough; pertussis
tos ferina whooping cough; pertussis
tos por fumar smoker's cough
toser to cough
tosferina whooping cough; pertussis
tostado *adj* suntanned

toxemia blood poisoning; septicemia; toxemia
toxemia del embarazo toxemia of pregnancy
toxicomanía (drug) addiction
toxicómano (drug) addict
trabajo de parto labor
tracción *f* traction
tracoma *m* conjunctivitis
traer carga *slang* to be carrying narcotic drugs
traficar *slang* to traffic in drugs
tragante *m, Chicano* esophagus
tragar to swallow
tragar humo to inhale (smoke)
trago swallow
trakes *m, fam* tracks
traques *m, fam* tracks
tramo flight of stairs
tranquilizante *m* tranquilizer
transferir (ie) to transfer
transfusión *f* tranfusion
tranfusión de sangre blood transfusion
transfusión sanguínea blood transfusion
transmisión *f* transmission
transmisión mediante contacto transmission by contact
transmisión mediante vector vector transmission
transmisión por gotillas droplet transmission
tráquea trachea
traqueostomía tracheostomy
trastorno alérgico allergic reaction
tratamiento therapy; treatment
tratamiento térmico heat therapy
trauma *m* trauma
traumatismo trauma
trementina turpentine
tremor *m* tremor
tricocéfalo trichocephalus
tricomonas trichomonas
triglicéridos elevados high triglycerides
trigueño *adj* olive-skinned (complexion)
trillizo triplet
trimo tetanus
tripa *fam* bowels
tripa ida blocked intestine
tripita *fam* appendix
triple *f* DPT vaccination
triquinosis *f* trichinosis
trismo lockjaw
trocisco lozenge
trombocito thrombocyte
tromboflebitis *f* thrombophlebitis
trombosis *f* thrombosis
trombosis coronaria coronary thrombosis
trompa tube; duct
trompa de eustaquio eustachian tube
trompa de Falopio fallopian tube
tronado *adj* drunk
tronar to smoke marijuana
trotador, trotadora *m/f* jogger
trotar to jog
tuberculina tuberculin test
tuberculosis *f* tuberculosis
tuberculoso *adj* tubercular
tubo catheter; tube
tubo de ensayo test tube
tubo de Falopio Fallopian tube
tubos Fallopian tubes

tuerto *adj* blind in one eye; one-eyed
tullido *adj* cripple
tumbar to have sexual relations
tumefacción swelling; tumefaction
tumor *m* swelling; tumor
tumorcito lump
turista *slang* diarrhea
turnio *adj* cross-eyed
turno appointment
úlcera canker; sore (wound); ulcer
   úlcera del estómago stomach ulcer
   úlcera gangrenosa canker sore
   úlcera gástrica gastric ulcer
   úlcera péptica peptic ulcer
   úlcera por decúbito bedsore
ulceración *f* canker sore
ultrasonda ultrasound
uncinaria uncinaria; hookworm
ungüento balsam; ointment; salve; unguent
   ungüento para los ojos eye salve
unto ointment
untos de Papanicolaou Pap smear
uña nail
   uña encarnada ingrown toenail
   uña enterrada ingrown toenail
uñero ingrown toenail
urea urea
uremia uremia
uréter *m* ureter
uretra urethra
uretritis *f* urethritis
   uretritis inespecífica nonspecific urethritis
   uretritis no específica nonspecific urethritis
   uretritis no gonococal nongonoccocal urethritis
urgencia emergency
urinálisis *m, inv* urinalysis
urobilina urobilin
urobilirrubina urobilirubin
urticaria hives; urticaria
urutar *Chicano* to burp
úrzula *Chicano* typhus fever
útero uterus; womb
úvula uvula
vaciar to empty
vacuna immunization vaccine
   vacuna oral contra el polio oral polio vaccine
   vacuna triple DPT vaccination
vacunación *f* vaccination
vacunar to vaccinate
vagina vagina
vaginal *adj* vaginal
vaginitis *f* vaginitis
vahído dizziness
válvula valve
   válvula del corazón heart valve

vapor *m* steam; vapor
várices *f, pl* varicose veins
varicela chicken pox
varicosidad *f* varicosity
varicoso *adj* varicose
vasectomía vasectomy
vaselina vaseline
vaso drinking glass
   vaso capilar capillary
   vaso sanguíneo blood vessel
vehículo vehicle
vejez *f* old aid
vejiga bladder; *Med* blister
   vejiga de la bilis gallbladder
   vejiga de la orina urinary bladder
vello hair; down (*soft hair on human body*)
   vello púbico pubic hair
velo del paladar soft palate; velum
vena vein
   vena dental dental vein
   vena varicosa vericose vein
venda bandage
vendaje *m* bandage; dressing
   vendaje abdominal binder
   vendaje de yeso gypsum cast
   vendaje elástico elastic bandage
veneno poison
   venenos aspirados inhaled poisons
   venenos comunes common poisons
   venenos inyectados injected poisons
   venenos tomados por la boca oral poisons
venenoso *adj* poisonous
venir to come
   venirse *slang* to ejaculate
ventaja advantage
ventana de la nariz nostril
ventanilla de la nariz nostril
ventosidad *f* flatulence
verdugón *m* weal (large welt)
verga *slang* penis
verme *m* intestinal worm
vermífugo *adj* vermifuge
verruga wart
   verruga genital genital wart
   verruga venérea genital wart
vértebra vertebra
vertiginoso *adj* dizzy
vértigo dizziness; fainting spell
vesícula bladder; blister
   vesícula biliar gallbladder
   vesícula seminal seminal vesicle
vestir(se) (i) to dress (oneself)
   vestirse (i) de bata de hospital to be gowned
vía *Anat* duct; passage; tube; tract
   vía aérea airway
   vía bucal, por orally; through the mouth; by mouth

vía de entrada route of entry
vías digestivas digestive tract
vía hipodérmica, por hypodermically
vía interna, por *Med* internally
vías respiratorias respiratory tract
vías urinarias urinary tract
vial *m* vial
víctima victim
vientre *m* abdomen; stomach
vinagre *m* vinegar
violación *f* rape
violeta de genciana gentian violet
viruela pock; smallpox
   viruelas locas *slang* chicken pox
virulo *adj, Chicano* one-eyed
virus *m* virus
   enfermedad por virus *f* virus disease
   Virus de (la) Inmunodeficiencia Humana Human Immunodeficiency Virus
   virus de papiloma humano human papilloma virus
vista vision
   vista borrosa blurred vision
   vista doble double vision
vitamina vitamin
vitíligo vitiligo
viveza alertness
voltear to turn around (over)
volver (ue) to return; to come back
vomitar to vomit
vomitivo *m, adj* emetic; vomitive
vómito vomit; vomiting
   vómito negro yellow fever
   vómitos de embarazo morning sickness
vulva vulva
xerosis *f* xerosis
yedo marijuana
yedra venenosa poison ivy
yema fleshy tip of the finger
yerba *slang* marijuana
yesca *slang* marijuana
yesco *slang* marijuana smoker
yeso cast; *slang* (drug) addict
   yeso mate plaster of Paris
yeyuno jejunum
yodo iodine
yoduro de potasio potassium iodide
yunque *m* anvil (incus)
zacate *m* marijuana (low-grade variety)
zambo *adj* twisted
zapeta *Mex.* diaper
zona shingles
zoster *f* shingles
zumaque venenoso *m* poison ivy
zumbido de oídos buzzing in the ears

Answer Key
Clave de respuestas

CHAPTER 2

▌ *CAPITULO*

Page 54:

Practice *Práctica*

1. me-di-ca-MEN-to
2. in-me-dia-ta-MEN-te
3. co-les-te-ROL
4. pa-LI-llo
5. A-gua
6. in-di-ges-TION
7. e-pi-LEP-sia
8. pe-RI-o-do
9. qui-mio-te-RA-pia
10. dia-BE-tes

¿Cómo se escribe?

1. te o ere ene i cu u e te e
2. e ene efe e ere eme e ere a
3. hache i ese te o ere i a ele
4. ese a ene ge ere e
5. jota e ere i ene ge a
6. eme u e ese te ere a
7. a ene te i be i o *con acento* te i ce o
8. efe a ere eme a ce i a

Correct Syllables

1. 4: e-pi-LEP-sia
2. 2: AS-ma
3. 4: o-be-si-DAD
4. 3: mu-ÑE-ca
5. 2: CIE-rre
6. 4: e-xa-mi-NAR
7. 3: a-GA-rra
8. 5: far-ma-CÉU-ti-co
9. 3: con-DUZ-ca
10. 4: neu-mo-NÍ-a

Practice *Práctica*

te-ra-PEU-ta	es-PE-jo	ra-dio-te-RA-pia	ven-DA-je	bo-RU-jo
en-jua-GAR	QUÍ-mi-ca	a-mo-NÍ-a-co	dre-NA-je	sa-ram-PIÓN
VUL-va	HOM-bro	i-no-cu-la-CIÓN	mu-LE-ta	LIEN-dra
om-BLI-go	a-na-TÓ-mi-co	dia-FRAG-ma	in-FAR-to	LEN-gua
man-DÍ-bu-la	pe-li-RRO-jo	la-va-TI-va	ca-rras-PE-ra	ru-BÉ-o-la

Page 55

READING EXERCISE *EJERCICIO DE LECTURA*

A doctor told me that I could not stay in this place and that I would have to sleep more, exercise more, and eat less.

"But, Doctor, where will I go to live like this [in this way]? I can't sleep so much if you awaken me early every day. And I don't like to entertain myself with sports."

San Roque's dog does not have a tail because Ramón Ramírez has cut it off.

Pages 57–58

A. Rewrite the following passages, inserting proper punctuation and capitals.
Escriba de nuevo los pasajes que siguen, insertando la punctuación correcta y las mayúsculas necesarias.

1. **¿Qué causa la alta presión arterial? El 90-95% de todos los casos de alta presión arterial es debido a una causa desconocida.**
   What causes high blood pressure? 90-95% of all cases of high blood pressure is due to an unknown cause.
2. **El tiempo en la sala de recuperación varía de una hora a 3 o 4 horas o más.**
   Time in the recovery room varies from an hour to 3 or 4 or more.
3. **La siguiente información es exigida por la Administración de Alimentos y Drogas de los Estados Unidos. La Píldora es el más eficaz de todos los anticonceptivos si sigue completamente las instrucciones sobre su uso.**
   The following information is required by the Food and Drug Administration of the United States. The Pill is the most effective of all the contraceptives if you are completely following the instructions about its use.
4. **Por favor, vaya a llamar al Dr. García del Departamento de Psiquiatría a ver si puede continuar con el examen.**
   Please, go call Dr. García from the Psych Department to see if you can continue the exam.
5. **Inglaterra tiene un sistema de la medicina socializada en que el gobierno paga los gastos médicos.**
   England has a system of socialized medicine in which the government pays for medical expenses.

B.

1. –¡Hola, Carlos! ¿Qué tal? ¿Cómo estás?
2. –Muy bien, gracias, ¿y tú?
3. –¿Cómo está usted, doctor?
4. –Estoy bien, gracias. ¿y Vd., señor?

CHAPTER 3

▌ *CAPITULO*

Page 77

IDENTIFICATION EXERCISES *EJERCICIOS DE IDENTIFICACION*

(Answers clockwise from the top. *Respuestas de arriba en la dirección de las agujas del reloj.*)

head	*cabeza*	kidneys	*riñones*	calf	*pantorrilla*	forearm	*antebrazo*
lungs	*pulmones*	coccyx	*cóccix*	heel	*talón*	back	*espalda*
armpit	*sobaco/axila*	buttock	*nalga*	hip	*cadera*	shoulder	*hombro*
humerus	*húmero*	rectum	*recto*	hand	*mano*	neck	*cuello*

Page 78

IDENTIFICATION EXERCISE   *EJERCICIO DE IDENTIFICACION*

(Answers clockwise from the top.   *Respuestas de arriba en la dirección de las agujas del reloj.*)

cranium	*cráneo*	knee	*rodilla*	groin	*ingle*
neck	*cuello*	leg	*pierna*	abdomen	*abdomen*
elbow	*codo*	ankle	*tobillo*	navel	*ombligo*
wrist	*muñeca*	foot	*pie*	thorax	*tórax*
flank	*costado*	toes	*dedos del pie*	breast/chest	*pecho*
palm	*palma*	lower extremity	*extremidad inferior*	shoulder	*hombro*
fingers	*dedos*	hand	*mano*	upper extremity	*extremidad superior*
thigh	*muslo*	genitals	*órganos genitales*	face	*cara*

Page 79

PARTS OF THE EYE AND EAR

PARTES DEL OJO Y DEL OIDO

IDENTIFY THE ITEMS ON THIS DIAGRAM   *PONGA LETREROS EN ESTE ESQUEMA:*

A.	optic nerve	*nervio óptico*	L.	middle ear	*oído medio*
B.	lens	*cristalino*	M.	auditory tube (eustachian tube)	*trompa auditiva (trompa de Eustaquio)*
C.	posterior chamber (vitreous humor)	*cámara posterior (humor vítreo)*	N.	hammer (malleus)	*martillo*
D.	cornea	*córnea*	O.	anvil (incus)	*yunque*
E.	sclera	*esclera/esclerótica*	P.	stirrup (stapes)	*estribo*
F.	choroid coat	*capa coroides*	Q.	external ear (auricle)	*oído externo (pabellón de la oreja)*
G.	anterior chamber (aqueous humor)	*cámara anterior (humor acuoso)*	R.	external auditory canal	*conducto auditivo externo*
H.	iris	*iris*	S.	eardrum (tympanic membrane)	*tímpano*
I.	ciliary body and muscle	*cuerpo y músculo ciliares*	T.	inner ear	*oído interno*
J.	fovea	*fóvea*	U.	cochlea	*caracol*
K.	retina	*retina*	V.	semicircular canals	*conductos semicirculares*

Page 80

INTERNAL ORGANS   *LOS ORGANOS INTERNOS*

Identify the items on this diagram   *Ponga letreros en este esquema*

1.	brain	*cerebro*	10. stomach	*estómago*
2.	spinal cord	*médula espinal*	11. gallbladder	*vesícula biliar*
3.	nose	*nariz*	12. large intestine	*intestino grueso*
4.	tongue	*lengua*	13. small intestine	*intestino delgado*
5.	trachea (windpipe)	*tráquea*	14. appendix	*apéndice*
6.	lungs	*pulmones*	15. bladder	*vejiga*
7.	diaphragm	*diafragma*	16. pancreas	*páncreas*
8.	esophagus	*esófago*	17. spleen	*bazo*
9.	liver	*hígado*		

Page 81

DIGESTIVE SYSTEM   *SISTEMA DIGESTIVO*

Identify the items on this diagram   *Ponga letreros en este esquema*

A.	esophagus	*esófago*	D.	small intestine	*intestino delgado*
B.	liver	*hígado*	E.	large intestine	*intestino grueso*
C.	stomach	*estómago*			

Page 82

GENITOURINARY SYSTEM   *SISTEMA GENITOURINARIO*

Identify the items on this diagram   *Ponga letreros en este esquema*

A.	testis	*testículo*	G.	prostrate gland	*glándula de la próstata*
B.	epidiymis	*epidídimo*	H.	urethra	*uretra*
C.	Cowper's gland	*glándula de Cowper*	I.	penis	*pene*
D.	seminal vesicle	*vesículo seminal*	J.	foreskin (prepuce)	*prepucio*
E.	sigmoid colon	*colon sigmoide*	K.	scrotum	*escroto*
F.	vas deferens	*conducto deferente*	L.	rectum	*recto*

M. anus   *ano*   P. Fallopian tube   *trompa de Falopio*
N. vagina   *vagina*   Q. uterus   *útero*
O. ovary   *ovario*   R. cervix   *cuello de la matriz*

Page 83

STRUCTURES OF THE MOUTH   *ESTRUCTURAS DE LA BOCA*

Identify the items on this diagram   *Ponga letreros en este esquema*

1. upper lip   *labio superior*   13. central incisor   *incisivo central*
2. gingiva   *encía*   14. lower lip   *labio inferior*
3. hard palate   *paladar duro*   15. gingiva   *encía*
4. soft palate   *paladar blando*   16. tongue   *lengua*
5. uvula   *úvula*   17. tonsil   *amígdala*
6. third molar   *muela del juicio*   18. second molar   *segundo molar*
7. second molar   *segundo molar*   19. first molar   *primer molar*
8. first molar   *primer molar*   20. second premolar/bicuspid *segundo bicúspide*
9. second premolar/bicuspid   *segundo diente premolar*   21. first premolar/bicuspid   *primer bicúspide*
10. first premolar/bicuspid   *primer diente premolar*   22. cuspid   *cúspide*
11. cuspid   *colmillo*   23. lateral incisor   *incisivo lateral*
12. lateral incisor   *incisivo lateral*   24. central incisor   *incisivo central*

Page 84

PARTS OF A TOOTH   *PARTES DE UN DIENTE*

Identify the items on this diagram   *Ponga letreros en este esquema*

1. enamel   *esmalte*   4. gum/gingiva   *encía*   7. root   *raíz*
2. dentine   *dentina*   5. capillaries   *capilares*   8. neck   *cuello del diente*
3. pulp   *pulpa*   6. nerve   *nervio*   9. crown   *corona*

Page 84

ADULT DENTITION   *DENTICION ADULTA*

Identify the items on this diagram   *Ponga letreros en este esquema*

A. central incisor   *incisivo central*   D. bicuspids   *bicúspides*
B. lateral incisor   *incisivo lateral*   E. molars   *molares*
C. cuspid (eyetooth)   *colmillo*   F. wisdom tooth   *muela del juicio*

Page 84

DECIDUOUS TEETH   *LOS DIENTES DE LECHE*

Identify the items on this diagram   *Ponga letreros en este esquema*

1. upper   *superior*   8. lower   *inferior*
2. central incisor   *incisivo central*   9. first permanent molar *primer molar permanente*
3. lateral incisor   *incisivo lateral*   10. second baby molar   *segundo molar temporal*
4. cuspid (eyetooth)   *colmillo*   11. first baby molar   *primer molar temporal*
5. first baby molar   *primer molar temporal*   12. cuspid (eyetooth)   *colmillo*
6. second baby molar   *segundo molar temporal*   13. lateral incisor   *incisivo lateral*
7. first permanent molar *primer molar permanente* 14. central incisor   *incisivo central*

CHAPTER 4
CAPITULO

Page 88

EXERCISES   *EJERCICIOS*

A.   Write out the cardinal numbers in Spanish.

1. un   5. catorce   8. veintiuna (veinte y una)
2. treinta y un   6. tres   9. treinta y seis
3. dieciséis (diez y seis)   7. cincuenta   10. setenta y dos
4. sesenta y cuatro

B.   Say the following in Spanish.

1. dos millones
2. diecisiete mil quinientos treinta y dos
3. ocho mil seiscientos cincuenta y tres
4. setecientos seis
5. novecientos once

6. mil cuatrocientos noventa y dos
7. ochocientos setenta y cinco
8. mil ochocientos doce
9. veinticinco dólares
10. dos mil quinientos ochenta y ocho

11. mil ciento veinticuatro
12. cien mil cuatrocientos
13. tres mil doscientos cuarenta y siete
14. trescientos sesenta y nueve
15. novecientos setenta mil noventa y siete

C.   Practice Saying the Following Years in Spanish:

1. mil cuatrocientos noventa y dos
2. mil setecientos setenta y seis
3. mil novecientos diez
4. mil novecientos cuarenta y dos

5. mil novecientos treinta y seis
6. mil novecientos setenta y uno
7. mil novecientos veintiocho

8. mil novecientos cincuenta y tres
9. mil quinientos doce
10. dos mil uno

Page 89

1. Colombia tiene treinta y tres millones ochocientos mil habitantes.
2. La población de Méjico es ochenta y cinco millones novecientos cincuenta mil habitantes.
3. Los Estados Unidos tienen veintinueve millones setecientos mil habitantes.
4. Cuba tiene once millones novecientos cincuenta mil habitantes.
5. Venezuela tiene diecinueve millones ochocientos mil habitantes.

Page 89

2. Answer in Spanish:

a. Argentina tiene dos millones quinientos veintiún mil habitantes más que Colombia.
b. Cuba tiene treinta y un mil quinientos setenta y dos menos habitantes que España.
c. Hay veintiocho millones trescientos mil habitantes hispanos en los Estados Unidos.

2. Conteste:

a. Hay ocho millones seiscientos sesenta y un mil habitantes hispanos en Texas, Florida e Illinois.
b. Illinois y Nueva York tienen (un total de) tres millones seiscientos setenta y cuatro mil habitantes hispanos.
c. Hay doce millones ciento sesenta y ocho mil habitantes hispanos en Nueva York y California.

Page 89

Answer the Questions using the Numbers as Cues:

1. La enfermera tiene veintisiete años.
2. El médico tiene cincuenta y cinco años.
3. La paciente tiene treinta y tres años.
4. Su/Mi dentista tiene sesenta y un años.
5. Su/Mi esposa tiene cuarenta y cinco años.

6. Su padre tiene ochenta y siete años.
7. El paciente tiene setenta y cinco años.
8. El especialista tiene treinta y nueve años.
9. La higienista tiene diecinueve años.
10. El camillero tiene veinticinco años.

Page 90

A. Calculate the Cost of the Following in Spanish:

1. sesenta pesos
2. cuatro pesos y un octavo
3. un peso y medio
4. cinco pesos y medio

B. Lea Estas Operaciones Aritméticas:

cinco más siete es igual a doce
cuarenta menos quince es igual a veinticinco

veinticuatro dividido por ocho es igual a tres
doce por doce es igual a ciento cuarenta y cuatro

Page 91

Practice Reading . . .:

1. (el) trescientos dieciséis cero nueve once sesenta y siete
    [tres dieciséis cero nueve once sesenta y siete]
    [tres uno seis cero nueve uno uno seis siete]
2. siete treinta y dos treinta y nueve treinta y ocho
    [siete tres dos tres nueve tres ocho]

3. ocho diez a dos cuarenta y ocho
4. cero cuarenta y uno veintiocho noventa y uno dieciséis
    [cero cuatro uno dos ocho nueve uno uno seis]
5. el seis cero cinco veintiuno

Page 94

A. Convert the Following:

1. 5 cm
2. .5 m / medio metro
3. 7.5 cm
4. .5m

B. Answer the following in Spanish.

1. Hay treinta y medio centímetros más o menos. [30.48]
2. Hay trescientos cuarenta y ocho milímetros.
3. Answers will vary.
4. La yarda es la unidad básica de medida más comúnmente usada para los estadounidenses.

5. El metro es la unidad básica de medida en el sistema métrico.
6. Hay treinta y seis pulgadas en una yarda. Hay treinta y nueve punto treinta y siete pulgadas en un metro.

Page 95

C. Solve the Following Problems:

1. 6'2" @ 1 cm = .4" [6'1" @ 1 cm = .393"]
2. 10 lbs @ 1 k = 2 lbs. [11.02 lbs. @ 1 k = 2.204 lbs.]

3. 3.2" × .8"
4. 90' @ 1 m = 3' [98.4' @ 1 m = 3.28']

EXERCISES

1. 325 mg; 500 mg

2. 20 cápsulas de 50 mg diarias; 10 cápsulas de 100 mg diarias

Page 98

Practice   *Práctica*

2:22   Son las dos y veintidós.
10:35 Son las once menos veinticinco.
5:45   Son las seis menos cuarto [menos quince].
7:55   Son las ocho menos cinco.
11:40 Son las doce menos veinte.
1:10   Es la una y diez.

3:24   Son las tres y veinticuatro.
7:56   Son las ocho menos cuatro.
1:50   Son las dos menos diez.
9:56   Son las diez menos cuatro.
7:00   Son las siete.
1:45   Son las dos menos cuarto [menos quince].

Page 99

Write Out These Times in Spanish:

1. Son las dos y cuarto (quince) de la tarde.
2. Son las ocho menos dieciocho de la mañana.
3. Es la una y diecinueve de la tarde.
4. Es la una menos doce de la madrugada.
5. Son las seis y diecisiete de la tarde / noche.
6. Son las ocho y dieciocho de la mañana.
7. Son las diez y media de la noche.
8. Es medianoche.

9. Son las cuatro y veintisiete de la madrugada.
10. Son las ocho menos cinco de la tarde / noche.
11. Son las tres y catorce de la madrugada.
12. Son las diez menos diez de la mañana.
13. Son las seis menos veintidós de la tarde.
14. Son las doce y veinte de la tarde.
15. Son las doce menos veintiuno de la mañana.

Page 101

EXERCISES   *EJERCICIOS*

A. Translate the following into Spanish.

1. Conchita nació el diecisiete de febrero de mil novecientos setenta y tres.
2. La operación va a costar / costará novecientos ochenta y cinco dólares.
3. ¿A qué hora llega aquí el técnico / la técnica?
4. Son las cuatro menos cuarto de la tarde el veintinueve de noviembre de mil novecientos ochenta y dos.
5. Doscientos muchachos están enfermos hoy.

6. Operan a las seis y media de la mañana.
7. No trabajamos los miércoles.
8. (Ella) Va al laboratorio todos los sábados.
9. El nene / La nena siempre tiene catarro en el invierno.
10. Siempre tengo turno con mi médico / médica los martes por la mañana a la clínica durante el verano. *or*
   Siempre tengo turno a la clínica con mi médico / médica cada martes por la mañana durante el verano.

B. Answer in Spanish.

1. Variable
2. Variable
3. Variable
4. Si hoy es lunes, mañana es martes.
5. Si hoy es lunes, ayer fue domingo.
6. Si hoy es jueves, mañana es viernes.
7. Si hoy es miércoles, ayer fue martes.
8. Si hoy es martes, pasado mañana es jueves.
9. Si hoy es martes, anteayer fue domingo.
10. Si hoy es domingo, pasado mañana es martes.

11. Los meses de la primavera son parte de marzo, abril, mayo, y parte de junio. Los meses del verano son parte de junio, julio, agosto, y parte de septiembre. Los meses del otoño son parte de septiembre, octubre, noviembre, y parte de diciembre. Los meses del invierno son parte de diciembre, enero, febrero, y parte de marzo.
12. Variable
13. Variable
14. Celebramos la Navidad en diciembre; celebramos la independencia de los Estados Unidos en julio.
15. Variable

C. Answer in Spanish.

1. Febrero es el mes que tiene veintiocho días. *or* Febrero tiene veintiocho días.
2. Abril, junio, septiembre, y noviembre tienen treinta días. *or* Abril, junio, septiembre, y noviembre son los meses que tienen treinta días.
3. Enero, marzo, mayo, julio, agosto, y octubre tienen treinta y un días. *or*

Los meses que tienen treinta y un días son enero, marzo, mayo, julio, agosto, y octubre.
4. Julio y agosto son dos meses del verano.
5. Mayo es un mes de la primavera.
6. Un mes del invierno que tiene treinta y un días es diciembre.
7. Noviembre es un mes del otoño que tiene treinta días.
8. Variable.

D. Item Substitution:

1. La farmacia está cerrada los sábados.
2. La farmacia está cerrada los domingos.
3. La farmacia está cerrada los días de fiesta.

4. La farmacia está abierta los días de fiesta.
5. La farmacia está abierta todos los días.
6. La clínica está abierta todos los días.

Page 102

PAIS	MES	ESTACION	PAIS	MES	ESTACION
Argentina	julio	invierno	Ecuador	junio	verano
Bolivia	agosto	invierno	Venezuela	marzo	verano
Illinois	diciembre	invierno	Honduras	enero	invierno
Paraguay	abril	otoño	Colombia	octubre	verano
Chile	febrero	verano	Perú	mayo	otoño
Uruguay	septiembre	primavera	Nueva York	noviembre	otoño

CHAPTER 5
CAPITULO

Page 111

THE ADMISSIONS OFFICE *LA OFICINA DE INGRESOS*

Preguntas:
1. El esposo de la señora Fernández la acompaña.
2. Ella tiene que llenar un formulario de entrada.
3. Su esposo puede visitarla desde las doce de la tarde hasta las ocho y media de la noche.

CHAPTER 6
CAPITULO

Page 118

D.
1. Buenos días, señora (Sra.) García.
2. Buenas tardes, Sr. (señor) Gómez.
3. Buenas noches, Dra. (doctora) Navas.
4. Buenas tardes, María Paz.
5. Buenas tardes, Srta. (señorita) Villarreal.
6. Buenos días, Dr. (doctor) Brown.

Page 121

C. Conversation
ENFERMERA: Buenos días. Soy María, su enfermera.
PACIENTE: Muy buenos. Soy la señora García.
ENFERMERA: Tanto gusto de conocerla.
PACIENTE: El gusto es mío.
ENFERMERA: ¿Cómo se siente hoy?

Page 125

A. Answer the questions using the cue given.
1. Soy el cirujano.
2. Soy la enfermera de guardia.
3. Soy la jefa de enfermeras.
4. Soy la enfermera diplomada.
5. Soy la ayudante de enfermera.
6. Soy el ayudante de hospital.
7. Soy el enfermero de guardia.
8. Soy la enfermera ambulante.
9. Soy el enfermero de salud pública.
10. Soy el camillero.

CHAPTER 7
CAPITULO

Page 135

PREGUNTAS:
1. Marcelina está resfriada. También sufre de un tremendo dolor del oído derecho, de dolor torácico, y de una temperatura de 102°F [39°C].
2. Necesita un (jarabe) expectorante y bebidas calientes como té hecho de hierba colorada así como unas gotas para el oído y un antibiótico para las infecciones.
3. Si la fiebre no baja, la familia debe llevarla al consultorio de la Dra. Poma el día siguiente por la tarde.

Page 137

PREGUNTAS:

1. El Sr. Gómez no se siente bien.
2. Cogió un fuerte resfriado. (Tiene catarro.)
3. Sí, ha perdido el apetito también.
4. Se siente indispuesto desde anoche. (Hace doce horas que se siente indispuesto.)
5. Llega al consultorio del Dr. Ortiz por taxi.

6. No, la señora Gómez no entra en la sala de reconocimientos.
7. Después de ver al médico, cuando aún no se siente mejor, el médico dice que tal vez le falta algo más fuerte contra un resfriado y dolor de cabeza.
8. Tiene que volver dentro de tres días si no se siente mejor.

Page 138

PRACTICE *PRACTICA*

Conteste Según el Modelo:

1. Le duele el codo izquierdo.
2. Le duelen los oídos.

3. Le duele el corazón.
4. Le duele el tobillo.

5. Le duele el estómago.

Page 139

PRACTICE *PRACTICA*

Conteste Según el Modelo:

1. Le duele la garganta a la niña cuando come.
2. Le duelen los pies cuando anda demasiado.
3. Me duele cuando hago ejercicios físicos.

4. Le duele cuando orina.
5. Le duele cuando corre.

Page 140

QUESTIONS:

1. He has a wound, and his whole leg hurts a lot.
2. When he returns home, his daughter can do his bandage.
3. He will have to change the dressing now and then again every two days.

PREGUNTAS:

1. Sufre de una herida y le duele un poquito toda la pierna.
2. Al volver a casa, la hija del paciente puede hacerle el vendaje.
3. Será preciso cambiar la venda ahora y entonces cada dos días.

CHAPTER 8

▌*CAPITULO*

Page 175

QUESTIONS:

1. Menstrual cycles are twenty-eight days on the average.
2. The ovary produces an egg each month.
3. The flow of blood lasts from three to five days.

Page 175

PREGUNTAS:

1. Los ciclos menstruales duran veintiocho días por lo regular.
2. Un ovario produce un óvulo cada mes.
3. El flujo sanguíneo dura de tres a cinco días.

CHAPTER 9

▌*CAPITULO*

Page 194

¿COMO SE DICE EN ESPAÑOL?

1. Por lo regular peso ciento sesenta y ocho libras.
2. Pablo bebe / toma dos botellas de cerveza cada día.
3. Nunca bebemos leche. / No bebemos nunca leche.
4. El hombre toma café descafeinado, pero (yo) bebo té.
5. Hace muchos años que fuman. / Fuman hace muchos años.
6. Ahora me levanto / me despierto a las seis y cuarto de la mañana.

7. Carlos se levanta / se despierta a medianoche porque trabaja por la noche.
8. ¿Fuma cigarrillos ahora?
9. ¿Por qué usa anfetaminas?
10. La viuda tiene siete hijos y una hija. / La viuda tiene ocho hijos.

CHAPTER 10

CAPITULO

Page 204

Preguntas:

1. Max tiene casi ocho años.
2. Tiene que llevar un parche porque sufre de estrabismo—tiene ojos con visión distorsionada.
3. Se llama «lazy eye.»
4. Parece que Max no los usa juntos.
5. Sí, parece que le falta la percepción de profundidad.
6. Tendrá que volver / regresar en seis meses.

Page 210

Questions:

1. Mrs. Peña is complaining about a slight burning when she urinates. She feels the need for frequent urination; she is unable to pass more than a few drops of urine.
2. A midstream urinalysis can determine if she has a kidney infection.
3. The perineum (perineal area) is located between the legs where you urinate, between the rectum and the urinary opening.
4. It is necessary to use a backward movement when wiping oneself to prevent further problems by introducing additional bacteria.
5. The flask should not be filled immediately upon urinating. It should be filled only after passing some urine first.
6. Only a small amount of urine is needed.

Preguntas:

1. La señora Peña se queja de ardor al orinar. Siente que tiene que orinar cada cinco minutos. [Le parece que tiene una urgencia para orinar.] No puede pasar más que unas gotitas al orinar.
2. Un análisis de la orina recogida a la mitad de la micción puede indicar si tiene o no una infección de los riñones o de la vejiga de la orina.
3. El perineo (el área perineal) es el área entre las piernas donde orina y está entre el recto y la abertura urinaria.
4. Es necesario usar un movimiento hacia el recto al limpiarse para no introducir bacterias (microbios) adicionales que podrían causar más problemas.
5. No debe llenar el frasco inmediatamente al orinar. Hay que pasar unas gotitas primero.
6. Sólo se necesita medio frasco de claro espécimen para esta prueba.

Page 214

Rewrite all commands from the musculoskeletal and neurological sections using alternatives:

1. Haga el favor de levantarse.
   Favor de levantarse.
   Tenga la bondad de levantarse.
   Sírvase levantarse.
2. Haga el favor de sentarse.
   Favor de sentarse.
   Tenga la bondad de sentarse.
   Sírvase sentarse.
3. Haga el favor de caminar un poco.
   Favor de caminar un poco.
   Tenga la bondad de caminar un poco.
   Sírvase caminar un poco.
4. Haga el favor de volver / regresar.
   Favor de volver /regresar.
   Tenga la bondad de volver / regresar.
   Sírvase volver / regresar.
5. Haga el favor de caminar hacia atrás.
   Favor de caminar hacia atrás.
   Tenga la bondad de caminar hacia atrás.
   Sírvase caminar hacia atrás.
6. Haga el favor de caminar sobre los dedos (del pie).
   Favor de caminar sobre los dedos (del pie).
   Tenga la bondad de caminar sobre los dedos (del pie).
   Sírvase caminar sobre los dedos (del pie).
7. Haga el favor de caminar sobre los talones.
   Favor de caminar sobre los talones.
   Tenga la bondad de caminar sobre los talones.
   Sírvase caminar sobre los talones.
8. Haga el favor de doblarse hacia adelante.
   Favor de doblarse hacia adelante.
   Tenga la bondad de doblarse hacia adelante.
   Sírvase doblarse hacia adelante.
9. Haga el favor de doblarse hacia atrás.
   Favor de doblarse hacia atrás.
   Tenga la bondad de doblarse hacia atrás.
   Sírvase doblarse hacia atrás.
10. Haga el favor de doblar el tronco hacia adelante todo lo que pueda.
    Favor de doblar el tronco hacia adelante todo lo que pueda.
    Tenga la bondad de doblar el tronco hacia adelante todo lo que pueda.
    Sírvase doblar el tronco hacia adelante todo lo que pueda.
11. Haga el favor de cerrar la mano.
    Favor de cerrar la mano.
    Tenga la bondad de cerrar la mano.
    Sírvase cerrar la mano.
12. Haga el favor de abrirla.
    Favor de abrirla.
    Tenga la bondad de abrirla.
    Sírvase abrirla.
13. Haga el favor de cerrar el puño.
    Favor de cerrar el puño.
    Tenga la bondad de cerrar el puño.
    Sírvase cerrar el puño.
14. Haga el favor de abrirlo.
    Favor de abrirlo.
    Tenga la bondad de abrirlo.
    Sírvase abrirlo.
15. Haga el favor de apretar mis manos con fuerza.
    Favor de apretar mis manos con fuerza.
    Tenga la bondad de apretar mis manos con fuerza.
    Sírvase apretar mis manos con fuerza.
16. Haga el favor de empujar mi mano tan fuerte como pueda.
    Favor de empujar mi mano tan fuerte como pueda.
    Tenga la bondad de empujar mi mano tan fuerte como pueda.
    Sírvase empujar mi mano tan fuerte como pueda.
17. Haga el favor de apretar fuerte mis dedos tanto como pueda.
    Favor de apretar fuerte mis dedos tanto como pueda.
    Tenga la bondad de apretar fuerte mis dedos tanto como pueda.
    Sírvase apretar fuerte mis dedos tanto como pueda.
18. Haga el favor de no dejarme mover su ____.
    Favor de no dejarme mover su ____.
    Tenga la bondad de no dejarme mover su ____.
    Sírvase no dejarme mover su ____.

19. Haga el favor de relajarse / relajar el cuerpo y dejarme mover su
    ____.
    Favor de relajarse / relajar el cuerpo y dejarme mover su ____.
    Tenga la bondad de relajarse / relajar el cuerpo y dejarme mover su
    ____.
    Sírvase relajarse / relajar el cuerpo y dejarme mover su ____.
20. Haga el favor de subir / levantar los brazos.
    Favor de subir / levantar los brazos.
    Tenga la bondad de subir / levantar los brazos.
    Sírvase subir / levantar los brazos.

21. Haga el favor de levantar / subir los brazos completamente.
    Favor de levantar / subir los brazos completamente.
    Tenga la bondad de levantar / subir los brazos completamente.
    Sírvase levantar / subir los brazos completamente.
22. Haga el favor de levantar / subir la pierna izquierda (derecha).
    Favor de levantar / subir la pierna izquierda (derecha).
    Tenga la bondad de levantar / subir la pierna izquierda (derecha).
    Sírvase levantar / subir la pierna izquierda (derecha).

CHAPTER 11

CAPITULO

Page 220

PRACTICE   *PRACTICA*

Translate into Spanish:

1. Vd. debe visitar a / consultar con un obstétrico / una obstétrica.
2. Mientras esté encinta / en estado, debe tomar una dieta balanceada.
3. ¿Cuándo va a dar luz?

4. El médico / La médica tiene los resultados de sus pruebas.
5. Debe evitar (cualquier) actividad vigorosa.
6. Tiene contracciones uterinas cada tres minutos.

Tradúzcase al inglés:

1. I have never had an abortion.
2. S/He has to breathe deeply.
3. I intend to nurse my baby.
4. You should see your obstetrician regularly.

5. The use of non-prescription drugs / The use of drugs not prescribed by your doctor harms the fetus.
6. There are no side effects.

Page 230

Preguntas:

1. El Sr. Rojas tiene hernia. Está en el hospital para una operación de hernia.
2. Piensan hacerle la operación mañana.
3. El Dr. Martínez es el anestesiólogo que le administrará la anestesia para la operación de su hernia. Le hace unas preguntas para conocerle y su historial mejor.
4. Sí, tiene alergia a la penicilina.
5. La condición cardíaca del Sr. Rojas es bastante seria, pero ahora no es crítica.
6. Toma muchas medicinas: veinte miligramos de Inderal cuatro veces al día, dos tabletas de ochenta miligramos de Lasix a las ocho de la mañana y otra tableta adicional a las dos de la tarde; y dos píldoras rosadas de Isordil cuando sufre un ataque de angina o cuando se encuentra en una situación que cree que le causará un ataque.
7. Al subir las escaleras tiene calambres o dolores en las piernas.
8. El anestesiólogo decide posponer la operación del Sr. Rojas hasta que se mejoren algunos aspectos de su salud.

9. No le darán el desayuno la mañana de la operación para prevenir la aspiración cuando se le anestesie—si come, le podrá venir a la boca todo lo que haya tomado que puede ser aspirado y alojado en los pulmones. Esto puede provocar la pulmonía y aun podrá ser fatal.
10. Puede comer y beber hasta medianoche.
11. Le recetará una inyección para hacerle dormir antes de bajarle a la sala de operaciones.
12. Van a ponerle la inyección o en el brazo o en la nalga.
13. El anestesiólogo piensa determinar el ritmo del corazón con los terminales del electrocardiograma.
14. Se dormirá casi en seguida al recibir pentotal de sodio.
15. La operación durará entre cuarenta y cinco minutos y una hora.
16. Siempre queda la posibilidad de efectos secundarios de la anestesia como un dolor de garganta y ronquera por unos días.
17. Las enfermeras en la sala de recuperación estarán al tanto de sus reacciones cada quince minutos y le aconsejarán que tosa y respire profundamente.

Page 243

Rewrite All Polite Commands:

35. Favor de guardar (almacenar) todas las medicinas y cosas peligrosas (tóxicas) fuera del alcance de los niños.
    Haga el favor de guardar (almacenar) todas las medicinas y cosas peligrosas (tóxicas) fuera del alcance de los niños.
    Tenga la bondad de guardar (almacenar) todas las medicinas y cosas peligrosas (tóxicas) fuera del alcance de los niños.
    Sírvase guardar (almacenar) todas las medicinas y cosas peligrosas (tóxicas) fuera del alcance de los niños.
36. Favor de guardar (almacenar) todas las medicinas y otros productos peligrosos en un gabinete cerrado con llave.
    Haga el favor de guardar (almacenar) todas las medicinas y otros productos peligrosos en un gabinete cerrado con llave.
    Tenga la bondad de guardar (almacenar) todas las medicinas y otros productos peligrosos en un gabinete cerrado con llave.
    Sírvase guardar (almacenar) todas las medicinas y otros productos peligrosos en un gabinete cerrado con llave.

37. Favor de nunca dejar ninguna medicina al alcance de la mano cuando vaya a contestar al teléfono o abrir la puerta.
    Haga el favor de nunca dejar ninguna medicina al alcance de la mano cuando vaya a contestar al teléfono o abrir la puerta.
    Tenga la bondad de nunca dejar ninguna medicina al alcance de la mano cuando vaya a contestar al teléfono o abrir la puerta.
    Sírvase nunca dejar ninguna medicina al alcance de la mano cuando vaya a contestar al teléfono o abrir la puerta.
38. Favor de darle al niño (a la niña) la cantidad recetada.
    Haga el favor de darle al niño (a la niña) la cantidad recetada.
    Tenga la bondad de darle al niño (a la niña) la cantidad recetada.
    Sírvase darle al niño (a la niña) la cantidad recetada.
39. Favor de leer cuidadosamente las etiquetas de las medicinas que se venden sin receta (remedios caseros; medicinas patentadas; medicinas auto-prescritas) y consultar a su farmacéutico (farmacéutica) o médico (médica) para saber si deben darse o no a los niños si Vd.

tiene alguna duda.

Haga el favor de leer cuidadosamente las etiquetas de las medicinas que se venden sin receta (remedios caseros; medicinas patentadas; medicinas auto-prescritas) y consultar a su farmacéutico (farmacéutica) o médico (médica) para saber si deben darse o no a los niños si Vd. tiene alguna duda.

Tenga la bondad de leer cuidadosamente las etiquetas de las medicinas que se venden sin receta (remedios caseros; medicinas patentadas; medicinas auto-prescritas) y consultar a su farmacéutico (farmacéutica) o médico (médica) para saber si deben darse o no a los niños si Vd. tiene alguna duda.

Sírvase leer cuidadosamente las etiquetas de las medicinas que se venden sin receta (remedios caseros; medicinas patentadas; medicinas auto-prescritas) y consultar a su farmacéutico (farmacéutica) o médico (médica) para saber si deben darse o no a los niños si Vd. tiene alguna duda.

40. Favor de pedir a su farmacéutico (farmacéutica) un envase de seguridad. . .
Haga el favor de pedir a su farmacéutico (farmacéutica) un envase de seguridad. . .
Tenga la bondad de pedir a su farmacéutico (farmacéutica) un envase de seguridad. . .
Sírvase pedir a su farmacéutico (farmacéutica) un envase de seguridad. . .

41. Favor de nunca decirle a un niño (una niña) que es un «dulce» o algo que le guste.
Haga el favor de nunca decirle a un niño (una niña) que es un «dulce» o algo que le guste.
Tenga la bondad de nunca decirle a un niño (una niña) que es un «dulce» o algo que le guste.
Sírvase nunca decirle a un niño (una niña) que es un «dulce» o algo que le guste.

CHAPTER 13

▌ *CAPITULO*

Pages 281

PREGUNTAS

1. Adela Mendoza tiene un diente de leche que tiene un absceso.
2. Le pregunta la edad de ella (¿Cuántos años tiene?), su peso (¿Cuánto pesa?), y si es alérgica a algunas medicinas.
3. La medicina se llama V-cillin K. Tiene que tomarla cuatro veces al día. (Debe tomar dos cucharaditas inmediatamente y después una

cucharadita cada cuatro horas hoy, y después una cucharadita después del desayuno, del almuerzo, de la cena, y al acostarse.)
4. Al volver a casa tiene que tomar dos cucharaditas de la medicina inmediatamente.

CHAPTER 15

▌ *CAPITULO*

Page 310

QUESTIONS:

1. Normal temperature is 98.6°F [37°C].
2. Yes, it fluctuates between 97.7°F and 98.6°F [36.5°C and 37°C].
3. No, an elevated temperature alone, without any other symptoms does not indicate a medical problem.
4. The little arrow on the thermometer shows the normal temperature limit which is 98.6°F [37°C].
5. Yes, there is a difference between the normal oral temperature, which is about 98.6°F [37°C], and the rectal one, which is 99.6°F [37.5°C].
6. It is necessary to be gentle when taking a rectal temperature in order not to harm the rectum.
7. About two minutes.

Pages 311–312

PREGUNTAS

1. Se considera normal una temperatura que oscila entre 97.7°F y 98.6°F [36.5°C y 37°C].
2. Sí, hay mucha variación de temperatura.
3. Una elevación de temperatura en sí, sin otros síntomas, no es señal de un problema médico.
4. La flechita muestra el límite de la temperatura normal, que es los 98.6°F [37°C].
5. Sí, la temperatura rectal normal generalmente es un grado más alto que la oral normal, es decir, los 99.6°F [37.5°C].
6. Es importante tener mucho cuidado al insertar un termómetro rectal para no dañar el recto del niño.
7. Unos dos minutos.

Page 320

PREGUNTAS:

1. Si no se trata la diabetes, puede causar invalideces, y hasta la muerte.
2. Algunas personas pueden controlar su diabetes solamente con insulina; otras pueden controlarla con dieta, ejercicios, y píldoras.
3. La diabetes insulino-dependiente a veces es llamada *diabetes de tipo I o diabetes (del principio) juvenil o precoz* porque ocurre en muchachos, adolescentes, y jóvenes que tienen menos de veinte años. En este tipo de diabetes, el páncreas no produce la insulina. Necesitan

una inyección de insulina todos los días. A diferencia es la *diabetes de tipo II o diabetes adquirida durante la madurez, o del adulto o de comienzo tardío.* Con este tipo de diabetes, el páncreas no produce *suficiente* cantidad de insulina para controlar el nivel de la glucosa en la sangre. Algunas personas con este tipo de diabetes pueden controlar el nivel de la glucosa en la sangre con dieta, ejercicio, y píldoras. Otras se inyectan diariamente con insulina.
4. Se puede sufrir de hipoglicemia.

Page 321

QUESTIONS:

1. Indigestion or heartburn, flatulence, nausea and belching, or regurgitation are early symptoms of gallbladder problems.
2. The problem is diagnosed from previous medical history, pain, or tenderness. A special gallbladder X-ray, a *cholecystogram*, makes the problem evident as does as ultrasound.
3. The doctor may suggest removing the gallstones surgically.

Page 322

PREGUNTAS:

1. Los síntomas de la enfermedad de la vesícula biliar incluyen la indigestión, o ardor epigástrico, después de comer alimentos fritos, legumbres ásperas, o fruta cruda, flatulencia, náusea y eructos, o vómitos.
2. Se diagnostican los cálculos biliares por medio de previo historial médico, dolor, y sensibilidad; una radiografía especial de la vesícula biliar, *un colecistograma*, o por medio de ondas ultrasónicas.
3. Un tratamiento para los cálculos biliares es la cirugía.

Page 323

QUESTIONS:

1. The kidneys filter the blood and remove unnecessary products from the body.
2. Kidney stones may block the flow of urine from the kidney to the urinary bladder, they may produce intense pain.
3. They may be treated surgically or with appropriate diet and drugs.

Page 324

PREGUNTAS:

1. Los riñones filtran la sangre y quitan del cuerpo todos los elementos que no sean necesarios.
2. Una obstrucción de la vía urinaria por un cálculo renal puede dañar a los riñones. También puede producir un dolor horrible.
3. Se pueden tratar los cálculos renales con cirugía, o con un régimen dietético y medicinas.

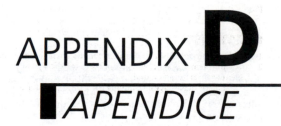

APPENDIX D
APENDICE

Selected Bibliography
Bibliografía selecta

Aday, L.A., Andersen, R.A. "A Framework for the Study of Access to Medical Care." *Health Serv Res* 1974; 9:208–220.

Aday, L.A., Anderson, R., Fleming, G.V. *Health Care in the U.S.: Equitable for Whom?* Beverly Hills: Sage Publications, 1980.

Aday, L.A., Anderson, R.M. "The National Profile of Access to Medical Care: Where Do We Stand?" *American Journal Public Health* 1984; 74:1331–1339.

Aguilar, I., Wood, V.N. "Aspects of Death, Grief and Mourning in the Treatment of Spanish-Speaking Mental Patients." *Journal of the National Association of Social Workers, Vol. 21 (1976), 49–54.*

Aguirre, S.T., Ito, K.L. *Maternal and Child Health Profile for Hispanics in California.* Sacramento, California: Health Officers Association of California, Border Maternal and Child Health Project, 1985.

Alcocer, A.M. "Alcohol Use and Abuse Among the Hispanic American Population." *In National Institute on Alcohol Abuse and Alcoholism.* Special Population Issues. Alcohol and Health Monograph No.4. DHHS Pub. No. ADM 82-1193. Washington, DC: Government Printing Office, 1982.

Alegria, D., Guerra, E., Martinez, C. Jr., Meyer, G.G. "El hospital invisible. A Study of *Curanderismo.*" Arch-Gen-Psychiatry 34 (11) (Nov. 1977) 1354–1357.

Andersen, R.M., Giachello, A.L., Aday, L.A. "Access of Hispanics to Health Care and Cuts in Services: A State of the Arts Overview." *Public Health Rep.* 101(3) (May-Jun. 1986) 238–252.

Angel, R., Guarnaccia, P.J. "Mind, Body, and Culture: Somatization among Hispanics." *Soc Sci Med* 1989; 28:1229–1238.

Angel, R., Worobey, J.L. "Acculturation and Material Reports of Children's Health: Evidence from the Hispanic Health and Nutrition Examination Survey." *Soc Sci Q* 1988; 69:707–721.

Angel, R., Worobey, J.L. "Single Motherhood and Children's Health." *Journal of Health and Social Behavior* 1988; 29:38–52.

Aponte, R. and Siles, M. *Latinos in the Heartland: The Browning of the Midwest.* Lansing, MI: Julian Samora Research Institute, November 1994.

Arce, C.H., Torres, D.L. "The Effects of Cultural Assimilation Y Education on Mexican American Workers' Earnings." *Economic Outlook USA,* v.10, n.4 (Autumn, 1983) 87–90.

Argüiro Martinez, R., ed. *Hispanic Culture and Health Care: Fact, Fiction, Folklore.* St. Louis: C.V. Mosby, 1978.

Arredondo, R., Weddige, R.L., Justice, C.L., Fitz, J. "Alcoholism in Mexican-Americans: Intervention and Treatment. *Hospital Community Psychiatry* 1987; 38:180–183.

Baca, J.E. "Some Health Beliefs of the Spanish Speaking." *American Journal of Nursing,* Vol. 69, No. 10, 2172–2176.

Bang, K.M., Gerge, P.J., Carroll, J. "Prevalence of Chronic Bronchitis among US Hispanics from the Hispanic Health and Nutrition Examination Survey, 1982–84." *American Journal of Public Health* 80(12): 1495–1497.

Baranowski, T., Bee, D.E., Rassin, D.K., Richardson, C.J., Brown, J.P., Guenther, N., Nader, P.R. "Social Support, Social Influence, Ethnicity and the Breastfeeding Decision." *Soc-Sci-Med* 17 (21) (1983) 1599–611.

Baumgartner, R.N., Roche, A.F., Guo, S., Chumlea, W.C., Ryan, A.S. "Fat Patterning and Centralized Obesity in Mexican American Children in the Hispanic Health and Nutrition Examination Survey (HHANES 1982–84)." *American Journal of Clinical Nutrition* 1990; 51:936S–943S.

Beals, R.L. *Cheran: A Sierra Tarascan Village.* Publications of the Institute of Social Anthropology, No. 2. Washington, DC: Smithsonian Institution, 1946.

Becerra, J.E., Hogue, C.J.R., Atrash, H. Pérez, N. "Infant Mortality among Hispanics." *Journal of the American Medical Association.* 1991; 265:217–221.

Berkanovic, E., Telesky, C. "Mexican-American, Black-American and White-American Differences in Reporting Illnesses, Disability and Physician Visits for Illnesses." *Soc. Sci-Med.* 20 (6) (1985) 567–77.

Black, S.A. & Markides, K.S. "Acculturation and Alcohol Consumption in Puerto Rican, Cuban-American, and Mexican-American Women in the United States." *American Journal of Public Health* 1993, 83, 890–893.

Boyoko, E.J., Keane, E.M., Marshall, J.A., Jamman, R.F. "Higher Insulin and C-Peptide Concentrations in Hispanic Population at High Risk for NIDDM." *Diabetes* 40:509–515.

Brook, J.S., Whiteman, M., Balka, E.B. & Hamburg, B.A. "African-American and Puerto Rican Drug Use: Personality, Familial, and Other Environmental Risk Factors." *Genetic, Social, and General Psychology Monographs* 1992, 118, 417–438.

Brown, J.P. "Dental Health Status and Treatment Needs among Mexican Americans," *Hispanic Health Status Symposium Proceedings* 1989.

Bruhn, J.G., Fuentes, R.G. "Cultural Factors Affecting Utilization of Services by Mexican Americans." *Psychiatric Ann* 1977; 7(12):608–613.

Burnam, A., Hough, R.L., Karno, M., Escobar, J.I., Tellese, C.A. "Acculturation and Lifetime Prevalence of Psychiatric Disorders among Mexican Americans in Los Angeles." *Journal of Health and Social Behavior* 1987; 28:89–102.

Burnside, M.A., Baer, P.E., McLaugh, R.J., Pokorny, A.D. "Alcohol Use by Adolescents in Disrupted Families." *Alcoholism* 1986; 10:274-8.

Burt, B.A., Ismail, A.I., Eklund, S.A. "Periodontal Disease, Tooth Loss, and Oral Hygiene among Older Americans." *Community Dental and Oral Epidemiology* 1985; 13:93–96.

Byers, T.E., Graham, S., Jaughey, B.P., Marshall, J.R., Swanson, M.K. "Diet and Lung Cancer Risk." Fundings from the Western New York Diet Study. *American Journal of Epidemiology* 1987; 125:351–363.

Caetano, R. "Self-Reported Intoxication among Hispanics in Northern California." *J-Study-Alcohol* 45(4) (Jul, 1984) 349–354.

Caetano, R. "Acculturation and Attitudes toward Appropriate Drinking among US Hispanics." *Alcohol* 1987; 22:427–433.

Caetano, R. "Acculturation and Drinking patterns among US Hispanics." *Br J Addict* 1987; 82: 789–799.

Caetano, R. "Acculturation, Drinking and Social Settings among US Hispanics." *Drug and Alcohol Dependence* 1987; 19:215–226.

Caetano, R. "Drinking Patterns and Alcohol Problems among Hispanics in the US. A Review." *Drug and Alcohol Depend* 1983; 12:37–59.

Caetano, R. "Hispanic Drinking Practices in Northern California." *Hispanic Journal of Behavioral Sciences* 1984; 6(4):345–364.

California Center for Health Statistics: *Diabetes among California Hispanics 1979-80.* Data Matters Topical Reports, No. 83-05079. Sacramento: State of California, 1983.

California Center for Health Statistics: *Health Status of Californians by Race/Ethnicity, 1970 and 1980.* Data matters, No. 84-02085. Sacramento: State of California, Health and Welfare Agency, 1984.

Cancer Facts and Figures for Minority Americans, Atlanta, GA: American Cancer Society, 1991.

Carrier, J.M. "Cultural Factors Affecting Urban Mexican Male Homosexual Behavior." *Archives of Sexual Behavior.* Vol. 5 (1976), 103–124.

Carrier, J.M. "Family Attitudes and Mexican Male Homosexuality." *Urban Life.* Vol. 5 (1976), 359–375.

Carroll, M.D., Sempos, C.T., Fullwood, R.F., *et al.* "Serum Lipids and Lipoproteins of Hispanics, 1982-84." National Center for Health Statistics. *Vital and Health Statistics.* 11(240). Washington, DC. Government Printing Office, 1990.

Carter-Pokras, O., Pirkle, J., Chavez, G., Gunter, E. "Blood Lead Levels of 4-11 Year Old Mexican American, Puerto Rican And Cuban Children." *Public Health Rep* 1990; 105:388–393.

Casas, J.M., Bimbela, A., Corral, C.V.,Yáñez, I., Swaim, R.C., Wayman, J.C. & Bates, S. "Cigarette and Smokeless Tobacco Use among Migrant and Nonmigrant Mexican American Youth, *Hispanic Journal of Behavioral Sciences.* 1998; 20(1):102–121.

Centers for Disease Control and Prevention. "Attempted Suicide among High School Students: United States, 1990." *Morbidity and Mortality Weekly Report,* Youth Risk Behavior Surveillance System, Vol. 40, No. 37, September 21, 1991.

Centers for Disease Control and Prevention. "Sexual Behavior among High School Students—United States, 1990" *Morbidity and Mortality Weekly Report.* Vol. 40, Nos. 51, 52. January 3, 1992.

Centers for Disease Control and Prevention. "Incidence and Impact of Selected Infectious Diseases in Childhood." *National Center for Health Statistics.* 1991: series 10, no. 180, October.

Centers for Disease Control and Prevention. *Impact of HIV/AIDS on Hispanics in the United States.* CDC Update, June 1998.

Chavez, E.L. & Swaim, R.C. "Hispanic Substance Use: Problems in Epidemiology." *Drugs and Society.* 1992, 6, 211–230.

Chavez, L.R., Cornelius, W.A., Jones, O.W. "Mexican Immigrants and the Utilization of U.S. Health Services: The Case of San Diego." *Soc. Sci Med.* 21 (1) (1985) 93–102.

Chavez, L.R. "The Power of the Imagined Community: The Settlement of Undocumented Mexicans and Central Americans in the United States." *American Anthropologist.* 96 (Mar. 1994). 52–73.

Chavez, L.R., Hubbell, F.A., McMullin, J.M., & Martinez, R.G. "Structure and Meaning in Models of Breast and Cervical Cancer Risk Factors: A Comparison of Perceptions among *Latinas,* Anglo Women, and Physicians. *Medical Anthropology Quarterly.* 1995; 9 (1):40–74.

Chavez, L.R., Hubbell, F.A., Mishra, S.I., & Burciaga Valdez, R. "The Influence of Fatalism on Self-Reported Use of Papanicolaou Smears." *American Journal of Preventive Medicine.* 1997; 13(6), 418–424.

Chavez, L.R., Hubbell, F.A., Mishra, S.I., Burciaga Valdez, R. "Undocumented *Latina* Immigrants in Orange County, California: A Comparative Analysis." *The International Migration Review.* 1997; 31(1), 88–107.

Chavez, L.R., Cornelius, W.A., & Jones, O.W. "Utilization of Health Services by Mexican Immigrant Women in San Diego," *Women & Health* 11(2), Summer 1986, 3–20.

Chesney, A.P., Chavira, J.A., Hall, R.P., Gary, H.E., Jr. "Barriers to Medical Care of Mexican-Americans: The Role of Social Classes, Acculturation, and Social Isolation." *Med-Care.* 20 (9) (Sep, 1982) 883–891.

Chesney, A.P., Thompson, B.L., Guevara, A., Vela, A., Schottstaedt, M.F. "Mexican-American Folk Medicine: Implications for the Family Physician." *J-Fam-Pract* 11(4) (Oct. 1980) 567–574.

Christian, C.M., Zobeck, T.S., Malin, H.J., Hitchcock, D.C. "Self-Reported Alcohol Use and Abuse among Mexican Americans: Preliminary Findings from the Hispanic Health and Nutrition Examination Survey Adult Sample Person Supplement." *In* Spiegler, D.L., Tate, D.A., Aitken, S.S., Christian, C.M. (eds). *Alcohol Use Among US Ethnic Minorities.* Proceedings of a Conference on the Epidemiology of Alcohol Use and Abuse among Ethnic Minority Groups, September 1985. Research Monograph No 18, National Institute on Alcohol Abuse and Alcoholism. DHHS Pub. No. ADM89-1435, Rockville, MD, 1989.

Cisernos, H.C., Di Angelis, A.J., Katz, R.V. "Oral Health Findings in a Minnesota Latino Population." *Northwest Dent* 1979; 58:7–11.

Clark, M. *Health in the Mexican American Culture.* 2nd ed. Berkeley: University of California Press, 1970.

Clark, M., Mendelson, M. "Mexican-American Aged in San Francisco: A Case Description." *Gerontologist,* Vol. 9 (1969), 90–95.

Clark, R. *Hispanic Attitudes on Cancer.* Prepared by Clark, Martire, and Bartolome. New York City: American Cancer Society, 1985.

Cobos, R. *A Dictionary of New Mexico and Southern Colorado Spanish.* Santa Fe: Museum of New Mexico Press, 1983.

Cockerham, W.C., Alster, J.M. "A Comparison of Marijuana Use Among Mexican-American and Anglo Rural Youth Utilizing a Matched-Set Analysis." *Int-J-Addict* 18(6) (Aug. 1983) 759–767.

Cohen, L.M. *Culture, Disease and Stress Among Latino Immigrants.* Research Institute on Immigration and Ethnic Studies Special Study. Washington, DC: The Catholic University of American, 1979.

Cohen, W.D., Friedman, L.A., Shapiro, J., Kyle, C.G., Franklin, S. "Diabetes Mellitus and Periodontal Disease: Two Year Longitudinal Observations." I.J. Periodontal 1970; 41:709–712.

Cooney, R. "Demographic Component of Growth in White, Black, and Puerto Rican Female Headed Families: A Comparison of the Cutright and Ross/Sawhill Methodologies." *Soc Sci Res* 1979; 8:144–158.

Costantino, G., Malgady, R.G., Rogler, L.H. "*Cuento* Therapy: A Culturally Sensitive Modality for Puerto Rican Children." *Journal Consult Clin Psychology.* 54 (5) (Oct. 1986), 639–645.

Council on Scientific Affairs. "Hispanic Health in the United States," *Journal of the American Medical Association.* 1991: 265:248–252.

Coultas, D.B., Harvard, C.A., Peake, G.T., Skipper, B.J., Samet, J.M. "Discrepancies Between Self-Reported and Validated Cigarette Smoking in a Community Survey of New Mexico Hispanics." *Am Rev Respir Dis* 1988; 137:810–814.

Cox, C. "Physician Utilization by Three Groups of Ethnic Elderly." *Med-Care.* 24 (8) (Aug. 1986) 667–676.

"The Culture of Illness," *U.S. News and World Report,* February 15, 1993, p. 76.

Currier, R.L. "The Hot-Cold Syndrome and Symbolic Balance in Mexican and Spanish-American Folk Medicine." *Ethnology,* Vol. 5 (1966), 251–263.

Daly, M., Osborne, C., Clark, G., McGuire, W. "Mexican-American Breast Cancer Patients Have a Worse Prognosis (Abstract)." *Proc Am Soc Clin Oncol* 1983; 2:C-18.

Dancy, B., Logan, B. "Culture and Ethnicity." *In* Bolander V. (ed.). *Sorensen and Luckmann's Basic Nursing* (3rd ed.) (pp. 331–342). Philadelphia: W.B. Saunders, 1994.

De La Rosa, M.R., H.J. Khalsa, and B.A. Rouse. "Hispanics and Illicit Drug Use: A Review of Recent Findings." *International Journal of Addiction.* 1990; 25:665–691.

De La Torre, A., Rush, L. "The Effects of Health Care Access on Maternal and Infant Health of California Migrant Seasonal Farm Worker Women." *Border Health* 1987; 3:18–25.

Delgado, J.L. and Treviño, F.M. "The State of Hispanic Health in the United States." In Obledo, M.G., (ed.): *The State of National Hispanic Center for Advanced Studies and Policy Analysis and the National Hispanic University,* 1985.

Diabetes Among Latinos. Washington, DC: National Council of La Raza, 1996.

Díaz, R. "Latino Gay Men and the Psycho-Cultural Barriers to AIDS Prevention," In Levine, M., Gagnon, J., Narde, P., (eds.). *A Plague of Our Own: The Impact of the AIDS Epidemic on Gay Men and Lesbians.* Chicago: University of Chicago Press, 1995.

Díz, R.M. *HIV Risk in Latino Gay/Bisexual Men: A Review of Behavioral Research.* San Francisco, CA: National Latino/a Lesbian and Gay Organization, 1995.

Díz, T., Buehler, J.W., Castro, K.G., et. al. "AIDS Trends among Hispanos in the United States," *American Journal of Public Health.* 1993: 83:504–509.

Dowling, P.T., Fisher, M. "Maternal Factors and Low Birthweight Infants: A Comparison of Blacks with Mexican Americans." *J Fam Pract* 1987; 25:153–158.

Dutton, D.B. "Explaining the Low Use of Health Services by the Poor: Costs, Attitudes, or Delivery Systems?" *Am Soc Rev* 1978; 43:348–368.

Eberstein, I.W., Pol, L.G. "Mexican American Ethnicity, Socioeconomic Status, and Infant Mortality: A County Level Analysis." *Soc Sci J.* 1982; 19:161–171.

Edgerton, R.B., Fernández, I. "*Curanderismo* in the Metropolis: The Diminishing Role of Folk-Psychiatry Among Los Angeles Mexican Americans." *American Journal of Psychotherapy.* 24 (1970), 124–134.

Eisenbruch, M. "Cross-Cultural Aspects of Bereavement: Ethnic and Cultural Variations in the Development of Bereavement Practices." *Culture, Medicine and Psychiatry.* 8(4)(Dec., 1984), 315–347.

Eklund, S.A., Ismail, A.I. "Time of Development of Occlusal and Proximal Lesions: Implications for Fissure Sealants." *J Public Health Dent* 1986; 46:114–121.

Escobedo, L.G., Remington, P.L., Anda, R.F. "Long-Term Age-Specific Prevalence of Cigarette Smoking among Hispanics in the United States." *Journal of Psychoactive Drugs.* 1989; 21:307–318.

Escobedo, L.G., Remington, P.L., Anda, R.F. "Long-Term Secular Trends in Initiation of Cigarette Smoking among Hispanics in the United States." *Public Health Rep* 1989; 104:583–587.

Escobedo, L.G., Remington, P.L. "Birth Cohort Analysis of Prevalence of Cigarette Smoking among Hispanics in the United States." *Journal of the American Medical Association.* 1989; 261:66–69.

Fanelli-Kuczmarski, M.T., Johnson, C.L., Elias, L. Najjar, M.F. "Folate Status of Mexican American, Cuban and Puerto Rican Women." *Am J Clin Nutr.* 1990; 52:368–372.

Fanelli-Kuczmarski, M. Woteki, C.E. "Monitoring the Nutritional Status of the Hispanic Population: Selected Findings for Mexican Americans, Cubans and Puerto Ricans." *Nutrition Today.* May-June 1990; 6–11.

Farge, E.J. "Medical Orientation Among a Mexican-American Population: An Old and a New Model Reviewed." *Soc-Sci-Med.* 12 (2A) (July, 1978), 277–282.

Fearon, Z. "Communication and the Medical Care Process." *Consumer Health Perspectives.* VII(5):1–7.

Firth, R. "Acculturation in Relation to Concepts of Health and Disease." *In* Goldstone, I. (ed.): *Medicine and Anthropology.* No. XXI of the New York Academy of Medicine Lectures to the Laity. New York: Books for Libraries Press, 1971.

Flegal, K.M., Ezzati, T.M., Harris, M.I., *et al.* "Prevalence of Diabetes in Mexican Americans, Cubans and Puerto Ricans from the Hispanic Health and Nutrition Examination Survey, 1982–84." *Diabetes Care.* 1991; 14(7):628–638.

Ford, E.S., Harel, Y., Heath, G., Cooper, R.S., Caspersen, C.J. "Test Characteristics of Self-Reported Hypertension Among the Hispanic Population: Findings from the Hispanic Health and Nutrition Examination Survey." *J Clin Epidemiol.* 1990; 43:159–165.

Foreman, J.T. "*Susto* and the Health Needs of the Cuban Refugee Population." *Topics in Clinical Nursing.* 1985; 7(3), 40–47.

Foster, G.M. "Relationships Between Spanish and Spanish-American Folk-Medicine." *Journal of American Folklore.* 66, (261) (1953), 201–217.

Foster, G.M., Rowe, J.H. "Suggestions for Field Recording of Information on the Hippocratic Classification of diseases and Remedies." *Kroeber Anthropological Society Papers.* Vol. V (1951), 1–3.

Fraser, D., Piacentini, J., Van Rossem, R., Hien, D., & Rotheram-Borus, M.J. "Effects of Acculturation and Psychopathology on Sexual Behavior and Substance Use of Suicidal Hispanic Adolescents," *Hispanic Journal of Behavioral Sciences,* 1998, 20 (1):83–101.

Fried, J. "Acculturation and Mental Health Among Indian Migrants in Peru." *In* Opler, M.K. (ed.): *Culture and Mental Health.* New York: Macmillan Co., 1959.

Friedman, L.A., Kimball, A.W. "Coronary Heart Disease Mortality and Alcohol Consumption in Framingham." *American Journal of Epidemiology.* 1986; 124:481–489.

Friis, R., Nanjundppa, G., Pedergast, T.J., Welsh, M. "Coronary Heart Disease Mortality and Risk Among Hispanics and Non-Hispanics in Orange County, California." *Public Health Rep.* 1981; 96:418–422.

Gali, H. *Hojas que curan.* Mexico City: Gómez Gómez Hermanos, 1985.

Gali, H. *Las hierbas del indio.* Mexico City: Gómez Gómez Hermanos, 1985.

Galli, N. "The Influence of Cultural Heritage on the Health Status of Puerto Ricans." *Journal of School Health.* 45 (1975), 10–16.

Garcia, J.A., Juarey, R.A. "Utilization of Dental Health Services by Chicanos and Anglos." *Journal of Health and Social Behavior.* 1978; 19:428–436.

Gardner, L.I., Jr., Stern, M.P., Haffner, S.M., *et al.* "Prevalence of Diabetes in Mexican Americans: Relationship to Percent of Gene Pool Derived from Native American Sources." *Diabetes.* 1984; 33:86–92.

Garrison, V. "The 'Puerto Rican Syndrome' in Psychiatry and Expiritismo." *In* Crapanzano, V. And Garrison, V. (eds.). *Case Studies in Spirit Possession.* New York: Wiley, 1977.

Gergen, P.J., Ezzati, T., Russell, H. "DTP Immunization Status and Tetanus Antitoxin Titers of Mexican American Children Ages 6 Months Through Eleven Years." *American Journal of Public Health.* 1988; 78:1446–1450.

Giachello, A.L. "Hispanics and Health Care." *In:* Cafferty, P.S.J. and McCready, (eds.). *Hispanics in the United States, a New Social Agenda.* NJ: Transaction Books, 1985.

Gilbert, M.J., Cervantes, R.C. "Patterns and Practices of Alcohol Use among Mexican Americans: A Comprehensive Review." *Hispanic Journal of Behavioral Science.* 1986; 8:1–60.

Gilbert, M.J., "Alcohol Consumption Patterns in Immigrant and Later Generation Mexican American Women." *Hispanic Journal of Behavioral Science.* 1987; 9:299–313.

Gillin, J. "Magical Fright." *Psychiatry.* Vol. 11 (1948), 387–400.

Gilman, S.C., Bruhn, J.G. "A Comparison of Utilization of Community Primary Health Care and School Health Services by Urban Mexican-American and Anglo Elementary School Children." *Med-Care.* 19 (2) (Feb. 1981) 223–232.

Gluck, G.M., Knox, C.D., Glass, R.L., Wolfman, M. "Dental Health of Puerto Rican Migrant Workers." *Health Services Rep.* 1972; 87:456–460.

Gómez, C.A. and Marin, B.V. "Gender, Culture, and Power: Barriers to HIV Prevention Strategies for Women," *Journal of Sex Research.* 1996; 33: 355–362.

González—Swafford, M.J., Gutiérrez, M.G. "Ethno-Medical Beliefs and Practices of Mexican-Americans." *Nurse-Pract.* 8 (10) (Nov-Dec., 1983) 29–30, 32, 34.

Graham, J. "The Role of the *Curandero* in the Mexican-American Folk Medicine System in West Texas." *American Folk Medicine: A Symposium Study of Comparative Folklore and Mythology. In* Hand, W.D. (ed.): U. of California Press, 1976.

Guendelman, S. "At Risk: Health Needs of Hispanic Children." *Health-Soc-Work.* 10 (3) (Summer, 1985) 183–90.

Guendelman, S., Abrams, B. "Dietary Intake among Mexican-American Women: Generational Differences and a Comparison with White Non-Hispanic Women." *American Journal of Public Health.* 1995; 85:20–25.

Guendelman, S., Schwalbe, J. "Medical Care Utilization by Hispanic Children. How does It Differ from Black and White Peers?" *Med. Care.* 24 (10) (Oct. 1986): 925–40.

Gurnack, A.M. *Access to Health in an Hispanic Community. In:* Hispanic Health Services Research Conference Proceedings. Washington, DC: Government Printing Office, 1980.

Gwinn, M.L., Webster, L.A., Lee, N.C., Layde, P.M., Rubin, G.L. "Alcohol Consumption and Ovarian Cancer Risk." *American Journal of Epidemiology.* 1986; 123:759–766.

Haffner, S.M., Fong, D., Stern, M.P., *et. al.,* "Diabetic Retinopathy in Mexican Americans and non-Hispanic Whites," *Diabetes.* 1988; 37:878–884.

Haffner, S.M., Knapp, J.A., Stern, M.P., Hazuda, H.P., Rosenthal, M., Franco, L.J. "Coffee Consumption, Diet, and Lipids." *American Journal of Epidemiology.* 1985; 122:1–12.

Haffner, S.M., Stern, M.P., Hazuda, H., *et al.* "Hyperinsulinemia in a Population at High Risk for Non-Insulin-Dependent Diabetes Mellitus." *New England Journal of Medicine.* 1986; 315:220–224.

Harris, M.I. "Epidemiological Correlates of NIDDM in Hispanics, Whites, and Blacks in the U.S. Population." *Diabetes Care* 14 (suppl. 3): 639–648, 1991.

Harwood, A. "Hot and Cold Theory of Disease." *Journal of the American Medical Association,* Vol. 216, No. 7 (Mary 17, 1971), 1153–1158.

Hayes-Bautista, D.E. "Coaches, Abritrators, and Access to Medical Care." *Journal of Health and Social Behavior.* 20(1) (Mar. 1979): 52–60.

Hayes-Bautista, D.E. "Chicano Patients and Medical Practitioners: A Sociology of Knowledges Paradigm of Lay—Professional Interaction." *Soc-Sci-Med.* 12(2A) (Mar. 1978) 83–90.

Hayes-Bautista, D.E. and Chapa, J., *"Latino* Terminology: Conceptual Bases for Standardized Terminology." *American Journal of Public Health.* 1987; 77:61–68.

Hazuda, H.P., Haffner, S.M., Stern, M.P., Eifler, C.W. "Effects of Acculturation and Socioeconomic Status on Obesity and Diabetes in Mexican Americans." *American Journal of Epidemiology.* 1988; 128:1289–1301.

Hazuda, H.P., Stern, M.P., Gaskill, S.P., Haffner, S.M., Gardner, L.I. "Ethnic Differences in Health Knowledge and Behaviors Related to the Prevention and Treatment of Coronary Heart Disease. The San Antonio Heart Study." *American Journal of Epidemiology.* 117 (6) (Jun. 1983) 717–728.

Hentges, K., Shields, C.E. & Catu, C. "Folk Medicine and Medical Practice." *Tex-Med.* 82 (10), (Oct, 1986), 27–29.

Hernández-Chávez, E., Cohen, A.D., Beltramo, A.F. *El Lenguaje de los Chicanos: Regional and Social Characteristics Used by Mexican Americans.* Virginia: Center for Applied Linguistics, 1975.

Hetherington, R.W., Hopkins, C.E. "Symptom Sensitivity: Its Social and Cultural Correlates." *Health Services Research* (Spring): 63–75. [1969]

Hidalgo, H., Hidalgo C.E. "The Puerto Rican Lesbian and the Puerto Rican Community." *Journal of Homosexuality,* 2 (2) (Winter 1976-77), 109–121.

Holck, S.F., Warren, C.W., Rochart, R.W., Smith, J.C. "Lung Cancer Mortality and Smoking Habits: Mexican American Women." *American Journal of Public Health.* 1982; 72:38–42.

Holland, W.R. "Mexican-American Medical Beliefs: Science or Magic?" *Arizona Medicine,* 20 (1963), 89–101.

Hoppe, S.K., Heller, P.L. "Alienation, Familism, and the Utilization of Health Services by Mexican-Americans." *Journal of Health and Social Behavior.* 16:304–314. [1975]

Howard, A. *Ethnicity and Medical Care.* Cambridge, MA: Harvard University Press, 1981.

Hubbell, F.A., Chavez, L.R., Mishra, S.I., Valdez, R. Burciaga. "Beliefs about Sexual Behavior and Other Predictors of Papanicolaou Smear Screening among *Latinas* and Anglo Women." *Archives of Internal Medicine.* 1996; 156(20), 2353–2358.

Hubbell, F.A., Chavez, L.R., Mishra, S.I., Valdez, R. Burciaga. "Differing Beliefs about Breast Cancer Among *Latinas* and Anglo Women." *The Western Journal of Medicine.* 1996; 164(5), 405–409.

Hubbell, F.A., Mishra, S.I., Chavez, L.R., Burciaga Valdez, R. "The Influence of Knowledge and Attitudes About Breast Cancer on Mammography Use among *Latinas* and Anglo Women." *Journal of General Internal Medicine.* 1997; 12(8), 505–508.

Hubbell, F.A., Waitzkin, H., Mishra, S.I., Dombrink, J, Chavez, L.R. "Access to Medical Care for Documented and Undocumented *Latinos* in a Southern California County." *The Western Journal of Medicine.* 1991; 154(4), 414–417.

Humble, C.G., Samet, J.M., Pathak, D.R. "Cigarette Smoking and Lung Cancer in Hispanic Whites and Other Whites in New Mexico." *American Journal of Public Health.* 75:145–148.

Humphrey, N.D. "Some Dietary and Health Practices of Detroit Mexicans." *Journal of American Folklore,* 58 (22): 255–258.

Hunsaker, A.C. "Chicano Drug Abuse Patterns: Using Archival Data to Test Hypotheses." Hispanic Journal of Behavioral Science. 1985; 7(1):93–104.

Ismail, A.I., Burt, B.A., Brunelle, J.A., Szpunar, S.M. *Dental Caries and Periodontal Disease among Mexican American Children from Five Southwestern States,* 1982–83. MMWR CDC Surveillance Summer. 1988; 37:33–45

Ismail, A.I., Burt, B.A., Brunelle, J.A. "Prevalence of Dental Caries and Periodontal Disease in Mexican American Adults: Results from Southwestern HHANES, 1982–83" *American Journal of Public Health.* 1987; 77:967–970.

Ismail, A.I., Szpunar, S.M. "Oral Health Status of Mexican Americans with Low and high Acculturation Status. Findings from Southwestern HHANES, 1982–84." *J Public Health Dent* 1990; 50:24–31.

Jarvis, D.C. *Folk Medicine.* New York: Holt, Rinehart & Winston, 1958.

Javitz, D.A. "Changes in Spanish Surname Cancer Rates Relative to Whites in the Denver Area 1969-71 to 1979-81." *American Journal of Public Health.* 1986; 76:1210–1215.

John, A.M., Martorell, R. "Incidence and Duration of Breast-Feeding in Mexican American Infants, 1970-82." *Am J Clin Nutr.* 1989; 50:868–874.

Johnson, C. "Mexican American Women in the labor Force and Lowered Fertility." *American Journal of Public Health.* 66 (12) (Dec. 1976), 1986-1988.

Johnson, C. "Nursing and Mexican American Folk Medicine." *Nursing Forum.* 3 (2) (1964), 104–113.

Jones, B.E., Gray, B.A., Parson, E.B. "Manic-Depressive Illness among Poor Urban Hispanics." *American Journal of Psychiatry.* 140(9) (Sep. 1983) 1208–10.

Kaplowitz, H., Martorell, R., Mendoza, F.S. "Fatness and Fat Distribution in Mexican American Children and Youths from the Hispanic Health and Nutrition Examination Survey." *American Journal of Human Biology.* 1989; 1:631–648.

Karno, M., and Edgerton, R.B. "Perception of Mental Illness in a Mexican American Community." *Archives of General Psychiatry.* Vol. 20 (1969), 233–238.

Karno, M., and Morales, A.A. "A Community Mental Health Service of Mexican Americans in a Metropolis." *Comprehensive Psychiatry.* Vol. 12 (1971), 116–121.

Karno, M., Ross, R.N., Caper, R.A. "Mental Health Roles of Physicians in a Mexican American Community." *Community Mental Health Journal.* Vol. 5 (1969), 62–69.

Keefe, S.E. "Acculturation and the Extended Family Among Urban Mexican Americans." *In* Padilla, A.M. (ed): *Acculturation Theory, Models and Some New Findings.* Boulder: Westview Press, 1980; 85–110.

Keefe, S.E. "Help Seeking Behavior among Foreign-Born and Native-Born Mexican Americans." *Soc-Sci-Med.* 16 (16) (1982) 1467–72.

Keefe, S.E. & Casas, J.M. "Mexican-Americans and Mental Health: A Selected Review and Recommendations for Mental Health Service Delivery." *Am-J-Community-Psychol* 8 (3) (Jun. 1980) 303–26.

Kiev, A. *Curanderismo: Mexican-American Folk Psychiatry.* New York: The Free Press, 1968.

Kiev, A. *Transcultural Psychiatry.* New York: The Free Press, 1972.

Klesges, R.C., Somes, G., Pascale, R.W., Klesges, L.M., Murphy, M. Brown, K., Williams, E. "Knowledge and Beliefs Regarding the Consequences of Cigarette Smoking and Their Relationships to Smoking Status in a Biracial Sample." *Health Psychol* 1988; 7:387–401.

Kovar, M.G., Johnson, C. *Design Effects from the Mexican American Portion of the Hispanic Health and Nutrition Examination Survey: A Strategy for Analysts. In* Proceedings of the Section on Survey Research Methodology of the American Statistical Association. Washington, DC: American Statistical Association, 1986; 396–399.

Krajewski, E.R. "Folk Healing among Mexican-American Families as a Consideration in the Delivery of Child Welfare and Child Health Care Services. *Child Welfare.* 70 (Mar./Apr. 1991), 157–167.

Kraus, J.F., Borhani, N.O., Franti, C.E. "Socioeconomic Status, Ethnicity, and Risk of Coronary Heart Disease." *American Journal of Epidemiology.* 1980; 111:407–414.

Kreisman, J.J. "The *Curandero's* Apprentice: A Therapeutic Integration of Folk and Medical Healing." *American Journal of Psychiatry,* Vol. 132 (1975), 81–83.

LaCroix, A.Z., Haynes, S.C., Savage, D.D., Havlik, R.J. "Rose Questionnaire: Angina Among United States Black, White, and Mexican American Women and Men. Prevalence and Correlates from the Second National and Hispanic Health and Nutrition Examination Surveys." *American Journal of Epidemiology.* 1989; 129:669–686.

Lagos, F. *Hierbas mexicanas: Secretos de curanderos mexicanos y plantas conocidas.* México: Impresora Lorenzana, 1992.

Landrine, H., Richardson, J.L. Klonoff, E.A. & Flay, B. "Cultural Diversity in the Predictors of Adolescent Cigarette Smoking: The Relative Influence of Peers." *Journal of Behavioral Medicine.* 1994, 17, 331–346.

Linn, M. W., Hunter, K. I., & Linn, B. S. "Self-Assessed Health, Impairment and Disability in Anglo, Black & Cuban Elderly." *Med-Care,* 18 (3) (Mar. 1980) 282–288.

Logan, M. H. "Humoral Medicine in Guatemala and Peasant Acceptance of Modern Medicine." *Human Organization,* Vol. 32 (Winter, 1973), 385–395.

Looker, A. C., Johnson, C. L., McDowell, M. A., Yetley, E. A. "Iron Status: Prevalence of Impairment in Three Hispanic Groups in the United States." *Am J Clin Nutr* 1989; 49:53–558.

Looker, A. C., Johnson, C. L., Underwood, B. A. "Serum Retinol Levels of Persons Aged 4–74 Years from Three Hispanic Groups." *Am J Clin Nutr* 1988; 48:1490–1496.

Looker, A. C., Johnson, C. L., Woteki, C. E., Yetley, E. A., Underwood, B. A. "Ethnic and Racial Differences in Serum Vitamin A Levels of Children Aged 4–11 Years." *Am J Clin Nutr* 1988; 47:247–252.

Looker, A. C., Sempos, C. T., Liu, K., Johnson, C. L., Gunter, E. W. "Within-Person Variance in Biochemical Indicators of Iron Status: Effects on Prevalence Estimates." *Am J Clin Nutr* 1990; 52:541–547.

Looker, A. C., Underwood, B. A., Wiley, J., Fulwood, R., Sempos, C. T. "Serum Alpha-Tocopherol Levels of Mexican Americans, Cubans, and Puerto Ricans Aged 4–74 Years." *Am J Clin Nutr* 1989; 50:491–496.

López Agueres, W., Kemp, B., Plopper, M. Staples, F. R., Brummel-Smith, K. "Health Needs of the Hispanic Elderly." *J-Am-Geriatr-Soc.* 32 (3) (March. 1984):191–8.

López-Aqueres, W., Kemp, B., Staples, F., Brummel-Smith, K. "Use of Health Care Services by Older Hispanics." *J Am Geriatr Soc* 32 (6) (Jun. 1984):435–440.

Loria, C. M., McDowell, M. A., Johnson, C. L., Wotecki, C. E. "Nutrient Data for Mexican American Foods: Are Current Data Adequate?" *J Am Diet Assoc* 1991, 91(8)919–922.

Lovato, C. Y., Litrownik, A. J., Elder, J., & Nunez-Liriano, A. "Cigarette and Alcohol Use among Migrant Hispanic Adolescents," *Family & Community Health.* 1994, 16, 18–31.

Lubchansky, I., Egri, I., Stokes, J. "Puerto Rican Spiritualists View Illness: The Faith Healer as a Paraprofessional." *American Journal of Psychiatry.* Vol. 127 (1970), 312–321.

Maddahian, E., Newcomb, M. D., Bentler, P. M. "Single and Multiple Patterns of Adolescent Substance Use: Longitudinal Comparisons of Four Ethnic Groups." *J Drug Educ* 1985; 15(4):311–326.

Madsen, M. C. "Development and Cross-Cultural Differences in the Cooperative and Competitive Behavior of Young Children." *Psychology.* Vol. 2 (1971), 365–371.

Madsen, W. "Health and Illness." *Society and Health in the Lower Rio Grande Valley.* Texas: Hogg Foundation of Mental Health, 1961.

Madsen, W. "Hot and Cold in the Universe of San Francisco Tecospa, Valley of Mexico." *Journal of American Folklore.* Vol. 68 (1955), 123–129.

Madsen, W. "Mexican-Americans and Anglo-Americans: A Comparative Study of Mental Health in Texas." *In* Ploy, S. C. and Edgerton, R. E. *(Eds.):* Changing Perspectives in Mental Illness. New York: Holt, Rinehart & Winston, 1969.

Madsen, W. "The Alcoholic Agringado." *American Anthropologist,* Vol. 66 (1964), 355–361.

Madsen, W. "Value Conflicts and Folk Psychiatry in South Texas." *In* Kiev A., (ed.): *Magic, Faith, and Healing.* New York: The Free Press, 1964.

Madsen, W. *The Mexican-Americans of South Texas.* 2nd ed. New York: Holt, Rinehart & Winston, 1973.

Maduro, R. "*Curanderismo* and Latino views of Disease and Curing." *The Western Journal of Medicine.* 139(6), 868–874. [1983]

Marcus, A. C., Crane, L. A. "Smoking Behavior Among US Latinos: An Emerging Challenge for Public Health." *Am J Public Health* 1985; 75:169–172.

Mardiros, M. "A View Toward Hospitalization: The Mexican American Experience." *J-Adv-Nurs.* (5) (Sep, 1984) 469–478.

Marín, B. V. O. *Analysis of AIDS Prevention among African Americans and Latinos in the United States.* Report prepared for the Office of Technology Assessment, 1995.

Marín, B. V. O. Gómez, C. A., & Hearst, N. "Multiple Heterosexual Partners and Condom Use among Hispanics and Non-Hispanic Whites." *Family Planning Perspectives.* 1993; 25: 170–174.

Marín, G., Pérez-Stable, E. & B. V. O. Marín, "Cigarette Smoking among San Francisco Hispanics: The Role of Acculturation and Gender," *American Journal of Public Health.* 1989, 79, 196–198.

Marín, B. V. O., Marín, G., Padilla, A. M. De La Rocha, C. "Utilization of Traditional and Non-Traditional Sources of Health Care Among Hispanics." *Hispanic J Beh Sci* 1983; 5(1);65–80.

Marin, G., Perez-Stable, E. J., Marin, B. V. O. "Cigarette Smoking Among San Francisco Hispanics: The Role of Acculturation and Gender." *Am J Public Health* 1989, 79:196–199.

Marin, G., Marin, B. V. O., Perez-Stable, E. J. *Prevalence and Smoking Behaviors of Hispanic in San Francisco.* Hispanic Smoking Cessation Research Project, Tech Report No. 18. San Francisco: University of California, 1987; 1–27.

Markides, K., Liang, J., Jackson, J. S. "Race, Ethnicity and Aging Conceptual and Methodological Issues," *In* Binstock, R. L., George, L. K. (eds): *Handbook of Aging and the Social Sciences,* 3rd Ed. New York: Academic Press, 1990.

Markides, K. S. "Mortality among Minority Populations: A Review of Recent Patterns and Trends." *Public Health-Rep* 98 (3) (May–Jun. 1983) 252–60.

Markides, K. S., Coreil, J. "The Health of Hispanics in the Southwestern United States: An Epidemiologic Paradox." *Public Health Rep.* 101 (3) (May–Jun. 1986) 253–65.

Markides, K. S., Krause, N. "Intergenerational Solidarity and Psychological Well-being among Older Mexican Americans: A Three Generational Study." *J-Gerontol.* 40 (3) (May, 1985) 390–392.

Markides, K. S., Vernon, S. W. "Aging, Sex-Role Orientation, and Adjustment: A Three-Generations Study of Mexican-Americans." *J. Gerontol.* 41 (4) (July 1986) 506–511.

Markides, K. S., Coreil, J., Ray, L. A. "Smoking among Mexican Americans: A Three-Generation Study." *Am J Public Health.* 1987; 77:708–711.

Markides, K. S., Hazuda, H. P. "Ethnicity and Infant Mortality in Texas Counties." *Soc Biol.* 1980; 27:261–271.

Markides, K. S., Krause, N., Mendes de Leon, D. F. "Acculturation and Alcohol Consumption among Mexican Americans: A Three-Generation Study." *Am J Public Health.* 1988; 78:1178–1181.

Markides, K. S., Levin, J. S., Ray, L. A. "Determinants of Physician Utilization among Mexican Americans: A Three-Generation Study." *Med Care.* 1985; 23:236–246.

Markides, K. S., Dickson, H. D., Pappas, C. "Characteristics of Dropouts in Longitudinal Research on Aging: A Study of Mexican Americans and Anglos." *Exp-Aging-Res.* 8 (3–4), (Fall–Winter, 1982) 163–167.

Marks, G., Solis, J., Richardson, J. L., Collins, L. M., Birba, L., Hisserich, J. C. "Health Behavior of Elderly Hispanic Women: Does Cultural Assimilation Make a Difference?" *Am J Public Health.* 1987; 77:1315–1319.

Martin, J., Juárez, L. "Cancer Mortality Among Mexican Americans and Other Whites in Texas, 1969–80." *Am J Public Health* 1987; 77:708–711.

Martínez, C., Martin, H. W. "Folk Diseases Among Urban Mexican-Americans: Etiology, Symptoms, and Treatment." *JAMA,* Vol. 196, No. 2 (April 11, 1966), 161–164.

Martínez, R. G., Chavez, L. R., Hubbell, F. A. "Purity and Passion: Risk and Morality in *Latina* Immigrants' and Physicians' Beliefs about Cervical Cancer." *Medical Anthropology.* 1996; 17(4), 337–362.

Moor, J. "The Chola Lifecourse: *Chicana* Heroin Users and the *Barrio* Gang." *International Journal of the Addictions.* 1994, 29(9), 115–1126.

Maurer, K. R., Everhart, J. E., Ezzati, T. M., Johannes, R. S., *et al:* "Prevalence of Gallstone Disease in Hispanic Populations in the United States." *Gastroenterology.* Feb 1989; 96:487–492 (erratum published 1989; 96:1630).

Maurer, K. R., Everhart, J. E., Knowler, W. C., Shawker, T. H., Roth, H. P. "Risk Factors for Gallstone Disease in the Hispanic Populations of the United States." *An J Epidemiol.* 1990; 131:836–844.

Mayers, R. S. "Use of Folk Medicine by Elderly Mexican-American Women." *Journal of Drug Issues.* 19 (Spring 1989), 283–295.

McKay, E. G. *The Changing Demographics of the Hispanic Family.* Washington, DC: National Council of La Raza, July, 1987.

McLemore, S. D. "Ethnic Attitudes Toward Hospitalization: An Illustrative Comparison of Anglos and Mexican Americans." *Southwestern Social Science Quarterly,* Vol. 43 (1963), 341–346.

McMullin, J. M., Chavez, L. R., Hubbell, F. A. "Knowledge, Power and Experience: Variation in Physicians' Perceptions of Breast Cancer Risk Factors." *Medical Anthropology.* 1996; 16(4), 295–317.

Mendes De Leon, C. F., Markides, K. S. "Alcohol Consumption and Physical Symptoms in a Mexican American Population." *Drug-Alcohol-Depend* 16 (4) (Feb. 1986) 369–379.

Mendoza, F. Ventura, S. J., Valdez, R. B. et al. "Selected Measures of Health Status for Mexican American, Mainland Puerto Rican and Cuban American Children." *JAMA.* 1991; 265.

Moscicki, E. K., Locke, B. Z., Rae, D. S., Boyd, J. H. "Depressive Symptoms Among Mexican Americans: The Hispanic Health and Nutrition Examination Survey." *Am J Epidemiol* 1989; 130:348–360.

Muñoz, E. "Care for the Hispanic Poor: A Growing Segment of American Society," *Journal of the American Medical Association.* 1988; 2600:2711–2712.

Murphy, S. P., Castillo, R. O., Martorell, R., Mendoza, F. S. "An Evaluation of Food Group Intakes by Mexican American Children." *J Am Diet Assoc.* 1990; 90:388–393.

Najjar, M. F., Kuczmarski, R. J. "Anthropometric Data and Prevalence of Overweight for Hispanics: 1982–1984". National Center for Health Statistics. *Vital and Health Statistics* 11(239). DHHS Pub No. PHS89-1689. Washington, DC: Government Printing Office, 1989.

Nall, F., Speilberg, J. "Social and Cultural Factors in the Responses of Mexican Americans to Medical Treatment." *Journal of Health and Social Behavior.* Vol. 8 (1967), 299–308.

Neff, J. A., & Dassori, A. M. "Age and Maturing Out of Heavy Drinking Among Anglo and Minority Male Drinkers: A Comparison of Cross-Sectional Data and Retrospective Drinking History Techniques," *Hispanic Journal of Behavioral Sciences.* 1998, 20(2), 225–240

Neff, J. A., Hoppe, S. K., Perea, P. "Acculturation and Alcohol Use: Drinking Patterns and Problems Among Anglo and Mexican American Male Drinkers." *Hispanic J Behav Sci.* 1987; 9:151–181.

Newsome, R. "*Curanderismo:* Barrier or Gateway to Health Care." In: *Barriers to Medical Care among Texas Chicanos.* Lubbock Texas: Project of the Southwest Medical Sociology Ad Hoc Committee, 1974.

Nikias, M. A., Fink, R., Sollecito, W. "Oral Health Status in Relation to Socioeconomic Status and Ethnic Characteristics of Urban Adults in the USA." *Community Dent Oral Epidemiol.* 1977; 5:200–206.

Norell, S. E., Ahlbom, A., Erwald, R., Jacobson, G., Lindaberg-Navier, I., Olin, R., Tornberg, B., Wiechel, K. "Diet and Pancreatic Cancer: A Case-Control Study." *Am J. Epidemiol.* 1986; 124:894–902.

Novello, A. C., Wise, P. H., Kleinman, D. V. "Hispanic Health: Time for Data, Time for Action." *JAMA* 1991; 265:253–255.

O'Nell, C. W. "An Investigation of Reported 'Fright' as a Factor in the Etiology of SUSTO, 'Magical Fright.' " *Ethos.* Vol. 3 (Spring, 1975), 41–63.

Padilla, A. M., Carlos, M. L., Keefe, S. E. "Mental Health Service Utilization by Mexican Americans." *In* Miranda, M. R. (ed.): *Psychotherapy with the Spanish-Speaking: Issues in Research and Service Delivery.* Los Angeles: University of California, Spanish Speaking Mental Health Center, Monograph No. 3, 1976.

Padilla, A. M. "The Role of Cultural Awareness and Ethnic Loyalty in Acculturation." *In* Padilla, A. M. (ed): *Acculturation: Theory, Models, and Some New Findings.* AAAS Selected Symposium 39. Boulder, CO: Westview Press, 1980.

Padilla, E. R. "The Relationship Between Psychology and Chicanos: Failures and Possibilities." *In* Hernández, C. A., Haug, M. J. and Wagner, N. N. (eds.): *Chicanos: Social and Psychological Perspectives.* 2nd ed. St. Louis: C. V. Mosby, 1976.

Padilla, E. R., Padilla, A. M., Morales, A., Olmedo, E. L., Ramírez, R. "Inhalant, Marijuana, and Alcohol Abuse Among Barrio Children and Adolescents." *Int J Addict.* 1979; 14:943–964.

Padrón, F. *El médico y el folklore.* San Luis Potosí, México: Talleres Gráficos de la Editorial Universitaria, 1956.

Page, J. B. "The Children of Exile: Relationships Between the Acculturation Process and Drug Use Among Cuban American Youth." *Youth and Society.* 1980; 11(4):431–447.

Pan American Health Organization. *Survey on Characteristics of Smokers in Latin America.* Washington DC. Scientific Pub. 337, 1997.

Parsons, T. "The Sick Role and the Role of the Physician Reconsidered." *The Milbank Memorial Fund Quarterly.* 53: 257–278. [1975]

Pérez, R., Padilla, A. M., Ramírez, A., Ramírez, R., Rodríguez, M. "Correlates and Changes Over Time in Drug and Alcohol Use Within a Barrio Population." *AM J Community Psychol.* 1980; 8(6)621–636.

Pérez-Arce, P. "Substance Use Patterns of Hispanics: Commentary." *International Journal of the Addictions.* 1994, 29, 1189–1199.

Pérez-Stable, E. J., Marin, B. V., Marin, G., Brody, D. J., Benowitz, N. L. "Apparent Underreporting of Cigarette Consumption Among Mexican American Smokers." *Am J Public Health.* 1990; 80:1057–1061.

Polednak, A. P. "Estimating Smoking Prevalence in Hispanic Adults." *Health Values.* 1994, 18, 32–40.

Putsch, III, R. W. "Cross-Cultural Communication: The Special Case of Interpreters in Health Care." *Journal of the American Medical Association.* 254 (23):3344–3348.

Quesada, G. M., Heller, P. L. "Sociocultural Barriers to Medical Care Among Mexican Americans in Texas: A Summary Report of Research Conducted by the Southwest Medical Sociology Ad Hoc COmmittee." *Med Care.* 1977; 15:93–101.

Quesada, G. M. "Language and Communication Barriers for Health Delivery to a Minority Group." *Soc Scie Med.* 1976; 10:323–327.

Ramos-MacKay, J., Comas-Díaz, L. and Rivera, L. "Puerto Ricans," in Comas-Díaz, L. and Griffith, E. H. (eds): *Clinical Guidelines in Cross-Cultural Mental Health.* New York: John Wiley & Sons, 1988.

Reinert, B. R. "The Health Care Beliefs and Values of Mexican-Americans." *Home Health Care Nurse.* Sept.-Oct. 86, 32–38.

Report of the Subcommittee of Chemical Dependency. *In* US Department of Health and Human Services: Report of the Secretary's Task Force on Black and Minority Health: Volume VII, Chemical Dependency and Diabetes. Washington, DC: DHHS, 1986.

Reyes-Acosta, V. "Folk Illnesses Reported to Physicians in the Lower Rio Grande Valley: A Binational Comparison," *Ethnology.* 24,3 (July, 1985), 229–236.

Richardson, J. L., Marks, G., Solis, J. M., Collins, L. C., Birba, L., Hisserich, J. C. "Frequency And Adequacy of Breast Cancer Screening among Elderly Hispanic Women." *Prev Med* 1987; 16:761–774.

Roberts, R. E., Lee E. S. "Medical Care Use by Mexican Americans: Evidence from the Human Population Laboratory Studies." *Med Care.* Mar. 1980; 18:267–281.

Roberts, R. E. "An Epidemiologic Perspective on the Mental Health of People of Mexican Origin." *In* Rodriquez, R., Coleman, M. T. (eds): *Mental Health Issues of the Mexican Origin Population in Texas.* Austin: Hogg Foundation for Mental Health, 1987.

Robertson, I. *Sociology: Cultural Responses to Illness* (3rd ed.). New York: Worth Publishing, 1987.

Robles, R., Martínez, R., Muscoso, M. "Drug Use among Public and Private Secondary School Students in Puerto Rico." *Int J Addic.* 1979; 14(2):243–258.

Roemer, M. I. "Medical Care and Social Class in Latin America." *The Milbank Memorial Fund Quarterly.* Vol. 42 (July, 1964), 54–64.

Rubel, A. J. *Across the Tracks.: Mexican Americans in a Texas City.* Austin: University of Texas Press, 1966.

Rubel, A. J. "Concepts of Disease in Mexican American Culture." *American Anthropologist,* Vol. 62, No. 5 (1960), 795–815.

Rubel, A. J. "The Epidemiology of a Folk Illness: *Susto* in Hispanic America." *Ethnology,* Vol. 3 (1964), 268–283.

Rubel, A. J. "Análisis functional y efectos negativos de algunas creencias acerca de la causación de enfermedades." *Anuario indigenista,* México, D.F., XXIX (1969), 269–275.

Rubel, A. J., O'Nell, C. W. *The Meaning of* Susto *(Magical Fright).* Paper presented at the XLI Internal Congress of Americanists, Mexico City, 1974.

Ruiz, P. "Cultural Barriers to Effective Medical Care among Hispanic-American Patients." *Annu-Rev-Med.* 36 (1985), 63–71.

Rust, G. S. "Health Status of Migrant Farmworkers: A Literature Review and Commentary." *American Journal of Public Health.* 1990; 9:1218-1224.

Sabagh, G. "Fertility Planning Status of Chicano Couples in Los Angeles." *American Journal of Public Health,* Vol. 70, No. 1 (Jan., 1980), 56–61.

Sabogal, F., Faigeles, B., Catania, J. A. "Multiple Sex Partners among Hispanics in the United States: The National AIDS Behavioral Surveys. *Family Planning Perspectives.* 1993; 25:257–262.

Salazar, J.G. "Socioeconomic Status and Alienation as Determinants of Attitudes Towards Illness." Ph.D. Dissertation, UCLA School of Public Health, University of California, Los Angeles, 1978.

Samet, J.M., Coultas, D.B., Howard, C.A., Skipper, B.J. "Respiratory Diseases and Cigarette Smoking in a Hispanic Population in New Mexico." *American Revised Respiratory Disease.* 1988. 137:815–819.

Samet, J.M., Schrag, S.D., Howard, C.A., Key, C.R., Pathak, D.R. "Respiratory Disease in a New Mexico Population Sample of Hispanic and Non-Hispanic Whites." *Annual Revised Respiratory Disease.* 1982; 125:152–157.

Samet, J.M., Wiggins, C.L., Key, C.R., Becker, T.M. "Mortality From Lung Cancer and Chronic Obstructive Pulmonary Disease in New Mexico, 1958–82." *American Journal of Public Health.* 1988; 78:1182–1186.

Samora, J. "Conceptions of Health and Disease Among Spanish Americans." *American Catholic Sociological Review.* Vol. XXII, No. 4 (1961), 314–323.

Sandler, A.P., Chan L.S. "Mexican-American Folk Belief in a Pediatric Emergency Room." *Medical Care.* 16 (9), (Sept. 1978) 778–784.

Sardo-Infirri, J., Barnes, D.E. "Epidemiology of Oral Diseases. Differences in National Problems." *Int Dent J.* 1979; 29:183–190.

Satariano, W.A. "Race, Socioeconomic Status, and Health: A Study of Age Differences in a Depressed Area." *American Journal of Preventive Medicine.* 2(1), 1–5. [1986]

Saunders, L. "Healing Ways in the Spanish Southwest." *In* Jaco, E.G. (ed.): *Patients, Physicians, and Illness.* Glencoe: The Free Press, 1958.

Saunders, L. *Cultural Difference and Medical Care.* New York: Russell Sage Foundations, 1954.

Saunders, L., Hewes, G.W. "Folk Medicine and Medical Practice." *Journal of Medical Education.* Vol. 28, No. 9 (1953), 43–46.

Schensul, S.L., *et. al.* "A Model of Fertility Control in a Puerto Rican Community." *Urban Anthropology.* 11,1 (Spring, 1982), 81–99.

Schulman, S., Smith, A.M. "The Concept of Health among Spanish-Speaking Villages of New Mexico and Colorado." *Journal of Health and Human Behavior.* 4:226–234. [1963]

Schur, C.L., Bernstein, A.B., Berk, M.L. "The Importance of Distinguishing Hispanic Subpopulations I the Use of Medical Care." *Medical Care.* 1987; 25:627–641.

Scriber, R., Dwyer, J. "Acculturation and Low Birth Weight Among Latinos in the Hispanic HHANES." *American Journal of Public Health*. 1989; 79:1263–1267.

Segall, A. "The Sick Role Concept: Understanding Illness Behavior." *Journal of Health and Social Behavior*. 17:163–170. [1976]

Selik, R.M., Castro, K.G., and Pappaioanou, M. "Birthplace and the Risk of AIDS among Hispanics in the United States." *American Journal of Public Health*. 1989; 79:836–839.

Shapiro, J. and Saltzer, E. "Cross-Cultural Aspects to Physician-Patient Communication Patterns." *Urban Health*. Dec. 1981, 1–15.

Shiono, P.H., Klebanoff, M.A., Graubard, B.I., Bernedes, H.W., Rhoads, G.G. "Birthweight Among Women of Different Ethnic Group." *Journal of American Medicine Association*. 1986; 225:48–52.

Silva, F.G.P. "*Tabaquismo* en México. *Bol Sanit Panam* 1986; 101:234–243. *Organización Pan-Americana de la Salud: Encuesta sobre las características del hábito de fumar en América Latina*. Washington, DC: Publicación científica 337, 1977.

Smith, K.W., McGraw, S.A. & Carillo, J.E. "Factors Affecting Cigarette Smoking and Intention to Smoke among Puerto Rican-American High School Students." *Hispanic Journal of Behavioral Sciences*. 1991, 13, 401–411.

Snow, L. "Folk Medical Beliefs and Their Implications for Care of Patients." *Annals of Internal Medicine*. Vol. 81 (1974), 82–96.

Sorlie, P.D., Garcia-Palmieri, M.R., Costas, R., Cruz-Vidal, M., Havlik, R. "Cigarette Smoking and Coronary Heart Disease in Puerto Rico." *Preventive Medicine*. 982; 11:304–316.

Spector, R.E. *Cultural Diversity in Health and Illness* (3rd ed.). East Norwalk, CT: Appleton and Lange, 1991.

Stoeckle, J., Zola, I.K., Davidson, G.E. "On Going to See the Doctor: The Contribution of the Patient to the Decision to Seek Medical Aid." *Journal of Chronic Diseases* 16:975–989. [1963]

Susenbury, L., Epstein, J.A., Botvin, G.J., & Díaz, T. "Social Influence Predictors of Alcohol Use among New York Latino Youth." *Addictive Behaviors*, 1994, 19, 363–372.

Szalay, L.B., Canino, G. & Vilov, S.K. "Vulnerabilities and Cultural Change: Drug Use among Puerto Rican Adolescents in the United States," *International Journal of the Addictions*, 1993, 28, 327–354.

Torres, E. *Green Medicine: Traditional Mexican-American Herbal Remedies*. Kingsville, Texas: Nieves Press, 1983.

Torres, E. *The Folk Healer: The Mexican American Tradition of "Curanderismo."* Kingsville, Texas: Nieves Press, 1984.

Treviño, F.M., Bruhn, J.G., Bunce, H III. "Utilization of Community Mental Health Services in a Texas-Mexico Border City." *Social Science and Medicine* 13A (3) (May, 1979) 331–4.

Treviño, F.M., Moss, A.J. "Health Indicators for Hispanic, Black, and White Americans." *Vital and Health Statistics* Series 10, No. 148. DHHS Pub. No. PHS 84-1576. Washington, DC: Public Health Service, National Center for Health Statistics, 1984.

Treviño, F.M., Moss, A.J. *Health Insurance Coverage and Physician Visits among Hispanic and Non-Hispanic People*. In: Health-United States, 1983. DHHS Pub. No. PHS 84-1232. Washington, DC: DHHS, PHS, NCHS, 1983; 45–48.

Treviño, F.M., Moyer, M., Baldez, B.V., Stroup-Benham, C.A. "Health Insurance Coverage and Utilization of Health Services by Mexican Americans, Mainland Puerto Ricans, and Cuban Americans." *Journal of American Medicine Association* 1991; 265:233–237.

Treviño, F.M., Ray, L. *Health Insurance Coverage and Utilization of Health Services by Mexican Americans in Texas and the Southwest*. In: Hispanic Health Status Symposium Proceedings, San Antonio, Texas: Center for Health Policy Development, 1988.

Trotter, R. *Curanderismo: Mexican American Folk Medicine*. 2nd Ed. Athens, GA: University of Georgia Press, 1997.

Trotter, R.T. "Folk Remedies as Indicators of Common Illnesses: Examples from the United States-Mexico Border," *Journal of Ethnopharmocology* 4 (2) (Sep 1981), 207–221.

Trotter, R.T. "Folk Medicine in the Southwest, Myths and Medical Facts." *Postgrad. Med*. 2D. 78(8) (Dec. 1985):167–170, 173–176, 179.

Turner, P.R., Turner, S. *Dictionary: Chontal to Spanish-English, Spanish to Chontal*. Tucson: University of Arizona Press, 1971.

Turner, P.R., ed. *Bilingualism in the Southwest*. Tucson: University of Arizona Press, 1973.

Uzzell, D. "*Susto* Revisited: Illness as a Strategic Role." *American Ethnologist*, Vol. 1 (May, 1974), 369–378.

Valdez, R.B., *et al*. "Insuring Latinos Against the Costs of Illness." *Journal of Medicine Association* 1993; 269.

Vega, W.A., Kolody, B; Valle, R., Hough, R. "Depressive Symptoms and Their Correlates among Immigrant Mexican Women in the United States." *Social Science and Medicine*. 22(6) (1986), 645–52.

Ventura, S.J., Taffel, S.M. "Childbearing Characteristics of US- and Foreign-Born Hispanic Mothers." *Public Health Report*. 1985; 100:647–652.

Villarreal, S.F., Martorell, R., Mendoza, F. "Sexual Maturation of Mexican American Adolescents." *American Journal of Human Biology*. 1989; 1:87–95.

Walker, G.M. "Utilization of Health Care: The Laredo Migrant Experience." *American Journal of Public Health*, Vol. 69, No. 7 (July, 1979), 667–671.

Weclew, R.V. "The Nature, Prevalence, and Level of Awareness of *Curanderismo* and Some of its Implications for Community Health." *Community Mental Health Journal*. 1975; 11(2);145–154.

Wells, K.B., Hough, R.L., Golding, J.M., Burnam, M.A., Karno, M. "Which Mexican Americans Underutilized Health Services?" *American Journal of Psychiatry*. 1987; 144;918–922.

Werner, D. *Donde no hay doctor*. 4th ed. México: Editorial Pax-México, 1980.

Williams, R.L., Binkin, N.J., Clingman, E.J. "Pregnancy Outcomes among Spanish-Surname Women in California." *American Journal of Public Health*. 1986; 76:387–391.

Woerner, L. "The Hispanic Elderly: Meeting the Needs of Special Population." *Civil Rights Digest*. 11 (3):2–11.

Woteki, C.E. "The Hispanic Health and Nutrition Examination Survey (HHANES 1982–84): Background and Introduction." *American Journal of Clinical Nutrition*. 1990; 51:897S–901S.

Yetley, E., Johnson, C. "Nutritional Applications of the Health and Nutrition Examination Surveys (HHANES)." *Annual Rev Nutr*. 1987; 7:441–463.

Zalamea, L. "The Modern Spirit of *Santería*." *Nuestro Magazine*, Vol. 2, No. 3 (1978), 61–63.

Zell, E.R., Dietz, V., Stevenson, J. Cochi, S., Bruce, R. "Low Vaccination Levels of US Preschool and School-Age Children." *Journal of American Medicine Association*. 1994; 271–833:839.

Zuckerman, M. "Some Dubious Premises in Research and Theory on Racial Differences: Scientific Social and Ethical Issues." *American Psychologist*. 45(19), 1297–1303. 1990.

Grammar Index
Indice Gramatical

ENGLISH

SPANISH

Index

Indice

ENGLISH

SPANISH